Neuro-Urology

Roger Dmochowski • John Heesakkers

Editors

Neuro-Urology

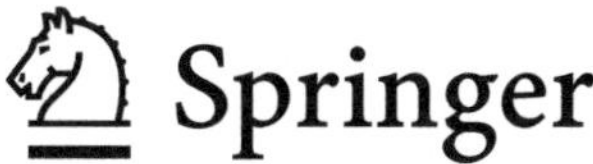 Springer

Editors
Roger Dmochowski
Department of Urology
Vanderbilt University Medical Center
Nashville, TN
USA

John Heesakkers
Department of Urology
Radboud University
Nijmegen
The Netherlands

ISBN 978-3-030-08152-2   ISBN 978-3-319-90997-4   (eBook)
https://doi.org/10.1007/978-3-319-90997-4

This Springer imprint is published by the registered company Springer Nature Switzerland AG
The registered company address is: Gewerbestrasse 11, 6330 Cham, Switzerland

This is dedicated to our families for their forbearance of our careers, our parents for the example in education that they provided us, our teachers who mentored us in the wonderful surgical specialty of urology, and our trainees who will carry on the care of those patients with neurourologic disease. We hope that the next generation will continue to advance this field for the betterment of patients impacted by these conditions and perhaps even find methods to reverse the disastrous consequences of these conditions and diseases.

Preface

This book represents our mutual attempt to provide an up-to-date, comprehensive, and summative review of the current status of neurourology from a global standpoint. The authors have been selected based on their reputational stance within the field of neurourology and also due to their acknowledged reputation and expertise in the topics on which they have graciously agreed to compose their chapters.

The subject matter of this book spans all aspects of neurourologic care and treatment, with an emphasis on summarizing areas of controversy and providing best evidence for proposed care paradigms and therapeutic interventions. The book has been divided into eight parts for ease of reference. Part I covers apropos aspects of anatomy, physiology, and pathophysiology as they pertain to the science of neurourology. Part II assesses specific clinical entities of neurourology and their associated consequences. Part III summarizes neurodiagnostics. Part IV evaluates specific urologic symptoms and their evaluation and treatment in neurourologic patients. Part V reviews the impacts of neurourologic conditions on bowel function and control. Part VI pertains to specific impacts on sexual function associated with neurourologic conditions. Part VII reviews the management of these disorders from a conservative approach. Finally Part VIII reviews surgical intervention as the ultimate aspect of neurourologic therapy.

We hope that you find this book not only informative and comprehensive but also practically useful and an easy reference for your daily practice and also for sharing knowledge with trainees in the next generation of neurourology.

Nijmegen, The Netherlands
Nashville, TN, USA
March 2018

John Heesakkers
Roger Dmochowski

Contents

Contributors

Maarten Albersen Department of Urology, University Hospitals, Leuven, Belgium

Riyad Taher Al-Mousa Department of Urology, King Fahad Specialist Hospital, Dammam, Saudi Arabia

Apostolos Apostolidis 2nd Department of Urology, Aristotle University of Thessaloniki, Thessaloniki, Greece

Paholo G. Barboglio Romo Division of Neurourology and Pelvic Reconstruction, Department of Urology, University of Michigan, Ann Arbor, MI, USA

Ivo de Blaauw Department of Surgery-Pediatric Surgery, Radboudumc-Amalia Children's Hospital, Nijmegen, The Netherlands

Bertil F. M. Blok Department of Urology, Erasmus MC, Rotterdam, The Netherlands

André J. A. Bremers Department of Surgery, Radboudumc, Nijmegen, The Netherlands

Shirley Budd Great Western Hospital Foundation Trust, Swindon, Wiltshire, UK

Emmanuel Chartier-Kastler Department of Urology, Academic Hospital Pitié Salpétrière, AP-HP, Médecine Sorbonne Université, Paris, France

Hanny Cobussen-Boekhorst Department of Urology, Radboudumc, Nijmegen, The Netherlands

Jacques Corcos Mcgill University, Montreal, QC, Canada

Francisco Cruz Faculty of Medicine of Porto, Department of Urology, Hospital de São João, Institute for Molecular and Cell Biology (IBMC), Porto, Portugal

Sophia Delpe Department of Urologic Surgery, Vanderbilt University Medical Center, Nashville, TN, USA

Roger Dmochowski Department of Urologic Surgery, Vanderbilt University Medical Center, Nashville, TN, USA

Hazel Ecclestone University College London Hospitals, London, UK

Yunliang Gao Department of Urology, The Second Xiangya Hospital, Central South University, Changsha, Hunan, China

Petros Georgopoulos 2nd Department of Urology, Aristotle University of Thessaloniki, Thessaloniki, Greece

David Ginsberg Department of Urology, Rancho Los Amigos National Rehabilitation Center, Downey, CA, USA

Department of Urology, Keck School of Medicine, University of Southern California, Los Angeles, CA, USA

Priyanka Gupta Division of Neurourology and Pelvic Reconstruction, Department of Urology, University of Michigan, Ann Arbor, MI, USA

Rizwan Hamid Department of Neurourology, Spinal Injuries Unit, Stanmore/London, UK

University College London Hospitals, London, UK

Hashim Hashim Southmead Hospital, Bristol Urological Institute, Bristol, UK

John Heesakkers Department of Urology, Radboudumc, Nijmegen, The Netherlands

Casey G. Kowalik Department of Urologic Surgery, Vanderbilt University Medical Center, Nashville, TN, USA

Helmut Madersbacher c/o Univ-Klinik Innsbruck/Tirol Kliniken, Innsbruck, Austria

Dominique Malacarne Pape Department of Urology, Female Pelvic Medicine and Reconstructive Surgery, NYU Langone Medical Center, New York, NY, USA

Frank M. J. Martens Department of Urology, Radboudumc, Nijmegen, The Netherlands

Uroš Milenković Department of Urology, University Hospitals, Leuven, Belgium

Konstantinos-Vaios Mytilekas 2nd Department of Urology, Aristotle University of Thessaloniki, Thessaloniki, Greece

Victor W. Nitti Department of Urology, Female Pelvic Medicine and Reconstructive Surgery, NYU Langone Medical Center, New York, NY, USA

Arndt van Ophoven Department of Neuro-Urology, Marien Hospital Herne, University Clinic Bochum, The Ruhr university Bochum, Herne, Germany

Jalesh N. Panicker Department of Uro-Neurology, The National Hospital for Neurology and Neurosurgery, UCL Institute of Neurology, London, UK

Mikolaj Przydacz Mcgill University, Montreal, QC, Canada

Muhammad Rasheed Department of Neuro-Urology, Marien Hospital Herne, University Clinic Bochum, The Ruhr University Bochum, Herne, Germany

Christine Reus Karolinska Institute, Department of Molecular Medicine and Surgery, Section of Urology, Stockholm, Sweden and Academic Hospital Pitié Salpétrière, Paris, France

Peter F. W. M. Rosier Department of Urology C.04.236, University Medical Center Utrecht, Utrecht, The Netherlands

J. L. H. Ruud Bosch Department of Urology, University Medical Center Utrecht, Utrecht, The Netherlands

Ryuji Sakakibara Department of Neurology, Internal Medicine, Sakura Medical Center, Toho University, Sakura, Japan

Melissa Sanford Department of Urology, Texas Tech University, Lubbock, TX, USA

Herjan J. J. van der Steeg Department of Surgery-Pediatric Surgery, Radboudumc-Amalia Children's Hospital, Nijmegen, The Netherlands

Paul W. Veenboer Department of Urology, University Medical Center Utrecht, Utrecht, The Netherlands

Part I

Neurourological Anatomy, Physiology and Pathology Relevant for the Urologist

Neuroanatomy Relevant for the Urologist

Bertil F. M. Blok

Introduction

Two components of the lower urinary tract (LUT) are essential for normal continence and micturition: (1) the reservoir is the urinary bladder with its urothelium, suburothelium, smooth detrusor muscle, and the serosa, and (2) the outlet is the urethra and its striated external urethral sphincter (EUS). The central nervous system (CNS) controls the bladder and the EUS via ascending and descending pathways during storage and periodically elimination of urine. The CNS maintains the bladder relaxed and the sphincter contracted during urine storage. When elimination of urine is required and safe to perform, the CNS contracts the bladder and relaxes the sphincter simultaneous via one unique descending pathway. This reciprocal or antagonistic coordinated action between the bladder and EUS is called synergy or synergic action and is controlled by a specific hierarchical network in the brain, spinal cord, and peripheral autonomic ganglia. The synergic coordination between the bladder and its sphincter is lost when this network is damaged between the brain and the spinal cord. Normal function of the LUT is no longer possible in spinal cord injury.

Peripheral Afferent Nerves and Their Central Projections

Afferent axons transmit information from the urinary bladder and urethra to interneurons in the lumbosacral spinal cord [1, 2]. Pelvic, hypogastric, and pudendal nerve afferents that innervate the bladder and urethra originate in lumbosacral

B. F. M. Blok
Department of Urology, Erasmus Medical Center, Rotterdam, The Netherlands
e-mail: b.blok@erasmusmc.nl

© Springer International Publishing AG, part of Springer Nature 2018   3
R. Dmochowski, J. Heesakkers (eds.), *Neuro-Urology*,
https://doi.org/10.1007/978-3-319-90997-4_1

dorsal root ganglia (DRG) and are divided into two populations: thin myelinated (Aδ) and unmyelinated C-fibers. The Aδ mechanoreceptor of the cat responds to both distension and contraction of the bladder and is silent when the bladder is empty [3]. The C-fiber afferents in cats are mechano insensitive and respond to cold stimuli or noxious stimuli [4, 5].

The Aδ nerves from the bladder wall convey bladder information via the pelvic and hypogastric nerves to the lumbosacral spinal cord. The afferent information from the bladder neck and urethra is conveyed via the pudendal and hypogastric nerves to the lumbosacral spinal cord [1, 6]. These lower urinary tract afferents terminate on interneurons in the lateral aspect of the dorsal horn and in the intermediate zone of the lumbosacral cord (Fig. 1). Most of the interneurons make intraspinal connections for proprioception, but other spinal interneurons send ascending fiber tracts to specific areas in the pons and midbrain. Some of these supraspinally projecting interneurons are involved in conveying information on bladder filling [6]. Other lumbosacral interneurons relay information to forebrain structures, including the thalamus and the hypothalamus [7]. The spinothalamic and spinohypothalamic tracts are thought not to play a specific role in the basic micturition reflex but are involved in sensory processes as sensation of urogenital pain, temperature, touch, and conscious awareness of bladder filling and voiding [8]. The sensory cortex is via the spinothalamic tract constantly informed about the filling state of the urinary bladder. In overactive bladder patients, there is too much awareness of bladder filling, which can be suppressed by therapies, like medication, pelvic floor physiotherapy, or sacral neuromodulation. In patients with complete spinal cord injury it is possible that the brain receives bladder filling information via the vagal nerve [9].

Central Projections that Control Micturition and Continence

In order to understand the role of the brain in the control of the urinary bladder and its sphincter, it is important to make a distinction between (1) areas and pathways which are intrinsic part of the micturition and continence reflex and (2) areas and pathways which modulate these micturition and continence areas. Most of the clinical therapies aimed at alleviating functional bladder disorders are not specifically targeted on the central reflex areas, like the pontine micturition center (PMC), but influence cortical and subcortical brain areas which, in turn, modulate the micturition reflex components. Examples of such therapies are pelvic floor physiotherapy, biofeedback, and medication which pass the blood-brain barrier, transcutaneous electrical nerve stimulation, posterior tibial nerve stimulation, and sacral neuromodulation. At this moment, there is probably no effective behavioral, electrical, or chemical treatments which work directly and specifically via the central components of the micturition reflex.

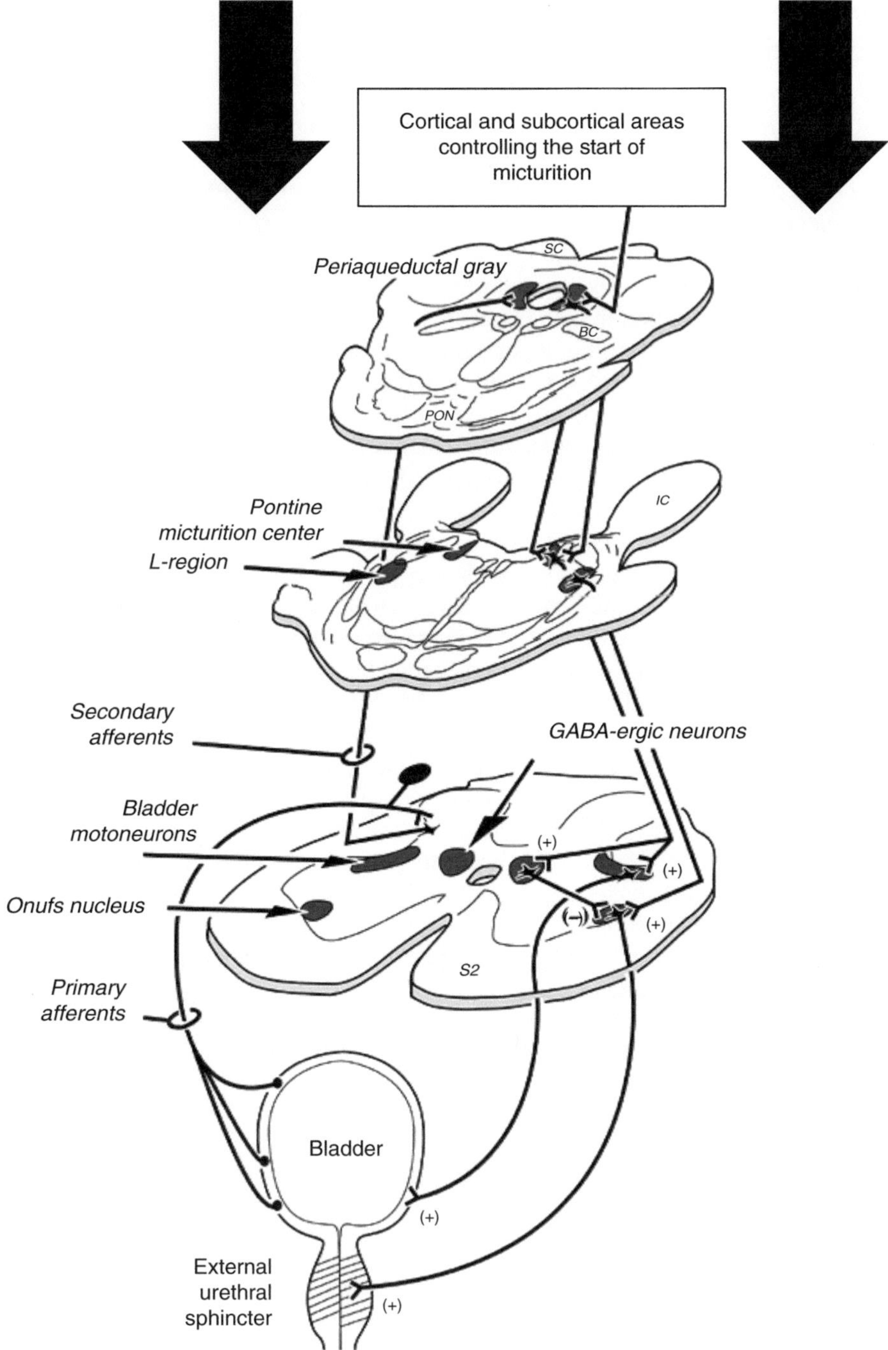

Fig. 1 Ascending and descending micturition pathways. L-region = pontine continence center (PCC)

Pontine Micturition Center (PMC) and its Descending Spinal Motor Pathway

In 1925 Barrington was the first to describe a pontine control center for micturition in the cat on the basis of bilateral lesion studies [10]. This region was localized in the dorsal pons and is now termed pontine micturition center (PMC), also known as Barrington's nucleus or M-region [11]. Later studies use more discrete lesions that abolished micturition and caused urinary retention in cats and rats [12, 13]. Lesions in humans as a result of stroke or multiple sclerosis in an analogous region similarly result in urinary retention in man [14, 15].

The PMC is located in the dorsal pons ventromedial to the rostral pole of the locus coeruleus (LC) in the rat but intermingled with neurons of the LC in the cat [16]. In humans, comparable regions in the pons have been demonstrated in the dorsal part of the pontine tegmentum, including the possible PMC [17]. The descending axons from the PMC have been described to project to the sacral cord [18]. These axons have excitatory terminal boutons in the intermediolateral cell column on parasympathetic preganglionic motoneurons [19], which, in turn, innervate the postganglionic neurons in the bladder wall. Activation of this PMC pathway results in contraction of the bladder muscle. However, contraction of the bladder muscle only is not sufficient for normal micturition. Stimulation of the PMC results in contraction of the bladder, which is preceded by a relaxation of the EUS.

This EUS relaxation by the PMC is realized via a direct descending collateral pathway to the intermediomedial cell column, also called dorsal gray commissure or lamina X, where it makes contact with inhibitory interneurons containing GABA and glycine [20, 21]. These inhibitory interneurons, in turn, project specifically to the motoneurons of the striated external urethral sphincter in the nucleus of Onuf [22]. Stimulation of the sacral intermediomedial cell column of the cat results in a strong relaxation of the external urethral sphincter, mimicking the relaxation of the sphincter during micturition [23, 24].

Together, the anatomical and physiological findings described above point to the PMC as being the command center or the switch during micturition for both the relaxation phase involving the external urethral sphincter and the contraction phase involving the smooth detrusor muscle of the urinary bladder (Fig. 1).

Pontine Continence Center (PCC) and Its Descending Spinal Motor Pathway

The bladder's function of urine storage requires detrusor relaxation accompanied by urethral sphincter contraction. Studies in the cat identified a pontine continence center (PCC) also termed the L(ateral)-region that is distinct from and lying ventrolateral to the PMC or M(edial)-region [11]. Neurons in this region project specifically to Onuf's nucleus in the sacral cord, which contains the external urethral sphincter motoneurons. Stimulation of this region stops micturition, excites the pelvic floor musculature, and contracts the urethral sphincter. Conversely, bilateral lesions of the PCC cause incontinence, excessive detrusor activity, an inability to store urine and relaxation of the urethral sphincter [11]. However, there is no anatomical evidence for connections between the PMC and the PCC, and it has been suggested that the PMC and PCC function independently [25]. Notably, the PCC has also been characterized by PET scanning in humans who try to start micturition [23, 24, 26] or orgasm [27] but fail to do so. The explanation for this failure is that the subjects tried to void or climax but because there is an unsafe (experimental) environment. Consequently, the forebrain does not pull the switch but increases the contraction of the urethral sphincter by stimulating the PCC.

The Role of the Sympathetic Outflow During Filling

Sympathetic preganglionic motoneurons in thoracolumbar segments T10 through L2 are involved in the relaxation of the bladder during filling. Efferent nerves travel within the hypogastric nerve via the thoracolumbar sympathetic ganglionic chain to the bladder wall. The sympathetic tone maintains the intravesical pressure low during bladder filling. The sympathetic nerves to the bladder only start to fire at about 60% of the bladder capacity [28]. The supraspinal control of the sympathetic nerves of the bladder is unknown.

Periaqueductal Gray

The mesencephalic periaqueductal gray (PAG) is main area in the caudal brainstem in the cat and probably also in humans which receives bladder information [29]. The PAG is a midbrain area known for its role in pain modulation [30]. In recent years, it has become clear that this dense neuronal matter around the aqueduct of Sylvius is essential for many vital basic functions, like respiration, aggression, mating, defecation, and micturition. The forebrain controls the PAG and the PMC like a switch. Complex behavior like micturition can be turned on or off instantly depending of the state of the individual [31]. In the cat, anterogradely labeled fibers from the lumbosacral spinal cord form a dense terminal field particularly in the lateral PAG [29]. Furthermore, bladder and pelvic nerve stimulation evokes activation of the PAG [32]. The importance of the PAG in the cat is exemplified by the observation that electrical stimulation of the lateral PAG results in the cat in micturition which includes an initial relaxation of the external urethral sphincter (EUS) followed by a bladder contraction [33, 34]. Furthermore, the lateral and, to a lesser extent, the dorsal PAG projects specifically to the PMC [33]. It has been proposed that the basic micturition reflex contains an ascending pathway from the lumbosacral cord to the PAG and PMC and a descending pathway from the PMC to the sacral cord. Lesions between the PAG-PMC and the sacral spinal cord will result in a disruption of the normal micturition reflex and cause bladder-sphincter dyssynergia. Lesions of rostral from the mesencephalic PAG will result in the loss of control of the timing of micturition, but the micturition reflex remains intact. Although these circuits are based on animal models, a pivotal role for both the PAG and PMC has been confirmed in man using positron emission tomography and functional magnetic imaging with and without a full bladder [23, 24, 26, 35–37].

The micturition reflex cycle consists of three phases controlled by separate central pathways: (1) pre-micturition phase during realization of a safe environment, (2) urethral relaxation phase during relaxation of the external urethral sphincter, and (3) urine expulsion phase during contraction of the detrusor muscle. Normal micturition does not take place without the onset of one of these phases. Phase 1—pre-micturition phase—is controlled via a forebrain (hypothalamic) pathway to the PAG and PMC which initiates micturition (see next paragraph); phase 2—urethral relaxation phase—is controlled via an excitatory descending PMC pathway to inhibitory sacral interneurons; and phase 3—the contraction phase—is controlled via the excitatory descending PMC pathway to sacral preganglionic bladder motoneurons.

Forebrain and Cortical Involvement

Hypothalamus

Suprapontine and supramesencephalic afferents to the PAG and PMC are important to initiate or withhold micturition (phase 1 or pre-micturition phase) and could be targets for modulating bladder function. The most prominent afferents in the cat and rat are the lateral hypothalamus and medial preoptic area [38–40].

The lateral hypothalamus is involved in defensive responses. Modulation of the PAG and PMC by the hypothalamic afferents likely plays a role in urination as a component of the defense response [41, 42]. A second major afferent to the PAG and PMC arises from the medial preoptic area [38]. The hypothalamus was activated with dynamic PET imaging during micturition in humans [23, 24, 26]. This area receives major projections from the dorsolateral prefrontal cortex and is thought to play a role in in the decision whether it is safe enough to start micturition via the PMC or unsafe and increase the contraction state of the urethral sphincter via the PCC [26].

Cortical Areas

The most common urinary symptoms in lesions of the cortical areas are urinary frequency and urgency urinary incontinence. Andrew and Nathan hypothesized on the basis of cerebral lesions in humans that disconnection of frontal or anterior cingulate gyrus from the hypothalamus results in involuntary start of micturition [43]. Indeed, the human prefrontal cortex and anterior cingulate gyrus are activated during micturition [20, 23, 24, 37].

Other Brain Areas

Cerebellum and Basal Ganglia

Several stimulation and lesioning studies in animals have shown that the cerebellum and basal ganglia have mainly an inhibitory action on the bladder during filling [1, 44, 45]. Cerebellar pathology in humans results in increased urinary frequency and urgency urine incontinence [46]. These overactive bladder symptoms are also found in Parkinson's disease [47]. Since there exist no direct projections from these areas to the PMC, the inhibitory influence is probably indirect via forebrain and midbrain structures.

References

1. De Groat WC, Griffiths D, Yoshimura N. Neural control of the lower urinary tract. Compr Physiol. 2015;5:327–96.
2. Morgan C, Nadelhaft I, De Groat WC. The distribution of visceral primary afferents from the pelvic nerve to Lissauer's Tract and the spinal gray matter and its relationship to the sacral parasympathetic nucleus. J Comp Neurol. 1981;201:415–40.
3. Satchell P, Vaughan C. Bladder wall tension and mechanoreceptor discharge. Pflugers Arch. 1994;426:304–9.
4. Fall M, Lindström S, Mazieres L. A bladder-to-bladder cooling reflex in the cat. J Physiol. 1990;427:281–300.
5. Häbler HJ, Jänig W, Koltzenburg M. Activation of unmyelinated afferent fibres by mechanical stimuli and inflammation of the urinary bladder in the cat. J Physiol. 1990;425:545–62.
6. Blok BF. Central pathways controlling micturition and urinary continence. Urology. 2002;59:13–7.
7. Blok BF. Sacral neuromodulation for the treatment of urinary bladder dysfunction. Bioelectron Med. 2018;1:85–94.
8. Chandler MJ, Hobbs SF, Fu QG, Kenshalo DR Jr, Blair RW, Foreman RD. Responses of neurons in ventroposterolateral nucleus of primate thalamus to urinary bladder distension. Brain Res. 1992;571:26–34.
9. Krhut J, Tintera J, Bilkova K, Holy P, Zachoval R, Zvara P, et al. Brain activity on fMRI associated with urinary bladder filling in patients with a complete spinal cord injury. Neurourol Urodyn. 2017;36:155–9.
10. Barrington FJ. The effect of lesion of the hind- and mid-brain on micturition in the cat. Quart J Exp Physiol. 1925;15:81–102.
11. Holstege G, Griffiths D, de Wall H, Dalm E. Anatomical and physiological observations on supraspinal control of bladder and urethral sphincter muscles in the cat. J Comp Neurol. 1986;250:449–61.

12. Satoh K, Shimizu N, Tohyama M, Maeda T. Localization of the micturition reflex center at dorsolateral pontine tegmentum of the rat. Neurosci Lett. 1978;8:27–33.
13. Tang PC. Levels of brain stem and diencephalon controlling micturition reflex. J Neurophysiol. 1955;18:583–95.
14. Cho H, Kang T, Chang J, Choi YR, Park MG, Choi KD, et al. Neuroanatomical correlation of urinary retention in lateral medullary infarction. Ann Neurol. 2015;77:726–33.
15. Komiyama A, Kubota A, Hidai H. Urinary retention associated with a unilateral lesion in the dorsolateral tegmentum of the rostral pons. J Neurol Neurosurg Psychiatry. 1998;65:953–4.
16. Valentino RJ, Pavcovich LA, Hirata H. Evidence for corticotropin-releasing hormone projections from Barrington's nucleus to the periaqueductal gray region and dorsal motor nucleus of the vagus in the rat. J Comp Neurol. 1995;363:402–22.
17. Blanco L, Yuste JE, Carillo-de Sauvage MA, Gomez F, Fernandez-Villalba E, Aviles-Olmos I, et al. Critical evaluation of the anatomical location of the Barrington nucleus: relevance for deep brain stimulation surgery of pedunculopontine tegmental nucleus. Neuroscience. 2013;247:351–63.
18. Loewy AD, Saper CB, Baker RP. Descending projections from the pontine micturition center. Brain Res. 1979;172:533–8.
19. Blok BF, Holstege G. Ultrastructural evidence for a direct pathway from the pontine micturition center to parasympathetic preganglionic motoneurons of the bladder of the cat. Neurosci Lett. 1997;222:195–8.
20. Blok BF, de Weerd H, Holstege G. The pontine micturition center projects to sacral cord GABA immunoreactive neurons in the cat. Neurosci Lett. 1997;233:109–12.
21. Sie JA, Blok BF, de Weerd H, Holstege G. Ultrastructural evidence for direct projections from the pontine micturition center to glycine-immunoreactive neurons in the sacral dorsal gray commissure in the cat. J Comp Neurol. 2001;429:631–7.
22. Konishi A, Itoh K, Sugimoto T, Yasui Y, Kaneko T, Takada M, et al. Leucine-enkephalin-like immunoreactive afferent fibers to pudendal motoneurons in the cat. Neurosci Lett. 1985;61:109–13.
23. Blok BF, Sturms LM, Holstege G. Brain activation during micturition in women. Brain. 1998;121:2033–42.
24. Blok BF, van Maarseveen JT, Holstege G. Electrical stimulation of the sacral dorsal gray commissure evokes relaxation of the external urethral sphincter in the cat. Neurosci Lett. 1998;249:68–70.
25. Blok BF, Holstege G. Two pontine micturition centers in the cat are not interconnected directly: implications for the central organization of micturition. J Comp Neurol. 1999;403:209–18.
26. Blok BF, Willemsen AT, Holstege G. A PET study on brain control of micturition in humans. Brain. 1997;120:111–21.
27. Huynh HK, Willemsen AT, Lovick TA, Holstege G. Pontine control of ejaculation and female orgasm. J Sex Med. 2013;10:3038–48.
28. Vaughan CW, Satchell PM. Role of sympathetic innervation in the feline continence process under natural filling conditions. J Neurophysiol. 1992;68:1842–9.
29. Blok BF, De Weerd H, Holstege G. Ultrastructural evidence for a paucity of projections from the lumbosacral cord to the pontine micturition center or M-region in the cat. J Comp Neurol. 1995;359:300–9.
30. Basbaum AI, Fields HL. Endogenous pain control systems: brainstem spinal pathways and endorphin circuitry. Annu Rev Neurosci. 1984;7:309–38.
31. Bandler R, Keay KA, Floyd N, Price J. Central circuits mediating patterned autonomic activity during active vs. passive emotional coping. Brain Res Bull. 2000;53:95–104.
32. Noto H, Roppolo JR, Steers WD, De Groat WC. Electrophysiological analysis of the ascending and descending components of the micturition reflex pathway in the rat. Brain Res. 1991;549:95–105.

33. Blok BF, Holstege G. Direct projections from the periaqueductal gray to the pontine micturition center (M-region). An anterograde and retrograde tracing study in the cat. Neurosci Lett. 1994;166:93–6.
34. Taniguchi N, Miyata M, Yachiku S, Kaneko S, Yamaguchi S, Numata A. A study of micturition inducing sites in the periaqueductal gray of the mesencephalon. J Urol. 2002;168:1626–31.
35. Griffiths D, Derbyshire S, Stenger A, Resnick N. Brain control of normal and overactive bladder. J Urol. 2005;174:1862–7.
36. Kavia RB, Dasgupta R, Fowler CJ. Functional imaging and the central control of the bladder. J Comp Neurol. 2005;493:27–32.
37. Michels L, Blok BF, Gregorini F, Kurz M, Schurch B, Kessler T, et al. Supraspinal control of urine storage and micturition in men: an fMRI study. Cereb Cortex. 2015;25:3369–80.
38. Holstege G. Some anatomical observations on the projections from the hypothalamus to brainstem and spinal cord: an HRP and autoradiographic tracing study in the cat. J Comp Neurol. 1987;260:98–126.
39. Kuipers R, Mouton LJ, Holstege G. Afferent projections to the pontine micturition center in the cat. J Comp Neurol. 2006;494:36–53.
40. Valentino RJ, Page ME, Luppi PH, Zhu Y, Van Bockstaele E, Aston-Jones G. Evidence for widespread afferents to Barrington's nucleus, a brainstem region rich in corticotropin-releasing hormone neurons. Neuroscience. 1994;62:125–43.
41. Fuchs SA, Edinger HM, Siegel A. The organization of the hypothalamic pathways mediating affective defense behavior in the cat. Brain Res. 1985;330:77–92.
42. Yardley CP, Hilton SM. The hypothalamic and brainstem areas from which the cardiovascular and behavioural components of the defence reaction are elicited in the rat. J Auton Nerv Syst. 1986;15:227–44.
43. Andrew J, Nathan PW. Lesions of the anterior frontal lobes and disturbances of micturition and defaecation. Brain. 1964;87:233–62.
44. Albanese A, Jenner P, Marsden CD, Stephenson JD. Bladder hyperreflexia induced in marmosets by 1-methyl-4-phenyl-1,2,3,6-tetrahydropyridine. Neurosci Lett. 1988;87:46–50.
45. Bradley WE, Teague CT. Cerebellar regulation of the micturition reflex. J Urol. 1969;101:396–9.
46. Zago T, Pea U, Fumagalli GL, Areta L, Marzorati G, Bianchi F. Cerebellar pathology and micturitional disorders: anatomotopographic and functional considerations. Arch Ital Urol Androl. 2010;82:177–80.
47. Pavlakis AJ, Siroky MB, Golstein I, Krane RJ. Neurourologic findings in Parkinson's disease. J Urol. 1983;129:80–3.

Pelvic Neurophysiology

Jalesh N. Panicker

Introduction

Neurophysiology testing involves the recording of bioelectrical activity from muscles and the nervous system to investigate nerve functions. Recordings from muscle (electromyography, EMG) and from nerves (conduction studies) provide information regarding the integrity of the neuromuscular input, as well as central neural pathways. The role of pelvic neurophysiology in the clinical assessment of patients reporting bladder, bowel and sexual dysfunction and/or pelvic floor complaints is debatable; however, there are clinical scenarios where tests may be useful in establishing a diagnosis (Table 1). This chapter provides an overview of the neurophysiology tests available for evaluating the pelvic nerves and their role in the evaluation of patients reporting unexplained pelvic organ or perineal complaints.

Electromyography

Electromyography (EMG) is a procedure that assesses the integrity of muscle functions and their innervation. This permits testing of muscles that are otherwise difficult to test clinically, such as those of the pelvic floor. Using a concentric needle electrode (CNE) is appropriate when recording from a specific muscle is required, but the discomfort from the needle itself is likely to influence relaxation of the pelvic floor muscles. Surface recording electrodes on the other hand record EMG signals from several pelvic floor muscle however may provide sufficient information to answer the clinical question being asked.

J. N. Panicker
Department of Uro-Neurology, The National Hospital for Neurology
and Neurosurgery, UCL Institute of Neurology, London, UK
e-mail: j.panicker@ucl.ac.uk

© Springer International Publishing AG, part of Springer Nature 2018

R. Dmochowski, J. Heesakkers (eds.), *Neuro-Urology*,
https://doi.org/10.1007/978-3-319-90997-4_2

Table 1 Examples of clinical scenarios where pelvic neurophysiology tests may be useful in establishing a neurological cause for pelvic organ/floor dysfunction

Clinical question	Tests	Abnormal findings	Interpretation
In a woman presenting with urinary retention, could this be due to a primary disorder of urethral sphincter relaxation (Fowler's syndrome)?	Urethral sphincter EMG	Decelerating bursts	Primary disorder of urethral sphincter relaxation (Fowler's syndrome)
In a patient presenting with a parkinsonian syndrome, could this patient be having multiple system atrophy (MSA)?	Anal sphincter EMG	Long-duration MUPs	Evidence for reinnervated motor unit potentials seen characteristically in, but not pathognomonic of, MSA
In a patient presenting with unexplained pelvic organ and perineal complaints, is there evidence for damage to the S2, S3 and S4 somatic innervation?	Anal sphincter EMG	High-amplitude MUPs, long-duration MUPs	Evidence for neurogenic damage (reinnervation)
	Bulbospongiosus EMG	Spontaneous activity (fibrillations, fasciculations, positive sharp waves)	Evidence for neurogenic damage (denervation)
		High-amplitude MUPs, long-duration MUPs	Evidence for neurogenic damage (reinnervation)
	Pudendal SEP	Delayed or absent response	Lesion of the afferent sensory pathway, e.g. S2, S3 and S4 root (see text)
	Bulbocavernosus reflex	Delayed or absent response	Lesion of the afferent or efferent pathway (see text)
In a patient presenting with numbness over the perineum or genitalia, is this due to nerve damage?	Pudendal SEP	Delayed or absent response	Lesion of the afferent pathway—pudendal nerve; S2, S3 and S4 root; sacral spinal cord; or posterior column of the spinal cord
	Bulbocavernosus reflex	Delayed or absent response	Lesion of the afferent or efferent pathways—pudendal nerve; S2, S3 and S4 root; or sacral spinal cord
In a patient presenting with obstructed voiding, is this due to detrusor–external sphincter dyssynergia?	Urethral sphincter EMG during uroflowmetry or pressure–flow study in cystometry	Continued motor unit activity during voiding	Non-relaxing striated urethral sphincter
Is there evidence for a pelvic autonomic (sympathetic) neuropathy?	Genital sympathetic skin response	Absent response	Lesion of the thoracolumbar sympathetic innervation

MUP motor unit potentials, *EMG* electromyography, *SEP* somatosensory evoked potentials

Kinesiological EMG

Pelvic floor EMG was first introduced as part of urodynamic studies to assess the extent of relaxation of the urethral sphincter during voiding, with the aim of recognising detrusor–sphincter dyssynergia. For this purpose, either surface or needle electrodes may be used. EMG allows an ongoing assessment of muscle activity during the entire urodynamic test; however, the test is performed less often nowadays because of increasing availability of fluoroscopy during urodynamic investigations, which provides a visual impression of dynamic changes at the bladder outlet during voiding and therefore is suitable for diagnosing detrusor–sphincter dyssynergia. Kinesiological EMG recordings may be useful during biofeedback, to help in the recognition of disturbances of pelvic floor muscle activity and enable patients to be actively involved in the treatment of their symptoms.

Non-kinesiological EMG

Concentric needle electrode EMG studies of the striated urethral and anal sphincter muscles, performed separately from urodynamics, have proven to be useful to assess the integrity of the innervation to individual pelvic floor muscles. The studies provide information on insertion activity, spontaneous activity, interference pattern and motor unit potentials. In health, sphincter EMG shows continuous "tonic" activity at rest, which may be increased voluntarily or reflexly. The number of motor units recorded depends upon the uptake area of the electrode. Using a CNE, activity from 1 to 5 motor units is usually recorded per site in the anal sphincter at rest. Electromyography has been used to demonstrate changes of reinnervation in the urethral or anal sphincter in a few neurological disorders [1]. Well-established values exist for the duration and amplitude of motor units recorded from the sphincter muscles in health.

Practical Applications of CNE EMG

Sphincter EMG in the Evaluation of Patients with Suspected Cauda Equina Lesions

Lesions of the cauda equina are an important cause for pelvic floor dysfunction and patients present with lower urinary tract (LUT) dysfunction and often sexual and bowel dysfunction. Most often, EMG of the external anal sphincter demonstrates changes of chronic reinnervation, characterised by reduced interference pattern with fewer motor units and enlarged polyphasic motor units (>1 mV amplitude), especially in patients with long-standing cauda equina syndrome [2]. EMG may demonstrate pathological spontaneous activity 3 weeks or more after injury; however, as the motor units of the sphincter are tonically firing, these changes of partial denervation (i.e. fibrillations and positive sharp waves) may become lost in the activity and may not be separately recognisable.

Sphincter EMG in the Diagnosis of Multiple System Atrophy

Multiple system atrophy (MSA), a variant of Parkinson's disease (PD), is a progressive neurodegenerative disease which often, particularly in its early stages, is mistaken for Parkinson's disease but is poorly responsive to antiparkinsonian treatment and is a fatal disease. Urinary incontinence occurs early in this condition, often appearing before the onset of neurologic features, and, not uncommonly, patients may present to the urologist initially [3]. Degenerative changes occur both in the brain and spinal cord resulting in LUT dysfunction. Neuropathological studies have shown that the anterior horn cells in the Onuf's nucleus are selectively lost in MSA, and this results in changes in the sphincter muscles that can be identified by EMG (Table 1). The anal sphincter is most often studied, and changes of chronic reinnervation in MSA result in prolonged duration of motor units which can be detected easily (Fig. 1).

The value of sphincter EMG in the differential diagnosis of Parkinsonism has been widely debated over the years. Technically, the MUPs recorded in MSA are quite prolonged and automated MUP analysis results in a tendency to chop these

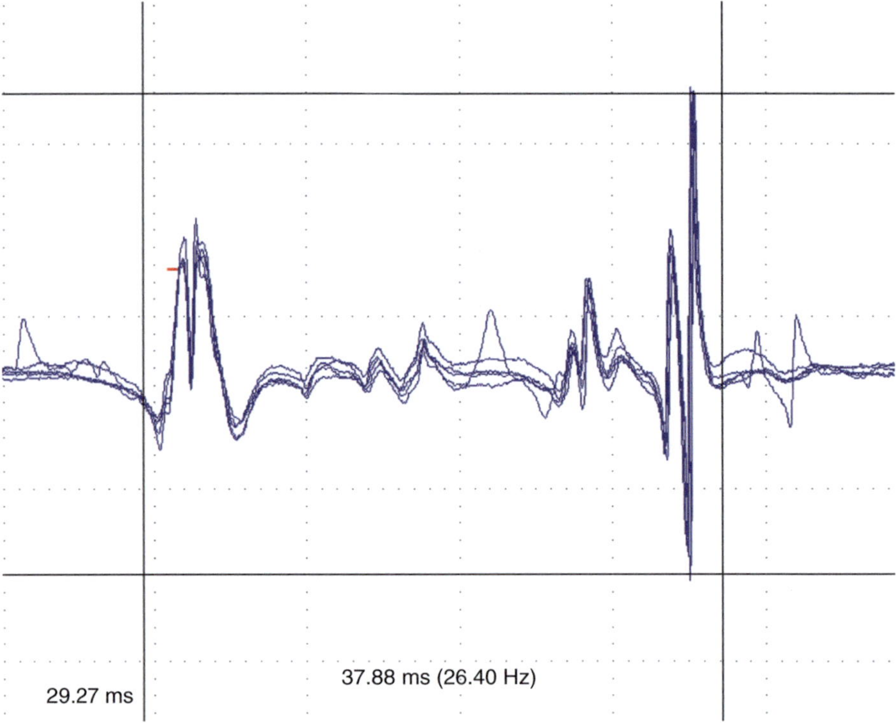

Fig. 1 Concentric needle EMG of the external anal sphincter from a middle-aged gentleman presenting with voiding difficulties on the background of a recent-onset parkinsonism syndrome. Duration of the recorded motor unit is 37.9 ms, which is prolonged and suggests chronic reinnervation. The mean duration of MUPs during the study was 19 ms (normal <10 ms), and the EMG was compatible with a diagnosis of multiple system atrophy (gain 200 μV/division, sweep speed 10 ms/division)

long polyphasic MUPs into individual components. The late components therefore might be missed when measuring the motor unit duration, and the duration of the MUP may by erroneously noted as being normal. It is advisable therefore to identify MUPs manually when performing the EMG for a patient with suspected MSA to avoid this pitfall. Moreover, the EMG changes are not specific to MSA, and similar changes of chronic reinnervation may be found in long-standing Parkinson's disease [1], other parkinsonian syndromes such as progressive supranuclear palsy [4] and dementia with Lewy bodies and other neurodegenerative conditions such as spinocerebellar ataxia type 3. Changes may be seen following obstetric injury with sphincter damage and cauda equina damage. Nevertheless, there is sufficient evidence to suggest that a highly abnormal result in a patient with mild Parkinsonism is of value in establishing a diagnosis of probable MSA [5]. A highly abnormal EMG in the absence of other obvious causes in a patient with suspected MSA in the first 5 years of the illness is significant [6].

Sphincter EMG in the Investigation of Urinary Retention in Young Women

Isolated urinary retention is uncommon in young women; however, there exists a group of women where neurological and urological investigations fail to identify a cause. A characteristic abnormality can be found on urethral sphincter EMG, consisting of decelerating bursts, a signal somewhat like myotonia, and complex repetitive discharges (CRD) (Table 1). It has been proposed that this abnormal spontaneous activity results in impairment of relaxation of the urethral sphincter, which may cause urinary retention in some women and obstructed voiding in others. This condition, nowadays known as Fowler's syndrome [7], is also characterised by elevated urethral pressures with values regularly in excess of 100 cmH_2O.

It is thought that the abnormal EMG activity prevents relaxation of the striated sphincter and abnormally high urethral pressure, and, through an exaggerated guarding reflex, poor bladder sensations and contractile function [8]. CRDs have been reported from other pelvic floor muscles in women presenting with isolated urinary retention [9] and in apparently asymptomatic women [10, 11]. Therefore the association between the abnormal EMG signal and voiding dysfunction requires to be further explored. Recently, EMG abnormalities have been shown to be associated with a pulsatile pattern in the UPP [12].

Sacral Reflexes

Reflex responses from the perineal and pelvic floor muscles can be assessed through neurophysiology testing to evaluate the integrity of the sacral (S2, S3 and S4) segments. The bulbocavernosus reflex and anal reflex involve both the sacral (S2, S3 and S4) roots and pudendal nerve in their reflex arc and are often elicited during the clinical examination. However, neurophysiology testing provides a more accurate and quantifiable assessment of these reflex responses.

The "bulbocavernosus" reflex (penilo-cavernosus reflex) assesses the afferent and efferent pathways consisting of the pudendal nerve, sacral roots and sacral spinal cord (S2, S3 and S4 segments). The dorsal nerve of the penis (or clitoris) is electrically stimulated, and recordings are made from the bulbospongiosus muscle or external anal sphincter, usually with a concentric needle. In those patients in whom the reflex is difficult to elicit, double electrical stimuli should be used [2]. In patients with a lesion at any point along the afferent or efferent pathways, the reflex may either be delayed or absent (Table 1). Testing may therefore be of value in the assessment of the sacral roots in patients with bladder dysfunction suspected to be secondary to cauda equina damage or damage to the lower motor neuron pathway. This test is however complementary to the clinically assessed response and the EMG examination of the pelvic floor muscles in patients with suspected peripheral nerve lesions [13]. Prolonged BCR latency may be valuable for distinguishing between MSA and PD in the early stages [14].

Continuous intraoperative recording of sacral reflex responses has been used in some spinal surgery centres when performing surgery of the cauda equina or conus [15], and patients with an absent bulbocavernosus reflex show poor recovery of bladder functions [16].

Evoked Potential Studies

Somatosensory Evoked Potentials

The recording of somatosensory evoked potentials (SEP) is a well-established method to assess the afferent sensory pathways from various parts of the body. Stimulation of a certain nerve (or sensory dermatome) elicits an electrical response, which can be measured along the spinal cord or over the cortex as an SEP with characteristic latency and amplitude measures. Gender differences have been noted, with longer response latencies reported in males [17].

Pudendal SEPs are typically recorded from the scalp through surface electrodes following electrical stimulation of the dorsal nerve of penis or clitoris (Fig. 2). The test assesses the integrity of the afferent sensory pathway in the pudendal nerve; S2, S3 and S4 nerve roots; sacral spinal cord; and posterior column of the spinal cord. The latency of the cortical response is influenced by the length of the neural pathway. However, rather surprisingly, the pudendal SEP is comparable in latency to the evoked potentials recorded following stimulation of the tibial nerve (tibial SEP). The reasons for this are not fully understood; however, the possibility exists that the cortical or spinal generators, or the spino-cortical pathways of the pudendal and tibial responses, differ [18]. Normative data has been published for women [19].

The SEP may be abnormal when a spinal cord lesion is the cause of sacral sensory loss or neurogenic detrusor overactivity (Table 1); however, such pathology is often apparent from the clinical examination. Additional recordings over the cauda

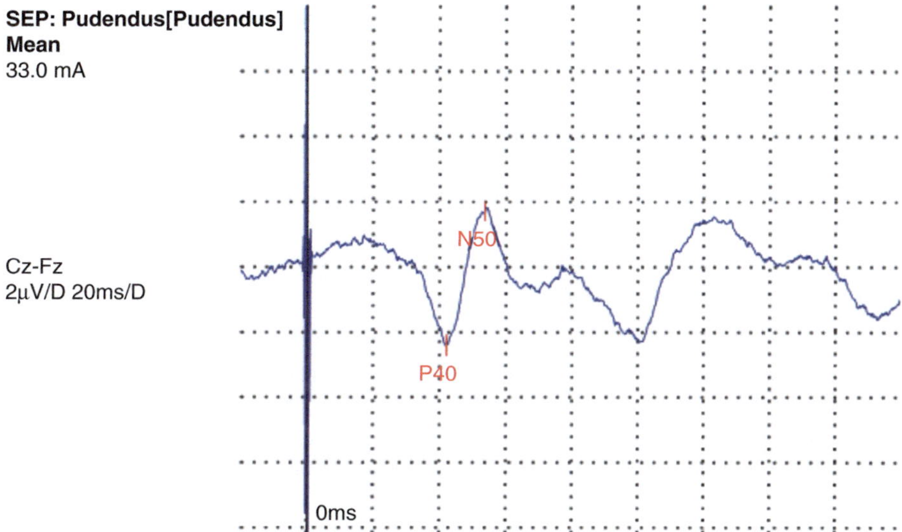

Fig. 2 Somatosensory evoked potential (SSEP) recorded at Cz–Fz during electrical stimulation of the dorsal penile nerve (33 mA) in a 50-year-old man presenting with genital numbness. The P40 waveform was of normal latency

equina and lumbosacral cord help in localising spinal lesions. The finding of a normal pudendal SEP can help to rule out a neurological cause in certain situations such as erectile dysfunction.

Tibial SEPs are more often abnormal than the pudendal SEP in multiple sclerosis, and only in exceptional cases is the pudendal SEP abnormal but the tibial SEP normal. Such findings would suggest an isolated lesion of the conus medullaris [20]. More recently, position-related reduction in SEP amplitudes has been observed, suggesting that dynamic SEP recordings may have a role in diagnosing pudendal nerve entrapment [21].

Recording of SEPs following clitoral stimulation has been reported as a valuable intraoperative monitoring method in patients undergoing surgery of the cauda equina or conus medullaris [22–24] and has become established in some spinal surgery centres, however requires further clinical investigations [25].

Motor Evoked Potentials

Following magnetic or electrical stimulation of the motor cortex, a response can be recorded from the pelvic floor. Motor evoked potentials (MEPs) can be recorded in the anal and urethral sphincters and bulbocavernosus [26] following electrical stimulation over the motor cortex of healthy subjects. These tests can be useful to localise lesions in the central nervous system, and indeed longer central conduction times are observed in patients with multiple sclerosis and spinal cord lesions with clinically recognisable cord disease. Recording MEPs has potential as a research tool to evaluate the central control of pelvic floor motor activity; however, its role in clinical practice is unclear. MEP recording may be useful for intraoperative monitoring [24].

Nerve Conduction Studies

Due to limited accessibility, the only test available to test motor nerve conductions of the pudendal nerve, the most important motor nerve innervating the pelvic floor, is the pudendal nerve terminal motor latency (PNTML). The pudendal nerve is stimulated either per rectally or vaginally adjacent to the ischial spine using the St. Mark's electrode, a finger-mounted stimulating device with a surface EMG recording electrode 7 cm proximal located around the base of the finger which records from the external anal sphincter [27]. Prolongation was initially considered evidence for pudendal nerve damage, although a prolonged latency is a poor marker of denervation. This test has not proved contributory in the investigation of patients with suspected pudendal neuralgia or faecal incontinence and can currently only be interpreted in combination with the results of other tests.

Autonomic Function Tests

The tests mentioned so far are restricted to evaluating the somatic innervation to the pelvic floor. Considering the significant autonomic innervation to the pelvic area responsible for bladder, bowel and sexual control, tests evaluating the sympathetic and parasympathetic nerves would be considered to be important. However, the only test available currently is recording of the sympathetic skin response (SSR) [28]. The SSR can be recorded from the genital area (Fig. 3), and this test provides an assessment of sympathetic innervation (Table 1). Although the responses are easily habituated and highly dependent on individual as well as environmental factors, the absence of a response from the perineum in an individual with otherwise recordable responses from the palms and soles would suggest a lesion affecting the perineal sympathetic innervation. The response has been shown to be of value: an absent response has been observed in individuals with neurogenic bladder neck incompetence in spinal cord-injured patients [29] and in female diabetic patients [30]. A significant association has been observed between pathological changes of reinnervation in the bulbocavernosus muscle and SSR latencies in the lower limb and penis in a cohort of men reporting erectile dysfunction [31].

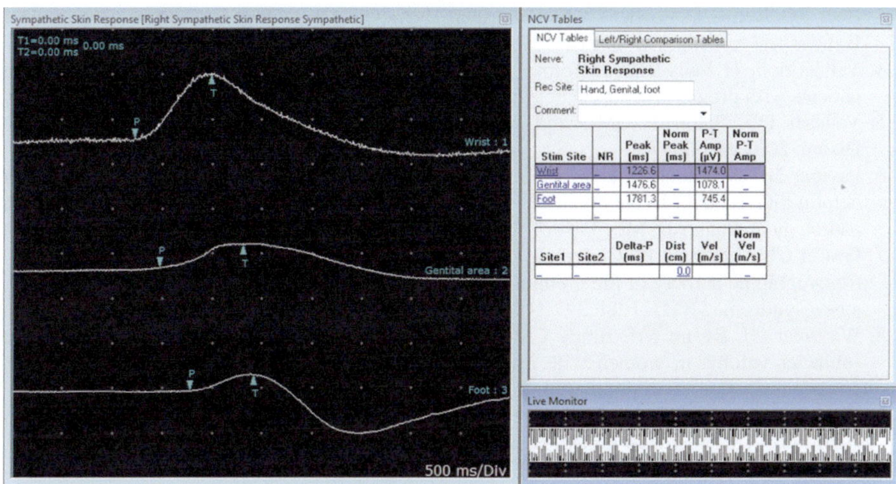

Fig. 3 Normal sympathetic skin response recorded from (top to bottom, respectively) the wrist, genital region and foot on the right side following electrical stimulation of the tibial nerve

Conclusion

Neurophysiological tests are important to better understand and diagnose the neurological lesions responsible for pelvic organ complaints. The currently available repertoire of tests provides a diagnostic assessment to evaluate the afferent and efferent somatic sacral segmental innervation. However, pelvic neurophysiology is technically demanding and often tests only a subset of nerves. Moreover, they require to be performed with care considering the sensitive nature of these tests, and patients must be put at ease during these tests for these to be successfully performed. It is anticipated that these tests will gain greater clinical relevance in the coming years for evaluating pelvic floor/ pelvic organ complaints.

Acknowledgements This work was undertaken at the UCLH/UCL Institute of Neurology which received a proportion of funding from the Department of Health's NIHR Biomedical Research Centres funding scheme.

References

1. Schwarz J, Kornhuber M, Bischoff C, Straube A. Electromyography of the external anal sphincter in patients with Parkinson's disease and multiple system atrophy: frequency of abnormal spontaneous activity and polyphasic motor unit potentials. Muscle Nerve. 1997;20:1167–72.
2. Podnar S, Trsinar B, Vodusek DB. Bladder dysfunction in patients with cauda equina lesions. Neurourol Urodyn. 2006;25:23–31.

3. Beck RO, Betts CD, Fowler CJ. Genitourinary dysfunction in multiple system atrophy: clinical features and treatment in 62 cases. J Urol. 1994;151:1336–41.
4. Valldeoriola F, Valls-Sole J, Tolosa ES, Marti MJ. Striated anal sphincter denervation in patients with progressive supranuclear palsy. Mov Disord. 1995;10:550–5.
5. Vodusek DB. Sphincter EMG and differential diagnosis of multiple system atrophy. Mov Disord. 2001;16:600–7.
6. Paviour DC, Williams D, Fowler CJ, Quinn NP, Lees AJ. Is sphincter electromyography a helpful investigation in the diagnosis of multiple system atrophy? A retrospective study with pathological diagnosis. Mov Disord. 2005;20:1425–30.
7. Fowler CJ, Christmas TJ, Chapple CR, Parkhouse HF, Kirby RS, Jacobs HS. Abnormal electromyographic activity of the urethral sphincter, voiding dysfunction, and polycystic ovaries: a new syndrome? BMJ. 1988;297:1436–8.
8. Wiseman OJ, Swinn MJ, Brady CM, Fowler CJ. Maximum urethral closure pressure and sphincter volume in women with urinary retention. J Urol. 2002;167:1348–51; discussion 1351–2.
9. Webb RJ, Fawcett PR, Neal DE. Electromyographic abnormalities in the urethral and anal sphincters of women with idiopathic retention of urine. Br J Urol. 1992;70:22–5.
10. Ramm O, Mueller ER, Brubaker L, Lowenstein L, Kenton K. Complex repetitive discharges—a feature of the urethral continence mechanism or a pathological finding? J Urol. 2012;187:2140–3.
11. Tawadros C, Burnett K, Derbyshire LF, Tawadros T, Clarke NW, Betts CD. External urethral sphincter electromyography in asymptomatic women and the influence of the menstrual cycle. BJU Int. 2015;116:423–31.
12. Sihra N, Malde S, Panicker J, Kightley R, Solomon E, Hamid R, et al. Does the appearance of the urethral pressure profile trace correlate with the sphincter EMG findings in women with voiding dysfunction? Neurourol Urodyn. 2018;37:751–7.
13. Tubaro A, Vodušek D, Amarenco R, Doumouchtsis S, DeLancey J, Fernando R, et al. Imaging, neurophysiological testing and other tests. Paris: ICUD-EAU; 2013.
14. Cai ZY, Niu XT, Pan J, Ni PQ, Wang X, Shao B. The value of the bulbocavernosus reflex and pudendal nerve somatosensory evoked potentials in distinguishing between multiple system atrophy and Parkinson's disease at an early stage. Acta Neurol Scand. 2017;136:195–203.
15. Deletis V, Vodusek DB. Intraoperative recording of the bulbocavernosus reflex. Neurosurgery. 1997;40:88–92; discussion 92–3.
16. Lee DG, Kwak SG, Chang MC. Prediction of the outcome of bladder dysfunction based on electrically induced reflex findings in patients with cauda equina syndrome: a retrospective study. Medicine (Baltimore). 2017;96:e7014.
17. Pelliccioni G, Piloni V, Sabbatini D, Fioravanti P, Scarpino O. Sex differences in pudendal somatosensory evoked potentials. Tech Coloproctol. 2014;18:565–9.
18. Opsomer RJ, Guerit JM, Wese FX, Van Cangh PJ. The contribution of electrophysiological tests in the assessment of paraplegia. Acta Urol Belg. 1991;59:61–2.
19. Cavalcanti GA, Bruschini H, Manzano GM, Nunes KF, Giuliano LM, Nobrega JA, et al. Pudendal somatosensory evoked potentials in normal women. Int Braz J Urol. 2007;33:815–21.
20. Rodi Z, Vodusek D, Denislic M. Clinical uro-neurophysiological investigation in multiple sclerosis. Eur J Neurol. 1996;3:574–80.
21. Ormeci B, Avci E, Kaspar C, Terim OE, Erdogru T, Oge AE. A novel electrophysiological method in the diagnosis of pudendal neuropathy: position-related changes in pudendal sensory evoked potentials. Urology. 2017;99:288.e1–7.
22. Vodusek D, Deletis V, Abbott R, et al. Prevention of iatrogenic micturition disorders through intraoperative monitoring. Neurourol Urodyn. 1990;9:444–5.
23. Cohen BA, Major MR, Huizenga BA. Pudendal nerve evoked potential monitoring in procedures involving low sacral fixation. Spine. 1991;16:S375–8.
24. Sala F, Squintani G, Tramontano V, Arcaro C, Faccioli F, Mazza C. Intraoperative neurophysiology in tethered cord surgery: techniques and results. Childs Nerv Syst. 2013;29:1611–24.

25. Eccher MA. Below the belt: sensory mapping and monitoring in the sacral-pudendal region. J Clin Neurophysiol. 2014;31:323–5.
26. Vodusek D, Zidar J. Perineal motor evoked responses. Neurourol Urodyn. 1988;7:236–7.
27. Kiff ES, Swash M. Slowed conduction in the pudendal nerves in idiopathic (neurogenic) faecal incontinence. Br J Surg. 1984;71:614–6.
28. Opsomer RJ, Boccasena P, Traversa R, Rossini PM. Sympathetic skin responses from the limbs and the genitalia: normative study and contribution to the evaluation of neurourological disorders. Electroencephalogr Clin Neurophysiol. 1996;101:25–31.
29. Rodic B, Curt A, Dietz V, Schurch B. Bladder neck incompetence in patients with spinal cord injury: significance of sympathetic skin response. J Urol. 2000;163:1223–7.
30. Secil Y, Ozdedeli K, Altay B, Aydogdu I, Yilmaz C, Ertekin C. Sympathetic skin response recorded from the genital region in normal and diabetic women. Neurophysiol Clin. 2005;35:11–7.
31. Valles-Antuna C, Fernandez-Gomez J, Escaf S, Fernandez-Gonzalez F. Sympathetic skin response in patients with erectile dysfunction. BJU Int. 2009;104:1709–12.

Systematic Neuro-urological Pathology

Helmut Madersbacher

When a neurological pathology in the brain, in the spinal cord or in the periphery affects the innervation of the lower urinary tract (LUT), the resulting dysfunction depends mainly on the location of the lesion, its extent, the underlying neurological pathology and the changes in the LUT occurring during the course of the neurological disease. Already in the 1960s of the last century, clinicians and pathologists tried to allocate urological symptoms to the underlying neurological pathology [1]. With the help of meticulous clinical investigations and correlating them with post-mortem studies, they were remarkably successful already in the past. Nowadays, modern functional neuroimaging including functional MRT and PET studies provided further insight in the complex innervation of the LUT and in the dysfunction which follows neurological disease or trauma.

For many decades, neuro-urological pathology has been divided into upper motor neuron lesions (UMNL), which included not only suprasacral spinal cord but also pontine and suprapontine cerebral lesions, and lower motor neuron lesions (LMNL), comprising sacral and subsacral (cauda equina and peripheral) nerve lesions.

Meanwhile, lesions are categorized into (1) cerebral, suprapontine and pontine lesions; (2) spinal suprasacral lesions; and (3) spinal sacral and subsacral nerve lesions.

H. Madersbacher
c/o Univ-Klinik Innsbruck/Tirol Kliniken, Innsbruck, Austria
e-mail: Helmut.Madersbacher@tirol-kliniken.at

© Springer International Publishing AG, part of Springer Nature 2018
R. Dmochowski, J. Heesakkers (eds.), *Neuro-Urology*,
https://doi.org/10.1007/978-3-319-90997-4_3

Cerebral Control of the Bladder Function

Cerebral Lesions and LUTS

There are areas and pathways in the brain which are an *intrinsic part* of the micturition and continence reflex, and there are areas and pathways which *modulate* them, e.g. the basal ganglia.

According to current knowledge, the micturition reflex cycle consists of three phases controlled by separate central pathways: (1) the pre-micturition phase controlled via a forebrain (hypothalamic) pathway to the PAG and PMC; (2) the urethral relaxation phase, controlled via an excitatory descending PMC pathway to inhibitory sacral interneurons; and (3) the contraction phase, controlled via an excitatory descending PMC pathway to sacral preganglionic bladder motor neurons.

The lower urinary tract afferent nerve pathways synapse primarily in the periaqueductal grey (PAG), sensation of the full bladder is registered in the insula, from there they are conveyed to the pre-frontal cortex, where the decision to void or not to void is made. Motor output from there is controlled by the anterior cingulate gyrus (ACG), which is part of the limbic system being responsible for our social behaviour, and when the ACG "agrees", motor output activates the pontine micturition centre (PMC) via the PAG. The PMC sends then motor output to the bladder and urethra [2, 3].

The Role of the Pontine Micturition Centre
and of the Pontine Continence Centre

The Pontine Micturition Centre (PMC)

In humans, a comparable region to the pontine micturition centre in cat was described in the dorsal part of the pontine tegmentum [4, 5]. In humans, lesions of the PMC (also called the M-region) e.g. caused by stroke or multiple sclerosis, result in urinary retention.

The Pontine Continence Centre (PCC)

The PCC is also called the L-region as it is located ventrolateral to the PMC, projects specifically to Onuf's nucleus in the sacral cord and fulfils the storage function of the bladder. Stimulation of the PCC stops micturition, excites the pelvic floor muscle and contracts the urethral sphincter. Bilateral lesions of the PCC cause incontinence, accompanied by excessive detrusor activity and relaxation of the urethral sphincter.

According to Blok et al. (1997) and Holstege et al. (1986), PMC and PCC function independently, no pathways between them were identified so far, but both are important and responsible for detrusor-sphincter synergia, responsible for coordinated micturition [6, 7].

The Periaqueductal Grey

The periaqueductal grey (PAG)—a dense neuronal matter around the aqueduct of Sylvius—is the main area for bladder control in the caudal brainstem. The forebrain controls the PAG and the PMC like a switch. It is assumed that the basic micturition reflex contains an ascending pathway from the lumbosacral cord to the PMC and PAG and a descending pathway from PAG via PMC to the sacral cord. Lesions between the PAG-PMC and the sacral spinal cord will result in a disruption of the normal micturition reflex causing detrusor-sphincter dyssynergia.

The role of the PAG and PMC has been described for the first time by Blok et al. (1997) and was again confirmed recently by Michels et al. (2015), using positron emission tomography (PET) and functional magnetic resonance imaging (MRI) with and without a full bladder [8, 9].

The Hypothalamus

The hypothalamus receives major projections from the prefrontal cortex and is obviously involved in the decision whether it is "safe enough" to start micturition. Already Andrew and Nathan (1964) assumed, on the basis of cerebral lesions in humans, that the connection of the prefrontal cortex and the anterior cingulate gyrus to the hypothalamus provides controllable micturition [10].

The Insula, Prefrontal Cortex and Anterior Cingulate Gyrus

Sensation of bladder fullness is registered in the insula, and from there afferent stimuli are conveyed to the prefrontal cortex, where the decision "to void or not to void" is made. Motor output from there is controlled by the anterior cingulate gyrus (ACG), which is part of the limbic system being responsible for our social behaviour, and normally only when the ACG "agrees", motor output activates the PMC via the PAG. The PMC sends then motor output to the bladder and urethra. It was shown by Blok et al. (1997, 1998) and Michels (2014) that the human pre-frontal cortex and the anterior cingulate gyrus are activated during micturition [8, 9, 11].

Cerebellum and Basal Ganglia

Animal studies have shown that also the cerebellum and the basal ganglia have mainly an inhibitory action on the bladder. Cerebellar pathology in humans causes urinary frequency and urge urinary incontinence [12]. This inhibitory influence is probably indirect via the forebrain and midbrain as no direct projections from these areas to the PMC could be identified. Overactive bladder symptoms are also found in Parkinson's disease. Sakakibara (2011) has designed a scheme showing the possible relation between the basal ganglia circuit and the micturition circuit, highlighting the role of GABA. GABA (gamma-aminobutyric acid) is a ubiquitous, inhibitory neurotransmitter in the CNS that can inhibit the micturition reflex on many points along the central pathways [13].

Functional Consequences of Brain Pathology on the Lower Urinary Tract

The net effect of the suprapontine areas of the brain on the micturition reflex is inhibitory. Lesions in the relevant areas cause symptoms of the overactive bladder. If the lesion is localized above the PMC/PAG, voiding remains coordinated (detrusor-sphincter synergia); in these patients, voiding is right, but timing is wrong. Lesions in the brainstem may cause detrusor overactivity but also underactivity depending on location and extent of the damage. With lesions in the pons, voiding may become uncoordinated due to cerebral detrusor-sphincter dyssynergia causing clinically, in addition to the storage symptoms, also voiding symptoms including post-void residual urine.

Also lesions in the areas and pathways which modulate the micturition and continence areas result in symptoms of the overactive bladder as shown in patients with Parkinson's disease in whom, due to dopamine deprivation, the inhibiting influence of the basal ganglia is lacking. Yamamoto et al. (2005) *have made a proposal on how the basal ganglia circuit interacts with the micturition reflex* [14].

Spinal Cord Control of Bladder Function

Suprasacral Spinal Cord Lesions

Afferent Spinal Pathways from the Lower Urinary Tract

Different sensations from the LUT are mediated by ascending spinal pathways located in different columns. In humans, the desire to void and pain from the bladder, urethra and lower ureteral end are conducted by the spinothalamic tracts of the lateral columns. According to Nathan and Smith (1951), the fibres are located opposite the dorsal lateral process of the anterior horn of the grey substance [15]. Fibres in the posterior columns convey sensations of touch, pressure or tension in the urethra. White et al. (1952) reported that the sensation of bladder distention is transmitted by these fibres because it was not affected by spinothalamic tractotomy which abolished among other sensations that of the desire to void [16].

Distribution of fibres subserving micturition and the lamellation of the long ascending and descending fibre tracts explain the appearance of characteristic clinical syndromes from trauma to the spinal cord in incomplete lesions.

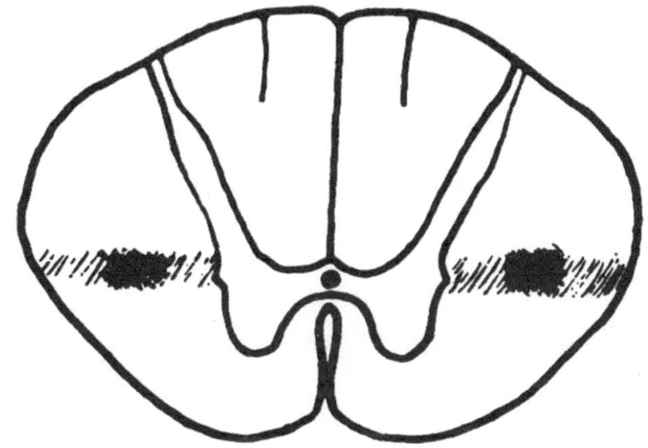

Fig. 1 The region within the spinal cord of the centrifugal pathway for micturition. The majority of the fibres probably lie within the region indicated by cross-hatching [19]

Efferent Spinal Cord Pathways from the Lower Urinary Tract

(a) *Spinal parasympathetic efferent pathways*

Efferent spinal cord pathways to the lower urinary tract convey stimuli from the PAG via the PMC to the intermediolateral region of the sacral spinal cord [17, 18].

The regions within the spinal cord of these efferent pathways for micturition are shown in Fig. 1 and are cross-hatched.

Both the corticospinal and the spinothalamic tracts are so lamellated that the sacral supply occupies the most superficial and the cervical supply the deepest position in the cord close to the grey matter, which again has implications on the clinical symptomatology of incomplete spinal cord lesions (see below).

When a central cord syndrome develops following injury, chiefly affecting the grey matter and the adjacent fibre tracts, the sacral supply will escape. Such patients characteristically retain their autonomic functions. When, on the other hand, an obstruction of the anterior spinal artery, e.g. causes degeneration of the lateral columns, supraspinal regulation of autonomic function ceases, and purely spinal reflex activity results which is characteristic for the anterior cord syndrome. When a hemisection of the cord is present, long afferents on one side and long efferents on the other side will escape, owing to the high crossing of the pyramidal efferent and the low segmental crossing of the afferent fibres. A Brown-Séquard syndrome is accompanied by precipitate micturition because of the reduction of supraspinal regulatory impulses.

(b) *Spinal sympathetic efferent pathways*

Sympathetic pathways to the lower urinary tract originate in the lumbosacral sympathetic chain ganglia as well as in the prevertebral inferior mesenteric ganglia. Sympathetic efferent input induce various effects including (1) inhibition of the detrusor muscle, (2) excitation of the bladder base and urethra [20] and (3) modulation of inhibition and facilitation in bladder parasympathetic ganglia [21–23].

(c) *Spinal somatic efferent pathways*

The efferent innervation of the urethral striated muscles originates from the motor cortex and is conveyed by the pyramidal tract on both sides to a circumscribed region of the lateral ventral horn that is called "Onuf's nucleus".

Effects of Lesions in the Spinal Cord

A spinal cord lesion above the lumbosacral level, depending on completeness of the lesion, may eliminate (complete lesions) or at least reduce (incomplete lesions) voluntary cerebral control of micturition leading to neurogenic spinal detrusor overactivity mediated by spinal reflex pathways. Once the bladder capacity is reached, afferent input from the bladder stimulates the nuclei of the parasympathetic nerves in the sacral cord as well as the Onuf's nucleus inducing a reflex contraction of the detrusor combined with a contraction of the sphincter at the same time. Therefore, this spinal detrusor overactivity has important disadvantages: reduced bladder capacity, detrusor-sphincter dyssynergia with post-void residual urine and a high intravesical pressure situation with a risk for lower and upper urinary tract deterioration. Moreover, detrusor-related incontinence is present. Clinical consequences of a spinal reflex bladder are not uniform but depend on the underlying pathophysiology: in traumatic lesions these spinal reflex bladders can be quite "aggressive" bearing a high risk for upper urinary tract deterioration, whereas the same spinal reflex bladder caused by multiple sclerosis is much less dangerous.

Incomplete Suprasacral Spinal Cord Lesions

In incomplete lesions with preserved proprioception, the patient may feel the urge to void but is unable to inhibit it adequately; thus, urge incontinence is possible. In about 30% of these patients, also DSD is present with all its consequences.

As mentioned above, lamellation of the long ascending and descending fibre tracts explains the appearance of four syndromes of incomplete spinal cord lesions which are important regarding the prognosis of future of bladder function: the central cord syndrome, the lateral syndrome, the anterior cord syndrome and the posterior cord syndrome.

The central cord syndrome (CCS, Schneider syndrome) [24, 25] is the most common form of cervical spinal cord injury, and the related motor impairment results from the pattern of lamellation of the corticospinal and spinal-thalamic tracts in the spinal cord which result from the stretch of the cord in the transverse axis by acute anterior-posterior compression. It is characterized by impairment with loss of motion and sensation in the arms and hands. Symptoms correlate with a lamellation of the long tracts in the lateral columns and the blood supply. Patients usually walk eventually. Sacral segments are the most lateral with lumbar-thoracic and cervical components arranged somato-typically, proceeding medially towards the central canal. Different types of LUT dysfunction were described such as detrusor underactivity/areflexia, detrusor overactivity and detrusor-sphincter dyssynergia. However, the prognosis for improvement or normalization of bladder, bowel and sexual function is good. Sensation is mostly preserved [26–28].

Lateral cord syndrome (LCS, Brown-Séquard): the classical hemisection of the cord as the result of e.g. a stab wound is characterized by the loss of motor function, impaired vibratory sense and proprioception, but preserved pain und temperature sense in the ipsilateral side. On the contralateral side, motor function is normal or almost normal, while temperature and pain perception are disturbed. Different LUT dysfunctions were described: urgency due to neurogenic detrusor overactivity, detrusor-sphincter dyssynergia or occasionally also detrusor areflexia [29].

Anterior cord syndrome (ACS): it results from injury or spontaneous occlusion of the anterior spinal artery involving the lateral columns including the autonomic pathway. Clinically activity is reduced or absent, as well as pain and temperature sensation. However, proprioception and bladder sensation may be spared if the dorsal columns are intact. Patients suffer from neurogenic detrusor overactivity; DSD is possible.

Posterior cord syndrome (PCS) can be seen in tabes dorsalis or diabetes. The disease causes changes in the posterior root ganglia, in the posterior roots and posterior columns. Clinically a large flaccid bladder develops, the bladder capacity increased, detrusor contractility impaired and post-void residual urine present. The loss of visceral sensation eventually includes bowel and sexual function manifested by the loss of desire to defecate and loss of libido and orgasm in women and erectile dysfunction in men.

Sacral and Subsacral Control of Bladder Function

Conus/Cauda Equina Lesions/Peripheral Neuropathy and LUTS

The lower urinary tract has autonomic innervation of the bladder and urethra and somatic innervation of the striated part of the urethral wall and of the striated peri-urethral sphincter (m. pubococcygeus).

The sacral parasympathetic outflow provides the majority of excitatory input to the urinary bladder. Cholinergic preganglionic neurons located in the intermediolateral region of the sacral spinal cord send axons via the pelvic nerves to ganglion cells in the pelvic plexus and in the wall of the bladder [17, 18].

Sympathetic pathways to the lower urinary tract originate in the lumbosacral sympathetic chain ganglia as well as in the prevertebral inferior mesenteric ganglia. They are conveyed to the bladder via hypogastric [30] and pelvic nerves [31]. Sympathetic efferent pathways induce various effects including (1) inhibition of the detrusor muscle, (2) excitation of the bladder base and urethra [20] and (3) modulation of inhibition and facilitation in bladder parasympathetic ganglia [21–23].

Spinal *somatic* efferent pathways originate primarily in the motor cortex, via the pyramidal tract; they are conveyed to a circumscribed region of the lateral ventral horn that is called "Onuf's nucleus". Sphincter motor neurons send their axons through the pudendal nerve stimulation sphincter muscles via the release of acetylcholine [32].

It is important to realize that patients with complete conus cauda equina or pelvic plexus injury are neurologically decentralized, but may not be completely denervated. These lesions allow possible afferent and efferent neuron interconnection at the level of the intramural ganglia in the detrusor muscle. The ganglia cells in turn excite bladder smooth muscle via the release of cholinergic (acetylcholine) and non-adrenergic, non-cholinergic transmitters (ATP and others) and also inhibit urethral smooth muscle via the release of nitric oxide [20]. This may also be the reason why also bladders with this type of lesion can develop a low compliance.

Lesions of the parasympathetic nerves to the bladder (*nn. pelvici*) will result in a neurogenic acontractile (or in incomplete lesion hypocontractile) bladder. Both the afferent and efferent arms of the micturition reflex are located in the pelvic nerves. Lesions of somatic nerves can influence voiding by changing the striated sphincter function; lesions of the sympathetic nerves (*nn. hypogastrici*) can alter tension in the bladder neck and the urethra. A characteristic finding in lesions of the sympathetic nerves is an open bladder neck. Sympathectomy on humans does not change the clinical pattern of voiding. However, peripheral local reflexes and feedback mechanisms can be disturbed also by peripheral neuropathies.

Both parasympathetic and somatic motor function can be compromised with peripheral neuropathies as observed in diabetes mellitus, chronic alcohol abuse or Guillain-Barré syndrome with the results of an underactive or areflexic detrusor and a flaccid paralysis of the external sphincter causing a detrusor-related overflow and, due to sphincter weakness, stress urinary incontinence.

The main complications of type 2 diabetes, responsible for the majority of peripheral neuropathies, are the vascular and the neurogenic ones, the latter being probably the most common. At the time when diabetes is discovered, neuropathy can already be seen in 10%; however, in patients with long-standing diabetes (more than 24 years), the prevalence of diabetic neuropathy is about 50%. The diabetic peripheral neuropathy can be separated into eight clinical syndromes known as diabetic neuropathy [33–35]. Autonomic neuropathy can cause neurogenic bladder dysfunction. It is often combined with one or the other syndrome, especially with the symmetric upper and lower limb distal polyneuropathy.

The clinical symptoms and findings in complete conus and cauda equina lesions are the loss of the sensation for the urge to void. Sensation for bladder fullness, may be present created by afferent input from the peritoneum which covers the bladder or by vertebral sympathetic nerves. No micturition is possible, and if adequate emptying is not provided in time, overflow incontinence may occur. Moreover, flaccid paralysis of the striated sphincter causes neurogenic stress urinary incontinence.

Herniated lumbar disc may cause cauda equina lesions. With lateral disc protrusion, it is very unlikely that the herniated disc compresses the cauda equina; however, with central disc protrusion, compressing of the cauda equina does occur.

Peripheral nerve lesions may be caused by radical surgery in the small pelvis. Mostly these lesions are incomplete resulting in partial decentralization of the bladder. The pudendal nerves are rarely affected because of their lateral anatomical location.

Mixed Lesions

Mixed lesions can occur especially with lesions in close proximity of the conus medullaris. Depending on the location and extent of the lesion, e.g. children with myelodysplasia can show different dysfunctional patterns of the LUT: one third of these children show a combination of an overactive detrusor with an overactive sphincter, and another third show a flaccid paresis of the detrusor combined with a flaccid paresis of the sphincter. However, there is a small group of children (around 10%) who have a combination of an overactive detrusor with a flaccid paresis of the sphincter or vice versa a spastic sphincter combined with an areflexic detrusor (see Fig. 2).

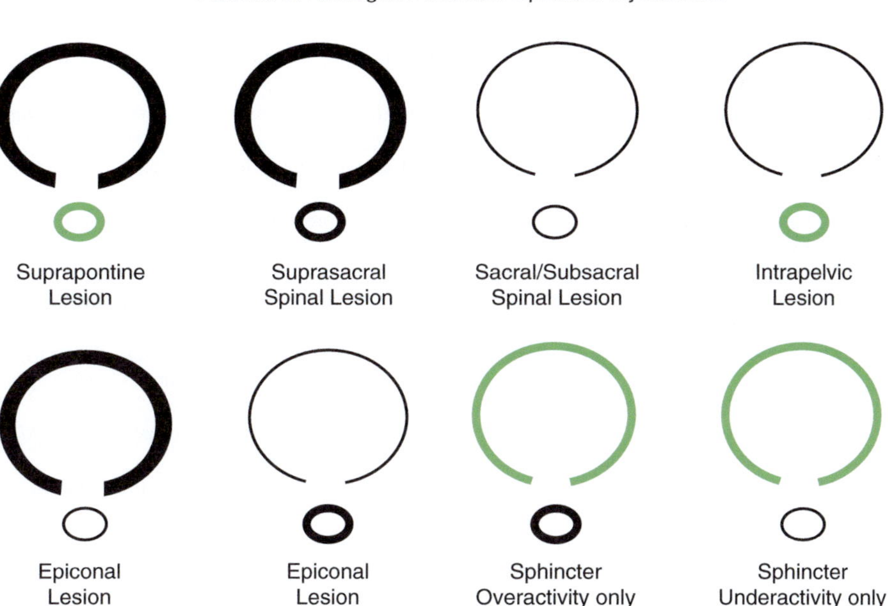

Fig. 2 Patterns of neurogenic detrusor-sphincter dysfunction [36]

Moreover, in degenerative diseases affecting not only the brain but also the spinal cord as in multisystem atrophy (MSA), degeneration in the brainstem may result in detrusor overactivity, and degeneration of the nuclei in the intermediolateral column causes parasympathetic failure with impaired detrusor contractility and incomplete emptying as well as a sympathetic failure by affecting the relevant nuclei in the thoracolumbar areas of the spinal cord. Characteristically an open bladder neck can be diagnosed during cystography or videourodynamics. At the same time, Onuf's nucleus atrophy can cause sphincter weakness.

Characteristics of Neurogenic Lower Urinary Tract (LUT) Dysfunction

Detrusor and sphincter may become overactive or underactive (acontractile) depending on the location and extent of the lesion. Mostly detrusor *and* sphincter are affected, from the same type or differently, normal function of the counterpart is possible (see Fig. 2). The same urodynamic pattern may have different clinical implications as shown on the example of the spinal reflex bladder (see above).

The term "neurogenic bladder" is misleading; mostly detrusor *and* sphincter are affected. A better term is "neurogenic (lower) urinary tract dysfunction".

References

1. Bors E, Comarr AE. Neurological urology. Basek, München, Paris, New York: S. Karger; 1971. p. 166.
2. Blok B. Central pathways controlling micturition and urinary continence. Urology. 2002;59:13–7.
3. De Groat W, Griffiths D, Yoshimura N. Neural control of the lower urinary tract. Compr Physiol. 2015;5:327–96.
4. Barrington F. The effect of lesion of the hind- and mid-brain on micturition in the cat. Quart J Exp Physiol. 1925;15:81–102.
5. Blanco L, Yuste J, Carillo-de Sauvage M. Critical evaluation of the anatomical location of the Barrington nucleus: relevance for deep brain stimulation surgery of pedunculopontine tegmental nucleus. Neuroscience. 2013;247:351–63.
6. Holstege G, Griffiths D, de Wall H, Dalm E. Anatomical and physiological observations on supraspinal control of bladder and urethral sphincter muscles in the cat. J Comp Neurol. 1986;250:449–61.
7. Blok B, de Weerd H, Holstege G. The pontine micturition center projects to sacral cord GABA immunoreactive neurons in the cat. Neurosci Lett. 1997;233:109–12.
8. Blok B, Willemsen A, Holstege G. A PET study on brain control of micturition in humans. Brain. 1997;120:111–21.
9. Michels L, Blok B, Gregorini F, Kurz M, Schurch B, Kessler T, Kollias S, Mehnert U. Supraspinal control of urine storage and micturition in men: an fMRI study. Cereb Cortex. 2015;25:3369–80.

10. Andrew J, Nathan P. Lesions of the anterior frontal lobes and disturbances of micturition and defaecation. Brain. 1964;87:233–62.
11. Blok B, Sturms L, Holstege G. Brain activation during micturition in women. Brain. 1998;121:2033–42.
12. Zago T, Pea U, Fumagalli G, Areta L, MArzorati G, Bianchi F. Cerebellar pathology and micturitional disorders: anatomotopographic and functional considerations. Arch Ital Urol Androl. 2010;82:177–80.
13. Sakakibara R, Kishi M, Ogawa E, Tateno F, Uchiyama T, Yamamoto T, Yamanishi T. Bladder, bowel, and sexual dysfunction in Parkinson's disease. Parkinsons Dis. 2011;2011:924605.
14. Yamamoto T, Sakakibara R, Hashimoto K, Nakazawa K, Uchiyama T, Liu Z, Ito T, Hattori T. Striatal dopamine level increases in the urinary storage phase in cats: an in vivo microdialysis study. Neuroscience. 2005;135:299–303.
15. Nathan P, Smith M. The centripetal pathway from the bladder and urethra within the spinal cord. J Neurol Neurosurg Psychiatry. 1951;14:262–80.
16. White J, Smitzwick R, Simeone F. The autonomic nervous system. Anatomy, physiology and surgical application. New York: MacMillan Co; 1952.
17. de Groat W, Ryall R. The identification and characteristics of sacral parasympathetic preganglionic neurones. J Physiol. 1968;196:563–77.
18. Nadelhaft I, de Groat W, Morgan C. Location and morphology of parasympathetic preganglionic neurons in the sacral spinal cord of the cat revealed by retrograde axonal transport of horseradish peroxidase. J Comp Neurol. 1980;193:265–81.
19. Nathan P, Smith M. The centrifugal pathway for micturition within the spinal cord. J Neurol Neurosurg Psychiatry. 1958;21:177–89.
20. Fry C, Kanai A, Roosen A, Takeda M, Wood D. Cell biology. In: Incontinence. 4th ed. Paris: Health Lublications Ltd; 2009. p. 113–66.
21. de Groat W, Saum W. Sympathetic inhibition of the urinary bladder and of pelvic ganglionic transmission in the cat. J Physiol. 1972;220:297–314.
22. de Groat W, Theobald R. Reflex activation of sympathetic pathways to vesical smooth muscle and parasympathetic ganglia by electrical stimulation of vesical afferents. J Physiol. 1976;259:223–37.
23. Keast J, Kawatani M, de Groat W. Sympathetic modulation of cholinergic transmission in cat vesical ganglia is mediated by alpha 1- and alpha 2-adrenoceptors. Am J Phys. 1990;258:R44–50.
24. Schneider R, Cherry G, Pantek H. The syndrome of acute central cervical spinal cord injury with special reference to the mechanisms involved in hyperextension injuries of cervical spine. J Neurosurg. 1954;11:546–77.
25. Schneider R. The syndrome of acute anterior spinal cord injury. J Neurosurg. 1955;12:95–122.
26. Molliqaj G, Payer M, Schaller K, et al. Acute traumatic central cord syndrome: a comprehensive review. Neurochirurgie. 2014;60:5–11.
27. Smith C, Kraus S, Nickell K, et al. Video urodynamic findings in men with the central cord syndrome. J Urol. 2000;164:2014–7.
28. Nath M, Wheeler J, Walter J. Urological aspects of tramatic central cord syndrome. J Am Paraplegia Soc. 1993;16:160–4.
29. Sakakibara R, Hattori T, Uchiyama T, et al. Urinary dysfunction in Brown_Sequard syndrome. Neurourol Urodyn. 2001;20:661–7.
30. Morgan C, Nadelhaft I, de Groat W. The distribution of visceral primary afferents from the pelvic nerve to Lissauer's tract and the spinal gray matter and its relationship to the sacral parasympathetic nucleus. J Comp Neurol. 1981;201:415–40.
31. Kuo D, Hisamitsu T, de Groat W. A sympathetic projection from sacral paravertebral ganglia to the pelvic nerve and to postganglionic nerves on the surface of the urinary bladder and large intestine of the cat. J Comp Neurol. 1984;226:76–86.
32. Thor K, de Groat W. Neural control of the female urethral and anal rhabdosphincters and pelvic floor muscles. Am J Phys Regul Integr Comp Phys. 2010;299:R416–38.

33. Dyck P, Low P, Stevens J. Diseases of peripheral nerves. In: Clinical neurology. Phildelphia: JB Lippincott; 1990. p. 1–126.
34. Adams RD, Vicotr M, Ropper A. Principles of neurology. 6th ed. New York: McGraw-Hil; 1997.
35. Thomas P, Tomlinson D. Diabetic and hypoglycemic neuropathy. In: Peripheral neuropathy. 3rd ed. Philadelphia: WB Saunders; 1993. p. 1219–50.
36. Madersbacher H. The various types of neurogenic bladder dysfunction: an update of current therapeutic concepts. Paraplegia. 1990;28(4):217–29.

Part II
Clinical Entities and Their Neuro-urological Consequences

Congenital Abnormalities (Meningomyelocele and Spinal Dysraphism)

Ryuji Sakakibara

Introduction

Malformations of the spinal cord are one of the most frequent in the embryo [1]. They have been described as spina bifida (SB) or spinal dysraphism (SD), most of which were myelomeningocele (MMC). SB is classified under the caudal group of neural tube defects, which also includes the rostral group such as Arnold-Chiari malformation, etc. SB involves a lack of fusion of one or several vertebral arches. The most common overt open, cystic form in infancy is MMC, found approximately in 1 per 1000 births, which needs early surgical closure to avoid infection [2]. After initial surgical management, walking with or without aids can be achieved in all patients with sacral levels and 95% with low lumbar lesions, while lower urinary tract (LUT) dysfunction tends to remain as large post-void residuals, high-pressure voiding, and urinary incontinence [2, 3]. In contrast, the incidence of occult SB remains uncertain. Most cases are asymptomatic and incidentally found during X-ray screening of low back pain. Some cases are accompanied by lipomeningomyelocele (lipoMMC), dermoid cyst, or thick filum terminale with minimum skin changes such as dimple and focal hypertrichosis [4]. In these instances, LUT dysfunction may present in late childhood or in adulthood, varying from nocturnal enuresis [5, 6] to urinary retention [7–9]. In these instances, bladder dysfunction appears as the sole initial manifestation or with minimum neurologic signs such as foot numbness.

R. Sakakibara
Department of Neurology, Internal Medicine, Sakura Medical Center,
Toho University, Sakura, Japan
e-mail: sakakibara@sakura.med.toho-u.ac.jp

© Springer International Publishing AG, part of Springer Nature 2018
R. Dmochowski, J. Heesakkers (eds.), *Neuro-Urology*,
https://doi.org/10.1007/978-3-319-90997-4_4

Embryology of Myelomeningocele (MMC) and Occult Spina Bifida (SB)

Many theories have been discussed (nonclosure, reopening, overgrowth, overdistension) for the generation of MMC [2, 10]. The nonclosure theory has gained almost universal acceptance, but there is no definitive evidence to refute the other theories. Numerous teratogenic agents and genetic disorders have been identified that act on specific parts of the neurulation sequence to produce neural tube defects. Folate deficiency has also been identified as one of the main causes of open SB and can be largely prevented by folate supplementation before conception and during the early stages of pregnancy. While it remains mostly unknown in humans, occult SB involves a mechanism clearly different from that which causes MMC. Detailed classification of SB is listed in Table 1 [11].

Table 1 Classification of spinal dysraphisms[a]

Classification	Description
Open spinal dysraphism	
Myelomeningocele	Protrusion of spinal cord segment and meninges through a bony defect in midline of the back
Myelocele	Myelomeningocele w/o expansion of underlying subarachnoid space
Hemimyelomeningocele	Myelomeningocele w/ associated SCM (defect of 1 hemicord)
Hemimyelocele	Myelocele w/ associated SCM (defect of 1 hemicord)
Closed spinal dysraphism w/ subcutaneous mass	
Lipomyelomeningocele	Large subcutaneous lipoma extending intraspinally; cord is tethered and lipoma-cord interface lies outside the spinal canal
Lipomyeloschisis	Large subcutaneous lipoma extending intraspinally; cord is tethered and lipoma-cord interface lies w/in or at edge of spinal canal
Terminal myelocystocele	Ependyma-lined cyst (dilation of terminal ventricle) bulging through a posterior spina bifida, causing herniation of meninges
Lumbosacral meningocele	Herniation of CSF-filled sac lined by dura and arachnoid through a posterior spina bifida
Cervical myelocystocele	Epithelial-lined cavity; only dorsal wall protrudes into meningocele
Cervical myelomeningocele	Fibroneurovascular stalk containing neurons, glia, and peripheral nerves traveling through a narrow dorsal dural opening; fans out into lining of meningeal sac; spinal cord remains in canal
Cervical meningocele	Herniation of CSF-filled sac lined by dura and arachnoid through a posterior spina bifida
Closed spinal dysraphism w/o subcutaneous mass	
Posterior spina bifida	Simple failure of fusion of the posterior vertebra
Intradural and intramedullary lipoma	Encapsulated mass w/ fibrous bundles residing in spinal canal
Tight filum terminate	Short, hypertrophic filum terminale resulting in tethering and impaired ascent of conus medullaris

Table 1 (continued)

Classification	Description
Abnormally long spinal cord	Absence of normally tapered conus medullaris
Persistent terminal ventricle	Cystic dilation of terminal ventricle; an ependyma-lined cavity in conus medullaris
Dorsal enteric fistula	Fistula connecting bowel w/ dorsal skin surface, traversing the spinal canal, spinal cord, neural arch, and subcutaneous tissue; involved segment of vertebral column and spinal cord is split around the fistula
Neurenteric cyst	Intradural cyst lined by mucin-secreting cuboidal or columnar epithelium that resembles gastrointestinal tract
Split cord malformation	Variations of splitting of spinal cord into two hemicords
Dermal sinus	Epithelium-lined fistula extending into the CNS; point of termination varies
Caudal regression syndrome	Family of anomalies representing total or partial agenesis of the spinal column, imperforate anus, genital anomalies, bilat renal dysplasia/aplasia, and pulmonary hypoplasia
Segmental spinal dysgenesis	Segmental agenesis/dysgenesis of lumbar/thoracolumbar spine, segmental abnormality of spinal cord and nerve roots, congenital paraplegia or paraparesis, and congenital lower-limb deformities

[a]Based in part on data from Tortori-Donati et al: *Neuroradiology* 42:471–491, 2000
Abbreviation: *SCM* split cord malformation

Innervation of the Lower Urinary Tract (LUT)

Central control of bladder function begins in the locus coeruleus of the pons, which is responsible for a reflex pathway that synchronizes bladder contraction with internal urethral sphincter relaxation during voiding (Fig. 1) [12, 13]. With appropriate training, cortical signals can voluntarily suppress this reflex. Infants who have not yet acquired this control have an uninhibited pontine reflex. Thus, the detrusor muscle contracts and the internal sphincter relaxes when a critical urine capacity is reached 65. Parasympathetic fibers are the primary innervation of the urinary bladder. Presynaptic fibers arise from neurons in the S2-S4 cord segments and travel via pelvic splanchnic nerves and the inferior hypogastric and vesical plexuses to the bladder. They form synapses with postsynaptic neurons that are found on or near the bladder wall. Parasympathetic fibers provide motor innervation to the detrusor muscle and inhibit the internal urethral sphincter. Sympathetic fibers arise from the T11-L3 cord segments, travel via lumbar splanchnic nerves, and synapse on the hypogastric system of plexuses. Sympathetic nerves have little role in bladder motor activity, but they do appear to heavily innervate the neck and trigone of the bladder. Sympathetic stimulation allows for bladder neck closure, which is crucial for bladder filling. Somatic fibers to the external urethral sphincter arise from motor neurons in the S2-S4 cord segments and travel to the bladder via the pudendal nerve. Although the external sphincter can be contracted voluntarily, it relaxes reflexively when micturition is initiated via cortical signals and the internal sphincter opens.

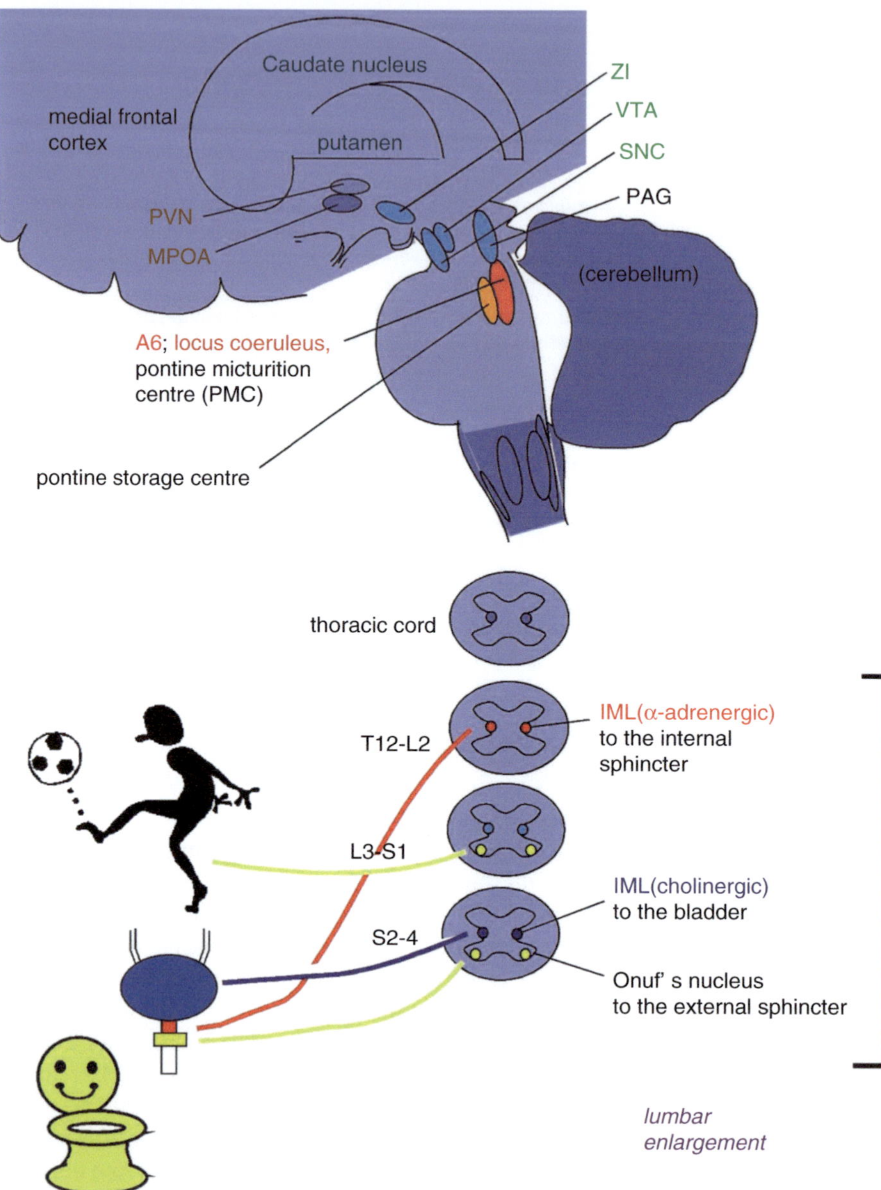

Fig. 1 Innervation of the lower urinary tract and the leg muscles. All of these segments are in the lumbar enlargement of the spinal cord, which may explain a combination of upper and lower motor neuron types of urinary and somatic nerve dysfunction in spinal bifida

Lower Urinary Tract Symptom (LUTS) in Cystic and Occult Spina Bifida (SB)

In the patient with cystic and occult SB, LUT dysfunction appears as the significant burden by the quality of life measure [14]. In a series of Veenboer et al. [15, 16], 120 cystic (postoperative)/occult SB patients with age > 18 years underwent urodynamics (UDS). Among these, 79.1% were wheelchair-bound or symptomatic. 35% underwent bladder replacement or augmentation cystoplasty. Clean intermittent catheterization (CIC) and anticholinergics were used in 40.8%. In these patients' cohort, 73.3% had subjective lower urinary tract (LUT) symptoms (LUTS). Incontinence was the most common (55%) while storage symptoms in 6.7% and voiding symptoms in 7.0%. Low percentage of LUTS other than incontinence might reflect bladder sensory impairment or depend on patients' age [15, 16]. In a series of patients by Sakakibara et al. [17], among 16 cystic (postoperative, 2–25 years) and 12 occult SB cases (7–32 years), all ambulatory, the most common LUTS in the cystic SB was urinary incontinence in 15 (94%) (urge type in 2 and undetermined type in 13), followed by voiding difficulty in 12 (75%), enuresis in 10 (63%), diurnal frequency in 5, nocturnal frequency in 2, urinary urgency in 2, and urinary retention in 3 patients (19%). Most common symptom in occult SB was voiding difficulty in eight (67%), urinary incontinence in eight (67%) (urge type in five, stress type in two, and undetermined type in one), and enuresis in eight (67%), followed by urinary urgency in seven, nocturnal frequency in four, diurnal frequency in four, and urinary retention in one. In both groups of patients, urinary incontinence and enuresis were commonly noted in any age. Four patients with the occult SB presented with urinary disorder as the sole initial complaint.

Urodynamics (UDS) in Cystic and Occult Spina Bifida (SB)

Urodynamics (UDS) provides a reliable way to evaluate the function of the LUT. Identification or confirmation of neurogenic bladder is an excellent use of UDSs, providing more specific and accurate information than imaging, neurological examination, and symptomatology alone [18, 19]. However, among various UDS measures, less invasive measures (free-flow, ultrasound post-void measurement) should start first. Some normative UDS values in infants and children are available [20]. Conservatively treated MMC may show UDS and upper urinary tract changes with time [21]. UDS in SB patients shows any combination of detrusor over- and underactivity and sphincter over- and underactivity.

Resting Phase

Sphincter electromyography (EMG) in cystic/occult SB reveals neurogenic change in the external sphincter, which may lead to sphincter weakness (intrinsic sphincter deficiency, type 3 stress urinary incontinence). Neurogenic motor unit potentials indicate external sphincter denervation reflecting lesions in the sacral Onuf's nucleus or its efferent fibers [17]. Torre et al. [22] undertook electrophysiological test in 28 children with SD and found that a combination of sphincter EMG and perineal evoked potentials yielded good predictive results. Urethral pressure profilometry showed low maximum urethral closure pressure (UPmax) in 56% of patients with cystic and in 17% of occult form [17] suggesting a peripheral type of hypogastric nerve dysfunction innervating the internal sphincter. External sphincter EMG activity during filling and voiding was completely silent in 25% of cystic form. Absent bulbocavernosus reflex was noted in 87% and in 56% and absent anal reflex in 100% and in 57% of each group, respectively [17], suggesting lower motor neuron lesion. These findings suggest that the combination of upper and lower neuron types of bladder and sphincter dysfunction is a feature of lumbosacral SB [2, 23]. In particular, lower neuron type of dysfunction was more common in cystic SB, which is in accordance with the neurological findings.

Again, considering the uro-neurological abnormalities, the location of lesions seems to be mostly in the lumbar enlargement, which contains sympathetic preganglionic neurons innervating the internal (smooth) sphincter at T12-L2 segments, motoneurons innervating leg muscles at L3-S1, parasympathetic preganglionic neurons innervating the bladder at S2-S4 segments, motoneurons (Onuf's nucleus) innervating the external (striated) sphincter at S2-S4 segments, and the descending and ascending pathways between these neurons and the pontine micturition regulatory centers (Fig. 1).

Filling Phase

Detrusor overactivity during filling, suggesting supranuclear type of pelvic nerve dysfunction, was noted in 38% of cystic SB and in 42% of occult SB [17]. Low bladder compliance, suggesting preganglionic type of pelvic nerve dysfunction, was noted in 81% and in 67% of each group. Detrusor overactivity and low-compliance detrusor are likely to represent an epiconus lesion and a conus/cauda equina lesion, respectively [12, 24], and the low-compliance detrusor is closely related to VUR via a high detrusor pressure during filling and voiding [2, 3]. A positive bethanechol test was noted in patients with the cystic/occult SB [17]. This finding indicates denervation supersensitivity of the detrusor [25], evidence of postganglionic type of pelvic nerve dysfunction either primarily or secondarily to transsynaptic degeneration. Some patients also showed impaired bladder sensation, suggestive of afferent nerve dysfunction in these disorders [26, 27].

Voiding Phase

On voiding, many SB patients with post-void residual show detrusor underactivity, suggesting nuclear/infranuclear type of pelvic nerve dysfunction. During filling, these patients have either detrusor overactivity, low-compliance bladder, or normal detrusor. To compare the urethral function in cystic and occult SB, detrusor-sphincter dyssynergia (DSD) was noted in 50% and in 27% of each group, respectively [17]. DSD could be considered as supranuclear type of pudendal nerve dysfunction, most probably reflecting an epiconus lesion [24, 28]. High-pressure voiding due to DSD is the problem that can lead to renal damage. Elevated bladder pressure leads to vesicoureteral reflux, hydronephrosis, and renal failure. In one study, up to 100% of children with untreated DSD together with high detrusor pressure have renal scarring [28].

Relation Between Bladder, Somatic Function and Neuroimaging in Cystic and Occult SB

It is generally thought that neurological disabilities in cystic SB are more extensive and severe than occult SB [2]. Motor weakness of the lower extremities was equally noted in cystic and occult SB with a combination of flaccid and spastic paresis. Hyperreflexia of patellar tendon reflex (upper motor neuron sign) was more common in occult SB. In contrast, absent Achilles tendon reflex (lower motor neuron sign) was more common in cystic SB [17]. Decreased superficial sensation particularly with higher segmental levels up to T5 was also more common in cystic SB [17]. In a report by Wyndaele and Sy [23], however, the level of intact skin sensation and the presence or absence of bulbocavernosus and anal reflexes could not significantly predict the function of the detrusor muscle, proximal urethra, and striated urethral sphincter. To sum up, the combination of flaccid and spastic paresis is a feature of lumbosacral SB [2, 17, 23], most probably reflecting lesions involving the spinal lumbar enlargement. This complex feature of SB is in contrast to other spinal cord diseases (cervicothoracic) [29, 30] where correlation between detrusor overactivity and DSD with upper motor neuron signs is found [31].

Most importantly, occult SB is often asymptomatic and incidentally found during X-ray screening of low back pain [27, 32]. Daytime urinary incontinence and/or nocturnal enuresis can become the sole initial complaint before the diagnosis was made. Cutaneous markers are associated with 43–95% of such patients [33–39]. Although MRI scan alone has a limited value [40, 41], the combination of uro-neurological assessment and the spinal MRI is helpful for young patients with urinary incontinence, enuresis, recurrent urinary tract infection, and large post-micturition residuals of unknown etiology [42].

Management and Care of Bladder/Kidney Function in Cystic and Occult SB

Medical management is determined by (1) post-void residual and high-pressure voiding with DSD, (2) incontinence due to detrusor overactivity and/or low compliance, and (3) sphincter weakness incontinence. This is because (1) post-void residual and high-pressure voiding leads to urinary tract infection and kidney damage [43, 44], (2) detrusor overactivity and/or low compliance leads to urge urinary incontinence, and (3) sphincter weakness leads to stress/total urinary incontinence. Among these, post-void residual and high-pressure voiding should be treated first in order to prevent adverse events [45].

Clean, Intermittent Self-Catheterization (CIC)

Clean, intermittent self-catheterization (CIC) is the treatment of choice, not only to avoid exacerbating kidney dysfunction due to high-pressure voiding and large residuals [46] but also to improve low-compliance bladder [47]. Saito et al. [47] reported their follow-up (18–100 months) results of 58 MD patients (16 males, 42 females, age 3 months–16 years). While the bladder compliance of 41 patients with CIC increased significantly from 5.1 to 11.1 mL/H$_2$O, that of 17 patients who underwent anti-reflux surgery failed to do so. Bladder overactivity also lessened or disappeared in 26 patients.

An approach for the treatment of LUT dysfunction in SB may require a combination of anticholinergics [48] and CIC for both filling and voiding disorders. Beginning CIC early in infancy conveys several advantages, including easier caregiver and patient adaptation to the routine and less need for augmentation cystoplasty [49–51]. As the children age and develop manual dexterity, they may be transitioned to CIC [44]. Credé maneuver is generally thought not to work in neurologic patients and not recommended because it can result in compression of the external urethral sphincter, causing high-pressure voiding or reflux in some patients, which is detrimental to the upper urinary tract [52].

Anticholinergic Drugs

In addition to CIC, oxybutynin (an anticholinergic) has been used to treat detrusor overactivity, low compliance, and high-pressure voiding [53–55]. Long-term studies demonstrated safety in children and infants and efficacy in lowering filling pressure, increasing bladder capacity, and preventing renal damage [44]. Anticholinergics can be administered orally or as an intravesical preparation in children with side effects or a poor response to the oral form [56]. The combined therapy of CIC and oxybutynin is successful in treating 90% of patients with LUTD. However, for those unresponsive to oxybutynin, propiverine or tolterodine is also available, but there is relatively little published information on efficacy in children [44]. Follow-up assessment includes ultrasound, UDS, cystography, urinalysis, or other tests [57]. The frequency of visits can be tapered from three per year in children up to age 3, two per year in school-age children, and annually in adults [44].

Botulinum A Toxin

Recent work has indicated that intravesical injection of botulinum A toxin may be a choice in children unresponsive to CIC and oxybutynin [58, 59] for the treatment of detrusor overactivity, low compliance, and high-pressure voiding.

Urologic Surgery

Urological surgery exists for the purpose of increasing bladder capacity and for urinary diversion in neurologic including SB children. These procedures include ureterostomy, vesicostomy, ileal conduit, and ileovesicostomy [60–62].

Neurosurgical Intervention for Bladder/Kidney Function in Cystic and Occult SB

SB is still a significant source of morbidity worldwide. Until the 1950s, the probability that an infant with MMC would survive to adulthood was low. Therapeutic advancements have changed the nature of SB. The focus of treatment is now shifting toward early recognition and surgical intervention, postoperative monitoring and management, and improvements in patient quality of life, particularly the lifelong LUT dysfunction. In fact, adults with MMC now account for greater health-care expenditures and more hospital admissions than children with this condition [63].

Fetal Surgery for Cystic SB

Studies regarding fetal surgery for open SB are available [64]. A long-term follow-up of 28 patients who underwent fetal MMC closure demonstrated a range of LUT dysfunctions (decreased bladder capacity, detrusor overactivity, and increased detrusor pressure) and no significant difference compared with those who underwent postnatal repair [65]. A limited number of studies have shown an improvement in UDS outcome, but there are minimal data to substantiate this [66].

Postnatal, Childhood, and Adulthood Surgery for Cystic and Occult SB (Untethering)

The initial goals for postnatal neurosurgical repair in cystic SB, often within the first few days of life, include elimination of cerebrospinal fluid leakage and prevention of infection, in addition to preservation of motor/sensory/LUT function and prevention of secondary tethering postoperatively [67].

Retethering rate is estimated in 3–40%, most frequently in patients with early repair of MMC and resection of lipoMMC [68–75]. In those patients, whether untethering is efficacious in ameliorating LUT dysfunction of occult SB remains controversial [76–78]. Keating et al. [76] reported pre-/postoperative UDS in 40 SB children (28 neonates/infants (average age 8.7 months), 12 older (age 11.7 years)). Preoperative UDS were normal in 18/28 (64%) in the younger group and 1/12 (8%) in the older group. Postoperative UDS returned to normal in 6/10 (60%) infants and 3/11 (27%) older group. They concluded that neuro-urologic abnormalities are potentially reversible, but this reversibility diminishes with age. Satar et al. [78] reported 21 patients with occult SB (age 3–46 years). Fourteen had incontinence and one urinary retention. Others had back pain or leg weakness. 18/21 patients had an abnormal neurological examination and 15 abnormal sphincter EMG. Imaging showed that nine had tethered cord, four had lipomeningocele and lipoma, two had bony spine abnormality, and one had thoracic meningocele and diastematomyelia. 19/21 patients underwent surgery. Postoperatively, neurological examination improved in 1 (5%) and unchanged in 18 (95%), while UDS improved in 3 (16%), unchanged in 11 (68%), and worsened in 5 (26%). Six deteriorated and required second surgery, which helped two (33%). They concluded that older children and adults with occult SB are more likely to be irreversible than younger children; therefore, treatment should start early. Khoury et al. [77] reported 31 occult SB (older than 5 years) with detrusor overactivity incontinence, which failed to respond to other treatment. After untethering, daytime incontinence resolved in 72%, detrusor overactivity disappeared in 59%, and bladder compliance improved in 66%. More recently, surgical intervention in occult SB ameliorated low back pain in three of four patients (75%). But in one patient, transient urinary incontinence appeared [79]. Sakakibara et al. [17] reported that, after untethering, all occult SB (lipoMMC) achieved neurological improvement in pain and leg weakness. However, voiding difficulty unchanged and urinary retention appeared in some, while urinary incontinence and enuresis improved in all.

More recently, Kumar et al. [80] reported, after untethering, among 25 SB patients (age 3 months–18 years, 10 cystic, 15 occult), LUTS improved in 42.8% with cystic and in 46.2% with occult SB. Wu et al. [81] had 43 patients who underwent early surgery for lipoMMC prior to manifestation of urological dysfunction; among them, 84% maintained stable function. Macejko et al. [82] described that lipoMMC was the poorest responder for untethering. Metcalfe et al. [83] reported 36 patients with occult SB. After untethering, LUTS improved in 72% and urinary incontinence disappeared in 42%. Tarcan et al. [84, 85] reported 56 patients with MMC. After untethering, using five tiers of urinary tract dilation, Grade 1–2 dilation disappeared in 33.3%, while Grade 3–4 dilation disappeared in none. Grade 1–3 vesicoureteral reflux (VUR) disappeared in 62.5%, while Grade 4–5 VUR disappeared in 33.3%, good in children with age <7. Abrahamsson et al. [86] reported, after untethering, in 20 SB patients, all with worsened UDS prior to surgery improved, while 90% with stable UDS prior to surgery unchanged. Dushi et al. [87] noted, after untethering, UDS improvement particularly in symptomatic LUTD. Palmer et al. reported, after untethering, 20 SB children showed no LUTS change, while subclinical UDS improvement in 75% of them. Maher et al. [88] showed improvement in LUT function in 71% of patients who underwent repeated untethering.

Conclusions

Cystic and occult spina bifida (SB) presents with a wide spectrum of urodynamic abnormalities including upper and lower neuron types of bladder and urethral dysfunction. Careful uro-neurological assessment and spinal MRI are important for diagnosing young adult patients with occult SB, because they may present with urinary symptoms as the sole initial symptom and have no other obvious neurological abnormalities. Despite consensus regarding the need for early urological management, controversy remains regarding the types of intervention. CIC, anticholinergics, botulinum A toxin, and reconstructive surgery have good outcomes for the primary goals, e.g., protection of renal function, improved urinary continence, and independence. Future studies are warranted to maximize bladder quality of life in the patients with SB.

References

1. Zerah M, Kulkarni AV. Spinal cord malformations. Handb Clin Neurol. 2013;112:975–91.
2. Welch K, Winston KR. Spina bifida. In: Myrianthopoulos NC, editor. Handbook of clinical neurology, Vol. 6 (50): malformations. Amsterdam: Elsevier Science Publishers BV; 1987. p. 477–508.

3. Kroovand RL, Bell W, Hart LJ, Benfield KY. The effect of back closure on detrusor function in neonates with myelomeningocele. J Urol. 1990;144:423–5.
4. James CCM, Lassman LP. Spinal dysraphism; spina bifida occulta. London: Butterworths; 1972.
5. Bourque PR, D'Alton JG, Russell NA, Gerridzen RG, Benoit BG. Congenital lumbosacral lipoma causing primary enuresis in an adult. CMAJ. 1986;135:1007–8.
6. Ritchey ML, Sinha A, DiPietro MA, Huang C, Flood H, Bloom DA. Significance of spina bifida occulta in children with diurnal enuresis. J Urol. 1994;152:815–8.
7. de Jong TP, Chrzan R, Klijn AJ, Dik P. Treatment of the neurogenic bladder in spina bifida. Pediatr Nephrol. 2008;23:889–96.
8. Fidas A, MacDonald HL, Elton RA, McInnes A, Chisholm GD. Neurological defects of the voiding reflex arcs in chronic urinary retention and their relation to spina bifida occulta. Br J Urol. 1989;63:16–20.
9. Snow-Lisy DC, Yerkes EB, Cheng EY. Update on urological management of spina bifida from prenatal diagnosis to adulthood. J Urol. 2015;194:288–96.
10. Kondo A, Kamihira O, Ozawa H. Neural tube defects: prevalence, etiology and prevention. Int J Urol. 2009;16:49–57.
11. Tortori-Donati P, Rossi A, Cama A. Spinal dysraphism: a review of neuroradiological features with embryological correlations and proposal for a new classification. Neuroradiology. 2000;42:471–91.
12. Fowler CJ, Griffiths D, de Groat WC. The neural control of micturition. Nat Rev Neurosci. 2008;9:453–66.
13. Sakakibara R. Lower urinary tract dysfunction in patients with brain lesions. Handb Clin Neurol. 2015;130:269–87.
14. Szymanski KM, Misseri R, Whittam B, Raposo SM, King SJ, Kaefer M, Rink RC, Cain MP. QUAlity of Life Assessment in Spina bifida for Adults (QUALASA): development and international validation of a novel healthrelated quality of life instrument. Qual Life Res. 2015;24:2355–64.
15. Veenboer PW, Ruud Bosch JL, de Kort LM. Assessment of bladder and kidney functioning in adult spina bifida patients by Dutch urologists: a survey. Neurourol Urodyn. 2014a;33:289–95.
16. Veenboer PW, Ruud Bosch JL, Rosier PFWM, Dik P, van Asbeck FWA, de Jong TPVM, de Kort LMO. Cross-sectional study of determinants of upper and lower urinary tract outcomes in adults with spinal dysraphism: new recommendations for urodynamic followup guidelines? J Urol. 2014b;192:477–82.
17. Sakakibara R, Hattori T, Uchiyama T, Kamura K, Yamanishi T. Uro-neurological assessment in patient with spinal bifida occulta and cystica. Neurourol Urodynam. 2003;22:328–34.
18. Drzewiecki BA, Bauer SB. Urodynamic testing in children: indications, technique, interpretation and significance. J Urol. 2011;186:1190–7.
19. Glazier DB, Murphy DP, Fleisher MH, Cummings KB, Barone JG. Evaluation of the utility of video-urodynamics in children with urinary tract infection and voiding dysfunction. Br J Urol. 1997;80:806–8.
20. Jansson UB, Hanson M, Sillén U, Hellström AL. Voiding pattern and acquisition of bladder control from birth to age 6 years—a longitudinal study. J Urol. 2005;174:289–93.
21. Almodhen F, Capolicchio JP, Jednak R, El Sherbiny M. Postpubertal urodynamic and upper urinary tract changes in children with conservatively treated myelomeningocele. J Urol. 2007;178:1479–82.
22. Torre M, Planche D, Louis-Borrione C, Sabiani F, Lena G, Guys JM. Value of electrophysiological assessment after surgical treatment of spinal dysraphism. J Urol. 2002;168:1759–62.
23. Wyndaele JJ, de Sy WA. Correlation between the findings of a clinical neurological examination and the urodynamic dysfunction in children with myelodysplasia. J Urol. 1985;133:638–9.
24. Blaivas JG. The neurophysiology of micturition; a clinical study of 550 patients. J Urol. 1982;127:958–63.

25. Lapides J, Friend CR, Ajemian EP, Reus WS. Denervation supersensibility as a test for neurogenic bladder. Surg Gyn Obst. 1962;114:241–4.
26. Giddens JL, Radomski SB, Hirshberg ED, Hassouna M, Fehlings M. Urodynamic findings in adults with the tethered cord syndrome. J Urol. 1999;161:1249–54.
27. Sutherland RS, Mevorach RA, Baskin LS, Kogan BA. Spinal dysraphism in children; an overview and an approach to prevent complications. Urology. 1995;46:294–304.
28. van Gool JD, Dik P, de Jong TP. Bladder-sphincter dysfunction in myelomeningocele. Eur J Pediatr. 2001;160:414–20.
29. Sakakibara R, Hattori T, Tojo M, Yamanishi T, Yasuda K, Hirayama K. The location of the paths subserving micturition; studies in patients with cervical myelopathy. J Autonom Nerv Syst. 1995;55:165–8.
30. Wyndaele JJ. Correlation between clinical neurological data and urodynamic function in spinal cord injured patients. Spinal Cord. 1997;35:213–6.
31. Nathan PW, Smith MC. The centrifugal pathway for micturition within the spinal cord. J Neurol Neurosurg Psychiatry. 1958;21:177–89.
32. Kaplan KM, Spivak JM, Bendo JA. Embryology of the spine and associated congenital abnormalities. Spine J. 2005;5:564–76.
33. Ackerman LL, Menezes AH. Spinal congenital dermal sinuses: a 30-year experience. Pediatrics. 2003;112:641–7.
34. Assaad A, Mansy A, Kotb M, Hafez M. Spinal dysraphism: experience with 250 cases operated upon. Childs Nerv Syst. 1989;5:324–9.
35. Gibson PJ, Britton J, Hall DM, Hill CR. Lumbosacral skin markers and identification of occult spinal dysraphism in neonates. Acta Paediatr. 1995;84:208–9.
36. Guggisberg D, Hadj-Rabia S, Viney C, Bodemer C, Brunelle F, Zerah M, et al. Skin markers of occult spinal dysraphism in children: a review of 54 cases. Arch Dermatol. 2004;140:1109–15.
37. Kanev PM, Lemire RJ, Loeser JD, Berger MS. Management and long-term follow-up review of children with lipomyelomeningocele, 1952–1987. J Neurosurg. 1990;73:48–52.
38. McAtee-Smith J, Hebert AA, Rapini RP, Goldberg NS. Skin lesions of the spinal axis and spinal dysraphism. Fifteen cases and a review of the literature. Arch Pediatr Adolesc Med. 1994;148:740–8.
39. Pierre-Kahn A, Lacombe J, Pichon J, Giudicelli Y, Renier D, Sainte-Rose C, et al. Intraspinal lipomas with spina bifida. Prognosis and treatment in 73 cases. J Neurosurg. 1986;65:756–61.
40. Mak V, Radomski SB. Value of magnetic resonance imaging of the lumbosacral spinal cord in patients with voiding dysfunction. J Urol. 1996;156:1421–3.
41. Salle JLP, Capolicchio G, Houle AM, Vernet O, Jednak R, O'Gorman AM, Montes JL, Farmer JP. Magnetic resonance imaging in children with voiding dysfunction; is it indicated? J Urol. 1998;160:1080–3.
42. Sadiq S, Faiq SM, Idrees MK. Lumbosacral dysraphism as cause of neurogenic bladder: magnetic resonance imaging based study from SIUT Pakistan. J Pak Med Assoc. 2015;65:501–5.
43. Madden-Fuentes RJ, McNamara ER, Lloyd LC, Wiener JS, Routh JC, Seed PC, Ross SS. Variation in definitions of urinary tract infections in spina bifida patients: a systematic review. Pediatrics. 2013;132:132–9.
44. Verpoorten C, Buyse GM. The neurogenic bladder: medical treatment. Pediatr Nephrol. 2008;23:717–25.
45. Snodgrass WT, Adams R. Initial urologic management of myelomeningocele. Urol Clin N Am. 2004;31:427–34.
46. Muller T, Arbeiter K, Aufricht C. Renal function in meningomyelocele: risk factors, chronic renal failure, renal replacement therapy and transplantation. Curr Opin Urol. 2002;12:479–84.
47. Saito M, Kato K, Goto M, Kondo A. Lower urinary tract function in myelomeningocele. Nippon Hinyokigakkai Zasshi. 1990;81:75–81.
48. Baskin LS, Kogan BA, Benard F. Treatment of infants with neurogenic bladder dysfunction using aticholinergic drugs and intermittent catheterisation. Br J Urol. 1990;66:532–4.

49. Edelstein RA, Bauer SB, Kelly MD, Darbey MM, Peters CA, Atala A, et al. The long-term urological response of neonates with myelodysplasia treated proactively with intermittent catheterization and anticholinergic therapy. J Urol. 1995;154(4):1500–4.
50. Kaefer M, Pabby A, Kelly M, Darbey M, Bauer SB. Improved bladder function after prophylactic treatment of the high risk neurogenic bladder in newborns with myelomeningocele. J Urol. 1999;162:1068–71.
51. Wu HY, Baskin LS, Kogan BA. Neurogenic bladder dysfunction due to myelomeningocele: neonatal versus childhood treatment. J Urol. 1997;157:2295–7.
52. Churchill BM, Abramson RP, Wahl EF. Dysfunction of the lower urinary and distal gastrointestinal tracts in pediatric patients with known spinal cord problems. Pediatr Clin N Am. 2001;48:1587–630.
53. Ferrara CM, D'aleo E, Tarquini S, Salvatore S, Salvaggio E. Side-effects of oral or intravesical oxybutynin chloride in children with spina bifida. BJU Int. 2001;87:674–8.
54. Kessler TM, Lackner J, Kiss G, Rehder P, Madersbacher H. Early proactive management improves upper urinary tract function and reduces the need for surgery in patients with myelomeningocele. Neurourol Urodyn. 2006;25:758–62.
55. Kessler TM, Lackner J, Kiss G, Rehder P, Madersbacher H. Predictive value of initial urodynamic pattern on urinary continence in patients with myelomeningocele. Neurourol Urodyn. 2006;25:361–7.
56. Buyse G, Verpoorten C, Vereecken R, Casaer P. Intravesical application of a stable oxybutynin solution improves therapeutic compliance and acceptance in children with neurogenic bladder dysfunction. J Urol. 1998;160:1084–7.
57. Tarcan T, Bauer S, Olmedo E, Khoshbin S, Kelly M, Darbey M. Long-term followup of newborns with myelodysplasia and normal urodynamic findings: is followup necessary? J Urol. 2001;165:564–7.
58. Hascoet J, Manunta A, Brochard C, Arnaud A, Damphousse M, Menard H, Kerdraon J, Journel H, Bonan I, Odent S, Fremond B, Siproudhis L, Gamé X, Peyronnet B, French Referral Network of Spina Bifida. Outcomes of intra-detrusor injections of botulinum toxin in patients with spina bifida: a systematic review. J Neurosurg Pediatr. 2016;18:150–63.
59. Kuo YC, Kuo HC. Botulinum toxin injection for lower urinary tract dysfunction. Int J Urol. 2013;20(1):40–55.
60. González R, Schimke CM. Strategies in urological reconstruction in myelomeningocele. Curr Opin Urol. 2002;12:485–90.
61. Westney OL. The neurogenic bladder and incontinent urinary diversion. Urol Clin North Am. 2010;37:581–92.
62. Wiener JS, Antonelli J, Shea AM, Curtis LH, Schulman KA, Krupski TL, et al. Bladder augmentation versus urinary diversion in patients with spina bifida in the United States. J Urol. 2011;186:161–5.
63. Ouyang L, Grosse SD, Armour BS, Waitzman NJ. Health care expenditures of children and adults with spina bifida in a privately insured U.S. population. Birth Defects Res A Clin Mol Teratol. 2007;79:552–8.
64. Holzbeierlein J, Pope JC IV, Adams MC, Bruner J, Tulipan N, Brock JW 3rd. The urodynamic profile of myelodysplasia in childhood with spinal closure during gestation. J Urol. 2000;164:1336–9.
65. Clayton DB, Tanaka ST, Trusler L, Thomas JC, Pope JC IV, Adams MC, et al. Long-term urological impact of fetal myelomeningocele closure. J Urol. 2011;186(4 Suppl):1581–5.
66. Carr MC. Fetal myelomeningocele repair: urologic aspects. Curr Opin Urol. 2007;17:257–62.
67. Tseng JH, Kuo MF, Tu YK, Tseng MY. Outcome of untethering for symptomatic spina bifida occulta with lumbosacral spinal cord tethering in 31 patients: analysis of preoperative prognostic factors. Spine J. 2008;8:630–8.
68. Balkan E, Kiliç N, Avşar I, Boyaci S, Aksoy K, Doğruyol H. Urodynamic findings in the tethered spinal cord: the effect of tethered cord division on lower urinary tract functions. Eur J Pediatr Surg. 2001;11:116–9.

69. Bowman RM, McLone DG, Grant JA, Tomita T, Ito JA. Spina bifida outcome: a 25-year prospective. Pediatr Neurosurg. 2001;34:114–20.
70. Dias MS. Neurosurgical management of myelomeningocele (spina bifida). Pediatr Rev. 2005;26:50–60.
71. Herman JM, McLone DG, Storrs BB, Dauser RC. Analysis of 153 patients with myelomeningocele or spinal lipoma reoperated upon for a tethered cord. Presentation, management and outcome. Pediatr Neurosurg. 1993;19:243–9.
72. Kang JK, Lee KS, Jeun SS, Lee IW, Kim MC. Role of surgery for maintaining urological function and prevention of retethering in the treatment of lipomeningomyelocele: experience recorded in 75 lipomeningomyelocele patients. Childs Nerv Syst. 2003;19:23–9.
73. Morimoto K, Takemoto O, Wakayama A. Spinal lipomas in children—surgical management and long-term follow-up. Pediatr Neurosurg. 2005;41:84–7.
74. Shurtleff DB, Duguay S, Duguay G, Moskowitz D, Weinberger E, Roberts T, et al. Epidemiology of tethered cord with meningomyelocele. Eur J Pediatr Surg. 1997;7(Suppl 1):7–11.
75. Tamaki N, Shirataki K, Kojima N, Shouse Y, Matsumoto S. Tethered cord syndrome of delayed onset following repair of myelomeningocele. J Neurosurg. 1988;69:393–8.
76. Keating MA, Rink RC, Bauer SB, Krarup C, Dyro FM, Winston KR, Shillito J, Fischer EG, Retik AB. Neurological implications of the changing approach in management of occult spinal lesions. J Urol. 1988;140:1299–301.
77. Khoury AE, Hendrik EB, McLorie GA, Kulkarni A, Churchill BM. Occult spinal dysraphism; clinical and urodynamic outcome after diversion of the filum terminale. J Urol. 1990;144:426–9.
78. Satar N, Bauer SB, Shefner J, Kelly MD, Darbey MM. The effects of delayed diagnosis and treatment in patients with an occult spinal dysraphism. J Urol. 1995;154:754–8.
79. Akay KM, Gonul E, Ocal E, Timurkaynak E. The initial treatment of meningocele and myelomeningocele lesions in adulthood: experiences with seven patients. Neurosurg Rev. 2003;26:162–7.
80. Kumar R, Singhal Gupta NM, Kapoor R, Mahapatra AK. Evaluation of clinico-urodynamic outcome of bladder dysfunction after surgery in children with spinal dysraphism—a prospective study. Acta Neurochir. 2008;150:129–37.
81. Wu HY, Kogan BA, Baskin LS, Edwards MS. Long-term benefits of early neurosurgery for lipomyelomeningocele. J Urol. 1998;160:511–4.
82. Macejko AM, Cheng EY, Yerkes EB, Meyer T, Bowman RM, Kaplan WE. Clinical urological outcomes following primary tethered cord release in children younger than 3 years. J Urol. 2007;178:1738–43.
83. Metcalfe PD, Luerssen TG, King SJ, Kaefer M, Meldrum KK, Cain MP, et al. Treatment of the occult tethered spinal cord for neuropathic bladder: results of sectioning the filum terminale. J Urol. 2006;176:1826–30.
84. Tarcan T, Önol FF, Ilker Y, Alpay H, Simsek F, Özek M. The timing of primary neurosurgical repair significantly affects neurogenic bladder prognosis in children with myelomeningocele. J Urol. 2006;176:1161–5.
85. Tarcan T, Onol FF, Ilker Y, Simsek F, Ozek M. Does surgical release of secondary spinal cord tethering improve the prognosis of neurogenic bladder in children with myelomeningocele? J Urol. 2006;176:1601–6. (Erratum in J Urol 176 (6 Pt 1):2749, 2006)
86. Abrahamsson K, Olsson I, Sillén U. Urodynamic findings in children with myelomeningocele after untethering of the spinal cord. J Urol. 2007;177:331–4.
87. Dushi G, Frey P, Ramseyer P, Vernet O, Meyrat BJ. Urodynamic score in children with lipomyelomeningocele: a prospective study. J Urol. 2011;186:655–9.
88. Maher CO, Bauer SB, Goumnerova L, Proctor MR, Madsen JR, Scott RM. Urological outcome following multiple repeat spinal cord untethering operations. Clinical article. J Neurosurg Pediatr. 2009;4:275–9.

Degenerative Diseases (Multiple Sclerosis, Parkinson's Disease)

Petros Georgopoulos, Konstantinos-Vaios Mytilekas, and Apostolos Apostolidis

Abbreviations

ASST	Actionable Bladder Symptom and Screening Tool
BOO	Bladder outlet obstruction
BPO	Benign prostatic obstruction
CIC	Clean Intermittent Catheterization
DO	Detrusor overactivity
DRE	Digital rectal examination
DSD	Detrusor sphincter dyssynergia
DUA	Detrusor underactivity
EAU	European Association of Urology
EDSS	Expanded Disability Status Scale
IPSS	International Prostate Symptom Score
ISC	Intermittent self-catheterization
LUTS	Lower urinary tract symptoms
MS	Multiple sclerosis
MSA	Multiple system atrophy
NLUTS	Neurogenic lower urinary tract symptoms
NMS	Non-motor symptoms
OAB	Overactive bladder
OR	Odds ratio
PD	Parkinson's disease
POP	Pelvic organ prolapse
PPMS	Primary progressive multiple sclerosis
PR	Progressive relapsing
PROMs	Patient-reported outcome measures

P. Georgopoulos · K.-V. Mytilekas · A. Apostolidis (✉)
2nd Department of Urology, Aristotle University of Thessaloniki, Thessaloniki, Greece

© Springer International Publishing AG, part of Springer Nature 2018
R. Dmochowski, J. Heesakkers (eds.), *Neuro-Urology*,
https://doi.org/10.1007/978-3-319-90997-4_5

PTNS   Percutaneous tibial nerve stimulation
PVR   Post-void residual
QoL   Quality of life
RRMS   Relapsing–remitting multiple sclerosis
SCI   Spinal cord injury
SNM   Sacral neuromodulation
SPMS   Secondary progressive multiple sclerosis
TUR-P   Transurethral resection of the prostate
UDS   Urodynamic study
UI   Urinary incontinence
UK   United Kingdom
UTIs   Urinary tract infections
UUI   Urge urinary incontinence

Multiple Sclerosis

Epidemiology

Multiple sclerosis (MS) is a chronic autoimmune inflammatory disease and is the most common cause of disability among young and middle-aged adults with a global prevalence of 30 per 100,000. The highest prevalence of the disease was observed in Northern Europe, North America (>100 per 100,000) and southern Australia and the lowest in Asia (2 per 100,000 in Japan) and Africa [1–4]. The onset of symptoms is between 25.3 and 31,8 years, and 50% of affected individuals will be unable to walk independently after 15 years [1, 4]. MS is more frequent among women than men (two females for every man) [1].

Multiple sclerosis is a demyelinating disorder characterized by spinal sparing, in the brain and spinal cord. Demyelinating plaques are prone to appear in the optic nerves, the periventricular white matter, the brainstem, the cerebellum and the spinal cord white matter [4]. The disorder is manifested by four different phenotypes: relapsing–remitting (RRMS), secondary progressive (SPMS), primary progressive (PPMS), and progressive relapsing (PRMS) [4, 5]. The vast majority of patients (85%) suffer from RRMS, and about 50% of them end up having the secondary progressive form of the disease within 11 years [6].

Pathophysiology of Bladder Dysfunction

The incidence of lower urinary tract symptoms (LUTS) in patients with MS varies and is associated with the spinal cord involvement and the degree of pyramidal symptoms in the lower limbs [7, 8]. The type of detrusor muscle dysfunction is functionally associated with the central nervous system localization of the lesion.

Patients with detrusor overactivity (DO) are more likely to have demyelinating plaques at subcortical white matter, whereas plaques at the spinal cord and pons result in DO with detrusor sphincter dyssynergia (DSD) and detrusor underactivity (DUA), respectively [6, 8, 9]. However, a variety of other disease-related factors may be also associated with LUT dysfunction, such as cognitive impairment, reduced mobility and general debilitation (often leading to functional incontinence), as well as some of the medications used for the complications of MS (e.g. opiates and tricyclic antidepressants). Classical urological conditions, such as anatomical bladder outlet obstruction, genuine stress incontinence and urinary tract infections, should also be investigated for possible causes of LUTS in MS patients [8].

LUTS in MS

The multiple locations of the MS lesions and the different phenotypes of the disease lead to a wide range of symptoms. The predominant MS symptoms include muscle weakness, sensory and visual abnormalities, fatigue, cognitive dysfunction and bladder–bowel dysfunction [6]. Only 10% of the individuals suffer from LUTS upon disease onset, and up to 80% of them develop LUTS with disease duration greater than 10 years [7]. Storage symptoms and urge urinary incontinence (UUI) are the most frequently reported (37–99%), secondary to detrusor overactivity: micturition frequency 31–85%, urgency 32–86% and UUI 37–72% [6, 7, 10]. Urinary urgency and urgency incontinence were thought to be the most bothersome symptoms [11]. Additionally, voiding symptoms affect 34–79% of the MS patient population usually secondary to DSD and/or detrusor bladder neck dyssynergia (DBND), with 25% of them resulting in urinary retention. It has been reported that 59% of men and 51% of women with MS suffer from both storage and voiding symptoms [7, 10].

However, a recent observational study carried out among 1052 MS participants revealed that post-micturition symptoms (post-micturition dribbling 64.9% and incomplete emptying 60.7%) and urgency (61.7%) were the most frequently reported symptoms [11]. It is noteworthy that 16% of patients had a post-void residual (PVR) greater than 100 mL without having a perception of inadequate bladder emptying. Nevertheless and for unknown reasons, deterioration of upper urinary tract function in MS patients is rare by contrast to patients with spinal cord injury (SCI) [12, 13].

The severity of the neurological condition and particularly the extent of demyelinated pyramid lesions are negative prognostic factors for the development of LUTS, but a strong correlation between radiological findings from the CNS and LUTS has not been clearly demonstrated. Two main factors affecting patient's LUTS are the duration/progression of MS and the patient's degree of physical disability [7]. Moreover, the prevalence of benign prostatic hyperplasia in MS men and urinary incontinence in MS women are at similar proportions as in the general population, but these conditions are highly demanding to be treated [7].

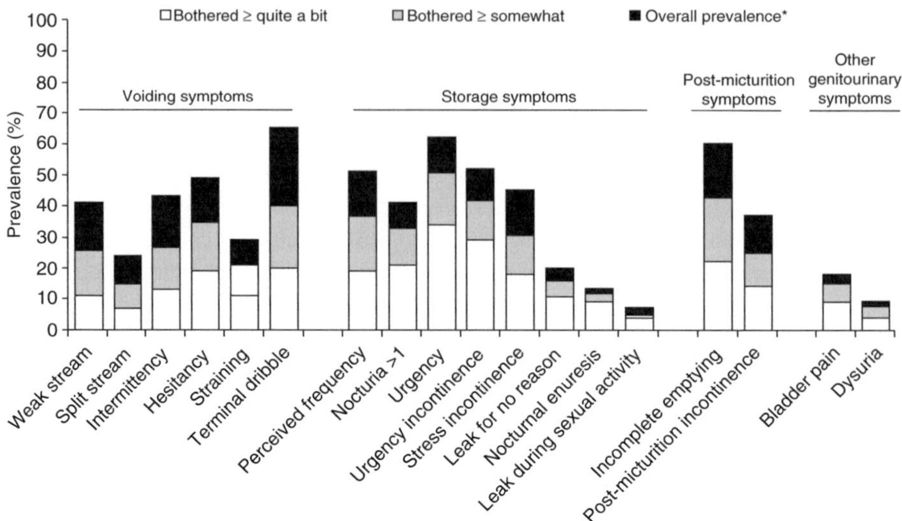

Fig. 1 Prevalence and bother associated with LUTS in MS patients (reproduced with permission from [11])

It is of great importance that healthcare professionals take into consideration the cognitive impairment of many MS patients. A large proportion of them suffer from language dysfunction, memory loss or apraxia; in addition they may have an intact bladder sensation. These conditions may not only lead to underestimation of their LUT dysfunction but may also render their symptoms refractory to treatment [10, 14] (Fig. 1).

Urological Complications

Complications from the urinary tract are the most common causes of hospitalization for an MS patient. The overall rate of such complications ranges between 0 and 40% in 18 years' follow-up; still, it is lower than the urological complication rate of other neurological disorders such as SCI or spina bifida [7, 10, 15]. Factors increasing the likelihood of complications are the presence of DO, elevated detrusor pressures (Pdet), low bladder compliance, DSD, indwelling catheter, post-void residual, older age, sex and duration of MS [7, 10, 16].

Urinary Tract Infections (UTIs)

UTIs are reported in 30% of MS patients and are associated with increased PVR, use of catheter (intermittent or indwelling) and female gender. A previous study has shown that patients with UTIs have an average PVR of 180 mL, while those without

UTIs have a lower PVR (approximately 119 mL). In addition, women with MS have higher rates of UTIs than men (42% vs. 17%) [15, 17]. Febrile infections, such as pyelonephritis, orchitis and prostatitis, are estimated to occur in 2–23% of patients (9% on average). Finally, UTIs are the main cause of morbidity in MS patients and can be a contributing factor to death [18].

Lower Urinary Tract Anatomical Complications

In an average 30% of MS patients, morphological alterations have been reported in the bladder (range 4–49%). Such alterations include reduced bladder compliance due to fibrosis, bladder diverticula, trabeculae and bladder wall thickening. The formation of bladder stones may render LUTS resistant to pharmacotherapy [7].

Bladder Cancer

The incidence of bladder cancer is higher among patients with MS by 0.29% compared to the general population, and it is almost equal to the incidence of bladder cancer among the SCI population. Particularly, MS patients who use intermittent self-catheterization (ISC) or have chronically indwelling catheters have increased likelihood to develop a bladder malignancy (by 0.7% and 0.23%, respectively). This risk is even higher among patients who have been treated with immunosuppressants like cyclophosphamide (incidence 5.7%) [7, 19]. The first sign of such complication is usually haematuria. An annual cystoscopy with bladder washing cytology and/or biopsy is suggested for the high-risk patients [7, 19].

Upper Urinary Tract Complications

The rate of any complication in the upper urinary tract is about 12% (0–25%), and it is higher among patients with long MS duration, indwelling catheter, high-pressure DO or high Pdet. Age over 50 years, presence of DSD and male gender constitute additional risk factors [7]. The incidence of kidney stones is 5%, same as the incidence of vesicoureteral reflux 5%. Although the rate of upper urinary tract dilatation is 8% (0–23%), the possibility of renal failure is estimated to be no different to the general population [7, 10, 20].

Mortality

There is a lack of studies predicting mortality rate in individuals with MS and vesico-urethral dysfunction. However, the early onset of urinary tract dysfunction can lead to an increased mortality rate. For instance, the rate was lower in patients who suffered from LUTS in the first 10 years after the diagnosis of MS (6.4% survivors) in comparison with ones who experienced the symptoms at a late stage (29.2% survivors) [7, 20].

Quality of Life of MS Patients with LUTS

Undoubtedly, LUTS can contribute to quality-of-life (QoL) impairment. They can limit physical and social activities of vulnerable individuals, with increasing level of embarrassment resulting in isolation and depression [21]. Nocturia has a negative effect on the QoL of MS patients, by reducing sleep quality. However, UI remains one of the main factors negatively affecting the daily living of patients with MS while having an additional major role in the cost of care; 70% of incontinent MS patients reported that UI had worsened their lives [8, 10, 17]. Finally, we have to take into consideration that bother from LUTS shows a strong negative association with patients' disability, being more bothersome to ambulant patients than those confined to a wheelchair [17].

Diagnostic Evaluation

Patient History and Questionnaires

Generally, all patients with MS should be assessed for the presence of LUT dysfunction. An extended history must be taken including LUTS and neurological, sexual and bowel symptoms. Among the wealth of tools used to assess patients' symptoms, only a few are validated in MS patients. The Actionable Bladder Symptom and Screening Tool (ASST) is a questionnaire validated in MS patients intended to reveal LUTS in this group of patients. It evaluates different aspects of vulnerable individuals such as social impact, embarrassment, work interference and the need for healthcare. Patients who report a score equal to or greater than 3 should be guided for further urologic evaluation [22, 23]. Furthermore, the Neurogenic Bladder Symptom Score (NBSS) is also used as a measure of LUTS among patients with MS, SCI and spina bifida. It assesses storage and voiding symptoms, severity of UI and urological complications [22, 24].

The Expanded Disability Status Scale for multiple sclerosis (EDSS) is the most widespread tool for quantifying neurological disability among individuals affected by MS [25]. The EDSS score varies between 0 (normal) and 10 (death from MS), and it is measured by the physician. It is based on measures of dysfunction in eight functional systems:

1. Pyramidal—limbs' mobility
2. Cerebellar—ataxia, loss of coordination or tremor
3. Brainstem—impaired speech, swallowing and persistence of nystagmus
4. Sensory—sensation impairment

Table 1 Validated questionnaires evaluating QoL (adapted from EAU Guidelines) [28]

Questionnaire	Underlying neurological disorder	Bladder	Bowel	Sexual function
FAMS	MS	X		X
FILMS	MS	X	X	
HAQUAMS	MS	X	X	X
IQOL	MS, SCI	X		X
MDS	MS	X	X	
MSISQ-15/MSISQ-19	MS	X	X	X
MSQLI	MS	X	X	X
MSQoL-54	MS	X	X	X
MSWDQ	MS	X	X	
NBSS	MS, SCI, congenital neurogenic bladder	X		
Qualiveen/ SF-Qualiveen	MS, SCI	X		X
RAYS	MS	X		X

5. Bowel and bladder dysfunction
6. Visual dysfunction
7. Cerebral (or mental) dysfunctions
8. Other

Measured scores over or equal to 4 indicate gait impairment, and scores below 4 indicate only functional system dysfunction. The EDSS is a widely used valid tool intended to evaluate MS patients' function and disability [25, 26].

Apart from these, the Qualiveen® (MAPI research trust, Lyon, France) is a questionnaire recommended by the European Association of Urology and validated for assessing the QoL of neurological patients [27, 28]. Symptoms' bother, patients' fears, different feelings and constraints constitute the different domains that are measured by this tool. The QoL-BM (Quality of Life—Bowel Management) is an additional questionnaire which can be used in MS and SCI patients in order to assess the QoL among patients with bowel dysfunction. QoL-assessing questionnaires may be valid tools for professionals providing healthcare to neurological patients not only upon baseline evaluation but also during treatment in order to follow the effectiveness of their management schemes [10, 25, 27, 28] (Table 1).

Physical Examination

The physical disabilities and mental status of the individual patient must be assessed. A neurological evaluation including sensation and reflexes assessment should be performed. In addition, females should be tested for pelvic organ prolapse (POP), and males should undergo a digital rectal examination (DRE) [28].

1. Asymptomatic patient

    The initial assessment of the patient who does not report any urological symptom includes [7]:

    (a) History and questionnaires.
    (b) Physical examination: LUTS, bowel symptoms, neurological symptoms and sexual dysfunction.
    (c) Urinalysis: It is used to detect any underlying urinary tract infection or haematuria.
    (d) Uroflowmetry and PVR.

2. Symptomatic patients (specific neurourological assessment)

    (a) History and questionnaires.
    (b) Physical examination: LUTS, bowel symptoms, neurologic symptoms and sexual dysfunction.
    (c) Measurement of creatinine clearance.
    (d) Urinalysis: It is used to detect any underlying urinary tract infection or haematuria.
    (e) Uroflowmetry.
    (f) Ultrasound of urinary tract and PVR measurement.
    (g) Urodynamic study (UDS).

The Role of UDS in Patients with MS

Urodynamic studies constitute a cornerstone in the urological evaluation of MS patients, and they are recommended in all patients with increased risk for upper urinary tract impairment. The risk of renal failure in MS patients is considerably low compared to patients with SCI or spina bifida. Consequently, UDS is not absolutely indicated in the asymptomatic patient or in the initial assessment as a routine. Urodynamic evaluation is indicated in patients with refractory LUTS or nonresponders to conservative treatment. It is additionally indicated in women with stress urinary incontinence and in those patients intended to undertake any invasive treatment [7, 8, 10, 17, 29].

Detrusor overactivity is the most common urodynamic finding in MS recorded in 34–99% of cases in reported series, and 30–65% of them have also DSD. The amplitude of detrusor contraction during filling cystometry is higher in MS patients compared to contractions in non-neurogenic DO [29]. The second most common UDS finding is detrusor underactivity in 25% [7, 8, 28, 30, 31]. Findings of MRI studies in association with urodynamic findings suggest that patients with DSD or DO display higher volume of demyelinated plaques in the brain, whereas patients with detrusor underactivity display higher number of thoracic plaques [32].

Cystoscopy

Cystoscopy and urine cytology are indicated on an annual basis in patients with increased risk for bladder cancer (gross haematuria, or chronic symptomatic UTI refractory to therapy—ICI 2016) [7, 17]. Otherwise, the use of indwelling catheter for at least 5 years is a strong determinant for annual bladder washing cytology after the 5th year, which should be combined with urethrocystoscopy after year 10 (ICI 2016). However, some researchers propose investigation with bladder washing cytology and urethrocystoscopy in patients suffering from neurogenic LUT dysfunction for at least 5 years [33].

Treatment

The treatment of lower urinary tract dysfunction in patients with MS requires a multidisciplinary approach including urologist, rehabilitation physicians, neurologists, gastroenterologists, psychiatrists, patient representatives, physiotherapists and continence nurses. A holistic approach is needed because the patients' mental status, environmental factors, level of disability, bowel symptoms, sexual dysfunction and urinary symptoms are strongly correlated [10].

Lifestyle Interventions

The daily need for fluid intake in this group of patients is about 1.5–2.5 L. Patients should be protected from dehydration that leads to exacerbation of constipation. Caffeine intake should be limited to lower than 100 mg per day. Caffeine restriction can contribute to the reduction of urinary urgency and micturition frequency [8, 10, 17].

Interestingly, the most popular management of LUTS among MS patients who sought healthcare professional advice was the reduction of fluid intake (32.2%) followed by pelvic floor exercises (24.1%), oral anticholinergic agents (22.6%), avoidance of alcohol or certain food consumption (20.9%). Fluid restriction and dietary modifications were the most common management scheme not only for incontinent MS patients but also among continent individuals [11].

Urological Rehabilitation

In a recent study, the percentage of MS patients who were treated with pelvic floor exercises and bladder training was 24.1% and 13.4%, respectively, and only 1.9% of them underwent electrical stimulation [11]. Pelvic floor rehabilitation can result in reduction of micturition frequency and UI episodes (from 2.8 ± 1.3 to 1.5 ± 1.5 per day) in females with MS. It can also contribute to an increase of mean cystometric capacity (from 173.8 ± 53.9 to 208.5 ± 57.6 mL after 1 month) [34]. Patients who participated in a pelvic floor muscle training (PFMT) programme with biofeedback and neuromuscular electrical stimulation had a greater benefit in their symptoms after 9 weeks (68%) compared to those who participated in a PFMT programme with biofeedback alone (45%) or PFMT programme alone (12%). The results of the treatment can be maintained up to 24 weeks [35]. Another study revealed that this combination therapy could reduce UI episodes by 85% compared to UI episodes before any intervention [36]. However, this therapeutic approach could be effective in patients with mental status and without any significant disability (low score in EDSS). Active neuromuscular electrical stimulation in combination with PFMT and biofeedback can be suggested as a first-line option in physically and mentally able patients [6, 34–36]. Finally, repetitive transcranial magnetic stimulation of the motor cortex for 5 days could be an alternative approach in these patients. It has been proposed that it improves LUTS in MS patients by reducing DO and relaxing the sphincter [37].

Pharmacotherapy

The goals of the treatment are the improvement of storage symptoms by alleviating DO and the reduction of voiding symptoms by ameliorating DSD, resulting in better emptying of the bladder.

1. Antimuscarinics

There are limited studies that evaluate the effectiveness of the treatment with contemporary antimuscarinic agents in MS patients [38, 39]. Nevertheless, antimuscarinics are used as first-line treatment for MS patients with LUTS in spite of the low level of evidence for their use [8, 10, 16, 17, 38]. The percentage of patients treated by antimuscarinics is about 22.6% [11]. Solifenacin 10 mg has been found to improve UDS parameters such as cystometric capacity as well as the quality of life of MS patients similarly to oxybutynin. The incidence of adverse events was low [39]. Another study demonstrated that solifenacin decreases urinary frequency (−2.2 episodes/day) and the number of pads per day (−1 pad/day) [40]. In addition, high doses of antimuscarinics in combination (combinations of oxybutynin, tolterodine and trospium) can contribute to a reduction of urinary incontinence episodes per day with good tolerability [41]. Intravesical atropine has also been demonstrated to improve LUTS in MS patients equally with oxybutynin, but its use requires administration in a clinic, a more complex procedure [42]. Finally, healthcare professionals should take into consideration the increased likelihood of cognitive impairment which can be caused in patients with MS by the use of antimuscarinics; therefore prescription of trospium and darifenacin may eliminate this side effect. These drugs are less likely to cross the brain–blood barrier [43].

2. Cannabinoids

Nabiximols is a specific extract of *Cannabis*, and it is a combination of the components tetrahydrocannabinol (THC) and cannabidiol (CBD). It has been approved in several countries as a drug for reducing spasticity in patients with MS. There are, additionally, a few studies demonstrating successful use of cannabinoid agonists in the treatment of the LUTS in MS patients [44–52]. It is shown that cannabinoids result in reduction of urinary frequency and nocturia, but its effect on UI is controversial [38, 48, 49]. Kavia et al. demonstrated that nabiximols can have a positive effect on nocturia and frequency of patients' voids, but it cannot alter the number of UI episodes. The most common side effect was confusion [44]. In other trials cannabinoid agonists decreased pad weight and bladder complaints [45, 49]. Such results together with animal research findings showing modulation of LUT function by cannabinoids suggest that this may be a promising treatment option not only for the spasticity of patients with MS but for the bladder dysfunction as well [38, 49].

3. Desmopressin

Treatment with desmopressin, a synthetic analogue of vasopressin, used orally or intranasally, can significantly reduce nocturia, urinary frequency and UI episodes within first 6–8 h in MS patients [10, 38, 53]. It has been used in a wide range of doses, from 10 to 100 µg, although all studies associated with this drug have short duration of active treatment and follow-up (6 weeks) [10, 53]. In addition, desmopressin not only can contribute to decreasing daytime urinary frequency for up to 6 h but can improve QoL of MS individuals as well [8, 53]. The most common side effects of the treatment were hyponatremia, related fluid retention (0–8%) and headache (3–4%), possibly limiting its use among elderly MS patients or among patients with low serum sodium level. Monitoring of the sodium level in serum is indicated before and after the use of desmopressin in all patients [6, 53].

4. Botulinum Neurotoxin Type A (BoNT-A) Intradetrusor Injection Therapy

BoNT-A in the onabotulinumtoxinA (BOTOX®) format has been licensed since 2012 in order to alleviate incontinence in MS patients not responding to first- and second-line treatment or having intolerable side effects from oral pharmacotherapy [10]. BoNT-A has been used both in the form of intradetrusor or sphincteric injections. Intradetrusor administration of BoNT-A (usually 30 injections delivered supratrigonally at 1 cm distance from each injection site), via rigid or flexible cystoscope, significantly decreases UI episodes (38% completely dry) and improves urodynamic parameters (increase of maximum cystometric capacity, volume during the first involuntary contraction and detrusor compliance) and consequently QoL in patients with MS regardless of the concomitant use of anticholinergics [6, 8, 10, 54–58]. The dose of 200 units of onabotulinumtoxinA was demonstrated to provide the best balance between efficacy and the lowest risk for need of ISC (30–35%) in this patients' group. It was found that the dose of 200 units is equally effective with the dose of 300 units, but the latter was associated with higher risk to increase the PVR (>200 mL) and the percentage of individuals initiating ISC (42%) [54–56]. A preliminary study using intradetrusor injection of 100 units of onabotulinumtoxinA showed improvements in both urodynamic parameters, such as maximum bladder capacity and maximum detrusor pressure, and bladder diary parameters, such as urinary frequency, urgency, UI and nocturia, while minimizing the risk for impaired bladder emptying [59]; results from ongoing studies in larger patient cohorts are eagerly awaited in order to establish the benefits of a lower-dose intravesical injection.

It is essential that each patient has agreed and been trained in the use of ISC prior to this kind of treatment; however the use of ISC does not affect QoL [8, 60]. The mean period until patients request retreatment is 42 weeks, and the most common adverse event is UTIs [6, 54, 56]. Published data suggest that the incidence of UTIs was higher among MS patients compared to the placebo arm (31% versus 16%), and it was considered to be a consequence of "de novo" use of ISC [6]. The percentage of nonresponders is about 23% after 3 months from the first injection, and the failure rates of those patients who continue the treatment with BoNT-A are 12.6%, 22.2% and 28.9% after 3, 5 and 7 years, respectively [6, 61, 62]. The main factor of discontinuation is the difficulty of using ISC [61]. Finally, the reduction of urethral leakage in end-stage MS patients with indwelling suprapubic catheter can be another possible benefit of intravesical BoNT-A [63].

Urethral BoNT-A injections can be an alternative treatment in quadriplegic patients not able to perform ISC. However, the studies related to sphincteric BoNT-A injections are of low level of evidence [38]. Available studies demonstrated that urethral BoNT-A injections can increase voided volume by a mean of 54% but failed to reduce PVR in MS patients. The main drawback of their use is the need for more frequent reinjections and possible temporary deterioration of incontinence [10, 38, 64, 65].

Neuromodulation Treatment

Tibial nerve stimulation (TNS): Electrical stimulation can be delivered via percutaneous (PTNS) or transcutaneous (TTNS) approach. It is demonstrated that PTNS can improve both clinical and urodynamic parameters [38]. It is an effective treatment option for MS-related storage symptoms such as frequency, UI episodes and nocturia while also improving urodynamic parameters such as bladder capacity, maximum flow rate and PVR. Such positive results are reflected in high MS patient satisfaction (up to 70% in 89% of them) and QoL improvement [10, 66–69]. In published schemes, PTNS is usually delivered for 30 min in weekly sessions over a 10–12-week period. Responders of PTNS treatment who follow a maintenance therapy have persistent efficacy at 24 months [6, 70]. According to recently published data (2017), long term (12 months) of PTNS achieved reduction of urinary frequency by 5.4 voids, UI by 3.4 episodes, urgency by 7.4 episodes, nocturia by 2.6 voids and improvement of voided volume by about 72 mL [71]. Transcutaneous tibial nerve stimulation can be an alternative, minimally invasive and cost-effective treatment option for neurogenic LUTS of MS patients reducing urinary frequency, urgency and UI and improving QoL [72].

Sacral neuromodulation (SNM): There are limited data and low level of evidence results to support the use of SNM in patients with MS; however published studies showed an improvement (reduction of frequency, UI and number of CIC) of LUTS among those individuals [38, 73, 74]. The need of repeated MRI assessment in MS patients could be a major limitation of SNM use in this group of individuals. It is proposed that SNM is a treatment option only in patients with MS who have not had any relapse for at least 2 years [10, 75].

Other routes of electrical stimulation: A number of studies have evaluated different ways of electrical stimulation aiming at eliminating neurogenic LUTS in patients with multiple sclerosis. The epidural continuous spinal cord stimulation, the epidural dorsal column stimulation and the intravaginal stimulation have shown improvement of patients' symptoms, but the long-term results are not satisfactory. Furthermore, dorsal penile or clitoral nerve stimulation is effective for a limited period of time [76–80].

Surgical Approaches

Surgery is a therapeutic option for patients with MS when conservative treatment has failed, the patient is not able to perform CIC or serious complications such as sepsis, fistulae, renal failure and severe UI have occurred [10]. Augmentation cystoplasty is the most invasive surgical approach in individuals able to perform CIC, and it can contribute to increasing bladder capacity refractory to less invasive treatment [81]. Cutaneous continent urinary diversion can be a treatment option in patients unable to perform CIC via urethra but with upper extremity dexterity (Mitrofanoff's or Monti principle) [10]. Ileal conduit can constitute a therapeutic approach in patients with quadriplegia, limited dexterity or severe cognitive impairment unable to perform CIC due to end-stage MS disease and complicated LUTS or UI [38, 82, 83]. Although the most invasive approaches result in high rates of urinary continence, the morbidity and complication rates are high (18.2% ileal conduit postoperative morbidity); therefore, both the UK consensus and EAU guidelines suggest that these operations should be done only with specific indications (upper urinary tract deterioration refractory to other treatment options) and by expert professionals [10, 38].

Clean Intermittent Catheterization (CIC)

According to the UK consensus, patients with multiple sclerosis should start CIC when PVR is higher than 100 mL although there is not an evidence-based cut-off PVR for this option. The percentage of patients who fail to perform CIC is about 13% and is related to numbers of lesions and to EDSS score; thus, a specialist nurse should teach all patients. It is noteworthy that it is independent from the course of the disease or cognitive impairment [84]. The use of CIC by vulnerable MS individuals contributes to reduction of UTIs, UI episodes and QoL improvement [85, 86].

Finally, PVR may be reduced in some MS patients by the use of selective alpha 1-adrenergic receptor antagonist like indoramin or by the use of tadalafil on a daily basis [87, 88]. Daily tadalafil may also result in improvement of both erectile dysfunction and LUTS in young men with MS [88].

Treatment Discontinuation

The main reason of conservative treatment discontinuation is its limited efficacy. Up to 29% of patients treated with fluid adjustment and 58% of those treated with urological rehabilitation discontinued the interventions due to their suboptimal efficacy. Up to 35% of MS patients using antimuscarinics ceased treatment due to either adverse events or limited efficacy. Finally, 28% of patients treated by CIC stopped their use due to adverse events, while another 32% discontinued their use due to LUTS resolution [11].

Parkinson's Disease

Epidemiology of LUTS in PD

Lower urinary tract symptoms (LUTS) seem to be quite prevalent among patients with Parkinson's disease (PD). It is estimated that neurogenic LUTS occur in almost 60% of PD patients [89]. In control-based studies, LUTS were found to be significantly more prevalent in PD patients (27–64%) than in healthy controls [90–94]. The prevalence of storage and voiding symptoms in PD were 35–83% and 17–27%, respectively [95–97]. A few studies have also reported different prevalence rates of micturition disorders in early and advanced PD [98, 99]. According to Barrero R et al., urinary symptoms correlate with rigidity severity and with the duration of PD [100]. By contrast, other researchers suggest that LUTS in PD, as other non-motor symptoms (NMS), may be dominant in the untreated and early phase of PD, causing a considerable burden [101].

Nocturia is considered to be the most prevalent of urinary symptoms in PD (>60%) [93, 94]. Nocturia as isolated symptom occurs in almost half of patients and according to Zhang and Zhang [102]. While nocturia was not related to the course of the disease, the number of nocturnal voids was positively associated with depression, anxiety, sleeping quality and severity of PD [102]. Latest data suggest that not only nocturia but generally LUTS in PS as many other NMS are highly correlated with anxiety and depression [102–104].

Among 107 patients with PD, frequency (IPSS: 71%) and urgency (IPSS: 68%) were the most frequently reported LUTS after exclusion of nocturia (IPSS = 86%). The most bothersome bladder storage symptom was urgency followed by nocturia and urgency incontinence [105].

According to Hattori et al., voiding symptoms although not predominant may exist without storage symptoms in almost 11% and with storage symptoms in another 21% of PD patients. On sum, one third of patients with PD have also bothersome voiding symptoms [89]. In the study by Sakakibara et al., PD patients had significantly higher rates of delay in initiating micturition (44% of men), prolongation/poor stream (70% of men) and straining (28% of women) compared with the control group [106]. Although they reported that males with PD and voiding symptoms have low post-void residuals (PVR), other researchers found pathologically increased PVR in 41% of males with PD [102].

Recent data suggest that the severity of LUTS in PD patients, as a part of the NMS, tends to become progressively worse with the course of the disease, while age is not related to the progression of those NMS [107].

LUTS in PD patients were also correlated with falls. Falls in patients with Parkinson's disease might be associated with urinary urgency, but not with the frequency of urination [108].

Urodynamic Observations

Detrusor overactivity (DO) appears to be a common urodynamic finding, being recorded in more than half of PD patients (51–58%) [99, 109]. Overactive bladder complex symptoms and increased bladder sensation (sensory urgency) were reported to affect almost 12% of PD patients [99]. Compared with non-neurogenic patients, PD patients with DO had a significantly lower median volume at first detrusor contraction [110]. During pressure-flow study, the most frequently reported urodynamic observation is detrusor underactivity (DU). In a study by Uchiyama et al., 50% of PD patients had DU with the combination of DO and DU to be the most frequent urodynamic diagnosis [99, 111]. According to Terayama et al., a weak detrusor in PD might have a central origin [112]. A wide range of bladder outlet obstruction (BOO) diagnosis has been reported—between 16% and 41.8% when only males with PD and voiding dysfunction were included [99, 113]. Detrusor sphincter dyssynergia (DSD), mainly impaired urethral relaxation, was noticed in 8% of cases [99].

Management of LUTS in PD Patients

Although LUTS are common in PD, few studies have assessed the management of LUTS specifically in patients with PD. Pilot studies have been small and often lacked a suitable control group making them vulnerable to the placebo effect [114].

Management of Benign Prostatic Obstruction (BPO)

PD is no longer an absolute contraindication for transurethral resection of the prostate (TUR-P) when PD males also suffer from benign prostatic obstruction (BPO) [115]. It is mandatory prior to TUR-P to exclude multiple systemic atrophy (MSA). Open bladder neck at the start of video cystomanometry, suggestive of internal sphincter denervation, was observed only in MSA patients, while an open bladder neck during the whole cystomanometry was noted in 31% of patients with PD compared to 87% of those with MSA. During invasive external sphincter EMG evaluation, motor unit potential analysis showed impaired motor unit potentials suggestive of external sphincter denervation in only 5% of patients with PD as opposed to 93% of those with MSA. As a conclusion TUR-P seems to be safe only in those PD patients with BPO with no evidence of denervated bladder neck during videourodynamic evaluation and without neurological sphincter motor unit potentials during invasive EMG [116].

Minimally invasive procedures for BPH: Due to the worries of post-prostatectomy incontinence in PD patients, it might be an idea to apply minimally invasive procedures for BPO in those patients. The prostatic urethral lift (UroLift®) and the upcoming radiofrequency-created thermal energy in the form of water vapour (Rezum), although not yet evaluated in this group of patients, might be a promising alternative to TUR-P [117]. Long-term studies already exist on UroLift showing either the noninferiority of the procedure against TUR-P in most of the evaluated parameters, including adverse events, or significant improvements in IPSS in controlled studies. Long-term results are awaited for Rezum.

Management of Storage Symptoms

Antimuscarinics are the first-line treatment of storage LUTS in patients with PD [106, 118]. Antimuscarinics are more effective than placebo in improving not only motor function in PD [119] but also neurogenic urinary incontinence. In a randomized, controlled trial, solifenacin was found to be superior to placebo in decreasing the number of micturitions per 24 h, the mean number of urinary incontinence episodes and the mean number of nocturia episodes per 24 h [120]. Neurogenic OAB symptoms also improved after antimuscarinic treatment in a pilot study evaluating both results from the OAB-q questionnaire and urodynamic studies in PD patients [121]. Close follow-up for changes in post-void residual is recommended by researchers but also because treatment with antimuscarinics may provoke the occurrence of neuropsychiatric and cognitive adverse events [106, 118, 119].

Sparse data exist on the use of α-blockers for the management of neurogenic LUTS due to PD [118]. A single study using doxazosin showed significant improvements in the total International Continence Society male short-form score, in the impact of LUTS on quality of life and the maximum urinary flow after doxazosin administration; however, the response to treatment seems to be dependent on the severity of neurological disability [122]. Anecdotal reports suggest that combination therapy with antimuscarinics and α-blockers is commonly used in PD patients with mixed neurogenic LUTS during everyday urological practice, but there are no placebo-controlled studies evaluating the efficacy and safety of such management.

Minimally Invasive Treatments

1. *Botulinum toxin A*

   Despite the scarcity of studies on first-line pharmaceutical treatments for LUTS in PD, there are increasing studies on treatments for refractory LUTS, suggesting a possible difficulty in effective management with oral pharmacotherapy. Doses of 100–200 U of onabotulinumtoxinA have been used for bladder injections in patients with PD and refractory to antimuscarinic neurogenic OAB symptoms or incontinence and were found to be both effective and safe [123–125]. In a study of 20 patients (12 men, 8 women), injection of 100 U of onabotulinumtoxinA resulted in moderate or marked symptom relief and at least 50% improvement of incontinence in 59% of patients, without a case of urinary retention [123]. Injection of 200 U of onabotulinumtoxinA resulted in major clinical (decreased micturition frequency, pad use and improved ICIQ scores) and urodynamic improvements (increased maximum cystometric capacity, volume at first and strong desire to void, decreased voiding detrusor pressures, elimination of DO in most patients) in another study of ten PD patients, with no patient requiring clean intermittent catheterization [124]. According to Giannantoni et al., an increase in post-void residual was noted in all PD patients treated with 200 U, but again none required clean intermittent catheterizations [125]. Interestingly, a significant increase in post-void residual ($36.7 \pm 32.4114.6 \pm 109$ mL, $p = 0.048$) was also recorded in a study of nine PD patients by Jiang et al. using 100 U of onabotulinumtoxinA. Despite improvements in the Urgency Severity Scale, the authors found no beneficial effects in the number of urgency or urgency incontinence episodes as per bladder diary, or in maximum cystometric capacity, while both maximum flow rate and detrusor pressures remained unchanged [126].

   Local anaesthesia is favoured in PD patients in order to avoid cognitive impairment from general anaesthesia [123, 127]. Available data suggest that intravesical botulinum toxin injections maybe helpful as a second-line treatment for neurogenic storage symptoms in PD patients, but due to the limited numbers of patients involved in these trials and the lack of a suitable control group, results can only be considered as indicative.

2. *Electrostimulation/magnetic stimulation*

   There is evidence that percutaneous tibial nerve stimulation (PTNS) may improve OAB symptoms (frequency, urgency and nocturia), reduce the number of urinary incontinence episodes per 24 h and increase the maximum cystometric capacity and the voided volume [67, 128].

   Several studies have investigated the effect of deep brain stimulation of the subthalamic nucleus (STN-DBS) on LUTS. Most studies showed improvements in both clinical symptoms and urodynamic parameters in PD patients with neurogenic LUTS after STN-DBS [129–131]. The increase in maximum cystometric capacity [129] was considered to be due to the improvement of increased bladder sensation [130] or the reduction of detrusor overactivity after the implantation [131]. By contrast, Winge K. et al. found that although there was an improvement in OAB symptoms, urodynamic parameters after the implantation of electrodes did not change significantly [132].

Future Therapies: Microbiota and Its Role in the Pathogenesis (and Treatment) of PD and Associated LUTS

Increasing evidence supports a role for the dysregulation of the brain–gut–microbiota axis in the pathogenesis of PD. Gastrointestinal dysfunction may precede or follow the central nervous system impairment, and it is thought that the gut may represent a gate for the entrance of environmental factors which may initiate the pathological process [133]. The gut microbiota seems to also play a role in the body homeostasis. Research is also evolving into the microbiota of the urinary tract which is now thought to have a role beyond urinary tract infections [134]. Further, it is believed that associations exist between the gut microbiota and certain urological diseases [134]. In this respect, it is possible that the gut microbiota modification could be explored as a novel therapeutic option in PD and associated LUTS.

References

1. World Health Organization. Atlas multiple sclerosis resources in the world 2008. Geneva: WHO Press; 2008.
2. Kingwell E, Marriott JJ, Jette N, Pringsheim T, Makhani N, Morrow SA, Fisk JD, Evans C, Beland SG, Kulaga S, Dykeman J, Wolfson C, Koch MW, Marrie RA. Incidence and prevalence of multiple sclerosis in Europe: a systematic review. BMC Neurol. 2013;13:128.
3. Howard J, Trevick S, Younger DS. Epidemiology of multiple sclerosis. Neurol Clin. 2016;34(4):919–39.
4. Noseworthy JH, Lucchinetti C, Rodriguez M, Weinshenker BG. Multiple sclerosis. N Engl J Med. 2000;343(13):938–52. Review
5. Lublin FD, Reingold SC, Cohen JA, Cutter GR, Sørensen PS, Thompson AJ, Wolinsky JS, Balcer LJ, Banwell B, Barkhof F, Bebo B Jr, Calabresi PA, Clanet M, Comi G, Fox RJ, Freedman MS, Goodman AD, Inglese M, Kappos L, Kieseier BC, Lincoln JA, Lubetzki C, Miller AE, Montalban X, O'Connor PW, Petkau J, Pozzilli C, Rudick RA, Sormani MP, Stüve O, Waubant E, Polman CH. Defining the clinical course of multiple sclerosis: the 2013 revisions. Neurology. 2014;83(3):278–86.
6. Sadiq A, Brucker BM. Management of neurogenic lower urinary tract dysfunction in multiple sclerosis patients. Curr Urol Rep. 2015;16(7):44.
7. de Sèze M, Ruffion A, Denys P, Joseph PA. Perrouin-Verbe B; GENULF. The neurogenic bladder in multiple sclerosis: review of the literature and proposal of management guidelines. Mult Scler. 2007;13(7):915–28. Epub 2007 Mar 15. Review

8. Panicker JN, Fowler CJ. Lower urinary tract dysfunction in patients with multiple sclerosis. Handb Clin Neurol. 2015;130:371–81.
9. Fowler CJ, Griffiths D, de Groat WC. The neural control of micturition. Nat Rev Neurosci. 2008;9(6):453–66.
10. Phe V, Chartier-Kastler E, Panicker JN. Management of neurogenic bladder in patients with multiple sclerosis. Nat Rev Urol. 2016;13:275–88.
11. Khalaf KM, Coyne KS, Globe DR, Armstrong EP, Malone DC, Burks J. Lower urinary tract symptom prevalence and management among patients with multiple sclerosis. Int J MS Care. 2015;17(1):14–25.
12. Kragt JJ, Hoogervorst EL, Uitdehaag BM, Polman CH. Relation between objective and subjective measures of bladder dysfunction in multiple sclerosis. Neurology. 2004;63(9):1716–8.
13. Wyndaele JJ, Castro D, Madersbacher H. Neurogenic and faecal incontinence. In: Abrams P, editor. Incontinence. Paris: Health Publications; 2005. p. 1059–162.
14. Blaivas JG, Kaplan SA. Urologic dysfunction in patients with multiple sclerosis. Semin Neurol. 1988;8(2):159–65.
15. Gallien P, Nicolas B, Robineau S, Le Bot MP, de Crouy AC, Durufle A, Edan G, Brissot R. Urological complications in multiple sclerosis: study of risk factors. Ann Readaptation Med Phys. 1998;41:155–8.
16. Groen J, Pannek J, Castro Diaz D, Del Popolo G, Gross T, Hamid R, Karsenty G, Kessler TM, Schneider M, 't Hoen L, Blok B. Summary of European Association of Urology (EAU) Guidelines on Neuro-Urology. Eur Urol. 2016;69:324–33.
17. Fowler CJ, Panicker JN, Drake M, Harris C, Harrison SC, Kirby M, Lucas M, Macleod N, Mangnall J, North A, Porter B, Reid S, Russell N, Watkiss K, Wells M. A UK consensus on the management of the bladder in multiple sclerosis. J Neurol Neurosurg Psychiatry. 2009;80:470–7.
18. Redelings MD, McCoy L, Sorvillo F. Multiple sclerosis mortality and patterns of comorbidity in the United States from 1990 to 2001. Neuroepidemiology. 2006;26:102–7.
19. De Ridder D, van Poppel H, Demonty L, D'Hooghe B, Gonsette R, Carton H, Baert L. Bladder cancer in patients with multiple sclerosis treated with cyclophosphamide. J Urol. 1998;159(6):1881–4.
20. Lawrenson R, Wyndaele JJ, Vlachonikolis I, Farmer C, Glickman S. Renal failure in patients with neurogenic lower urinary tract dysfunction. Neuroepidemiology. 2001;187:138–43.
21. Ouslander JG. Management of overactive bladder. N Engl J Med. 2004;350(8):786–99. Review
22. Clark R, Welk B. Patient reported outcome measures in neurogenic bladder. Transl Androl Urol. 2016;5(1):22–30.
23. Burks J, Chancellor M, Bates B, Denys P, MacDiarmid S, Nitti V, et al. Development and validation of the actionable bladder symptom screening tool for multiple sclerosis patients. Int J MS Care Winter. 2013;15(4):182–92.
24. Welk B, Morrow S, Madarasz W, Baverstock R, Macnab J, Sequeira K. The validity and reliability of the neurogenic bladder symptom score. J Urol. 2014;192(2):452–7.
25. Kurtzke JF. Rating neurologic impairment in multiple sclerosis: an expanded disability status scale (EDSS). Neurology. 1983;33(11):1444–52.
26. Kurtzke JF. On the origin of EDSS. Mult Scler Relat Disord. 2015;4(2):95–103.
27. Bonniaud V, Jackowski D, Parratte B, Paulseth R, Grad S, Margetts P, Guyatt G. Quality of life in multiple sclerosis patients with urinary disorders: discriminative validation of the English version of Qualiveen. Qual Life Res. 2005;14(2):425–31.
28. Blok B, Padilla-Fernández B, Pannek J, Castro-Diaz D, Del Popolo G, Groen J, Hamid R, Karsenty G, Kessler TM, Guidelines Associates: Ecclestone H, Musco S, Padilla-Fernández B, Phé V, Sartori A, 't Hoen L. Guidelines on neuro-urology 2018. European Association of Urology. https://uroweb.org/guideline/neuro-urology/.
29. Campbell, MF, Wein AJ, Kavoussi LR. In: Wein AJ, Kavoussi LR, editors. Campbell-Walsh urology. Philadelphia: Elsevier/Saunders; 2012.

30. Allio BA, Peterson AC. Urodynamic and physiologic patterns associated with the common causes of neurogenic bladder in adults. Transl Androl Urol. 2016;5(1):31–8.
31. Litwiller SE, Frohman EM, Zimmern PE. Multiple sclerosis and the urologist. J Urol. 1999;161(3):743–57. Review
32. Ukkonen M, Elovaara I, Dastidar P, Tammela TL. Urodynamic findings in primary progressive multiple sclerosis are associated with increased volumes of plaques and atrophy in the central nervous system. Acta Neurol Scand. 2004;109:100–5.
33. Sammer U, Walter M, Knüpfer SC, Mehnert U, Bode-Lesniewska B, Kessler TM. Do we need surveillance urethro-cystoscopy in patients with neurogenic lower urinary tract dysfunction? PLoS One. 2015;10(10):e0140970.
34. De Ridder D, Vermeulen C, Ketelaer P, Van Poppel H, Baert L. Pelvic floor rehabilitation in multiple sclerosis. Acta Neurol Belg. 1999;99(1):61–4.
35. McClurg D, Ashe RG, Marshall K, Lowe-Strong AS. Comparison of pelvic floor muscle training, electromyography biofeedback, and neuromuscular electrical stimulation for bladder dysfunction in people with multiple sclerosis: a randomized pilot study. Neurourol Urodyn. 2006;25(4):337–48.
36. McClurg D, Ashe RG, Lowe-Strong AS. Neuromuscular electrical stimulation and the treatment of lower urinary tract dysfunction in multiple sclerosis—a double blind, placebo controlled, randomised clinical trial. Neurourol Urodyn. 2008;27(3):231–7.
37. Centonze D, Petta F, Versace V, Rossi S, Torelli F, Prosperetti C, Rossi S, Marfia GA, Bernardi G, Koch G, Miano R, Boffa L, Finazzi-Agrò E. Effects of motor cortex rTMS on lower urinary tract dysfunction in multiple sclerosis. Mult Scler. 2007;13(2):269–71.
38. Çetinel B, Tarcan T, Demirkesen O, Özyurt C, Şen İ, Erdoğan S, Siva A. Management of lower urinary tract dysfunction in multiple sclerosis: a systematic review and Turkish consensus report. Neurourol Urodyn. 2013;32(8):1047–57.
39. Amarenco G, Sutory M, Zachoval R, Agarwal M, Del Popolo G, Tretter R, Compion G, De Ridder D. Solifenacin is effective and well tolerated in patients with neurogenic detrusor overactivity: results from the double-blind, randomized, active- and placebo-controlled SONIC urodynamic study. Neurourol Urodyn. 2017;36(2):414–21.
40. van Rey F, Heesakkers J. Solifenacin in multiple sclerosis patients with overactive bladder: a prospective study. Adv Urol. 2011;2011:834753.
41. Amend B, Hennenlotter J, Schäfer T, Horstmann M, Stenzl A, Sievert KD. Effective treatment of neurogenic detrusor dysfunction by combined high-dosed antimuscarinics without increased side-effects. Eur Urol. 2008;53(5):1021–8.
42. Fader M, Glickman S, Haggar V, Barton R, Brooks R, Malone-Lee J. Intravesical atropine compared to oral oxybutynin for neurogenic detrusor overactivity: a double-blind, randomized crossover trial. J Urol. 2007;177(1):208–13. discussion 213
43. Panicker JN, Fowler CJ, Kessler TM. Lower urinary tract dysfunction in the neurological patient: clinical assessment and management. Lancet Neurol. 2015;14:720–32.
44. Kavia RB, De Ridder D, Constantinescu CS, Stott CG, Fowler CJ. Randomized controlled trial of Sativex to treat detrusor overactivity in multiple sclerosis. Mult Scler. 2010;16(11):1349–59.
45. Freeman RM, Adekanmi O, Waterfield MR, Waterfield AE, Wright D, Zajicek J. The effect of cannabis on urge incontinence in patients with multiple sclerosis: a multicentre, randomised placebo-controlled trial (CAMS-LUTS). Int Urogynecol J Pelvic Floor Dysfunct. 2006;17(6):636–41. Epub 2006 Mar 22
46. Wade DT, Makela P, Robson P, House H, Bateman C. Do cannabis-based medicinal extracts have general or specific effects on symptoms in multiple sclerosis? A double-blind, randomized, placebo-controlled study on 160 patients. Mult Scler. 2004;10(4):434–41.
47. Brady CM, DasGupta R, Dalton C, Wiseman OJ, Berkley KJ, Fowler CJ. An open-label pilot study of cannabis-based extracts for bladder dysfunction in advanced multiple sclerosis. Mult Scler. 2004;10(4):425–33.
48. Andersson KE. Current and future drugs for treatment of MS-associated bladder dysfunction. Ann Phys Rehabil Med. 2014;57(5):321–8.

49. Koppel BS, Brust JC, Fife T, Bronstein J, Youssof S, Gronseth G, Gloss D. Systematic review: efficacy and safety of medical marijuana in selected neurologic disorders: report of the Guideline Development Subcommittee of the American Academy of Neurology. Neurology. 2014;82(17):1556–63.
50. Podda G, Constantinescu CS. Nabiximols in the treatment of spasticity, pain and urinary symptoms due to multiple sclerosis. Expert Opin Biol Ther. 2012;12(11):1517–31.
51. Ruggieri MR Sr. Cannabinoids: potential targets for bladder dysfunction. Handb Exp Pharmacol. 2011;202:425–51.
52. Tyagi P, Tyagi V, Yoshimura N, Chancellor M. Functional role of cannabinoid receptors in urinary bladder. Indian J Urol. 2010;26(1):26–35.
53. Bosma R, Wynia K, Havlikova E, et al. Efficacy of desmopressin in patients with multiple sclerosis suffering from bladder dysfunction: a meta-analysis. Acta Neurol Scand. 2005;112:1–5.
54. Cruz F, Herschorn S, Aliotta P, Brin M, Thompson C, Lam W, Daniell G, Heesakkers J, Haag-Molkenteller C. Efficacy and safety of onabotulinumtoxinA in patients with urinary incontinence due to neurogenic detrusor overactivity: a randomised, double-blind, placebo-controlled trial. Eur Urol. 2011;60(4):742–50.
55. Ginsberg D, Gousse A, Keppenne V, Sievert KD, Thompson C, Lam W, Brin MF, Jenkins B, Haag-Molkenteller C. Phase 3 efficacy and tolerability study of onabotulinumtoxinA for urinary incontinence from neurogenic detrusor overactivity. J Urol. 2012;187(6):2131–9.
56. Rovner E, Dmochowski R, Chapple C, Thompson C, Lam W, Haag- Molkenteller C. OnabotulinumtoxinA improves urodynamic outcomes in patients with neurogenic detrusor overactivity. Neurourol Urodyn. 2013;32:1109–15.
57. Ginsberg D, Cruz F, Herschorn S, Gousse A, Keppenne V, Aliotta P, et al. OnabotulinumtoxinA is effective in patients with urinary incontinence due to neurogenic detrusor overactivity regardless of concomitant anticholinergic use or neurologic etiology. Adv Ther. 2013;30(9):819–33.
58. Sussman D, Patel V, Del Popolo G, Lam W, Globe D, Pommerville P. Treatment satisfaction and improvement in health-related quality of life with onabotulinumtoxinA in patients with urinary incontinence due to neurogenic detrusor overactivity. Neurourol Urodyn. 2013;32(3):242–9.
59. Mehnert U, Birzele J, Reuter K, Schurch B. The effect of botulinum toxin type a on overactive bladder symptoms in patients with multiple sclerosis: a pilot study. J Urol. 2010;184:1011–6.
60. Kalsi V, Gonzales G, Popat R, Apostolidis A, Elneil S, Dasgupta P, Fowler CJ. Botulinum injections for the treatment of bladder symptoms of multiple sclerosis. Ann Neurol. 2007;62(5):452–7.
61. Joussain C, Popoff M, Phé V, Even A, Falcou L, Chartier-Kastler E, Schurch B, Denys P. Long-term real life efficacy of onabotulinum toxin A for the treatment of neurogenic detrusor overactivity in a population using intermitten self-catheterization. Ann Phys Rehabil Med. 2016;59S:e105.
62. Deffontaines-Rufin S, Weil M, Verollet D, Peyrat L, Amarenco G. Botulinum toxin A for the treatment of neurogenic detrusor overactivity in multiple sclerosis patients. Int Braz J Urol. 2011;37(5):642–8.
63. Lekka E, Lee LK. Successful treatment with intradetrusor botulinum-A toxin for urethral urinary leakage (catheter bypassing) in patients with endstaged multiple sclerosis and indwelling suprapubic catheters. Eur Urol. 2006;50:806–10.
64. Mahfouz W, Karsenty G, Corcos J. Injection of botulinum toxin type A in the urethral sphincter to treat lower urinary tract dysfunction: review of indications, techniques and results: 2011 update. Can J Urol. 2011;18:5787–95.
65. Gallien P, Reymann JM, Amarenco G, Nicolas B, de Sèze M, Bellissant E. Placebo controlled, randomized, double blind study of the effects of botulinum A toxin on detrusor sphincter dyssynergia in multiple sclerosis patients. J Neurol Neurosurg Psychiatry. 2005;76:1670–6.
66. Kabay S, Kabay SC, Yucel M, Ozden H, Yilmaz Z, Aras O, Aras B. The clinical and urodynamic results of a 3-month percutaneous posterior tibial nerve stimulation treatment in

patients with multiple sclerosis-related neurogenic bladder dysfunction. Neurourol Urodyn. 2009;28(8):964–8.

67. Kabay SC, Kabay S, Yucel M, Ozden H. Acute urodynamic effects of percutaneous posterior tibial nerve stimulation on neurogenic detrusor overactivity in patients with Parkinson's disease. Neurourol Urodyn. 2009;28(1):62–7.

68. Kabay SC, Yucel M, Kabay S. Acute effect of posterior tibial nerve stimulation on neurogenic detrusor overactivity in patients with multiple sclerosis: urodynamic study. Urology. 2008;71(4):641–5.

69. Gobbi C, Digesu GA, Khullar V, El Neil S, Caccia G, Zecca C. Percutaneous posterior tibial nerve stimulation as an effective treatment of refractory lower urinary tract symptoms in patients with multiple sclerosis: preliminary data from a multicentre, prospective, open label trial. Mult Scler. 2011;17(12):1514–9.

70. Zecca C, Digesu GA, Robshaw P, Singh A, Elneil S, Gobbi C. Maintenance percutaneous posterior nerve stimulation for refractory lower urinary tract symptoms in patients with multiple sclerosis: an open label, multicenter, prospective study. J Urol. 2014;191(3): 697–702.

71. Canbaz Kabay S, Kabay S, Mestan E, Cetiner M, Ayas S, Sevim M, Ozden H, Karaman HO. Long term sustained therapeutic effects of percutaneous posterior tibial nerve stimulation treatment of neurogenic overactive bladder in multiple sclerosis patients: 12-months results. Neurourol Urodyn. 2017;36(1):104–10.

72. de Sèze M, Raibaut P, Gallien P, Even-Schneider A, Denys P, Bonniaud V, Gamé X, Amarenco G. Transcutaneous posterior tibial nerve stimulation for treatment of the overactive bladder syndrome in multiple sclerosis: results of a multicenter prospective study. Neurourol Urodyn. 2011;30(3):306–11.

73. Ruud Bosch JL, Groen J. Treatment of refractory urge urinary incontinence with sacral spinal nerve stimulation in multiple sclerosis patients. Lancet. 1996;348:717–9.

74. Minardi D, Muzzonigro G. Sacral neuromodulation in patients with multiple sclerosis. World J Urol. 2012;30:123–8.

75. Chaabane W, Guillotreau J, Castel-Lacanal E, Abu-Anz S, De Boissezon X, Malavaud B, Marque P, Sarramon JP, Rischmann P, Game X. Sacral neuromodulation for treating neurogenic bladder dysfunction: clinical and urodynamic study. Neurourol Urodyn. 2011;30(4):547–50.

76. Read DJ, Matthews WB, Higson RH. The effect of spinal cord stimulation on function in patients with multiple sclerosis. Brain. 1980;103:803–33.

77. Primus G. Maximal electrical stimulation in neurogenic detrusor hyperactivity: experiences in multiple sclerosis. Eur J Med. 1992;1:80–2.

78. Hawkes CH, Fawcett D, Cooke ED Emson PC, Paul EA, Bowcock SA. Dorsal column stimulation in multiple sclerosis: Effects on bladder, leg blood flow and peptides. Appl Neurophysiol. 1981;44:62–70.

79. Berg V, Bergmann S, Hovdal H, Hovdal H. The value of dorsal column stimulation in multiple sclerosis. Scand J Rehabil Med. 1982;14:183–91.

80. Fjorback MV, Rijkhoff N, Petersen T, Nohr M, Sinkjaer T. Event driven electrical stimulation of the dorsal penile/clitoral nerve for management of neurogenic detrusor overactivity in multiple sclerosis. Neurourol Urodyn. 2006;25(4):349–55.

81. Zachoval R, Pitha J, Medova E, Heracek J, Lukes M, Zalesky M, Urban M. Augmentation cystoplasty in patients with multiple sclerosis. Urol Int. 2003;70:21–6.

82. Legrand G, Rouprêt M, Comperat E, Even-Schneider A, Denys P, Chartier-Kastler E. Functional outcomes after management of end-stage neurological bladder dysfunction with ileal conduit in a multiple sclerosis population: a monocentric experience. Urology. 2011;78(4):937–41.

83. Guillotreau J, Panicker JN, Castel-Lacanal E, Viala F, Roumiguié M, Malavaud B, Marque P, Clanet M, Rischmann P, Gamé X. Prospective evaluation of laparoscopic assisted cystectomy and ileal conduit in advanced multiple sclerosis. Urology. 2012;80(4):852–7.

84. Vahter L, Zopp I, Kreegipuu M, Kool P, Talvik T, Gross-Paju K. Clean intermittent self-catheterization in persons with multiple sclerosis: the influence of cognitive dysfunction. Mult Scler. 2009;15(3):379–84.
85. Kornhuber HH, Schutz A. Efficient treatment of neurogenic bladder disorders in multiple sclerosis with initial intermittent catheterization and ultrasound- controlled training. Eur Neurol. 1990;30:260–7.
86. Castel-Lacanal E, Gamé X, De Boissezon X, Guillotreau J, Braley-Berthoumieux E, Terracol C, Gasq D, Labrunee M, Viala F, Rischmann P, Clanet M, Marque P. Impact of intermittent catheterization on the quality of life of multiple sclerosis patients. World J Urol. 2013;31(6):1445–50. https://doi.org/10.1007/s00345-012-1017-8. Epub 2013 Jan 6
87. O'Riordan JI, Doherty C, Javed M, Brophy D, Hutchinson M, Quinlan D. Do alpha-blockers have a role in lower urinary tract dysfunction in multiple sclerosis? J Urol. 1995;153(4):1114–6.
88. Francomano D, Ilacqua A, Cortese A, Tartaglia G, Lenzi A, Inghilleri M, Aversa A. Effects of daily tadalafil on lower urinary tract symptoms in young men with multiple sclerosis and erectile dysfunction: a pilot study. J Endocrinol Invest. 2017;40(3):275–9.
89. Hattori T, Yasuda K, Kita K, Hirayama K. Voiding dysfunction in Parkinson's disease. Jpn J Psychiatry Neurol. 1992;46(1):181–6.
90. Benli E, Özer FF, Kaya Y, Özcan TŞ, Ayyıldız A. Is there a difference between Parkinson disease patients and a control group in terms of urinary symptoms and quality of life? Turk J Med Sci. 2016;46(6):1665–71.
91. Araki I, Kuno S. Assessment of voiding dysfunction in Parkinson's disease by the international prostate symptom score. J Neurol Neurosurg Psychiatry. 2000;68(4):429–33.
92. Lemack GE, Dewey RB Jr, Roehrborn CG, O'Suilleabhain PE, Zimmern PE. Questionnaire-based assessment of bladder dysfunction in patients with mild to moderate Parkinson's disease. Urology. 2000;56(2):250–4.
93. Campos-Sousa RN, Quagliato E, da Silva BB, et al. Urinary symptoms in Parkinson's disease: prevalence and associated factors. Arq Neuropsiquiatr. 2003;61(2B):359–63.
94. Sakakibara R, Shinotoh H, Uchiyama T, Sakuma M, Kashiwado M, Yoshiyama M, et al. Questionnaire-based assessment of pelvic organ dysfunction in Parkinson's disease. Auton Neurosci. 2001;92(1–2):76–85.
95. Yeo L, Singh R, Gundeti M, Barua JM, Masood J. Urinary tract dysfunction in Parkinson's disease: a review. Int Urol Nephrol. 2012;44:415–24.
96. Barone P, Antonini A, Colosimo C, et al. The PRIAMO study: A multicenter assessment of nonmotor symptoms and their impact on quality of life in Parkinson's disease. Mov Disord. 2009;24:1641–9.
97. Ragab MM, Mohammed ES. Idiopathic Parkinson's disease patients at the urologic clinic. Neurourol Urodyn. 2011;30:1258–61.
98. Winge K, Nielsen KK. Bladder dysfunction in advanced Parkinson's disease. Neurourol Urodyn. 2012;31:1279–83.
99. Uchiyama T, Sakakibara R, Yamamoto T, et al. Urinary dysfunction in early and untreated Parkinson's disease. J Neurol Neurosurg Psychiatry. 2011;82:1382–6.
100. Barrero R, Mir P, Cayuela A, et al. Urinary symptoms and urodynamic findings in Parkinson's disease. Neurologia. 2007;22(2):93–8.
101. Zis P, Martinez-Martin P, Sauerbier A, et al. Non-motor symptoms burden in treated and untreated early Parkinson's disease patients: argument for non-motor subtypes. Eur J Neurol. 2015;22(8):1145–50.
102. Li-Mei Z, Xu-Ping Z. Investigation of urination disorder in Parkinson's disease. Chin Med J (Engl). 2015;128(21):2906–12.
103. Baig F, Lawton M, Rolinski M, et al. Delineating nonmotor symptoms in early Parkinson's disease and first-degree relatives. Mov Disord. 2015;30(13):1759–66.
104. Jiang SM, Yuan YS, Tong Q, et al. The association between clinically relevant anxiety and other non-motor symptoms in Parkinson's disease. Neurol Sci. 2015;36(11):2105–9.

105. Winge K, Skau AM, Stimpel H, Nielsen KK, Werdelin L. Prevalence of bladder dysfunction in Parkinson's disease. Neurourol Urodyn. 2006;25(2):116–22.
106. Sakakibara R, Tateno F, Kishi M, Tsuyuzaki Y, Uchiyama T, Yamamoto T. Pathophysiology of bladder dysfunction in Parkinson's disease. Neurobiol Dis. 2012;46(3):565–71.
107. Ou R, Yang J, Cao B, et al. Progression of non-motor symptoms in Parkinson's disease among different age populations: a two-year follow-up study. J Neurol Sci. 2016;360:72–7.
108. Sakushima K, Yamazaki S, Fukuma S, et al. Influence of urinary urgency and other urinary disturbances on falls in Parkinson's disease. J Neurol Sci. 2016;360:153–7.
109. Krygowska-Wajs A, Weglarz W, Szczudlik ZD. Micturition disturbances in Parkinson's disease. Clinical and urodynamic evaluation. Neurol Neurochir Pol. 2002;36(1):25–32.
110. Defreitas GA, Lemack GE, Zimmern PE, et al. Distinguishing neurogenic from non-neurogenic detrusor overactivity: a urodynamic assessment of lower urinary tract symptoms in patients with and without Parkinson's disease. Urology. 2003;62(4):651–5.
111. Liu Z, Uchiyama T, Sakakibara R, Yamamoto T. Underactive and overactive bladders are related to motor function and quality of life in Parkinson's disease. Int Urol Nephrol. 2015;47(5):751–7.
112. Terayama K, Sakakibara R, Ogawa A, et al. Weak detrusor contractility correlates with motor disorders in Parkinson's disease. Mov Disord. 2012;27(14):1775–80.
113. Xue P, Wang T, Zong H, Zhang Y. Urodynamic analysis and treatment of male Parkinson's disease patients with voiding dysfunction. Chin Med J (Engl). 2014;127(5):878–81.
114. McDonald C, Winge K, Burn DJ. Lower urinary tract symptoms in Parkinson's disease: prevalence, aetiology and management. Parkinsonism Relat Disord. 2017;35:8–16.
115. Roth B, Studer UE, Fowler CJ, Kessler TM. Benign prostatic obstruction and Parkinson's disease—should transurethral resection of the prostate be avoided? J Urol. 2009;181(5):2209–13.
116. Sakakibara R, Hattori T, Uchiyama T, Yamanishi T. Videourodynamic and sphincter motor unit potential analyses in Parkinson's disease and multiple system atrophy. J Neurol Neurosurg Psychiatry. 2001;71(5):600–6.
117. Sievert KD, Kunit T. Emerging techniques in 'truly' minimal-invasive treatment options of benign prostatic obstruction. Curr Opin Urol. 2017;27(3):287–92.
118. Ogawa T, Sakakibara R, Kuno S, Ishizuka O, Kitta T, Yoshimura N. Prevalence and treatment of LUTS in patients with Parkinson disease or multiple system atrophy. Nat Rev Urol. 2017;14(2):79–89.
119. Katzenschlager R, Sampaio C, Costa J, Lees A. Anticholinergics for symptomatic management of Parkinson's disease. Cochrane Database Syst Rev. 2003;2:CD003735.
120. Zesiewicz TA, Evatt M, Vaughan CP, et al. Non-motor working group of the Parkinson Study Group (PSG) randomized, controlled pilot trial of solifenacin succinate for overactive bladder in Parkinson's disease. Parkinsonism Relat Disord. 2015;21(5):514–20.
121. Palleschi G, Pastore AL, Stocchi F, et al. Correlation between the Overactive Bladder questionnaire (OAB-q) and urodynamic data of Parkinson disease patients affected by neurogenic detrusor overactivity during antimuscarinic treatment. Clin Neuropharmacol. 2006;29(4):220–9.
122. Gomes CM, Sammour ZM, Bessa Junior JD, et al. Neurological status predicts response to alpha-blockers in men with voiding dysfunction and Parkinson's disease. Clinics (Sao Paulo). 2014;69(12):817–22.
123. Anderson RU, Orenberg EK, Glowe P. OnabotulinumtoxinA office treatment for neurogenic bladder incontinence in Parkinson's disease. Urology. 2014;83(1):22–7.
124. Knüpfer SC, Schneider SA, Averhoff MM, et al. Preserved micturition after intradetrusor onabotulinumtoxinA injection for treatment of neurogenic bladder dysfunction in Parkinson's disease. BMC Urol. 2016;16(1):55.
125. Giannantoni A, Rossi A, Mearini E, et al. Botulinum toxin A for overactive bladder and detrusor muscle overactivity in patients with Parkinson's disease and multiple system atrophy. J Urol. 2009;182(4):1453–7.

126. Jiang YH, Liao CH, Tang DL, Kuo HC. Efficacy and safety of intravesical onabotulinum-toxinA injection on elderly patients with chronic central nervous system lesions and overactive bladder. PLoS One. 2014;9(8):e105989.
127. Kulaksizoglu H, Parman Y. Use of botulinim toxin-A for the treatment of overactive bladder symptoms in patients with Parkinsons's disease. Parkinsonism Relat Disord. 2010;16(8):531–4.
128. Kabay S, Canbaz Kabay S, Cetiner M, et al. The clinical and urodynamic results of percutaneous posterior tibial nerve stimulation on neurogenic detrusor overactivity in patients with Parkinson's disease. Urology. 2016;87:76–81.
129. Shimizu N, Matsumoto S, Mori Y, Yoshioka N, Uemura H, Nakano N, Taneda M. Effects of deep brain stimulation on urodynamic findings in patients with Parkinson's disease. Hinyokika Kiyo. 2007;53(9):609–12.
130. Seif C, Herzog J, van der Horst C, et al. Effect of subthalamic deep brain stimulation on the function of the urinary bladder. Ann Neurol. 2004;55(1):118–20.
131. Finazzi-Agrò E, Peppe A, D'Amico A, et al. Effects of subthalamic nucleus stimulation on urodynamic findings in patients with Parkinson's disease. J Urol. 2003;169(4):1388–91.
132. Winge K, Nielsen KK, Stimpel H, Lokkegaard A, Jensen SR, Werdelin L. Lower urinary tract symptoms and bladder control in advanced Parkinson's disease: effects of deep brain stimulation in the subthalamic nucleus. Mov Disord. 2007;22(2):220–5.
133. Mulak A, Bonaz B. Brain-gut-microbiota axis in Parkinson's disease. World J Gastroenterol. 2015;21(37):10609–20.
134. Whiteside SA, Razvi H, Dave S, Reid G, Burton JP. The microbiome of the urinary tract—a role beyond infection. Nat Rev Urol. 2015;12(2):81–90.

Traumatic Lesions

Frank M. J. Martens

Introduction

Urinary storage and periodically micturition are regulated by several areas in the brain and spinal cord with extensive tracts between them that involve autonomic (mediated by sympathetic and parasympathetic nerves) and somatic (mediated by pudendal nerves) efferent pathways. The sympathetic innervation of the bladder by the hypogastric nerve arises from the thoracolumbar level of the spinal cord (T10–L2), whereas the parasympathetic innervations by the pelvic nerve originate in the sacral segments of the spinal cord (S2–S4). Somatic efferent nerves for voluntary control of the external urethral sphincter arise in S2–S4 motor neurons in Onuf's nucleus and reach the periphery through the pudendal nerves. Sensations of bladder fullness are conveyed to the spinal cord by the pelvic and hypogastric afferent nerves, whereas sensory input from the bladder neck and the urethra is carried in the pudendal and hypogastric afferent nerves [1].

Normal function of the lower urinary tract is not possible anymore when trauma causes damage to this extensive network of innervation at any level due to head injury, spinal cord injury and peripheral nerve injury. Traumatic injury origins from a wide range of causes, for example, traffic accidents, work accidents, sports and recreation accidents, falls (especially in the elderly) and violence (mainly penetrating trauma). Theoretically, suprasacral spinal cord injury will result in detrusor overactivity with or without detrusor sphincter dyssynergia. Injury to or below the sacral level will cause acontractility of the detrusor muscle.

F. M. J. Martens
Department of Urology, Radboudumc, Nijmegen, The Netherlands
e-mail: frank.martens@radboudumc.nl

Epidemiology

Incidence rates of most published reports on spinal cord injury count only those persons who are admitted to the hospital [2]. Most of the studies are from developed countries (none from South America or from Africa and relatively few from Eastern Europe/Asia), and incidence ranges differ per region [3]. The global estimate of spinal cord injury incidence lies between 10.4 per million per year and 83 per million per year when only patients that survived before hospital admission were included [3].

Most spinal cord injury patients are young men in the beginning of their 30s, and the mean sex distribution between men and women is 3.8/1 (range, 2.5–5.8/1) [3]. The sex distribution decreased compared to the past. About one-third of patients are reported to be tetraplegic and about half to have complete spinal cord injury [3].

Morbidity and Mortality

Life expectancy of patients with traumatic spinal cord injury has increased [4–6]. Median survival in traumatic spinal cord injury ranges from 35.4 days in a study including prehospital death to 35.6 years in a study including only tetraplegics, whereas in non-traumatic spinal cord injury, median survival varied from 2.9 months in individuals with malignant spinal cord compression to 29 years in individuals with intervertebral disc herniation [6]. Despite a decrease in mortality due to renal diseases, mortality due to diseases of the urinary system remains higher than in the general population [4, 7]. Overall mortality in traumatic spinal cord injury is between 1.47 and 2.8 times higher than in the general population [6]. Lower survival rates are associated with older age at lesion onset, higher neurological levels and completeness of spinal cord injury, as well as with earlier decades of injury [5, 6]. For example, a median survival time of 38 years post-injury, with 43% surviving at least 40 years, was predicted from a retrospective cohort, all of whom sustained a spinal cord injury between the ages of 25 and 34 years and between 1945 and 1990 [5].

Although mortality decreased and urologic and medical management improved, morbidity and patient well-being are still important issues in spinal cord injury patient management, including vesicoureteral reflux, urinary tract infections, urolithiasis and urinary incontinence [8–10]. Bladder cancer, with a higher incidence of squamous cell carcinoma and higher rate of muscle invasive bladder cancer compared to the general population, is more prevalent in spinal cord injury patients [11]. Long-lasting indwelling catheters seem to increase the risk for bladder cancer compared to other bladder-emptying methods.

Autonomic Dysreflexia

Autonomic dysreflexia is a syndrome resulting from upper thoracic or cervical spinal cord injury above T6, elicited by a stimulus in the field of distribution of the autonomous sympathetic nucleus, characterized by unregulated sympathetic function below the lesion and compensatory autonomic responses [12]. The exact pathophysiology of autonomic dysreflexia is not completely understood [13].

Clinical hallmark of autonomic dysreflexia is a sudden increase in blood pressure defined as 20–40 mmHg above baseline blood pressure, typically but not often accompanied by a bradycardia (Liu 2015) [13, 14]. Other symptoms are, for example, headache, flushing, piloerection, nasal congestion, sweating above the level of the neurologic lesion, vasoconstriction below the level of the lesion or dysrhythmias [13, 15, 16]. In case of asymptomatic autonomic dysreflexia, there is only an increase of blood pressure without any other symptoms [12].

Generally autonomic dysreflexia cannot occur until after spinal shock has resolved and reflexes return. However, it was presented in several cases that autonomic dysreflexia can even be present immediately after spinal injury during the spinal shock phase [17]. The majority of autonomic dysreflexia occurs in spinal cord injury patients with injury at or above T6 spinal cord level but can also occur in patients with injury below T6 [14]. Autonomic dysreflexia is more prevalent in cervical spinal cord injury than in thoracic spinal cord injury, and blood pressure increases more for those with cervical lesions [14]. There is no significant difference regarding the frequencies of autonomic dysreflexia between C1–C5 and C6–C8 spinal cord injury patients [18]. Autonomic dysreflexia does not only occur in complete spinal cord injury but also incomplete spinal cord injury [14, 19]. However, the relationship between completeness of injury and autonomic dysreflexia remains controversial [16].

In most cases autonomic dysreflexia is triggered by events located in the lower urinary tract, commonly iatrogenic factors like urodynamic investigations, cystoscopy and transurethral procedures [16]. To detect this potential life-threatening complication, routine blood pressure monitoring during urological procedures is highly recommended.

It is important to prevent this potentially life-threatening event. If autonomic dysreflexia occurs, proper recognition and acute treatment are needed [13, 15]. In order to prevent further blood pressure increase, the patient needs to be placed in the upright, sitting position. The next measure is a rapid survey of possible triggering factors and resolving them. If the elevated blood pressure does not start to decline or the cause cannot be determined, then symptomatic treatment to lower blood pressure is essential, e.g. calcium channel antagonist like nifedipine, ACE-inhibitor like captopril or nitrates [13, 15].

Neurological Classification of Spinal Cord Injury and Severity

Neurological function in spinal cord injury is generally assessed by the International Standards for Neurological and Functional Classification of Spinal Cord Injury, according to the American Spinal Injury Association (ASIA) [20]. It determines the neurological level of injury, being the most caudal segment with normal motor and sensory function, and assigns a classification as a measure of severity according to the ASIA impairment scale (AIS). In complete spinal cord injury (AIS A), there is an absence of sensory and motor function in the lowest sacral segments S4–S5. To the contrary, incomplete injuries (AIS B–D) comprise preservation of any sensory and/or motor function below the neurological level that includes the lowest sacral segments S4–S5, the so-called sacral sparing. Sensory sacral sparing includes sensation preservation (intact or impaired) at the anal mucocutaneous junction (S4–S5 dermatome) on one or both sides for light touch or pinprick or deep anal pressure. Motor sacral sparing includes the presence of voluntary contraction of the external anal sphincter upon digital rectal examination. AIS E patients have normal sensory and motor function.

Most difficult tasks are the correct determination of motor levels and motor incompleteness [21]. Moreover, AIS can spontaneously change over time [22]. Up to 30% of AIS A patients convert during the first year after spinal cord injury to incomplete injury, mainly into AIS B. Only a few of them became motor incomplete (AIS C or D). Of the initial incomplete lesions, only 22.5% of AIS B and 10.9% of AIS C remained the same, while for AID 89.8% AIS did not change at 12 months follow-up.

Urological Classification of Neurogenic Bladder Dysfunction

Dysfunction of the lower urinary tract in patients with traumatic lesions of the nerve system will depend on the site, the extent and the evolution of the lesion. Systematic neuro-urologic pathology is described in Chap. 3 of the previous section, including specific syndromes, like central cord syndrome, Brown-Sequard syndrome, anterior cord syndrome, conus medullaris syndrome and cauda equina syndrome. Clinical urological implications will be described below.

Spinal Shock Phase

Spinal shock is the period just after injury with depressed spinal reflexes caudal to spinal cord injury and can last up to 12 months after injury but mainly resolves within several months [23]. This results in initial detrusor acontractility and requires adequate bladder drainage by an indwelling catheter and preferably intermittent catheterization as soon as possible thereafter. The recovery of bladder function usually follows that of skeletal muscle reflexes. It is important to determine when the patient is out of the spinal shock phase to schedule further evaluation of the bladder function by urodynamics.

Traumatic Brain Injury

In a study of 57 patients with severe traumatic brain injury which resulted in temporary coma, 85.9% of patients reported urinary symptoms, 61.2% had overactive bladder symptoms, 14.3% had symptoms of the voiding phase, and 24.5% had both. Most frequent overactive bladder symptoms were urgency and increased daytime frequency, and 52.6% of patients complained of urge incontinence. Urodynamics showed normal detrusor activity in 49.1%, detrusor overactivity in 49.1% and acontractility in 1.8%. No detrusor sphincter dyssynergia was found. Detrusor overactivity was found to be associated with the presence of right hemispheric damage, while impaired contractility was associated with left hemispheric damage [24].

Traumatic Spinal Cord Injury

In a study in which spinal cord injury level or levels were determined by CT or MRI, most patients (94.9%) with suprasacral injuries demonstrated detrusor overactivity with or without detrusor sphincter dyssynergia. In comparison, 14.3% of patients with sacral injuries and 69.7% of patients with combined suprasacral and sacral injuries had detrusor overactivity with or without dyssynergia. 3.1% with suprasacral injuries had acontractility, and all of these patients had lumbar injuries. Acontractility was found in 85.7% and 27.3% of patients with sacral injuries and combined suprasacral and sacral injuries, respectively. No significant differences in voiding dysfunction patterns between the completeness of injury classifications per level of injury were found. All patients with complete (AIS A) suprasacral injuries had detrusor overactivity with or without detrusor sphincter dyssynergia. Patients with incomplete (AIS B, C, and D) suprasacral injuries had a slightly lower frequency (93.8%) of detrusor overactivity with or without dyssynergia. All patients with complete sacral injuries had detrusor acontractility compared to 75% in patients with incomplete sacral injury [25].

Also other studies indicate that although there is a general correlation between the neurological level of injury and the expected vesicourethral function, it is neither absolute nor specific [26–29]. Kaplan et al. reported a positive predictive value for positive sacral cord signs and detrusor acontractility of 87% and for negative sacral cord signs and detrusor overactivity with or without detrusor-external sphincter dyssynergia of 81% [27]. Another study with traumatic spinal cord injury patients showed detrusor overactivity with or without detrusor sphincter dyssynergia in 81.5% and 20% in patients with suprasacral and with sacral injuries, respectively [26]. In suprasacral lesions, detrusor overactivity with or without detrusor sphincter dyssynergia is more prevalent and detrusor hypo- or acontractility less frequent in patients with lesions above the lumbar spinal cord compared to patients with lesions at the level of the lumbar spinal cord [28, 29]. Detrusor overactivity and preservation of the bladder-filling sensation were more frequent in C1–C5 than C6–C8 spinal cord injury patients [18].

No differences in cystometric bladder capacities and leak point intravesical pressures at terminal detrusor overactivity were demonstrated between complete (AIS A) and incomplete (AIS B–E) spinal cord injury patients, being equally unfavourable for both groups [30].

Detrusor Sphincter Dyssynergia

Detrusor sphincter dyssynergia is characterized by concurrent involuntary contractions of the urethral and/or periurethral striated muscle during detrusor contractions, occasionally preventing flow altogether [12]. As a result, high intravesical pressures, elevated residual urine, bladder wall changes and vesicoureteral reflux will occur with consequently renal failure if not treated adequately, especially in case of concomitant urinary tract infections. Detrusor sphincter dyssynergia occurs in suprasacral spinal cord lesions [31]. Patients with supracervical neurologic lesions have synergistic function of their detrusor and sphincter due to intact pontine to sacral pathways [31–33].

Traumatic Peripheral Nerve Damage

Peripheral nerves can be damaged by surgical procedures in the pelvis, like abdominoperineal resection for rectal cancer and hysterectomy, resulting in detrusor hypocontractility. Nerve sparing procedures have shown to reduce the risk of voiding difficulties and should be encouraged to prevent iatrogenic causes of bladder dysfunction and burden for the patients [34, 35].

Management of the Neurogenic Bladder

Besides a specific urological history, including, for example, management of bladder emptying, incontinence and urinary tract infections, history should also be focused on the comorbidity of the patient. While these patients are managed with a multidisciplinary approach, one should inform himself about the sexual function, faecal function and general functioning including autonomy during daily activities.

Heath-related quality of life in neurogenic patients can be assessed by several questionnaires, like Qualiveen and SF-36 [36–38]. In addition, frequency-volume charts or voiding/catheterization diaries can be used.

Physical examination including neurological tests for bulbocavernosus reflex and perianal sensations alone is insufficient in accurately classifying bladder behaviour in spinal cord injury patients [29, 39]. Examination of physical function of the patient is important, for instance, to determine whether the patient is able to perform self-catheterization or will depend on other caregivers.

A working group of the Urodynamics Committee of the International Continence Society (ICS) analysed the available evidence-based literature leading to a Delphi consensus formation by the members of the working group and reviewed by all the members of the ICS Urodynamics Committee on spinal cord injury core panel. It was concluded that urodynamics are highly recommended for patients with spinal cord injury after a proper initial assessment. Regular urodynamic follow-up is recommended to avoid upper urinary tract damage. There is limited evidence on how frequently urodynamic control should be performed [40].

First urodynamics should be done as soon as possible after the end of the spinal shock phase. Video-urodynamics are the gold standard for neurogenic bladder patients, which combines anatomical and functional information of the urinary tract. If video-urodynamics are not available, voiding urethrocystography should be done in addition to filling and voiding cystometry. Video-urodynamics or urodynamics with voiding urethrocystography should be combined with electromyography for the diagnosis of detrusor-external sphincter dyssynergia [41].

In non-neurogenic patients, patients indicate that their symptoms are better represented by ambulatory urodynamics than video-urodynamics [42]. Ambulatory urodynamics at physiological bladder-filling rate has a higher detection rate of detrusor overactivity than conventional urodynamics at supraphysiological filling rates [42–44]. On the other hand, higher rates might be caused by a higher false-positive rate in non-neurogenic as well as spinal cord injury patients [45–47]. Even in non-symptomatic volunteers, detrusor overactivity has been detected in considerable rates with a higher rate for ambulatory urodynamics compared to conventional urodynamics [48]. As a consequence of the false positivity, the sensitivity of ambulatory urodynamics is overestimated, and the actual sensitivity will be lower. Ambulatory urodynamics do not seem necessary for the diagnosis and risk assessment in spinal cord injury patients suspected for detrusor overactivity when conventional urodynamics are done properly [45].

Regarding follow-up of the neuro-urological patient, regular patient assessment with, for instance, urinalysis, renal function, ultrasonography of the kidneys and urethrocystoscopy, is recommended. However, there is a lack of high-level evidence studies, and guidelines are mainly based on expert opinions [49].

One of the major goals in the management of patients with a neurogenic bladder is protection of the upper urinary tract to preserve renal function. This should be accomplished by ensuring detrusor pressures within safe limits and prevention of urinary tract infections. High detrusor leak point pressures (>40 cmH$_2$O), especially sustained high pressures, are a risk factor for renal deterioration, which has been studied in myelodysplastic patients [50, 51]. Patients with detrusor leak point pressures over 40 cmH$_2$O presented more renal scars and vesicoureteral reflux than their counterparts [50]. Also spinal cord injury patients with detrusor pressures >40 cmH$_2$O have an increased risk for renal damage [52]. Maximum detrusor pressure in spinal cord injury patients with a neurogenic bladder is significantly higher in case of abnormal upper tracts than in those with normal kidneys [53]. Patients with sacral or below sacral spinal cord injury and detrusor acontractility have the best bladder status associated with less upper tract deterioration [54].

Neurogenic detrusor overactivity with concomitant high intravesical pressures is not only a risk factor for upper urinary tract deterioration but also for urinary incontinence. Incontinence is a social and hygienic burden. Moreover, incontinence increases the risk of complications in spinal cord injury patients, like pressure ulcers and poor wound healing.

Proper bladder emptying is preferably done by intermittent catheterization or indwelling catheter if intermittent catheterization is not possible [55–57]. Conservative treatment of neurogenic detrusor overactivity consists of anticholinergics [58]. Higher dosages or combinations of anticholinergics might be useful in neurogenic patients [59, 60]. Probably beta-3 agonist can also be of importance for use in neurogenic patients, probably with a synergistic effect when used in combination with anticholinergics [61, 62]. The main surgical interventions for patients who are refractory to conservative treatment include botulinum toxin detrusor injections, sacral neuromodulation for both neurogenic detrusor overactivity and hypocontractility, bladder augmentation or a dorsal rhizotomy of the sacral roots [63–67]. If the latter is combined with sacral anterior root stimulation, the so-called Brindley procedure, stimulation enables bladder and bowel emptying [68].

References

1. Fowler CJ, Griffiths D, De Groat WC. The neural control of micturition. Nat Rev Neurosci. 2008;9(6):453–66.
2. Sekhon LHS, Fehlings MG. Epidemiology, demographics, and pathophysiology of acute spinal cord injury. Spine. 2001;26:S2–S12.
3. Wyndaele M, Wyndaele JJ. Incidence, prevalence and epidemiology of spinal cord injury: what learns a worldwide literature survey? Spinal Cord. 2006;44(9):523.
4. Geisler WO, Jousse AT, Wynne-Jones M, Breithaupt D. Survival in traumatic spinal cord injury. Paraplegia. 1983;21:364–73.
5. McColl MA, Walker J, Stirling P, Wilkins R, Corey P. Expectations of life and health among spinal cord injured adults. Spinal Cord. 1997;35:818–28.
6. Van den Berg MEL, Castellote JM, De Pedro-Cuesta J, Mahillo-Fernandez I. Survival after spinal cord injury: a systematic review. J Neurotrauma. 2010;27:1517–28.
7. Soden RJ, Walsh J, Middleton JW, et al. Causes of death after spinal cord injury. Spinal Cord. 2000;38(10):604–10.
8. Ku JH, Choi WJ, Lee KY, Jung TY, Lee JK, Park WH, Shim HB. Complications of the upper urinary tract in patients with spinal cord injury: a long-term follow-up study. Urol Res. 2005;33:435–9.

9. Selzman AA, Hampel N. Urologic complications of spinal cord injury. Urol Clin North Am. 1993;20(3):453–64.

10. Van Kerrebroeck PE, Koldewijn EL, Scherpenhuizen S, Debruyne FM. The morbidity due to lower urinary tract function in spinal cord injury patients. Paraplegia. 1993;31(5):320–9.

11. Ismail S, Karsenty G, Chartier-Kastler E, Cussenot O, Compérat E, Rouprêt M, Phé V. Prevalence, management, and prognosis of bladder cancer in patients with neurogenic bladder: a systematic review. Neurourol Urodyn. 2018;37:1386–95.

12. Gajewski JB, Schurch B, Hamid R, Averbeck M, Sakakibara R, Agrò EF, Dickinson T, Payne CK, Drake M, Haylen B. An international continence society (ICS) report on the terminology for adult neurogenic lower urinary tract dysfunction (ANLUTD). Neurourol Urodyn. 2018;37:1152–61.

13. Karlsson AK. Autonomic dysreflexia. Spinal Cord. 1999;37:383–91.

14. Huang Y, Bih L, Chen G, Lin C, Chen S, Chen W. Autonomic dysreflexia during urodynamic examinations in patients with suprasacral spinal cord injury. Arch Phys Med Rehabil. 2011;92:1450–4.

15. Khastgir J, Drake MJ, Abrams P. Recognition and effective management of autonomic dysreflexia in spinal cord injuries. Expert Opin Pharmacother. 2007 May;8(7):945–56.

16. Liu N, Zhou M, Biering-Sørensen F, Krassioukov AV. Iatrogenic urological triggers of autonomic dysreflexia: a systematic review. Spinal Cord. 2015;53:500–9.

17. Silver J. Early autonomic dysreflexia. Spinal Cord. 2000;38:229–33.

18. Sayilir S, Ersöz M, Yalçin S. Comparison of urodynamic findings in patients with upper and lower cervical spinal cord injury. Spinal Cord. 2013;51:780–3.

19. Giannantoni A, Di Stasi SM, Scivoletto G, Mollo A, Silecchia A, Fuoco U, Vespasiani G. Autonomic dysreflexia during urodynamics. Spinal Cord. 1998;36:756–60.

20. Kirshblum SC, Burns SP, Biering-Sorensen F, Donovan W, Graves DE, Jha A, Johansen M, Jones L, Krassioukov A, Mulcahey MJ, Schmidt-Read M, Waring W. International standards for neurological classification of spinal cord injury (revised 2011). J Spinal Cord Med. 2011;34(6):535–46.

21. Schuld C, Franz S, Van Hedel HJ, Moosburger J, Maier D, Abel R, van de Meent H, Curt A, Weidner N, EMSCI Study Group, Rupp R. International standards for neurological classification of spinal cord injury: classification skills of clinicians versus computational algorithms. Spinal Cord. 2015;53:324–31.

22. Spiess MR, Müller RM, Rupp R, Schuld C, EM-SCI Study Group, Van Hedel HJ. Conversion in ASIA Impairment Scale during the first year after traumatic spinal cord injury. J Neurotrauma. 2009;26:2027–36.

23. Ditunno JF, Little JW, Tessler A, Burns AS. Spinal shock revisited: a four-phase model. Spinal Cord. 2004;42:383–95.

24. Giannantoni A, Silvestro D, Siracusano S, Azicnuda E, D'ippolito M, Rigon J, Sabatini U, Bini V, Formisano R. Urologic dysfunction and neurologic outcome in coma survivors after severe traumatic brain injury in the postacute and chronic phase. Arch Phys Med Rehabil. 2011;92:1134–8.

25. Weld KJ, Dmochowski RR. Association of level of injury and bladder behaviour in patients with post-traumatic spinal cord injury. Urology. 2000;55(4):490–4.

26. Agrawal M, Joshi M. Urodynamic patterns after traumatic spinal cord injury. J Spinal Cord Med. 2015;38(2):128–33.

27. Kaplan SA, Chancellor MB, Blaivas JG. Bladder and sphincter behaviour in patients with spinal cord lesions. J Urol. 1991;146(1):113–7.

28. Wyndaele JJ. A critical review of urodynamic investigations in spinal cord injury patients. Paraplegia. 1984;22:138–44.

29. Wyndaele JJ. Correlation between clinical neurological data and urodynamic function in spinal cord injured patients. Spinal Cord. 1997;35:213–6.

30. Moslavac S, Dzidic I, Kejla Z. Neurogenic detrusor overactivity: comparison between complete an incomplete spinal cord injury patients. Neurourol Urodyn. 2008;27(6):504.

31. Blaivas JG, Sinha HP, Zayed AA, Labib KB. Detrusor-external sphincter dyssynergia. J Urol. 1981;125(4):542–4.
32. Rudy DC, Awad SA, Downie JW. External sphincter dyssynergia: an abnormal continence reflex. J Urol. 1988;140(1):105–10.
33. Siroky MB, Krane RJ. Neurologic aspects of detrusor-sphincter dyssynergia, with reference to the guarding reflex. J Urol. 1982;127(5):953–7.
34. Kneist W, Wachter N, Paschold M, Kauff DW, Rink AD, Lang H. Midterm functional results of taTME with neuromapping for low rectal cancer. Tech Coloproctol. 2016;20:41–9.
35. Long Y, Yao DS, Pan XW, Ou TY. Clinical efficacy and safety of nerve-sparing radical hysterectomy for cervical cancer: a systematic review and meta-analysis. PLoS One. 2014;9(4): e94116.
36. Costa P, Perrouin-Verbe B, Colvez A, Didier J, Marquis P, Marrel A, Amarenco G, Espirac B, Leriche A. Quality of life in spinal cord injury patients with urinary difficulties. Development and validation of qualiveen. Eur Urol. 2001;39(1):107–13.
37. Forchheimer M, McAweeney M, Tate DG. Use of the SF-36 among persons with spinal cord injury. Am J Phys Med Rehabil. 2004;83(5):390–5.
38. Ku JH. Health-related qulaity of life in patients with spinal cord injury: review of the short form 36-health questionnaire survey. Yonsei Med J. 2007;48(3):360–70.
39. Shenot PJ, Rivas DA, Watanabe T, Chancellor MB. Early predictors of bladder recovery and urodynamics after spinal cord injury. Neurourol Urodyn. 1998;17:25–9.
40. Schurch B, Iacovelli V, Averbeck M, Stefano C, Altaweel W, Agro EF. Urodynamics in patients with spinal cord injury: a clinical review and best practice paper by a working group of the international continence society urodynamics committee. Neurourol Urodyn. 2018;37:581–91.
41. De EJB, Patel CY, Tharian B, Westney OL, Graves DE, Hairston J. Diagnostic discordance of electromyography (EMG) versus voiding cystourethrogram (VCUG) for detrusor-external sphincter dyssynergy (DESD). Neurourol Urodyn. 2005;24:616–21.
42. Radley SC, Rosario DJ, Chapple CR, Farkas AG. Conventional and ambulatory urodynamic findings in women with symptoms suggestive of bladder overactivity. J Urol. 2001;166(6):2253–8.
43. Pannek J, Pieper P. Clinical usefulness of ambulatory urodynamics in the diagnosis and treatment of lower urinary tract dysfunction. Scand J Urol Nephrol. 2008;42(5):428–32.
44. Van Waalwijk van Doorn ES, Remmers A, Janknegt RA. Extramural ambulatory urodynamic monitoring during natural filling and normal daily activities: evaluation of 100 patients. J Urol. 1991;146(1):124–31.
45. Martens FM, Van Kuppevelt HJ, Beekman JA, Heijnen IC, D'Hauwers KW, Heesakkers JP. No primary role of ambulatory urodynamics for the management of spinal cord injury patients compared to conventional urodynamics. Neurourol Urodyn. 2010;29(8):1380–6.
46. Salvatore S, Khullar V, Cardozo L, et al. Evaluating ambulatory urodynamics: a prospective study in asymptomatic women. BJOG. 2001;108(1):107–11.
47. Salvatore S, Khullar V, Anders K, Cardozo LD. Reducing artefacts in ambulatory urodynamics. Br J Urol. 1998;81(2):211–4.
48. Robertson AS. Behaviour of the human bladder during natural filling: the Newcastle experience of ambulatory monitoring and conventional artificial filling cystometry. Scand J Urol Nephrol Suppl. 1999;201:19–24.
49. Averbeck MA, Madersbacher H. Follow-up of the neuro-urological patient: a systematic review. BJU Int. 2015;115:S39–46.
50. Bruschini H, Almeida FG, Srougi M. Upper and lower urinary tract evaluation of 104 patients with myelomeningocele without adequate urological management. World J Urol. 2006;24:224–8.
51. McGuire EJ, Woodside JAAR, Borden TA, Weiss RM. Prognostic value of urodynamic testing in myelodysplastic patients. J Urol. 1981;126(2):205–9.
52. Jamil F, Williamson M, Ahmed YS, Harrison SC. Natural-fill urodynamics in chronically catheterized patients with spinal-cord injury. BJU Int. 1999;83(4):396–9.

53. Gerridzen RG, Thijssen AM, Dehoux E. Risk factors for upper tract deterioration in chronic spinal cord injury patients. J Urol. 1992;147:416–8.
54. Hackler RH. A 25-year prospective mortality study in the spinal injured patient: comparison with the long-term living paraplegic. J Urol. 1977;117:486–8.
55. Feifer A, Corcos J. Contemporary role of suprapubic cystostomy in treatment of neuropathic bladder dysfunction in spinal cord injured patients. Neurourol Urodyn. 2008;27:475–9.
56. Weld KJ, Dmochowski RR. Effect of bladder management on urological complications in spinal cord injured patients. J Urol. 2000b;163(3):768–72.
57. Wyndaele JJ, Madersbacher H, Kovindha A. Conservative treatment of the neuropathic bladder in spinal cord injured patients. Spinal Cord. 2001;39:294–300.
58. Chancellor MB, Anderson RU, Boone TB. Pharmacotherapy for neurogenic detrusor overactivity. Am J Phys Med Rehabil. 2006;85:536–45.
59. Amend B, Hennenlotter J, Schäfer T, Horstmann M, Stenzl A, Sievert KD. Effective treatment of neurogenic detrusor dysfunction by combined high-dosed antimuscarinics without increased side-effects. Eur Urol. 2008;53:1021–8.
60. Horstmann M, Schaefer T, Aguilar Y, Stenzl A, Sievert KD. Neurogenic bladder treatment by doubling the recommended antimuscarinic dosage. Neurourol Urodyn. 2006;25:441–5.
61. Wada N, Shimizu T, Takai S, Shimizu N, Tyagi P, Kakizaki H, Yoshimura N. Neurourol Urodyn. 2017;36:1039–45.
62. Wöllner J, Pannek J. Initial experience with the treatment of neurogenic detrusor overactivity with a new ß-3 agonist (mirabegron) in patients with spinal cord injury. Spinal Cord. 2016;54(1):78–82.
63. Ginsberg D, Gousse A, Keppenne V, Sievert KD, Thompson C, Lam W, Brin MF, Jenkins B, Haag-Molkenteller C. J Urol. 2012;187(6):2131–9.
64. Hohenfellner M, Pannek J, Böte U, Dahms S, Pfitzenmaier J, Fichtner J, Hutschenreiter G, Thüroff JW. Sacral bladder denervation for treatment of detrusor hyperreflexia and autonomic dysreflexia. Urology. 2001;58(1):28–32.
65. Mehta S, Hill D, McIntyre A, Foley N, Hsieh J, Ethans K, Reasell R, Loh E, Welk B, Wolfe D. Meta-analysis of botulinum toxin A detrusor injections in the treatment of neurogenic detrusor overactivity after spinal cord injury. Arch Phys Med Rehabil. 2013;94(8):1473–81.
66. Quek ML, Ginsberg DA. Long-term urodynamics follow-up of bladder augmentation for neurogenic bladder. J Urol. 2003;169:195–8.
67. Wöllner J, Krebs J, Pannek J. Sacral neuromodulation in patients with neurogenic lower urinary tract dysfunction. Spinal Cord. 2016;54(2):137–40.
68. Brindley GS. The first 500 patients with sacral anterior root stimulator implants: general description. Paraplegia. 1994;32(12):795–805.

Metabolic Problems: In Particular Diabetic Neuropathy

Apostolos Apostolidis

Epidemiology of Diabetes

The prevalence of diabetes mellitus (DM) is on the rise worldwide following the increase of the risk factors for the metabolic syndrome. The US epidemiological data constitute an obvious example of this new "epidemic." It has been estimated that about 1 of every 14 Americans has DM (7% of the population or 20.8 million people in 2005, estimates by the US Centers for Disease Control and Prevention; see review by [1]), with roughly 30% of them being undiagnosed. The prevalence is significantly higher among African-Americans—almost one of every seven—and among senior citizens ($\geq$65 years old): 21.8% of residents of nursing homes were found to suffer from DM in a multinational study conducted in eight countries (the Services and Health for Elderly in Long TERm care (SHELTER) project) [2]. The problem is becoming alarming, as the incidence of type 2 DM has increased by 33% in less than a decade (1990–1998), with warning signs among younger ages as the incidence increase reached 75% among those 30–39 years of age [1].

Diabetes and Lower Urinary Tract Dysfunction (LUTD)

Earlier literature [3, 4] suggests significant prevalence of LUTS in diabetic patients—up to 59%. The development of LUTD is even more prevalent among diabetics with peripheral neuropathy: 75–100% of those will develop LUTD [5]. For decades, "diabetic cystopathy," characterized by impaired bladder sensation, increased bladder capacity, infrequent urination, and impaired bladder emptying,

A. Apostolidis
2nd Department of Urology, Aristotle University of Thessaloniki, Thessaloniki, Greece

© Springer International Publishing AG, part of Springer Nature 2018
R. Dmochowski, J. Heesakkers (eds.), *Neuro-Urology*,
https://doi.org/10.1007/978-3-319-90997-4_7

has been considered as the most identifiable type of LUTD associated with DM; it has been estimated to occur in 43–87% of insulin-dependent diabetics, independent of sex or age [6], and in about 25% of patients on oral hypoglycemic agents [7]. Other studies, however, have produced very different epidemiological data. In a Scandinavian study of patients who have had diabetes for 10 years, the prevalence of diabetic cystopathy in those who were insulin-dependent was 2–4 per 1000 and in those on oral hypoglycemic agents was 1–3 per 1000. Nephropathy, by contrast, was much more frequently seen (30–40% of cases) [4]. Longer duration of diabetes and inadequate glycemic control have traditionally been associated with poorer voiding efficiency [5].

However, in the last two decades, urodynamic studies have drawn attention to a broad range of findings, supporting the notion that LUT dysfunctions in patients with DM comprise both storage and voiding problems. In a retrospective analysis of urodynamic traces from 182 diabetic patients, detrusor overactivity (DO) was the most common disorder (55%), while impaired contractility was found in 23% of cases, including 10% of asystolic patients [8]. In another study, evidence of diabetic cystopathy (increased volume at first desire to void, impaired detrusor contractility, and increased post-void residual) were combined with DO in 25% of cases [9]. In a urodynamic study of 84 diabetics, urinary urgency, DO, and increased bladder sensation were seen in 55%, 42%, and 14%, respectively, further to large post-void residuals and decreased sensation. However, the prevalence of DO was independent of the duration of diabetes [10]. Larger series [11] have identified a 40–80% risk of urgency incontinence and a 30–80% risk of overflow incontinence in diabetics. Finally, there are studies which found temporal associations between urodynamic findings and duration of diabetes: clinical and urodynamic evidence of "diabetic cystopathy" (impaired bladder sensation, detrusor underactivity, and impaired emptying) were more likely to characterize diabetics presenting relatively late with severe LUTS, while DO and urgency incontinence are more likely to be diagnosed in those seeking medical advice at earlier stages [12].

Diabetes and Urinary Incontinence

Several large prospective studies have identified associations between DM and incontinence: the Diabetes Control and Complications Trial (DCCT; 1983–1993) and its observational follow-up study, the Epidemiology of Diabetes Interventions and Complications study (EDIC; 1994-present) [13], the Diabetes and Aging Study, the NHANES [14], and the Services and Health for Elderly in Long TERm care (SHELTER) project [2]. In women, particularly, DM has been found to be a risk factor for incontinence together with prolapse and gynecological surgery [2, 15, 16], even after adjusting for age, body mass index, parity, and history of urinary tract infections [17]. Diabetes increases the risk for all types of UI: any UI (OR 1.99; 95% CI 1.44–2.74), urgency UI (OR 2.23; 95% CI 1.38–3.61), and stress UI (OR 1.54; CI 1.07–2.22) [17]. The Nurses' Health Study I and II conducted among women with type 2 DM showed that the longer the duration of diabetes, the more increased are the odds for prevalent UI [18]. Diabetes duration and treatment type as well as the presence of diabetic complications (peripheral neuropathy, retinopathy) were again identified as negative predictors of severe UI in another study, even after adjustment for multiple factors such as age, education, and history of UTI [19]. Further studies have confirmed that treatment type is associated with UI. Insulin-dependent diabetes as opposed to non-insulin-dependent diabetes increased the risk for UI in a study of women at least 50 years of age [20], while in another study in frail older diabetics, both insulin (OR 2.62, 95% CI 1.67–4.13) and oral therapy (OR 1.81, 95% CI 1.33–2.45) were associated with UI [21]. Finally, gestational DM has been found to be an independent risk factor for all types of UI (odds ratio 1.97 [1.56–2.51], 3.11 [2.18–4.43], and 2.73 [1.70–4.40] for stress, urgency, and mixed UI, respectively) and to be associated with more severe UI postpartum compared with women without gestational DM [22].

Glycemic Control and the Risk of UI: Is There a Potential in Long-Term Lifestyle and Therapeutic Interventions?

Several studies suggest that glycemic control may be associated with UI, but the literature may be controversial. In women with type 1 DM who participated in the DCCT and its observational follow-up study, the EDIC, the association of incident UI (weekly urinary incontinence present at EDIC year 17 but not at EDIC year 10) with comorbid prevalent conditions and glycemic control was investigated [13]. Results showed that incident UI was associated with higher HbA1c levels, independent of other recognized risk factors, suggesting the potential for women to modify their risk of UI with improved glycemic control [13]. Other studies have shown a variety of results. In a study of diabetic women, increases in HbA1c were associated with significant increases in the risk for any UI (13% increased odds for each one-unit increase of HbA1c) and for stress UI (34% increased odds, respectively), but not for urgency UI or mixed UI [14]. In another study, however, higher HbA1c levels were found to be associated with the presence of OAB (odds ratio 1.24, 95% confidence interval 1.06–1.45), urgency UI (odds ratio 1.20, 95% confidence interval 1.00–1.45), and nocturia (odds ratio 1.17) [23]. In a third study, women with type II DM had an increased prevalence of both stress and urgency UI compared to women with normal HbA1c (52.5% vs 38.6% and 40.3% vs 21.7%, respectively, each $p < 0.001$). Both glycemic control and insulin resistance were significantly associated with UI, but this was not reproduced in multivariate analysis after adjusting for patient body mass index [24]. Finally, there have been studies, including the Diabetes and Aging Study, which failed to show an association between UI and HbA1c levels [21, 25].

Large prospective studies, such as the Diabetes Prevention Program Outcomes Study and the Look AHEAD trial, have demonstrated a positive effect of long-term improvement of glycemic control on UI in both genders, suggesting a potential to such interventions. The former study randomized 1778 diabetic women to intensive lifestyle intervention, metformin therapy, or placebo and found a modest positive but lasting impact of intensive lifestyle intervention on UI [26]. In the latter trial, overweight/obese men with type 2 DM were randomly assigned to diabetes support and education [27]. After 1 year, intensive lifestyle intervention was superior to the other interventions as it reduced the prevalence of UI from 11.3% to 9.0% as opposed to an increase from 9.7% to 11.6% in the diabetes support and education group. Intensive lifestyle intervention group also doubled the chances for complete cure of UI (OR 1.93, 95% CI 1.04–3.59, $p = 0.04$ and 56.0% vs 40.7%, $p = 0.03$) compared to the diabetes support and education group [27].

Pathophysiology of Bladder Dysfunction in DM

Animal and human research has produced a wealth of findings over the years, and theories have developed to explain the pathophysiological basis of LUT dysfunction in diabetes. In bladder biopsies from patients with severe insulin-dependent diabetes, acetylcholinesterase (AChE) and S100 immunohistochemical expression were found to be significantly altered when compared to control specimens [28]. The decrease in AChE activity was attributed to axonal degeneration, while the increase in S100 immunostaining was thought to be due to Schwann cell proliferation as a regeneration attempt after demyelination or axonal degeneration. The authors proposed that the combination of decreased AChE activity with S100 increase was highly suggestive of diabetic cystopathy, which might respond to early symptomatic treatment.

Altered NGF activity in patients with DM and poor glycemic control may also contribute to the development of diabetic bladder dysfunction [29, 30].

Animal studies have proposed a range of mechanisms to explain bladder dysfunction in diabetes. A recent study using a rat model of streptozotocin-induced type I diabetes showed enhancement of the TRPA1-dependent mechanism involved in detrusor contractility in diabetic rats. This is thought to be due to the general inflammatory reaction caused by diabetes and may be part of a cascade that leads to an increase in cyclooxygenase-2-dependent prostaglandin synthesis, enhanced functional coupling between the tachykinin and prostanoid systems, and the concomitant increase of their impact on detrusor contractility in response to TRPA1 activation [31]. Other researchers proposed that alterations in the number and function of interstitial cells in the detrusor muscle (ICs-DM) may contribute to detrusor contractility dysfunction in later phase diabetic bladders [32]. ICs were found to play a role as mediators of muscarinic receptor-induced phasic contractions in diabetic rat bladders [33]. Further research showed that loss of caveolae and caveolin-3 together with a decrease in hyperpolarization-activated cyclic nucleotide-gated (HCN) channels in ICs-DM may play a role in the development of weak detrusor contractility in diabetic cystopathy [34].

A temporal theory has been proposed to explain the functional changes of the bladder in diabetes as well as the mixed clinical and urodynamic findings [1]. According to this, early and late myogenic and neurogenic alterations signify diabetic bladder dysfunction. Early-stage changes may be attributed to the hyperglycemia-induced osmotic polyuria which leads to compensatory bladder hypertrophy and increased detrusor contractility, while late-stage changes were proposed to be due to the accumulation of oxidative stress products resulting from prolonged hyperglycemia, which lead to decompensation of bladder function. A key factor proposed to stimulate the oxidative stress in diabetes is the increased mitochondrial production of reactive oxygen species [35], which may be related to a wide range of pathways such as auto-oxidations of glucose, glycated proteins, stimulations of cytochrome P450-like activity, alterations of NADPH/NADP ratio by excess glucose going through the polyol pathway, increased production of superoxide dismutase, and increased production of lipid peroxidation [35, 36]. They may have neurotoxic effects which could explain the associations between diabetic cystopathy and peripheral neuropathy. Electrophysiological studies in type 2 diabetic women found reduced sensitivity of unmyelinated C-fiber afferents at the distal extremities in parallel with vesical C-fiber neuropathy; thus the authors proposed C-fiber dysfunction at the distal extremities to be an indicator of early-stage diabetic bladder dysfunction [37].

Several studies support the association between peripheral neuropathy and diabetic cystopathy. Twice as many patients with cystopathy compared to diabetic patients without cystopathy did not have bladder sensation during the ice water (25% vs. 12.5%, respectively) [38]. A study evaluating sympathetic skin response in correlation with cystometry found that patients without or with lower amplitude of sympathetic skin responses had increased residual urine and decreased detrusor contraction pressure compared to controls [9]. These changes could be noted as early as 1 year from the diagnosis of diabetes. The presence of peripheral neuropathy in diabetic patients was found to be a strong predictor of increased post-void residual urine [39], after exclusion of comorbidities.

Novel theories explore the role of circadian disorders and of diabetes as part of the metabolic syndrome (MetS) in diabetic LUT dysfunction [40]. Circadian disorders have been associated with impaired glucose tolerance in nondiabetics and poor glycemic control in patients with DM. In addition, glycosuria is the main cause of nocturnal polyuria in diabetic patients via an increase in solute diuresis. Several factors and disturbances such as insufficient sleep, periodic limb movement disorders during sleep, narcolepsy, insomnia, obstructive sleep apnea syndrome, shift work, and nocturia may contribute to sleep disorders. However, multiple pathophysiological mechanisms, such as changes in food intake and physical activity, levels of leptin and ghrelin, inflammation, oxidative stress, and increased sympathetic activity, seem to connect these factors also to metabolic disorders such as obesity, DM, and hypertension. Moreover, there are known associations between sleep deficiencies and LUTS. Thus, associations between sleep disorders, urine production, and bladder dysfunction may be the basis for the explanation of the relationship between metabolic disorders and LUTS, but this needs to be further researched.

Another possible pathway linking diabetes to LUTS is via the development of low testosterone levels or late-onset hypogonadism, which is also associated with LUTS. Intervention with hormone replacement therapy (the HIM study) may correct hypogonadism and decrease the odds for "prostate disease" [41]. Also, in diabetic hypogonadal men, long-term testosterone therapy improved risk factors of the MetS [42] but with unknown effect on LUTS. Importantly, the Osteoporotic Fractures in Men study demonstrated that physical activity can normalize steroid hormone and insulin levels, also resulting in reduced risk for LUTS in older men [43].

Finally, an impressively high prevalence of multiple cerebral infarctions was seen in diabetic patients with DO in a brain MRI study (76.5%), suggesting that, further to peripheral, central pathophysiological mechanisms may be involved in the generation of urinary urgency in diabetic cystopathy [1].

Clinical and Urodynamic Manifestations of LUTD in DM

The clinical manifestations of diabetic cystopathy, as mentioned above, include reduced sensation of bladder fullness, decreased frequency of voiding, weak urinary stream, and difficulty in voiding due to impaired detrusor contraction. Impaired bladder emptying is also common in diabetic cystopathy and is thought to be related to the development of urinary tract infections (UTIs). Moreover, poor glycemic control seems to be associated with increased frequency of UTI. In women with type 1 DM, an increase by 1% in HbA1c level results in a 21% increase in the incidence of UTI [44].

However, a combination of storage and voiding LUTS may also be common in diabetic patients. Several controlled and cross-sectional surveys to date confirm that OAB symptoms are significantly more prevalent (24.2–28%) and severe in diabetics compared to the general population [23, 45, 46]. The presence of diabetic peripheral neuropathy [45, 47] and the duration of diabetes [46] showed significant correlations with the risk for development of OAB and with higher OAB-q scores. Urodynamic studies confirm the basis for such symptoms: in a series of female diabetics, urodynamic traces demonstrated increased bladder sensation, followed by DO [48]. Interestingly, patients with OAB were more likely to also have impaired voiding function.

The temporal theory of pathophysiological changes could apply to explain mixed LUT dysfunction, with clinical evidence provided by a study of 181 women with type 2 DM, which showed a time-dependent progression trend in the development of bladder dysfunction: earlier findings included stress incontinence (in women suffering from DM for 6.8 ± 2.8 years) followed by DO and/or increased bladder sensation (7.3 ± 6.5 years duration of DM), while impaired voiding function was seen in the more advanced stages (10.4 ± 8.3 years of DM duration) [49]. Urodynamic studies have demonstrated negative associations of both DM duration and HbA_{1c} level with parameters related to detrusor contractility (Q_{max}, $P_{det}@Q_{max}$, and bladder contractility index—BCI) [50]. All three parameters were lower in the DM group compared to controls. Poor glycemic control appears to be associated with increased odds of larger PVR ($\geq$100 mL) [10, 51].

Controlled studies showed different urodynamic characteristics of DO between diabetics and age-matched controls; the amplitude and volume of first overactive contraction, as well as Pdetmax, were greater in diabetics compared with controls (16.00 cmH$_2$O vs. 9.00 cmH$_2$O, 309.00 mL vs. 167.00 mL, and 76.48 cmH$_2$O vs. 55.41 cmH$_2$O, respectively) [10, 52].

Management of LUTD in Diabetics: Does Diabetes Affect the Outcome of LUTS Treatment?

There are no specific recommendations concerning the treatment of LUTD in patients with diabetic LUT dysfunction. The International Consultation on Incontinence proposes that general rules as for the other bladder conditions with impaired detrusor contractility should be followed [5]. More specifically, the Neurogenic Committee recommends, albeit with low grades of recommendation (mostly C):

- The measurement of post-void residual and check for UTIs by urine dipstick with the optional use of urine culture in diabetic patients on a yearly basis
- Prompted voiding in cases of increased post-void residual
- The use of intermittent catheterizations in cases of acontractile bladder

An important query is whether the presence of DM constitutes a negative factor for the success of various treatments for LUTS/UI. Most available studies to date suggest a negative effect of diabetes on the outcomes of LUTS treatment. Lower cure rates have been reported for mid-urethral sling procedures in diabetic women suffering from stress UI [53], as well as for OAB symptoms after treatment with antimuscarinics [54]. Also, diabetic patients treated with intravesical botulinum toxin A injection for intractable OAB symptoms were found to be at increased risk of large PVR urine volumes and general weakness compared to nondiabetic age-matched controls, despite similar efficacy at 6 months [55]. Nevertheless, diabetic patients seem to suffer more bothersome OAB symptoms and present higher persistence and adherence rates to OAB medication compared to non-DM patients [56]. By contrast, when using sacral neuromodulation to treat LUTD in diabetics, long-term success rates were found to be similar as in nondiabetic patients [57].

Conclusions

Diabetic bladder dysfunction, either in its most traditionally identifiable form, that of diabetic cystopathy, or in the form of a mixed LUTS syndrome, is highly prevalent among diabetic patients. A wealth of epidemiological evidence confirms strong associations between diabetes and urinary incontinence, particularly in insulin-dependent diabetes mellitus, while mounting data show increased prevalence and severity of OAB in diabetes. Poor glycemic control and/or longer duration of diabetes, as well as the presence of peripheral neuropathy, seem to be the strongest negative predictors for the development of diabetic bladder dysfunction, as proven by urodynamic, epidemiological, and pathophysiological studies. Animal and human research confirms neurogenic and myogenic alterations associated with diabetic bladder dysfunction, and several pathogenetic mechanisms have been proposed, including mitochondrial dysfunction, circadian changes, interstitial cell dysfunction, and hormonal deficiencies.

Poor glycemic control seems to be associated with damaging effects on the contractile properties of the detrusor and a higher risk of increased post-void residual and of urinary tract infections. There is, however, mounting evidence from long-term studies that intensive lifestyle intervention can have a positive impact on LUTS/urinary incontinence in diabetics further to the improvement of glycemic control. A strong recommendation, thus, has been given by the ICI to consult patients with diabetes about the positive effect and consequent need for lifestyle intervention and good glycemic control on LUTS. Further to such interventions, there are no currently specific recommendations as to the treatment diabetic bladder dysfunction. However, single studies suggest that the presence of diabetes may negatively affect the outcomes of surgical treatment for stress UI and pharmacotherapy/BOTOX for OAB, thus bearing further warning when consulting patients pretreatment. Further research is required to more specifically explore the effect of type I vs. type II diabetes as well as gender effects on bladder function and the management of urinary tract infections and to provide results of pharmacotherapy and minimally invasive and more invasive surgery on the therapeutic outcomes of LUTS/UI in diabetics.

References

1. Daneshgari F, Liu G, Birder L, Hanna-Mitchell AT, Chacko S. Diabetic bladder dysfunction: current translational knowledge. J Urol. 2009;182(6 Suppl):S18–26.
2. Szczerbinska K, Topinkova E, Brzyski P, van der Roest HG, Richter T, Finne-Soveri H, et al. The characteristics of diabetic residents in European nursing homes: results from the SHELTER study. J Am Med Dir Assoc. 2015;16(4):334–40.
3. Ellenberg M. Development of urinary bladder dysfunction in diabetes mellitus. Ann Intern Med. 1980;92(2 Pt 2):321–3.
4. Frimodt-Moller C. Diabetic cystopathy: epidemiology and related disorders. Ann Intern Med. 1980;92(2 Pt 2):318–21.
5. Drake M, Apostolidis A, Emmanuel A, Gazewski J, Harrison S, Heesakkers J, et al. Neurologic urinary and faecal incontinence. In: Abrams P, Cardozo L, Khoury S, Wein AJ, editors. Incontinence. 5th ed. Paris: ICUD-EAU 2013; 2013. p. 827–1000.
6. Hampel C, Gillitzer R, Pahernik S, Melchior S, Thuroff JW. Diabetes mellitus and bladder function. What should be considered? Urologe A. 2003;42(12):1556–63.
7. Bradley WE. Diagnosis of urinary bladder dysfunction in diabetes mellitus. Ann Intern Med. 1980;92(2 Pt 2):323–6.
8. Kaplan SA, Te AE, Blaivas JG. Urodynamic findings in patients with diabetic cystopathy. J Urol. 1995;153:342–4.

9. Ueda T, Yoshimura N, Yoshida O. Diabetic cystopathy: relationship to autonomic neuropathy detected by sympathetic skin response. J Urol. 1997;157(2):580–4.

10. Yamaguchi C, Sakakibara R, Uchiyama T, Yamamoto T, Ito T, Liu Z, et al. Overactive bladder in diabetes: a peripheral or central mechanism? Neurourol Urodyn. 2007;26(6):807–13.

11. Brown JS, Nyberg LM, Kusek JW, Burgio KL, Diokno AC, Foldspang A, et al. Proceedings of the national institute of diabetes and digestive and kidney diseases international symposium on epidemiologic issues in urinary incontinence in women. Am J Obstet Gynecol. 2003;188(6):S77–88.

12. Bansal R, Agarwal MM, Modi M, Mandal AK, Singh SK. Urodynamic profile of diabetic patients with lower urinary tract symptoms: association of diabetic cystopathy with autonomic and peripheral neuropathy. Urology. 2011;77(3):699–705.

13. Lenherr SM, Clemens JQ, Braffett BH, Dunn RL, Cleary PA, Kim C, et al. Glycaemic control and risk of incident urinary incontinence in women with type 1 diabetes: results from the diabetes control and complications trial and epidemiology of diabetes interventions and complications study (DCCT/EDIC). Diabet Med. 2016;33(11):1528–35.

14. Wang R, Lefevre R, Hacker MR, Golen TH. Diabetes, glycemic control, and urinary incontinence in women. Female Pelvic Med Reconstr Surg. 2015;21(5):293–7.

15. Saadia Z. Urinary problems amongst gynecological consultations. Association between prolapse, gynecological surgery and diabetes. Med Arch. 2015;69(5):315–8.

16. Karter AJ, Laiteerapong N, Chin MH, Moffet HH, Parker MM, Sudore R, et al. Ethnic differences in geriatric conditions and diabetes complications among older, insured adults with diabetes: the diabetes and aging study. J Aging Health. 2015;27(5):894–918.

17. Bani-Issa W, Almomani F, Eldeirawi K. Urinary incontinence among adult women with diabetes in Jordan: epidemiology, correlates and perceived impact on emotional and social Wellbeing. J Clin Nurs. 2014;23(17–18):2451–60.

18. Devore EE, Townsend MK, Resnick NM, Grodstein F. The epidemiology of urinary incontinence in women with type 2 diabetes. J Urol. 2012;188(5):1816–21.

19. Jackson SL, Scholes D, Boyko EJ, Abraham L, Fihn SD. Urinary incontinence and diabetes in postmenopausal women. Diabetes Care. 2005;28(7):1730–8.

20. Lewis CM, Schrader R, Many A, Mackay M, Rogers RG. Diabetes and urinary incontinence in 50- to 90-year-old women: a cross-sectional population-based study. Am J Obstet Gynecol. 2005;193(6):2154–8.

21. Hsu A, Conell-Price J, Stijacic Cenzer I, Eng C, Huang AJ, Rice-Trumble K, et al. Predictors of urinary incontinence in community-dwelling frail older adults with diabetes mellitus in a cross-sectional study. BMC Geriatr. 2014;14:137.

22. Chuang CM, Lin IF, Horng HC, Hsiao YH, Shyu IL, Chou P. The impact of gestational diabetes mellitus on postpartum urinary incontinence: a longitudinal cohort study on singleton pregnancies. BJOG. 2012;119(11):1334–43.

23. Chiu AF, Huang MH, Wang CC, Kuo HC. Higher glycosylated hemoglobin levels increase the risk of overactive bladder syndrome in patients with type 2 diabetes mellitus. Int J Urol. 2012;19(11):995–1001.

24. Weinberg AE, Leppert JT, Elliott CS. Biochemical measures of diabetes are not independent predictors of urinary incontinence in women. J Urol. 2015;194(6):1668–74.

25. Lee SJ, Karter AJ, Thai JN, Van Den Eeden SK, Huang ES. Glycemic control and urinary incontinence in women with diabetes mellitus. J Womens Health (Larchmt). 2013;22(12):1049–55.

26. Phelan S, Kanaya AM, Ma Y, Vittinghoff E, Barrett-Connor E, Wing R, et al. Long-term prevalence and predictors of urinary incontinence among women in the diabetes prevention program outcomes study. Int J Urol. 2015;22(2):206–12.

27. Breyer BN, Phelan S, Hogan PE, Rosen RC, Kitabchi AE, Wing RR, et al. Intensive lifestyle intervention reduces urinary incontinence in overweight/obese men with type 2 diabetes: results from the look AHEAD trial. J Urol. 2014;192(1):144–9.

28. Van Poppel H, Stessens R, Van Damme B, Carton H, Baert L. Diabetic cystopathy: neuropathological examination of urinary bladder biopsies. Eur Urol. 1988;15(1–2):128–31.

29. Pittenger G, Vinik A. Nerve growth factor and diabetic neuropathy. Exp Diabesity Res. 2003;4(4):271–85.
30. Cheng JT, Tong YC. Alterations of nerve-growth factor and p75(NTR) expressions in urinary bladder of fructose-fed obese rats. Neurosci Lett. 2008;441(1):25–8.
31. Philyppov IB, Paduraru ON, Gulak KL, Skryma R, Prevarskaya N, Shuba YM. TRPA1-dependent regulation of bladder detrusor smooth muscle contractility in normal and type I diabetic rats. J Smooth Muscle Res. 2016;52:1–17.
32. Chen W, Jiang C, Jin X, Shen W, Song B, Li L. Roles of stem cell factor on loss of interstitial cells of Cajal in bladder of diabetic rats. Urology. 2011;78(6):1443.e1–6.
33. Vahabi B, McKay NG, Lawson K, Sellers DJ. The role of c-kit-positive interstitial cells in mediating phasic contractions of bladder strips from streptozotocin-induced diabetic rats. BJU Int. 2011;107(9):1480–7.
34. Dong X, Song Q, Zhu J, Zhao J, Liu Q, Zhang T, et al. Interaction of Caveolin-3 and HCN is involved in the pathogenesis of diabetic cystopathy. Sci Rep. 2016;6:24844.
35. Brownlee M. The pathobiology of diabetic complications: a unifying mechanism. Diabetes. 2005;54(6):1615–25.
36. Rolo AP, Palmeira CM. Diabetes and mitochondrial function: role of hyperglycemia and oxidative stress. Toxicol Appl Pharmacol. 2006;212(2):167–78.
37. Lee WC, Wu HC, Huang KH, Wu HP, Yu HJ, Wu CC. Hyposensitivity of C-fiber afferents at the distal extremities as an indicator of early stages diabetic bladder dysfunction in type 2 diabetic women. PLoS One. 2014;9(1):e86463.
38. Ishigooka M, Hashimoto T, Hayami S, Suzuki Y, Ichiyanagi O, Nakada T. Thermoreceptor mediated bladder sensation in patients with diabetic cystopathy. Int Urol Nephrol. 1997;29(5):551–5.
39. Beylot M, Marion D, Noel G. Ultrasonographic determination of residual urine in diabetic subjects: relationship to neuropathy and urinary tract infection. Diabetes Care. 1982;5(5):501–5.
40. Denys MA, Anding R, Tubaro A, Abrams P, Everaert K. Lower urinary tract symptoms and metabolic disorders: ICI-RS 2014. Neurourol Urodyn. 2016;35(2):278–82.
41. Mulligan T, Frick MF, Zuraw QC, Stemhagen A, McWhirter C. Prevalence of hypogonadism in males aged at least 45 years: the HIM study. Int J Clin Pract. 2006;60(7):762–9.
42. Haider A, Yassin A, Doros G, Saad F. Effects of long-term testosterone therapy on patients with "diabesity": results of observational studies of pooled analyses in obese hypogonadal men with type 2 diabetes. Int J Endocrinol. 2014;2014:683515.
43. Parsons JK, Messer K, White M, Barrett-Connor E, Bauer DC, Marshall LM. Obesity increases and physical activity decreases lower urinary tract symptom risk in older men: the osteoporotic fractures in men study. Eur Urol. 2011;60(6):1173–80.
44. Lenherr SM, Clemens JQ, Braffett BH, Cleary PA, Dunn RL, Hotaling JM, et al. Glycemic control and urinary tract infections in women with type 1 diabetes: results from the DCCT/EDIC. J Urol. 2016;196(4):1129–35.
45. Ikeda M, Nozawa K. Prevalence of overactive bladder and its related factors in Japanese patients with diabetes mellitus. Endocr J. 2015;62(9):847–54.
46. Palleschi G, Pastore AL, Maggioni C, Fuschi A, Pacini L, Petrozza V, et al. Overactive bladder in diabetes mellitus patients: a questionnaire-based observational investigation. World J Urol. 2014;32(4):1021–5.
47. Karoli R, Bhat S, Fatima J, Priya S. A study of bladder dysfunction in women with type 2 diabetes mellitus. Indian J Endocrinol Metab. 2014;18(4):552–7.
48. Ho CH, Tai HC, Yu HJ. Urodynamic findings in female diabetic patients with and without overactive bladder symptoms. Neurourol Urodyn. 2010;29(3):424–7.
49. Lin TL, Chen GD, Chen YC, Huang CN, Ng SC. Aging and recurrent urinary tract infections are associated with bladder dysfunction in type 2 diabetes. Taiwan J Obstet Gynecol. 2012;51(3):381–6.

50. Shin YS, On JW, Kim MK. Clinical significance of diabetes mellitus on detrusor functionality on stress urinary incontinent women without bladder outlet obstruction. Int Urogynecol J. 2016;27(10):1557–61.
51. Appa AA, Brown JS, Creasman J, Van Den Eeden SK, Subak LL, Thom DH, et al. Clinical predictors and significance of postvoid residual volume in women with diabetes. Diabetes Res Clin Pract. 2013;101(2):164–9.
52. Golabek T, Kiely E, O'Reilly B. Detrusor overactivity in diabetic and non-diabetic patients: is there a difference? Int Braz J Urol. 2012;38(5):652–9. discussion 60
53. Bohlin KS, Ankardal M, Pedroletti C, Lindkvist H, Milsom I. The influence of the modifiable life-style factors body mass index and smoking on the outcome of mid-urethral sling procedures for female urinary incontinence. Int Urogynecol J. 2015;26(3):343–51.
54. Schneider T, Marschall-Kehrel D, Hanisch JU, Michel MC. Does concomitant diabetes affect treatment responses in overactive bladder patients? Int J Clin Pract. 2013;67(11):1138–43.
55. Wang CC, Liao CH, Kuo HC. Diabetes mellitus does not affect the efficacy and safety of intravesical onabotulinumtoxinA injection in patients with refractory detrusor overactivity. Neurourol Urodyn. 2014;33(8):1235–9.
56. Liao CH, Wang CC, Jiang YH. Intravesical OnabotulinumtoxinA injection for overactive bladder patients with frailty, medical comorbidities or prior lower urinary tract surgery. Toxins (Basel). 2016;8(4):91.
57. Daniels DH, Powell CR, Braasch MR, Kreder KJ. Sacral neuromodulation in diabetic patients: success and complications in the treatment of voiding dysfunction. Neurourol Urodyn. 2010;29(4):578–81.

Clinical Entities and Their Neuro-urological Consequences: Infections

Mikolaj Przydacz and Jacques Corcos

Introduction

Neurogenic bladder (NB) or neurogenic lower urinary tract dysfunction of the urinary bladder and urethra, due to central and/or peripheral nervous system diseases, is one of the most challenging problems in urology. Various disorders affecting the nervous system may cause chronic bladder dysfunction, which type depends on central or peripheral nervous system damage level and intensity. Infections of the nervous system pose a unique challenge to physicians, due to both the potential morbidity and mortality that they cause and the inherent difficulties involved in patients' treatment, recovery, and future quality of life. Neurological infections can significantly affect bladder functions. However, heterogeneity of pathophysiology leads to different clinical presentations and treatment options. Moreover, a part of NB-related pathogens has predisposition to patients with immune deficiencies, thus the management should be usually provided by strong concerted efforts of different specialists.

In this chapter, we will focus on the pathophysiology, epidemiology, symptom presentation, urodynamic findings, and treatment of the urological sequelae following neurological infections.

Pathophysiology

Infections of the nervous system leading to NB involve peripheral and/or central nervous system resulting in peripheral neuropathy, central neuropathy, or both of them simultaneously. A wide variety of pathogens, including bacteria, viruses, fungus, or prions, may affect the nervous system.

M. Przydacz (✉) · J. Corcos
Mcgill University, Montreal, QC, Canada
e-mail: jcorcos@uro.jgh.mcgill.ca

© Springer International Publishing AG, part of Springer Nature 2018
R. Dmochowski, J. Heesakkers (eds.), *Neuro-Urology*,
https://doi.org/10.1007/978-3-319-90997-4_8

Peripheral Neuropathies

Peripheral neuropathy is a rare but significant cause of storage and voiding dysfunction. The infection mechanism involves autoimmune reaction to peripheral nerves and/or roots or spreading of the infection from cutaneous nerve endings to the corresponding dorsal root ganglia. The neuropathy affecting the bladder often takes the form of an autonomic neuropathy, which may involve both the sympathetic and the parasympathetic, as well as afferent and efferent innervation of the bladder and urethra, leading to alteration of bladder sensation, the sacral reflex arc, detrusor-sphincter synergy, and detrusor contractility [1]. The most common infection-related peripheral neuropathies that may lead to voiding dysfunctions are lumbosacral herpes zoster (varicella-zoster virus, VZV), genitourinary herpes simplex (herpes simplex virus, HSV), tabes dorsalis (*Treponema pallidum*), and Guillain-Barré syndrome (GBS).

VZV-related bladder dysfunction is thought to be a result of sensory neuropathy from inflammatory reaction in the dorsal nerve roots and ganglia, which spreads proximally and distally to the sacral segments of the cord, with interruption of the micturition reflex [2]. Further involvement of the sacral micturition center or even lumbar and thoracic segments is often seen and could predispose to symptom exacerbation [3, 4]. Moreover, virus particles and neurotropic factors have been identified in neurons and supporting satellite cells in the sensory ganglia and within the peripheral sensory nerves of the corresponding dermatomes [5].

Whereas HSV type 1 is known to infect about 95% of the human population, it rarely involves the genitals and bladder. Anogenital type 2 of HSV is a more common cause of neural bladder impairment. The pathogenesis of HSV-related voiding dysfunctions involves localized lumbosacral meningomyelitis with commitment of sacral nerve roots or infectious neuritis that affects the pelvic nerves [6].

Of note, both VZV and HSV are characterized by a feature called neurotropism (becoming dormant in the dorsal root ganglia after the initial infection). It was proven by demonstration of viral proteins and perineural/intraneural inflammation within the cutaneous nerve afferent to the infected ganglia [7]. These studies also presented that neurotropic factors may be transported between cutaneous nerve endings and the corresponding dorsal root ganglia, which explain the dermatomal distribution of neuralgia and dermatological symptoms.

Tabes dorsalis is a neurological presentation of syphilis, a sexually transmitted disease caused by the spirochete *Treponema pallidum*. The mechanism of micturition dysfunction includes demyelination, and it mainly occurs in advanced stages of the disease (tertiary syphilis) [1]. This demyelinating atrophy of the dorsal spinal cord affects the posterior column and can result in impaired bladder innervation.

GBS is commonly parainfectious. Two-thirds of people with GBS have experienced an infection before the onset of the condition, and it is usually considered as a gastroenteritis or a respiratory tract infection [8]. The pathophysiologic mechanism of GBS is an autoimmune destruction of myelin by antiganglioside antibodies.

Activated T cells, macrophages, and increased matrix metalloproteinases may also play a role [9]. The lumbosacral spinal roots and thoracolumbar sympathetic chain may be involved resulting in lower urinary tract dysfunction [10].

Central Neuropathies

Central neuropathy describes damage or injury to the central nervous system, which is composed of the brain, brain stem, and spinal cord. Infections of the central nervous system can result in acute or chronic bladder dysfunctions. The most important infection-related central neuropathies predisposing to NB are progressive multifocal leukoencephalopathy (JC virus, JCV), tropical spastic paraparesis (human T-cell lymphotropic virus type 1, HTLV-1), poliomyelitis (poliovirus, PV), and transverse myelitis.

Progressive multifocal leukoencephalopathy is an infectious demyelinating brain disease (with a special predisposition to oligodendrocytes) caused by the JCV and associated with significant morbidity and mortality in the immunocompromised host [11]. Following asymptomatic primary infection, the virus becomes latent in bone marrow, spleen, tonsils, and other tissues. Periodically, the virus reactivates, and then it can be demonstrated in circulating peripheral lymphocytes. In cases of impaired immunity, it strongly affects brain functions. The role of other polyomaviruses, especially BK virus, in pathophysiology of progressive multifocal leukoencephalopathy is still unclear [12].

Tropical spastic paraparesis is a condition associated with and probably caused by the retrovirus HTLV-1 with special affinity for CD4 T cells [13, 14]. More importantly, meningomyelitis with demyelination and axonal loss (particularly focused on the corticospinal tracts) is usually present. These findings are most prominent in lower thoracic and upper lumbar regions [15]. In rare cases, peripheral nerves may be involved as well [16].

Poliomyelitis, often called polio or infantile paralysis, is an infectious disease caused by the PV. The mechanisms by which PV spreads to the central nervous system and provokes a local inflammatory response are poorly understood [17]. PV propagates along certain nerve fiber pathways, preferentially replicating in and destroying motor neurons within the spinal cord, brain stem, or motor cortex.

Transverse myelitis, similarly to GBS, is a clinical parainfectious syndrome, where an immune-mediated process causes a neural injury to the spinal cord. Thus, its etiology can be viral, bacterial, parasitic, tuberculosis, or idiopathic [11]. Of note, transverse myelitis may exist as a part of a multifocal disease of the central nervous system (e.g., multiple sclerosis), multisystemic disease (e.g., systemic lupus erythematosus), or as an isolated, idiopathic entity. Both gray and white matter of spinal cord are involved. Despite the fact that the central nervous system is mainly affected, peripheral part may be involved in some cases as well.

Central and Peripheral Neuropathies

Multisystemic disorders affect both central and peripheral parts of the nervous system. Among them, human immunodeficiency virus/acquired immune deficiency syndrome (HIV/AIDS) and Lyme disease should be taken into special consideration.

AIDS is a spectrum of conditions caused by infection with the HIV. The main mechanism of action includes depletion of CD4 T cells which results in strong weakness of the immune system. Impaired micturition becomes more common with disease progression and can occur as a part of a global neurologic dysfunction (mainly demyelination) or due to other opportunistic infections within nervous system (usually caused by HTLV-1, HSV, cytomegalovirus, toxoplasmosis) [18]. Moreover, in some cases, voiding dysfunctions can occur as a result of spinal cord compression by metastatic lymphoma or tuberculoma.

Lyme disease is an infectious disease caused by bacteria of the *Borrelia* type. Micturition disorders can occur because the spirochete directly invades the urinary bladder or more importantly they are related to neuroborreliosis, such as meningoencephalopathy, transverse myelitis, myeloradiculitis, and demyelinating lesions of the spinal cord [11].

Others

Tuberculosis represents different mechanism of NB pathophysiology. Mycobacterium tuberculosis rarely affects bladder innervation; however, it can influence the bones and joints, in particular the vertebral column. The lower thoracic and upper lumbar vertebrae are the areas of the spine most often affected. Progressing necrosis can lead to vertebral collapse and spinal damage resulting in impaired bladder innervation.

Epidemiology

NB incidence and prevalence caused by neural infections are difficult to establish, as epidemiological reports are few and far between. They mainly include case reports or case series with a small number of patients. Moreover, existent data are sometimes limited to a single study. Until now, only AIDS-related voiding dysfunctions have been reliably estimated to affect 16–45% of patients with neurological complications of this disease [19]. Moreover, neurogenic voiding dysfunction in AIDS patients portends poor prognosis. Broseta et al. tried to estimate urological manifestation of VZV infection [20]. Although they concluded that up to one-quarter of VZV-infected patients with sacral presentation may suffer from NB, their analysis included only 57 cases. Chen et al. estimated the incidence of VZV-related neurogenic voiding dysfunctions as 4% in a group of 423 patients, which increased to almost 9% when excluding those with cranial nerve rather than spinal involvement [21]. Further analysis of lumbosacral dermatome-involved patients revealed voiding dysfunctions in almost 30% of these patients. Greenstein et al. investigated the prevalence of NB dysfunction in patients with anogenital HSV infection [22]. They concluded that this condition is rare and occurs in less than 1% of cases. Sakakibara et al. described urologic findings in 28 patients with GBS [23]. Voiding symptoms were seen in 25% of patients. Murphy et al. performed a cross-sectional analysis of HTLV-seropositive subjects who were detected from five blood donor centers in the United States [24]. Myelopathy was confirmed in 4 of 166 (2.4%) HTLV-1-positive subjects, and all 4 patients were found to have detrusor-sphincter dyssynergia. Howard et al. investigated urological symptoms in a group of 203 patients affected by poliomyelitis [25]. They reported an 11% prevalence of retention during the acute polio episode, whereas 34% of patients had chronic urinary symptoms persisting after resolution of the acute episode. In turn, Johnson et al. evaluated 330 completed questionnaires mailed randomly to subjects in West Texas with a history of polio and reported that up to 93% of patients notified different urological symptoms [26]. Acute transverse myelitis has an incidence of one to four new cases per million people per year affecting individuals of all ages with bimodal peaks between the ages of 10 and 19 years and 30 and 39 years [27, 28]. When the maximal level of deficit is reached, virtually all patients have bladder dysfunctions. The prevalence of neuroborreliosis has been investigated by numerous studies and established as 19–71% of *Borrelia*-infected patients [29, 30]. However, none of these studies conducted a subgroup analysis for patients presenting only with neurological voiding dysfunctions. Micturition disturbances related to neurosyphilis had a high prevalence in the prepenicillin era. Fortunately, improvements in medical care have made neurosyphilis a rare entity with urological sequelae even less prevalent. Similarly, backbone tuberculosis complicated by bladder dysfunctions is currently a rare finding. On the other hand, the use of more potent immunosuppression in transplantations (administration of natalizumab in particular) and the AIDS pandemic have coincided with a significant increase in the prevalence of JCV-related progressive multifocal leukoencephalopathy in the past few decades [31]. Thus, a great deal of interest has been stimulated in this previously obscure viral demyelinating disease.

The main factors that can increase the risk of NB development in neural infections include immune deficiency, malnutrition, diabetes, older age, and previous transplantation surgery with immunosuppressive therapy [1, 11, 32].

Clinical Presentation

Presented pathogens usually involve multiple organ systems and appear with constellations of their own signs and symptoms. To make things worse, symptoms may appear in different time intervals and in different order. Despite the involvement of the bladder innervation, presented infections may be accompanied by the following:

- Skin or mucous lesions (circumscribed painful vesicular eruption in VZV and HSV; infectious children dermatitis in HTLV-1; acrodermatitis chronica atrophicans, lymphadenosis benigna cutis, or erythema migrans in Lyme disease)
- Sensation disturbances (reduced or absent sensations in VZV and HSV; paresthesia of the hands and feet in GBS; diminished vibration sense in HTLV-1; numbness, paresthesias, or band-like dysesthesias in transverse myelitis; tingling or numbness in the extremities or facial palsy (paralysis) in Lyme disease)
- Visual impairment (uveitis or cerebellar type dysfunction of eye movements in HTLV-1; visual changes in JCV and Lyme disease)
- Musculoskeletal disorders (arthritis, polymyositis, and muscle weakness in HTLV-1; muscle weakness in PV; juvenile and adult arthritis in Lyme disease)
- Gastrointestinal disorders (nausea, vomiting, abdominal pain, constipation, or diarrhea in PV)
- Cardiac involvement (carditis and arrhythmias in Lyme disease)
- Respiratory tract infections (sore throat and fever in PV and Lyme disease)
- General symptoms (symmetric ascending weakness of the limbs and gait disorders in GBS; progressive weakness with speech and personality changes in JCV; cerebellar syndrome with ataxia/gait disturbance and intention tremor in HTLV-1; inability to move with spastic paralysis and seizures in PV; weakness in transverse myelitis; severe fatigue with a stiff, aching neck and headaches sometimes accompanied by cognitive, mental disorders in Lyme disease)
- Autonomic neuropathy (labile blood pressure and cardiac arrhythmias in GBS; bowel incontinence or constipation in transverse myelitis)
- Other disorders (adult T-cell leukemia/lymphoma in HTLV-1)

Micturition dysfunction can appear as an initial symptom or as a later-stage symptom. Patients may report storage problems (frequency, urgency, nocturia, bladder pain, incontinence) or voiding difficulties (hesitancy, straining, poor and intermittent flow, incomplete emptying, post-micturition dribble, dysuria). Simultaneous occurrence of storage and emptying symptoms can also be detected. Presented urological symptoms depend on underlying urodynamic pathology: detrusor underactivity, detrusor overactivity, or sphincter abnormalities. Thus, patients usually present with retention or incontinence with frequency and urgency.

Retention

Urinary retention due to bladder underactivity or sphincter overactivity, usually with reduced or absent bladder sensations, is the most common finding in the infection-related neurogenic bladder dysfunctions. It afflicts 3.5% of patients with active herpes zoster infection and is most commonly seen in the infection of the sacral dorsal root ganglia (78%), followed by thoracolumbar (11%) and higher thoracic levels (11%) [20]. The urinary retention typically presents concurrently with or within a few days following the onset of the rash which occurred in a sacral dermatomal distribution, typically affecting one or more of adjacent S2, S3, or S4 areas [33]. The lesions can be either unilateral or bilateral. However, all urodynamic changes are reversible and usually resolve within 4–8 weeks. Similarly, urinary retention is the most common urological finding in patients with anogenital herpes infection. However, in view of special distribution of HSV type 2 rash in genital area, most cases of retention are due to severe dysuria caused by direct contact of urine with the blistering urethral mucosa. True neurogenic urinary retention in anogenital HSV infection is rare and occurs in less than 1% of infected patients [22]. In these cases, the onset of bladder dysfunction occurs typically 1–2 weeks after the onset of a vesicular and painful rash in the anogenital region. Similarly to herpes zoster, urodynamic findings are fully reversible, often within 4–8 weeks, but sometimes it may take months [34, 35]. Elevated post-void residual volume due to detrusor underactivity is also typical for neurosyphilis. However, in contrast to previous disorders, first symptoms of bladder impairment usually occur long time after primary infection, even up to 20 years after the primary bacterial invasion [1]. Bladder function often improves with time after treatment with penicillin but may not return entirely to normal [36]. Bladder dysfunction characterized by detrusor underactivity (rarely by detrusor-sphincter dyssynergia) and impaired sensation with large post-void residuals is seen in patients affected by GBS but improves gradually and simultaneously with patients' recovery [37, 38]. Similar clinical presentation and future prognosis are typical and characteristic for acute phase of poliomyelitis [39]. A variety of neurologic symptoms including acute urinary retention (mainly in mechanism of detrusor-sphincter dyssynergia) and sacral sensory loss may appear in HIV patients at the time of seroconversion [19, 40, 41]. In AIDS patients with neural involvement, bladder underactivity may appear in up to 45% of cases. Impaired micturition becomes more common with disease progression [18, 42]. Data on prevalence of retention in patients with transverse myelitis varies. Studies present conflicting results indicating this condition as a common or rare finding [43, 44]. Elevated post-void residual volume may also be seen in tropical spastic paraparesis (due to detrusor underactivity or high urethral activity), tabes dorsalis (due to detrusor-sphincter dyssynergia), or neuroborreliosis (due to underactive detrusor) [45, 46].

Incontinence

Incontinence, frequency, and urgency most commonly appear as a result of neurogenic detrusor overactivity. Overactive detrusor is the most typical urodynamic finding in HTLV-1-associated myelopathy with tropical spastic paraparesis (up to 70% of patients) [47–49]. Nevertheless, detrusor-sphincter dyssynergia with elevated post-void residual volume is either a common finding [46]. Thus, both storage (detrusor overactivity) and voiding (detrusor-sphincter dyssynergia) symptoms usually coexist in patients with HTLV-1 associated myelopathy. Storage symptoms may be reported by up to 75% of patients, with the greatest prevalence of increased daytime frequency, urgency, nocturia, and urge urinary incontinence. On the other hand, 40% of the patients may report voiding symptoms: slow stream, feeling of incomplete emptying, or intermittent stream. Urological symptoms in the HTLV-1-infected individuals usually begin simultaneously with progressive paraparesis and back pain. In some cases, urological symptoms can persist and progress with a tendency for urinary dysfunction to become worse as the primary disease progresses [50]. Similarly, combination of storage and voiding symptoms is typical for patients with transverse myelitis, and residual bladder dysfunction usually has a tendency to persist for a long time [51]. However, no consensus exists whether detrusor overactivity or detrusor-sphincter dyssynergia occurs more often [52, 53]. Whereas acute phase of poliomyelitis is usually characterized by retention, patients affected by post-polio syndrome (progressive functional deterioration occurring years after an acute episode of poliomyelitis) often suffer from detrusor overactivity [26]. Urodynamic evaluation of patients with neuroborreliosis usually reveals neurogenic detrusor overactivity. Neurologic and urological symptoms in patients with Lyme disease are slow to resolve, and convalescence is usually protracted [54, 55]. Detrusor overactivity may also occur in tabes dorsalis or HIV-infected patients [1, 41]. Advanced stages of AIDS disease may be demonstrated by detrusor overactivity in up to one-quarter of patients [19]. Overactive detrusor is a rare finding in GBS or in the acute phase of poliomyelitis [38, 39].

Until now, there is a lack of data for urodynamic presentation of progressive multifocal leukoencephalopathy.

Diagnosis

The diagnosis can be clinched from the history, symptoms (both urological and non-urological), and serologic tests (ELISA, immunoblot, PCR) which type depends on suspected pathology. Midstream urine usually should be collected to exclude bacterial infection, and appropriate investigations should be performed if any sexually transmitted diseases are suspected. To define the common diagnosis of neurogenic bladder, urodynamic study (UDS) or video UDS should be performed. The study of UDS is useful for establishing the bladder pattern and choosing the best therapeutic approach. This evaluation identifies the storage pressures, the residual volume, and voiding dysfunctions, which are important for the treatment planning. Underlying pathophysiology may enforce implementation of diagnostic imaging, usually computed tomography or magnetic resonance imaging. However, it should be noted that some of discussed pathogens might be difficult to identify, even with multiple diagnostic measures (e.g., progressive multifocal leukoencephalopathy, JCV infection). On the other hand, some of the presented disorders have established sets of diagnostic criteria, for instance, transverse myelitis [56]. These sets were proposed to avoid the confusion that inevitably results when investigators use differing criteria. They ensure a common language of classification and lay the groundwork necessary for multicenter clinical trials. Counseling with other specialists is often advised as non-urological symptoms may help in the final diagnosis. Physicians should also be aware about possible complications of NB as urological symptoms may be underestimated by patients or isolated for a long time. Thus, ultrasound, cystoscopy, or other medical imaging should be performed in cases suspected for hydronephrosis, vesicoureteral reflux, ureteral dilatation, kidney stones, or cancer. As a general comment, the best treatment often depends on a timely and accurate diagnosis. Because majority of presented disorders are relatively rare, delayed and incomplete work-up often occurs. Rapid and accurate diagnosis will ensure appropriate treatment. Future studies with establishment of diagnostic algorithms will likely lead to improved care, although it is recognized that the entire evaluation may not be performed for every patient.

Treatment

All discussed disorders should be appropriately treated accordingly to underlying pathology. That indicates the use of systemic antiviral, antibacterial, or antifungal drug therapy as it may help in partial or complete relief of urological symptoms [1, 11]. It should be conducted with relevant guidelines and in cooperation with other physicians representing specific fields of medicine as concomitant non-urological dysfunctions are common. Thus, additional opinion should be sought at the outset so that adequate management for non-urological symptoms can be instituted to prevent development of other complications. Of note, prophylactic and therapeutic interventions for some of presented diseases are limited by our current understanding of their pathogenesis. Clinical trials are limited by small numbers of patients affected with clinically significant disease, lack of defined risk factors and disease definitions, no proven effective treatment, and the overall significant morbidity and mortality associated with these diseases [57].

It is important to point out that NB dysfunction is an uncommon complication of nervous system infection. Thus, any patient, especially young who presents with unexplained bladder dysfunction, should be investigated for other neurologic pathologies, some of which include multiple sclerosis, lumbosacral disc prolapse, lumbar canal stenosis, spinal cord or brain tumors, other forms of sacral radiculo-myelitis, spina bifida occulta, primary bladder neck obstruction, Fowler's syndrome, or immunodeficiency disorders. Furthermore, hospitalization and patient monitoring may be required, in particular for patients with GBS. Monitoring of respiratory function and elective endotracheal intubation for impending respiratory failure may become necessary. With respect to autonomic neuropathy, cardiac monitoring or strict bowel regime may be necessary for arrhythmias or constipation.

Management of neurogenic bladder caused by a nervous system infection is a serious challenge due to lack of strong recommendations and well-proved evidence. Thus, conservative neurogenic bladder management guided by urodynamic evaluation is recommended. Appropriate bladder treatment will allow to avoid possible future complications of neurogenic bladder, in particular urinary tract infections and renal damage.

Management of urinary retention consists of simple analgesics and clean intermittent catheterization or the use of an indwelling catheter. Indwelling catheterization should be discontinued as early as reasonably possible. Depending on suspected underlying pathology, patients should be informed that the voiding dysfunction is transient, and full return to normal detrusor behavior is expected, or micturition disturbances may persist and evolve to a more fixed disorder.

Urinary incontinence due to detrusor overactivity should be managed by bladder retraining (e.g., prompted voiding for at least 6 weeks), optimized access to technical facilities (e.g., easy access to the toilet, use of handheld urinals, access to a call bell, easy to remove clothing), fluid restrictions, and pelvic floor muscle training. Clean intermittent or indwelling catheterization for those with additional detrusor-sphincter dyssynergia might be necessary to implement.

Physiotherapy for overactive bladder and urinary incontinence has been confirmed as a good option, rendering satisfactory results in patients with urinary symptoms of idiopathic or neurogenic origin through the use of behavioral therapy and kinesiotherapy. A recently published study proved that physiotherapy for neurogenic bladder in HTLV-1-infected patients improved clinical and urinary complaints, increased the strength of the perineal muscles, and improved patients' quality of life [58].

Drug treatment is usually necessary. However, there is no strong evidence of anticholinergic management in patients with neural infections. Lack of prospective or even retrospective studies with a large number of patients deteriorates management planning [59]. Moreover, numerous side effects of anticholinergics may limit their usefulness. Thus, anticholinergic drugs should be used according to general practice of treatment of neurogenic detrusor overactivity. Application of alpha-blockers in bladder dysfunctions due to nervous system infection has been reported by single cases [60]. Any superimposed urine infection should be treated, but prophylactic antibiotics are not necessary.

Evaluation of the usefulness of sacral nerve stimulation and botulinum toxin A injections in patients with infection-related NB has not been investigated. Chartier-Kastler et al. assessed clinical and urodynamic results of sacral nerve stimulation for patients with neurogenic (spinal cord diseases) urge incontinence and detrusor overactivity resistant to parasympatholytic medications [61]. However, only one of nine included patients was diagnosed with viral myelitis. Nevertheless, all patients had clinically significant improvement of incontinence. In view of these promising results, more research is warranted. Wosnitzer et al. reported the first case of GBS patient with persistent urinary retention successfully treated with sacral neuromodulation [62]. Immediately following neuromodulator placement, the patient voided spontaneously and has had no voiding dysfunction or post-void residual after 5 months of follow-up. Both sacral neuromodulation and botulinum toxin injections should be indicated when patients are refractory to conventional treatment.

Management with urinary diversion has been reported only by individual cases of Lyme disease or transverse myelitis with schistosomal myelopathy [44, 63].

Conclusion

Infections of the nervous system can significantly affect bladder function as a result of peripheral and/or central neuropathy. Due to a wide variety of possible pathogens, clinical presentation varies. Both urological and non-urological symptoms may appear. Retention is the most common bladder dysfunction, followed by urinary incontinence with frequency and urgency. Treatment should be implemented as soon as reasonably possible and tailored to underlying pathology. Strong concerted efforts of multiple specialists should aim to improve these patients' prognosis.

References

1. Tse V, Stone A. Other peripheral neuropathies (lumbosacral herpes zoster, genitourinary herpes, tabes dorsalis, Guillain–Barré syndrome). In: Corcos J, Ginsberg D, Karsenty G, editors. Textbook of the neurogenic bladder. 3rd ed. Boca Raton: CRC Press; 2016. p. 260–4.
2. Gibbon N. A case of herpes zoster with involvement of urinary bladder. Br J Urol. 1956;28:417–21.
3. Rankin JT, Sutton RA. Herpes zoster causing retention of urine. Br J Urol. 1969;41:238–41.
4. Kendall AR, Karafin L. Classification of neurogenic bladder disease. Urol Clin N Am. 1974;1:45.
5. Bastian FO, Rabson AS, Yee CL, Tralka TS. Herpesvirus varicellae: isolated from human dorsal root ganglia. Arch Pathol. 1974;97:331–3.
6. Yamanishi T, Yasuda K, Sakakibara R, et al. Urinary retention due to herpes virus infections. Neurourol Urodyn. 1998;17:613–9.
7. Worrell JT, Cockerell CJ. Histopathology of peripheral nerves in cutaneous herpes virus infection. Am J Dermatopathol. 1997;19:133–7.
8. van den Berg B, Walgaard C, Drenthen J, Fokke C, Jacobs BC, van Doorn PA. Guillain-Barré syndrome: pathogenesis, diagnosis, treatment and prognosis. Nat Rev Neurol. 2014;10(8):469–82.
9. Pascuzzi R, Fleck J. Acute peripheral neuropathy in adults. Neurol Clin. 1997;15(3):529–48.
10. Honavar M, Tharakan JKJ, Hughes RAC, et al. A clinicopathological study of the Guillain–Barré syndrome; nine cases and literature review. Brain. 1991;114:1245–69.
11. Hanus T. Other diseases (transverse myelitis, tropical spastic paraparesis, progressive multifocal leukoencephalopathy, Lyme's disease). In: Corcos J, Ginsberg D, Karsenty G, editors. Textbook of the neurogenic bladder. 3rd ed. Boca Raton: CRC Press; 2016. p. 260–4.
12. Bratt G, Hammarin AL, Grandien M, et al. BK virus as the cause of meningoencephalitis, retinitis and nephritis in a patient with AIDS. AIDS. 1999;13(9):1071–5.
13. Gessaia A, Barin F, Vemant JC, et al. Antibodies to human T-lymphotropic virus type-1 in patients with tropical spastic paraparesis. Lancet B. 1985;407–9(16):5.
14. Cruickshank JK, Rudge P, Dalgkish AG, et al. Tropical spastic paraparesis and human T cell lymphotropic virus type l in the United Kingdom. Brain. 1989;112:1057–90.
15. Iwasaki Y. Pathology of chronic myelopathy associated with HTLV1 infection (HAM/TSP). Neurol Sci. 1990;6:103–23.
16. Carod-Artal FJ, Del-Negro MC, Vargas AP, Rizzo I. Cerebellar syndrome and peripheral neuropathy as manifestations of infection by HTLV-I human T-cell lymphotropic virus. Rev Neurol. 1999;29(9):932–5.
17. Duintjer Tebbens RJ, Pallansch MA, Chumakov KM, et al. Expert review on poliovirus immunity and transmission. Risk Anal. 2013;33(4):544–605.

18. Gyrtrup HJ, Kristiansen VB, Zachariae CO, Krogsgaard K, Colstrup H, Jensen KM. Voiding problems in patients with HIV infection and AIDS. Scand J Urol Nephrol. 1995;29:295–8.
19. Staiman VR, Lowe FC. Urologic problems in patients with acquired immunodeficiency syndrome. ScientificWorldJournal. 2004;4(Suppl 1):427–37.
20. Broseta E, Osca JM, Morera J, et al. Urological manifestations of herpes zoster. Eur Urol. 1993;24:244–7.
21. Chen PH, Hsueh HF, Hong CZ. Herpes zoster-associated voiding dysfunction: a retrospective study and literature review. Arch Phys Med Rehabil. 2002;83(11):1624–8.
22. Greenstein A, Matzkin H, Kaver I, Braf Z. Acute urinary retention in herpes genitalis infection. Urology. 1988;31(5):453–6.
23. Sakakibara R, Hattori T, Kuwabara S, et al. Micturitional disturbance in patients with Guillain–Barré syndrome. J Neurol Neurosurg Psychiatry. 1997;63:649–53.
24. Murphy EL, Fridey J, Smith JW, et al. HTLV-associated myelopathy in a cohort of HTLV-I and HTLV-II-infected blood donors. Neurology. 1997;48:315–20.
25. Howard RS, Wiles CM, Spencer GT. The late sequelae of poliomyelitis. Q J Med. 1988;66:219–32.
26. Johnson VY, Hubbard D, Vordermark JS. Urologic manifestations of post-polio syndrome. J Wound Ostomy Continence Nurs. 1996;23:218–23.
27. Krishnan C, Kaplin AI, Pardo CA, Kerr DA, Keswani SC. Demyelinating disorders: update on transverse myelitis. Curr Neurol Neurosci Rep. 2006;6(3):236–43.
28. Oliveira P, Castro NM, Muniz AL, et al. Prevalence of erectile dysfunction in HTLV-1–infected patients and its association with overactive bladder. Urology. 2010;75:1100–3.
29. Christova I, Komitova R. Clinical and epidemiological features of Lyme borreliosis in Bulgaria. Wien Klin Wochenschr. 2004;116(1–2):42–6.
30. Nygarg K, Bransaeter AB, Mehl A. Disseminated and chronic Lyme borreliosis in Norway, 1995–2004. Euro Surveill. 2005;10(10):83–5.
31. Aksamit AJ. Review of PML and natalizumab. Neurologist. 2006;12(6):293–8.
32. Kobylecki C, Lee L, Kellett M. Cerebral palsy, cerebellar ataxia, AIDS, phacomatosis, neuromuscular disorders, and epilepsy. In: Corcos J, Ginsberg D, Karsenty G, editors. Textbook of the neurogenic bladder. 3rd ed. Boca Raton: CRC Press; 2016. p. 260–4.
33. Cohen LM, Fowler JF, Owen LG, Callen JP. Urinary retention associated with herpes zoster infection. Int J Dermatol. 1993;32(1):24–6.
34. Clason AE, McGeorge A, Garland C, Abel BJ. Urinary retention and granulomatous prostatitis following sacral herpes zoster infection. Br J Urol. 1982;54:166–9.
35. Riehle RA Jr, Williams JJ. Transient neuropathic bladder following herpes simplex genitalis. J Urol. 1979;122(2):263–4.
36. Wheeler JS Jr, Culkin DJ, O'Hara RJ, Canning JR. Bladder dysfunction and neurosyphilis. J Urol. 1986;136:903–5.
37. Kogan BA, Soloman MH, Diokno AC. Urinary retention secondary to Landry–Guillain–Barré syndrome. J Urol. 1981;126:643–4.
38. Grbavac Z, Gilja I, Gubarev N, Bozicevic D. Neurologic and urodynamic characteristics of patients with Guillain–Barré syndrome. Lijec Vjesn. 1989;111(1–2):17–20.
39. Timmermans L, Bonnet F, Maquinay C. Urological complications of poliomyelitis and their treatment. Acta Urol Belg. 1965;33:409–26.
40. Menendez V, Valls J, Espuna M, Perez A, Barranco MA, Carretero P. Neurogenic bladder in patients with acquired immunodeficiency syndrome. Neurourol Urodyn. 1995;14:253–7.
41. Hermieu JF, Delmas V, Boccon-Gibod L. Micturition disturbances and human immunodeficiency virus infection. J Urol. 1996;156:157–9.
42. Zeman A, Donaghy M. Acute infection with human immunodeficiency virus presenting with neurogenic urinary retention. Genitourin Med. 1991;67:345–7.
43. Kalita J, Shah S, Kapoor R, Misra UK. Bladder dysfunction in acute transverse myelitis: magnetic resonance imaging and neurophysiological and urodynamic correlations. J Neurol Neurosurg Psychiatry. 2002;73(2):154–9.

44. Leroy-Malherbe V, Sebire G, Hollenberg H, Tardieu M, Landrieu P. Neurogenic bladder in children with acute transverse myelopathy. Arch Pediatr. 1998;5(5):497–502.
45. Chancellor MB, Dato VM, Yang JY. Lyme disease presenting as urinary retention. J Urol. 1990;143(6):1223–4.
46. Troisgros O, Barnay JL, Darbon-Naghibzadeh F, Olive P, René-Corail P. Retrospective clinic and urodynamic study in the neurogenic bladder dysfunction caused by human T cell lymphotrophic virus type 1 associated myelopathy/tropical spastic paraparesis (HAM/TSP). Neurourol Urodyn. 2016;36(2):449–52.
47. Sakiyama H, Nishi K, Kikukawa H, Ueda S. Urinary disturbance due to HTLV-1 associated myelopathy. Nippon Hinyokika Gakkai Zasshi. 1992;83(12):2058.
48. Yamashita H, Kumazawa J. Voiding dysfunction: patients with human T-lymphotropic-virus-type-1-associated myelopathy. Urol Int. 1991;47(Suppl 1):69–71.
49. Imamura A. Studies on neurogenic bladder due to human T-lymphotropic virus type-I associated myelopathy (HAM). Nippon Hinyokika Gakkai Zasshi. 1994;85(7):1106–15.
50. Nomata K, Nakamura T, Suzu H, et al. Novel complications with HTLV-1-associated myelopathy/tropical spastic paraparesis: interstitial cystitis and persistent prostatitis. Jpn J Cancer Res. 1992;83(6):601–8.
51. Ganesan V, Borzyskowski M. Characteristics and course of urinary tract dysfunction after acute transverse myelitis in childhood. Dev Med Child Neurol. 2001;43(7):473–5.
52. Sakakibara R, Hattori T, Yasuda K, Yamanishi T. Micturition disturbance in acute transverse myelitis. Spinal Cord. 1996;34(8):481–5.
53. Berger Y, Blaivas JG, Oliver L. Urinary dysfunction in transverse myelitis. J Urol. 1990;144(1):103–5.
54. Chancellor MB, McGinnis DE, Shenot PJ, Kiilholma P, Hirsch IH. Urinary dysfunction in Lyme disease. J Urol. 1993;149(1):26–30.
55. Chancellor MB, McGinnis DE, Shenot PJ, Hirsch IH, Kiilholma PJ. Lyme cystitis and neurogenic bladder dysfunction. Lancet. 1992;339(8803):1237–8.
56. Transverse Myelitis Consortium Working Group. Proposed diagnostic criteria and nosology of acute transverse myelitis. Neurology. 2002;59:499–505.
57. Roskopf J, Trofe J, Stratta RJ, Ahsan N. Pharmacotherapeutic options for the management of human polyomaviruses. Adv Exp Med Biol. 2006;577:228–54.
58. Andrade RC, Neto JA, Andrade L, et al. Effects of physiotherapy in the treatment of neurogenic bladder in patients infected with human T-Lymphotropic virus 1. Urology. 2016;89:33–8.
59. Tsiodras S, Kelesidis T, Kelesidis I, Voumbourakis K, Giamarellou H. Mycoplasma pneumoniae-associated myelitis: a comprehensive review. Eur J Neurol. 2006;13(2):112–24.
60. Olivares JP, Pallas F, Ceccaldi M, et al. Lyme disease presenting as isolated acute urinary retention caused by transverse myelitis: an electrophysiological and urodynamical study. Arch Phys Med Rehabil. 1995;76(12):1171–2.
61. Chartier-Kastler EJ, Rudd Bosch JL, Perrigot M, et al. Long-term results of sacral nerve stimulation (S3) for the treatment of neurogenic refractory urge incontinence related to detrusor hyperreflexia. J Urol. 2000;164(5):1476–80.
62. Wosnitzer MS, Walsh R, Rutman MP. The use of sacral neuromodulation for the treatment of non-obstructive urinary retention secondary to Guillain-Barré syndrome. Int Urogynecol J Pelvic Floor Dysfunct. 2009;20(9):1145–7.
63. Hattori T, Yasuda K, Kita K, Hirayama K. Disorders of micturition in tabes dorsalis. Br J Urol. 1990;65(5):497–9.

Clinical Entities and Their Neuro-urological Consequences: Stroke

Mikolaj Przydacz and Jacques Corcos

Introduction

Undisturbed functioning of the central nervous system, in particular the cerebral cortex and the pons, is necessary for urinary continence, voiding reflex, bladder control, and sexual functions. Cerebrovascular accidents (or strokes) may lead to disintegration of this system and result in dysfunctions of the urinary tract. Brain neural control of micturition can become affected by the stroke, and this is of utmost importance to urologists in their day-to-day clinical practice in terms of patients' quality of life and protection of renal function.

Among a wide spectrum of urological consequences following cerebrovascular accidents, storage and voiding dysfunctions are the most common. They usually include urinary incontinence, urinary retention, frequency, and urgency. Uncontrollable urinary incontinence has the highest prevalence among them with the greatest impact on patients' quality of life. Urological symptoms following a stroke strongly correlate with disability and economic deprivation. Therefore, appropriate diagnosis and management could help to avoid complications leading to further health improvement and better quality of life.

In this chapter, we will focus on the epidemiology, pathophysiology, symptoms, impact on patients' quality of life, and treatment of the urological sequelae following cerebrovascular accidents.

M. Przydacz (✉) · J. Corcos
Mcgill University, Montreal, QC, Canada
e-mail: jcorcos@uro.jgh.mcgill.ca

© Springer International Publishing AG, part of Springer Nature 2018
R. Dmochowski, J. Heesakkers (eds.), *Neuro-Urology*,
https://doi.org/10.1007/978-3-319-90997-4_9

Epidemiology

Global stroke epidemiology is changing rapidly. Although age-adjusted rates of stroke mortality have decreased worldwide in the past two decades, the absolute numbers of people who develop a stroke every year and live with the consequences or die from it are increasing [1]. Stroke is often of a lower priority to health service and research than other diseases with a similar or lower public health impact leading to difficulties in epidemiological assessment [2]. There is a considerable variability between countries and regions, presumably because of differences in exposure to environmental, genetic, and other risk factors, lifestyle differences, stroke management strategies, and differences in methodology used to report these statistics. Epidemiological data are fully available from well-developed countries, whereas from the developing and emerging regions of the world, data are rather sparse. It should be noted that two-thirds of all strokes in the world occur in developing countries [1]. This explains the huge variation in stroke incidence rates ranging from 41 to 316 per 100,000 persons per year. Some regions have three- to fivefold greater incidence of stroke than other countries.

Cerebrovascular accidents are the fifth leading cause of death in developed countries, behind diseases of the heart, cancer, chronic lower respiratory diseases, and unintentional injury [3]. Each year approximately one million US people experience a stroke. Seventy-seven percent are initial episodes, whereas the remainder are recurrent strokes [4]. Ischemic type occurs seven times more often than hemorrhagic. However, the latter is characterized by up to four times higher risk of death [5].

Stroke is a leading cause of a serious long-term disability in the United States [6]. Among patients discharged from the hospital after stroke, almost half return directly home, one-fourth is discharged to inpatient rehabilitation facilities, and the rest are discharged to skilled nursing facilities. More specifically, of the survivors, 10% have no residual effects, 40% have mild disability, 40% have significant disability, and 10% require nursing home care [7].

High prevalence of disability caused by stroke and population aging process have significant health-care financial implications. It has been estimated that approximately 26 million stroke survivors are currently alive around the world [1]. Nowadays, total direct medical stroke-related costs in the United States are projected to triple, from USD 72 billion to 184 billion dollars [6]. Moreover, the number of incidence of stroke among adolescents and young adults has been growing. Approximately 10% of all strokes occur in individuals 18–50 years of age leading to a serious problem in human resources and workforces [8].

As cerebrovascular accidents have the highest prevalence and incidence among the elderly, preexisting urological problems are common in the population of stroke patient. Prostatic disorders, overactive bladder, and stress urinary incontinence are often seen in these patients and may influence the clinical presentation [7]. It should be noted that prevalence of urinary incontinence in general population has been estimated as 6%; however, for the elderly it can range from 11% to 29% [9]. After stroke, up to 79% of patients may struggle with this condition. Likewise, uninhibited detrusor contractions can be observed in 30% of elderly men and women [10]. Stroke can increase this observation in up to 90% of patients [11].

Pathophysiology

The two major mechanisms causing brain damage in stroke are ischemia and/or hemorrhage. In the first type, also called embolic or thrombotic, decreased or absent blood circulation deprives neurons of necessary energetic substrates. Intracerebral hemorrhage originates from deep penetrating vessels and causes injury to brain tissue by disrupting connecting pathways and causing localized pressure injury with the mass effect. Voiding dysfunctions in patients after stroke may be produced by different mechanisms. First, the direct impairment of higher cortical centers, especially located in frontal lobes, usually leads to disorders in contractions of bladder detrusor. Second, immobility and loss of initiative/cognition, especially decreased sensations and awareness of bladder filling, can produce significant functional disabilities. Therefore, stroke patients can present a wide variety of urological symptoms and urodynamically identified dysfunctions.

The normal function of the bladder, alternating filling and emptying, is secured by several systems placed at different levels in the central nervous system. The most important are located at the cerebral cortex (anterior cingulate gyrus), pons, and spinal cord [7]. Intact function of all of them is required to normal voiding. After emerging of the need to void, the urethral sphincter can be allowed to relax, whereas the detrusor is able to contract reflexively and initiates the voiding process. During storage phase, there is a net inhibitory effect by the CNS on the detrusor contractions.

Cerebral Cortex

Micturition is regulated voluntarily by cortical centers at the level of the frontal lobes and premotrice area (paracentral lobule) [12]. The frontal cortex contains cognitive centers of voiding control. The main inhibitory input on the detrusor function during filling phase derives from this structure [13]. Any decision regarding initiation of voiding is made through the frontal lobes [14]. Possible damage of this system after stroke may lead to detrusor overactivity and urge incontinence [15].

Pons

Central regulation, coordination, and control of voiding occur in the pontine micturition center [16]. It is located in the dorsal pontine tegmentum and responsible for relaxation of the urinary sphincter with coordinated detrusor contractions, thus initiating micturition [13, 17]. Ablation of this area causes urinary retention by disabilities in sphincter relaxation and detrusor contractions [18]. In patients with pons affected by stroke, similar results have been demonstrated with clinical presentation of retention [19].

Spinal Cord

Cerebrovascular accidents within brain very rarely influence micturition mechanisms in spinal cord. However, stroke as a general condition affects the whole organism. Post-ischemic inflammation in the brain, represented either by blood cells and chemical compounds distributed in the whole organism, could influence crucial steps of the tissue injury/repair cascade [20]. Systemic response to stroke could influence various organs via different corticospinal pathways [21]. The impact of cerebrovascular incidents on voiding mechanisms in spinal cord has not been well investigated; thus, more research has to be done on this phenomenon.

Clinical Presentation

The effects of stroke depend on several factors, including the type, severity, location, and number of episodes. Physical poststroke conditions include paralysis, vision and speech problems, behavioral style changes, cognitive impairment, decreased self-care ability, and deficits in volitional control of voiding. Loss of bladder control is considered as one of the most affecting factors on health-related quality of life in poststroke patients [22]. The prevalence of urological symptoms in stroke patients ranges from 11% to almost 80% [11]. Urinary incontinence is the most common sequela of stroke affecting more than a third of stroke patients admitted to hospital with up to a quarter of these patients remaining incontinent at 1 year [7, 23]. Poststroke urinary incontinence is a strong predictor of higher rates of mortality, greater institutionalization, and increased disability [23]. However, reports on the frequency other urological symptoms are few and far between. Among them, significant numbers of incidences are reported in nocturia (36–79%), frequency (17.5–36%), urgency (19–29%), difficulty in voiding (25%), straining (3.5%), and pain (2.5%) [9, 24, 25]. However, it should be noted that the prevalence of all above-mentioned symptoms depends on a stroke phase.

Acute Phase

In the acute phase of cerebrovascular accidents, patients often present with urinary retention. Mechanism of this condition has not been well established. The retention could be connected with neurological effect of brain infarct (called as a "cerebral shock") presented as detrusor underactivity or detrusor-sphincter dyssynergia [7]. However, overdistention of the bladder that resulted in the inability to void may also be caused by impaired consciousness, restricted mobility, and an inability to communicate [26]. Preexisting bladder dysfunction or medications may also have a role in urinary retention in the acute poststroke period [27]. Studies on correlation between the site of brain injury and bladder dysfunctions have shown that retention appears to be more commonly associated with cortical infarcts in the frontal lobe or cerebellum. Burney et al. showed an 85% incidence rate of this condition related to bladder underactivity in patients with hemorrhagic strokes of the frontal lobe [28]. In comparison only 10% of the patients with ischemic infarcts had retention. However, the authors were unable to explain this phenomenon. They hypothesized that the type of infarct may determine the results of urinary dysfunction in the early poststroke period. As hemorrhagic variant is associated with a higher risk of death and other stroke-related complications than ischemic, even after adjustment for age, sex, initial stroke severity, and relevant cardiovascular risk factors, it could result in more retention. Han et al. confirmed that the hemorrhage patients are more predisposed to have detrusor underactivity than overactivity [29]. A recently published study by Cho et al. stated that interruption of the descending pathways from the pontine micturition center to the sacral spinal cord in the lateral medulla may be responsible for the development of urinary retention [30]. Nevertheless, they clearly added that more research is warranted.

Data from prospective studies of lower urinary tract symptoms in stroke patients have showed prevalence of urinary retention from 29% up to 67% within 2 weeks of the stroke incident [28, 31–33]. The higher percentages of retention were observed within the first 3 days of brain injury. Retention resolved in almost all patients within 2 months after discharge. It correlates with other studies where changes in detrusor behavior from underactivity to overactivity with time have been described [34]. Possible related risk factors of retention were reported such as diabetes, cognitive impairment, aphasia, and decreased functional status. More recently, Kim et al. confirmed these factors as the danger of retention [33].

As mentioned previously, urinary incontinence is the most common urological symptom among stroke patients, and it could also be recognized in the early recovery period. However, there is considerable variation in the reported prevalence rates [26, 27, 35]. Brittain et al. identified rates of this condition at hospital admission following stroke ranging from 32% to 79% based on data from nine hospital-based studies [36]. Thomas et al. reported incontinence in 40–60% of patients admitted to hospital after a stroke, with 25% still having problems on hospital discharge, and approximately 15% remaining incontinent at 1 year [37]. Amelioration of urinary incontinence in 25–45% of patients may reflect improvement of both functional component (cognition and mobility) and neurological constituent of the bladder dysfunction. Kolominsky-Rabas et al. conducted a community-based study over a 4-year period, which included almost 700 patients presenting with a new stroke [38]. They reported that 35% of previously continent patients were incontinent at 7 days following a stroke. Patel et al. evaluated the rate of incontinence among a half thousand patients after the same time period [39]. They found that 39% of survivors demonstrated urinary incontinence, which has also been found as a negative prognostic factor for higher mortality. These results were connected with the premorbid urinary dysfunctions, overall size of the stroke, and affected area of the brain. Wilson et al. published similar results. They analyzed data from the UK National Sentinel Stroke Audit between 1998 and 2004 and identified urinary incontinence rates of 39–44% at 1 week [40]. Recently published study by Kuptniratsaikul et al. noted bladder/bowel dysfunction in 31.5% of patients among 327 poststroke survivors who started rehabilitation [41]. This variation in prevalence rates could be caused by different definitions of urinary incontinence, failures of assessment in the premorbid condition, different time points of measurement, and disparities among population samples [23].

Chronic Phase

Although some resolution of micturition problems occurs with time, a significant number of patients do not present normal voiding. There appears to be a persistent urinary incontinence or an evolution from retention to a more fixed dysfunction, usually manifested by incontinence, frequency, and urgency [7]. Patel et al. explored the natural history of urinary incontinence in 235 participants through personal interviews and postal questionnaires over a 2-year period [42]. They reported the following prevalence rates: 19% at 3 months, 15% at 1 year, and 10% at 2 years. Brocklehurst et al. presented similar results [35]. They found a low (12%) rate of incontinence several months post CVA. Data from a prospective study confirmed these findings. Rotar et al. evaluated 100 patients presenting with a first ever stroke for the presence of lower urinary tract dysfunction using a questionnaire and ultrasound scan [43]. At 72 h, more than 50% of the population experienced symptoms, but at 1 year the symptoms persisted in 9% of stroke survivors. However, due to different definitions of urinary incontinence, assessment methods, and analyzed populations, data on reported prevalence can vary. For instance, in a study by Tsuchida et al., frequency, urgency, and urge incontinence were seen in 67% of patients 19 months after a stroke [44]. Another study of voiding complaints in elderly patients (over 75 years) after a cerebrovascular accident found a 79% rate of urinary incontinence [45]. Despite these disparities, we can state that the incidences of urinary incontinence among stroke patients decrease with time.

Possible related risk factors of urinary incontinence in poststroke patients have been analyzed. Williams et al. discovered that increasing age, female sex, and stroke severity were independent predictors of urinary incontinence at 12 months [25]. Another research conducted by Patel et al. specified that patients aged 75 and older are less likely to regain continence [39]. Furthermore, they investigated that hemorrhagic or ischemic etiology of stroke did not appear to have a significant effect on patients remaining incontinent or regaining continence at 3 months. Studies on correlations between the location of the stroke, its size, and the risk of urinary incontinence in recovery period showed very interesting results. Gelber et al. prospectively investigated the bladder function of 51 patients with unilateral hemispheric stroke

[27]. They found a significant correlation between large infarcts involving both cortical and subcortical regions and the development of urinary incontinence. Cognitive and/or language barriers caused by such strokes may indirectly affect continence and provoke or exaggerate voiding dysfunctions. Moreover, the authors reported that no correlation was evident between the location of the stroke lesion and the development of urinary incontinence. Further research presented similar results and suggested that the size of the stroke lesion is a better predictor of the development of incontinence than its location [27, 39, 46, 47].

Urodynamics

When incontinence occurs after a cerebrovascular accident and patient's condition is enough stabilized to diagnose and cure voiding dysfunctions, the main urodynamic finding is usually detrusor overactivity. Detrusor underactivity can also be seen, especially in patients with cerebellar lesions or in the acute phase related to the cerebral shock. However, the early phase of stroke usually does not allow to perform urodynamic assessment due to an unstable patient condition and evolution of voiding dysfunctions.

The mechanism of poststroke detrusor overactivity seems not to be established. Detrusor overactivity has been described in patients with different locations of lesions in the central nervous system but is also seen in survivors without clear neurologic involvement. It is believed that the micturition reflex is under tonic inhibitory influence [48, 49] from the central cholinergic [50] and dopaminergic pathways [51]. Their failure as an effect of the stroke may lead to detrusor overactivity. No statistically significant correlations have been demonstrated between lesion site and urodynamic findings [52, 53]. However, patients with frontal lobe lesions often present uninhibited sphincter relaxation with detrusor overactivity [24, 28, 44]. Therefore, disrupted higher cortical control systems of the external sphincter could predispose to more profound urine loss and reduced awareness. In multiple clinical studies, the presence of sphincteric dysfunction ranges from 8.3% to 17% [24, 28, 44].

Pizzi et al. performed urodynamic studies on 106 ischemic stroke patients at admission and repeated in 63 patients after 30 days. Urodynamic studies, performed during admission, showed normal bladder function in 15%, detrusor overactivity in 56%, detrusor overactivity with impaired contractility in 14%, and detrusor underactivity in 15%. After 1 month urodynamic assessment showed normal studies in 30%, overactive detrusor in 48%, detrusor overactivity with impaired contractility in 6%, and underactive detrusor in 16% [54]. Similar results were presented by Gelber et al. They reported detrusor overactivity in 37%, underactive detrusor in 21%, and detrusor-sphincter dyssynergia in 5% among 19 patients at 3 weeks of cerebrovascular accident [27]. Of note, detrusor-sphincter dyssynergia is a rare finding after a cerebrovascular accident and is usually confused with pseudodyssynergia [55]. True dyssynergia usually implies a contemporaneous cord lesion occurring with the cortical lesion. Khan et al. demonstrated detrusor overactivity without detrusor-sphincter dyssynergia in 79% of 33 poststroke patients with lower urinary tract symptoms. Majority of patients were studied within 3 months of the stroke [56]. Similarly, a study done by Nitti et al. of 38 symptomatic stroke men showed overactive detrusor in 82% and outlet obstruction in 63% patients [57]. Mean interval from cerebrovascular accident to urodynamic evaluation was 32 months.

Stroke Location and Possible Urological Outcomes

The location of the stroke can predispose to some voiding dysfunctions. However, data on this topic are very limited. The majority of studies have described micturition problems as a result of defects in frontal lobes, brain stem, and cerebellum. Based on them, lesions of the anteromedial frontal lobe and the basal ganglia are mainly responsible for bladder dysfunctions after stroke. There are no clear reports of voiding dysfunctions as a consequence of a single/focal deficit in the parietal, temporal, or occipital lobe.

Frontal Lobes

Correlations between frontal lobes impairment and lower urinary tract dysfunction have been described most accurate. Study done by Khan et al. [56] reported significant interdependence between voiding problems and frontal cortex and/or internal capsular lesions. Bogousslavsky and Regli presented similar results; they showed that frontal lobes may be the hypothetical center of poststroke voiding dysfunctions [58]. Sakakibara et al. looked at CT and magnetic resonance imaging findings in patients within 3 months of their stroke [24]. The rate of urinary symptoms was 53%, and patients affected by them were significantly more likely to have frontal lobe and frontoparietal-temporal and frontoparietal-occipital lesions than temporal, parietal, and occipital lesions. This study again showed the importance of the frontal lobe in the pathogenesis of voiding problems in poststroke patients. When it comes to urodynamic assessment of patients with affected frontal lobes, detrusor overactivity and sphincter relaxation are the most common findings [28].

Brain Stem

Brain stem strokes are also associated with a high incidence of urinary symptoms. In a study of 39 patients with brain stem strokes, Sakakibara et al. found a 49% rate of urinary symptoms [19]. In addition, they found a higher rate of obstructive symptoms and urinary retention than incontinence. Recently conducted study by Yum et al. analyzed 30 brainstem infarction cases [59]. They found micturition dysfunctions in 70% of patients with storage disorders occurring two times more often than emptying. Moreover, storage disorder was found only in pontine lesions. On the other hand, emptying disorder was more common in medullary lesions.

Cerebellum

The role of cerebellum in the pathogenesis of neurogenic bladder has not been established. It is known that cerebellum plays a role in voiding coordination between the cortical centers and detrusor nuclei in the brain stem [15]. Burney et al. reported that patients with cerebellar infarctions are highly predisposed to detrusor underactivity with normal function of the sphincter [28]. However, in another study using fMRI, the cerebellum was found to be involved in the inhibition of the micturition reflex [60]. Moreover, Nardulli et al. stated that cerebellar strokes are strongly correlated with overactive detrusor [61]. Thus, it is clear that more research in this area is warranted.

Sidedness

It has not been established whether the sidedness of the cerebrovascular accident is correlated with possible urological outcomes. Kuroiwa et al. reported that urgency, frequency, and incontinence were more common in right-sided lesions [62]. Their results agree with findings presented by Griffiths, who perform comprehensive investigations with SPECT brain scanning [63]. These data are consistent with PET study, which confirm that the right hemisphere is involved in voluntary voiding [13]. However, Gelber et al. also analyzed lesion sidedness and found no correlation between the side of the lesion and incontinence [27]. Burney et al. presented the same conclusions [64].

To summarize, stroke location has an effect on the presented voiding dysfunctions. Affection of frontal lobes usually leads to incontinence and detrusor overactivity, whereas brain stem lesions are often connected with retention and obstructive symptoms.

Effects on Stroke Outcomes

The forwardness of voiding dysfunctions following a stroke has been strongly associated with increased mortality rates, poor functional outcomes, and worse health-related quality of life.

John et al. have demonstrated that poststroke urinary incontinence is independently associated with higher mortality rates [65]. Through pooled meta-analysis with almost 25,000 patients, they proved this association at any time point of the follow-up, after both hemorrhagic and ischemic stroke. This stresses the importance of diagnosis and specific care for stroke patients suffering from urinary incontinence. Similarly, Barer et al. found that stroke outcomes were better in those patients who regained continence or remain continent [43]. Premorbid urinary incontinence has also been associated with poor poststroke prognosis. Jawad et al. reported that almost 80% of patients who died within 6 months of the cerebrovascular accident were premorbidly incontinent [66].

Patients who are able to regain continence have a better functional status with lower institutionalization and disability rates than those who remain incontinent. Patel et al. examined this relationship with a multiple logistic regression analysis and found that persistent incontinence was independently associated with worse outcomes, with an institutionalization rate of 27% compared to 9% in the continent group [39]. Another study reported even higher institutionalization rates of 45% at 1 year with a fourfold higher risk compared with those who regained continence [38]. Poor functional outcomes of patients with poststroke urinary incontinence are usually associated with an inability to participate in stroke rehabilitation therapy and incontinence-related depression [67].

Urinary symptoms also play a major role in the quality of life and overall well-being of patients after stroke. According to a population-based study with 10,000 community members, Brittain et al. found a significant relationship between severity of urinary symptoms and both decreased quality of life and difficulties with activities of daily living [9]. Moreover, regaining of continence was connected with improvement in quality of life [22].

Interventions

Treatment of voiding dysfunctions in poststroke patients is a challenge. Medical management of symptoms can be difficult and surgical treatment can be fraught with complications and limitations [7, 68]. Even though 12 randomized controlled trials on different treatment strategies with a total of 724 participants have been completed, evidence-based interventions are limited [23]. All of these trials had a relatively small sample size with wide confidence intervals, and nine did not specify if patients with premorbid incontinence had been excluded. Current data are insufficient to make strong recommendations, but a structured assessment and specialist continence nursing are likely to reduce rates of poststroke micturition problems.

In the acute phase, usually accompanied by detrusor underactivity with overflow incontinence, intermittent catheterization and the use of an indwelling catheter are acceptable strategies [7]. Indwelling catheterization should be discontinued as early as reasonably possible. Bowel management strategies should also be employed [69]. Drugs exacerbating symptoms have to be stopped, if possible (i.e., diuretics).

Detrusor overactivity with urge incontinence, occurring both in the acute and chronic phase, should be followed by bladder retraining (e.g., prompted voiding for at least 6 weeks), optimized access to technical facilities (e.g., easy access to the toilet, use of handheld urinals, access to a call bell, easy to remove clothing), fluid restrictions, and pelvic floor muscle training [23].

The use of medications is usually required. However, due to multiple side effects, it is often limited. Alpha-blockers can cause hypotension or dizziness with further implications in patient functioning and rehabilitation. Anticholinergics may have negative impact on cognitive functions [70]. Nevertheless, until now, positive results have been reported in propiverine, oxybutynin, imidafenacin, and tolterodine [71–74]. Also, other drug groups can be used in the treatment of urological symptoms in poststroke patients: tricyclic antidepressants (imipramine), serotonin-norepinephrine reuptake inhibitors (duloxetine), and central acetylcholinesterase inhibitors (donepezil) [75, 76].

For patients with persistent urge incontinence, intravesical botulinum type A toxin (Botox) injections may be a treatment option. Kuo applied 200 U of botulinum A toxin in 12 patients with detrusor overactivity due to stroke [77]. He found 50% achievement of continence but yet in comparison with 90% success rate in spinal cord injured patients. It is clear that more research is warranted, based on these promising results.

Electroacupuncture has shown an improvement in urinary incontinence after stroke with increase of bladder capacity and amelioration of bladder emptying [78, 79]. Sacral neuromodulation is another possible option of treatment. However, it has not been approved yet for patients with neurologic disease and may not be as effective [80].

Conservative neurogenic bladder therapy may be efficient, especially if treatment is introduced in early stage of the disease. However, in front of refractory incontinence with poor urodynamic changes, augmentation cystoplasty or urinary diversion can provide a safe functional reservoir for urinary continence and prevention of upper tract deterioration [7].

Conclusion

Storage and voiding dysfunctions following stroke are common and complex disorders with multifactorial components. It is well established that they are associated with poor functional outcomes, higher rates of disability, institutionalization, and mortality. Detriments in emotional well-being and social relationships are not rare. Management of these patients is a challenge. However, strong concerted efforts allow to change these patients' prognosis and to improve their quality of life.

References

1. Feigin VL, Krishnamurthi RV, Parmar P, Norrving B, Mensah GA, Bennett DA, et al. Update on the global burden of ischemic and hemorrhagic stroke in 1990-2013: the GBD 2013 study. Neuroepidemiology. 2015;45(3):161–76.
2. Thrift AG, Cadilhac DA, Thayabaranathan T, Howard G, Howard VJ, Rothwell PM, et al. Global stroke statistics. Int J Stroke. 2014;9(1):6–18.

3. Centers for Disease Control and Prevention, National Center for Health Statistics [Internet]; Life Stages and Populations, Deaths and Mortality. Publicated: 2014 [Cited: 2014 November]. Available from: http://www.cdc.gov/nchs/fastats/deaths.htm

4. Writing Group Members, Mozaffarian D, Benjamin EJ, Go AS, Arnett DK, Blaha MJ, et al. Executive summary: heart disease and stroke statistics – 2016 update: a report from the American Heart Association. Circulation. 2016;133(4):447–54.

5. Andersen KK, Olsen TS, Dehlendorff C, Kammersgaard LP. Hemorrhagic and ischemic strokes compared: stroke severity, mortality, and risk factors. Stroke. 2009;40(6):2068–72.

6. Writing Group Members, Mozaffarian D, Benjamin EJ, Go AS, Arnett DK, Blaha MJ, et al. Heart disease and stroke Statistics-2016 update: a report from the American Heart Association. Circulation. 2016;133(4):e38–360.

7. Osborn DJ, Reynolds WS, Dmochowski RR. Cerebrovascular accidents, intracranial tumors, and urologic consequences. In: Corcos J, Ginsberg D, Karsenty G, editors. Textbook of the neurogenic bladder. 3rd ed. Boca Raton: CRC Press; 2016. p. 260–4.

8. Nedeltchev K, der Maur TA, Georgiadis D, Arnold M, Caso V, Mattle HP, et al. Ischaemic stroke in young adults: predictors of outcome and recurrence. J Neurol Neurosurg Psychiatry. 2005;76:191–5.

9. Brittain KR, Perry SI, Peet SM, Shaw C, Dallosso H, Assassa RP, et al. Prevalence and impact of urinary symptoms among community-dwelling stroke survivors. Stroke. 2000;31(4):886–91.

10. Pfisterer MH, Griffiths DJ, Rosenberg L, Schaefer W, Resnick NM. The impact of detrusor overactivity on bladder function in younger and older women. J Urol. 2006;175(5):1777–83. discussion 1783

11. Ruffion A, Castro-Diaz D, Patel H, Khalaf K, Onyenwenyi A, Globe D, et al. Systematic review of the epidemiology of urinary incontinence and detrusor overactivity among patients with neurogenic overactive bladder. Neuroepidemiology. 2013;41(3–4):146–55.

12. Saad Aldousari Jacques Corcos. Simplified anatomy of the vesicourethral functional unit. In: Corcos J, Ginsberg D, Karsenty G, editors. Textbook of the neurogenic bladder. 3rd ed. Boca Raton: CRC Press; 2016. p. 260–4.

13. Blok BF, Willemsen AT, Holstege G. A PET study on brain control of micturition in humans. Brain. 1997;120(Pt 1):111–21.

14. Fukuyama H, Matsuzaki S, Ouchi Y, Yamauchi H, Nagahama Y, Kimura J, et al. Neural control of micturition in man examined with single photon emission computed tomography using 99mTc-HMPAO. Neuroreport. 1996;7(18):3009–12.

15. Bradley WE, Sundin T. The physiology and pharmacology of urinary tract dysfunction. Clin Neuropharmacol. 1982;5(2):131–58.

16. Carlsson CA. The supraspinal control of the urinary bladder. Acta Pharmacol Toxicol (Copenh). 1978;43(Suppl 2):8–12.

17. De Groat WC. Nervous control of the urinary bladder of the cat. Brain Res. 1975;87(2–3):201–11.

18. Kavia RB, Dasgupta R, Fowler CJ. Functional imaging and the central control of the bladder. J Comp Neurol. 2005;493(1):27–32.

19. Sakakibara R, Hattori T, Yasuda K, Yamanishi T. Micturitional disturbance and the pontine tegmental lesion: urodynamic and MRI analyses of vascular cases. J Neurol Sci. 1996;141(1–2):105–10.

20. Mirabelli-Badenier M, Braunersreuther V, Viviani GL, Dallegri F, Quercioli A, Veneselli E, et al. CC and CXC chemokines are pivotal mediators of cerebral injury in ischaemic stroke. Thromb Haemost. 2011;105(3):409–20.

21. Reinkensmeyer DJ, Guigon E, Maier MA. A computational model of use-dependent motor recovery following a stroke: optimizing corticospinal activations via reinforcement learning can explain residual capacity and other strength recovery dynamics. Neural Netw. 2012;29-30:60–9.

22. Tapia CI, Khalaf K, Berenson K, Globe D, Chancellor M, Carr LK. Health-related quality of life and economic impact of urinary incontinence due to detrusor overactivity associated with a neurologic condition: a systematic review. Health Qual Life Outcomes. 2013;11:13.

23. Mehdi Z, Birns J, Bhalla A. Post-stroke urinary incontinence. Int J Clin Pract. 2013;67(11):1128–37.
24. Sakakibara R, Hattori T, Yasuda K, Yamanishi T. Micturitional disturbance after acute hemispheric stroke: analysis of the lesion site by CT and MRI. J Neurol Sci. 1996;137(1):47–56.
25. Williams MP, Srikanth V, Bird M, Thrift AG. Urinary symptoms and natural history of urinary continence after first-ever stroke--a longitudinal population-based study. Age Ageing. 2012;41(3):371–6.
26. Borrie MJ, Campbell AJ, Caradoc-Davies TH, Spears GF. Urinary incontinence after stroke: a prospective study. Age Ageing. 1986;15(3):177–81.
27. Gelber DA, Good DC, Laven LJ, Verhulst SJ. Causes of urinary incontinence after acute hemispheric stroke. Stroke. 1993;24(3):378–82.
28. Burney TL, Senapati M, Desai S, Choudhary ST, Badlani GH. Acute cerebrovascular accident and lower urinary tract dysfunction: a prospective correlation of the site of brain injury with urodynamic findings. J Urol. 1996;156(5):1748–50.
29. Han KS, Heo SH, Lee SJ, Jeon SH, Yoo KH. Comparison of urodynamics between ischemic and hemorrhagic stroke patients; can we suggest the category of urinary dysfunction in patients with cerebrovascular accident according to type of stroke? Neurourol Urodyn. 2010;29(3):387–90.
30. Cho HJ, Kang TH, Chang JH, Choi YR, Park MG, Choi KD, et al. Neuroanatomical correlation of urinary retention in lateral medullary infarction. Ann Neurol. 2015;77(4):726–33.
31. Kong KH, Young S. Incidence and outcome of poststroke urinary retention: a prospective study. Arch Phys Med Rehabil. 2000;81(11):1464–7.
32. Garrett VE, Scott JA, Costich J, Aubrey DL, Gross J. Bladder emptying assessment in stroke patients. Arch Phys Med Rehabil. 1989;70(1):41–3.
33. Kim TG, Chun MH, Chang MC, Yang S. Outcomes of drug-resistant urinary retention in patients in the early stage of stroke. Ann Rehabil Med. 2015;39(2):262–7.
34. Arunabh, G.H. Badlani urologic problems in cerebrovascular accidents D.F. Paulson (Ed.), Problems in urology, vol. 7, J. B. Lippincott Co., Philadelphia (1993), pp. 41–53 1.
35. Brocklehurst JC, Andrews K, Richards B, Laycock PJ. Incidence and correlates of incontinence in stroke patients. J Am Geriatr Soc. 1985;33:540–2.
36. Brittain KR, Peet SM, Castleden CM. Stroke and incontinence. Stroke. 1998;29:524–8.
37. Thomas LH, Barrett J, Cross S, French B, Leathley M, Sutton C, et al. Prevention and treatment of urinary incontinence after stroke in adults. Cochrane Database Syst Rev. 2005;3:CD004462.
38. Kolominsky-Rabas PL, Hilz MJ, Neundoerfer B, Heuschmann PU. Impact of urinary incontinence after stroke: results from a prospective population based stroke register. Neurourol Urodyn. 2003;22:322–7.
39. Patel M, Coshall C, Lawrence E, Rudd AG, Wolfe CD. Recovery from poststroke urinary incontinence: associated factors and impact on outcome. J Am Geriatr Soc. 2001;49(9):1229–33.
40. Wilson D, Lowe D, Hoffman A, Rudd A, Wagg A. Urinary incontinence in stroke: results from the UK National Sentinel Audits of stroke 1998–2004. Age Ageing. 2008;37:542–6.
41. Kuptniratsaikul V, Kovindha A, Suethanapornkul S, Manimmanakorn N, Archongka Y. Complications during the rehabilitation period in thai patients with stroke. A multicenter prospective study. Am J Phys Med Rehabil. 2009;88(2):92–9.
42. Patel M, Coshall C, Rudd AG, Wolfe CDA. Natural history and effects on 2-year outcomes of urinary incontinence after stroke. Stroke. 2001;32:122–7.
43. Rotar M, Blagus R, Jeromel M, Skrbec M, Trsinar B, Vodusek DB. Stroke patients who regain urinary continence in the first week after acute first-ever stroke have better prognosis than patients with persistent lower urinary tract dysfunction. Neurourol Urodyn. 2011;30:1315–8.
44. Tsuchida S, Noto H, Yamaguchi O, Itoh M. Urodynamic studies on hemiplegic patients after cerebrovascular accident. Urology. 1983;21:315–8.
45. Kalra L, Smith DH, Crome P. Stroke in patients aged over 75 years: outcome and predictors. Postgrad Med J. 1993;69:33–6.
46. Badlani GH, Vohra S, Motola JA. Detrusor behavior in patients with dominant hemispheric strokes. Neurourol Urodyn. 1991;10:119–23.

47. Feder M, Heller L, Tadmor R, Snir D, Solzi P, Ring H. Urinary continence after stroke: association with cystometric profile and computerised tomography findings. Eur Neurol. 1987;27:101–5.
48. Fowler CJ, Griffiths D, de Groat WC. The neural control of micturition. Nat Rev Neurosci. 2008;9(6):453–66.
49. Birder L, Drake M. Neural control. In: Abrams P, Cardozo L, Khoury S, et al., editors. Incontinence. Paris: Health Publications Ltd; 2009. p. 167–254.
50. Masuda H, Chancellor MB, Kihara K, Sakai Y, Koga F, Azuma H, et al. Effects of cholinesterase inhibition in supraspinal and spinal neural pathways on the micturition reflex in rats. BJU Int. 2009;104(8):1163–9.
51. Sakakibara R, Panicker J, Fowler CJ, Tateno F, Kishi M, Tsuyusaki Y, et al. "Vascular incontinence" and normal-pressure hydrocephalus: two common sources of elderly incontinence with brain etiologies. Curr Drug Ther. 2012;7:67–76.
52. Gupta A, Taly AB, Srivastava A, Thyloth M. Urodynamics post stroke in patients with urinary incontinence: is there correlation between bladder type and site of lesion? Ann Indian Acad Neurol. 2009;12(2):104–7.
53. Yoo KH, Lee SJ, Chang SG. Predictive value of the ischemic stroke lesion to detrusor function. Neurourol Urodyn. 2010;29(7):1355–6.
54. Pizzi A, Falsini C, Martini M, Rossetti MA, Verdesca S, Tosto A. Urinary incontinence after ischemic stroke: clinical and urodynamic studies. Neurourol Urodyn. 2014;33(4):420–5.
55. Wein A, Barrett DM. Etiologic possibilities for increased pelvic floor electromyography activity during cystometry. J Urol. 1982;127:949–52.
56. Khan Z, Starer P, Yang WC, Bhola A. Analysis of voiding disorders in patients with cerebrovascular accidents. Urology. 1990;35(3):265–70.
57. Nitti VW, Adler H, Combs AJ. The role of urodynamics in the evaluation of voiding dysfunction in men after cerebrovascular accident. J Urol. 1996;155(1):263–6.
58. Bogousslavsky J, Regli F. Anterior cerebral artery territory infarction in the Lausanne stroke registry. Clinical and etiologic patterns. Arch Neurol. 1990;47(2):144–50.
59. Yum KS, Na SJ, Lee KY, Kim J, Oh SH, Kim YD, et al. Pattern of voiding dysfunction after acute brainstem infarction. Eur Neurol. 2013;70(5–6):291–6.
60. Zhang H, Reitz A, Kollias S, Summers P, Curt A, Schurch B. An fMRI study of the role of suprapontine brain structures in the voluntary voiding control induced by pelvic floor contraction. NeuroImage. 2005;24:174–80.
61. Nardulli R, Monitillo V, Losavio E, Fiore P, Nicolardi G, Megna G. Urodynamic evaluation of 12 ataxic subjects: neurophysiopathologic considerations. Funct Neurol. 1992;7(3):223–5.
62. Kuroiwa Y, Tohgi H, Ono S, Itoh M. Frequency and urgency of micturition in hemiplegic patients: relationship to hemisphere laterality of lesions. J Neurol. 1987;234(2):100.
63. Griffiths D. Clinical studies of cerebral and urinary tract function in elderly people with urinary incontinence. Behav Brain Res. 1998;92:151–5.
64. Burney TL, Senapati M, Desai S, Choudhary ST, Badlani GH. Effects of cerebrovascular accident on micturition. Urol Clin North Am. 1996;23:483–90.
65. John G, Bardini C, Mégevand P, Combescure C, Dällenbach P. Urinary incontinence as a predictor of death after new-onset stroke: a meta-analysis. Eur J Neurol. 2016;23(10):1548–55.
66. Jawad SH, Ward AB, Jones P. Study of the relationship between premorbid urinary incontinence and stroke functional outcome. Clin Rehabil. 1999;13:447–52.
67. Brittain KR, Stroke RD. Urinary symptoms and depression in stroke survivors. Age Ageing. 1998;27(suppl 1):P72-c.
68. Marinkovic SP, Badlani G. Voiding and sexual dysfunction after cerebrovascular accidents. J Urol. 2001;165:359–70.
69. Roe B, Williams K, Palmer M. Bladder training for urinary incontinence in adults. Cochrane Database Syst Rev. 2004;1:CD001308.

70. Bottiggi KA, Salazar JC, Yu L, Caban-Holt AM, Ryan M, Mendiondo MS, et al. Long-term cognitive impact of anticholinergic medications in older adults. Am J Geriatr Psychiatry. 2006;14:980–4.
71. McKeage K. Propiverine: a review of its use in the treatment of adults and children with overactive bladder associated with idiopathic or neurogenic detrusor overactivity, and in men with lower urinary tract symptoms. Clin Drug Investig. 2013;33(1):71–91.
72. Gelber DA, Swords L. Treatment of post-stroke urinary incontinence (abstract). J Neurol Rehabil. 1997;11:131.
73. Sakakibara R, Tateno F, Yano M, Takahashi O, Sugiyama M, Ogata T, et al. Imidafenacin on bladder and cognitive function in neurologic OAB patients. Clin Auton Res. 2013;23(4):189–95.
74. Sakakibara, Tateno F, Yano M, Takahashi O, Sugiyama M, Ogata T, et al. Tolterodine activates the prefrontal cortex during bladder filling in OAB patients: a real-time NIRS-urodynamics study. Neurourol Urodyn. 2014;33(7):1110–1115.
75. Hunsballe JM, Djurhuus JC. Clinical options for imipramine in the management of urinary incontinence. Urol Res. 2001;29:118–25.
76. Sakakibara R, Ogata T, Uchiyama T, Kishi M, Ogawa E, Isaka S, et al. How to manage overactive bladder in elderly individuals with dementia? A combined use of donepezil, a central acetylcholinesterase inhibitor, and propiverine, a peripheral muscarine receptor antagonist. J Am Geriatr Soc. 2009;57(8):1515–7.
77. Kuo HC. Therapeutic effects of suburothelial injection of botulinum a toxin for neurogenic detrusor overactivity due to chronic cerebrovascular accident and spinal cord lesions. Urology. 2006;67:232–6.
78. Song FJ, Jiang SH, Zheng SL, Ye TS, Zhang H, Zhu WZ, et al. Electroacupuncture for post-stroke urinary incontinence: a multi-center randomized controlled study. Zhongguo Zhen Jiu. 2013;33(9):769–73.
79. Yu KW, Lin CL, Hung CC, Chou EC, Hsieh YL, Li TM, et al. Effects of electroacupuncture on recent stroke inpatients with incomplete bladder emptying: a preliminary study. Clin Interv Aging. 2012;7:469–74.
80. Amundsen CL, Romero AA, Jamison MG, Webster GD. Sacral neuromodulation for intractable urge incontinence: are there factors associated with cure? Urology. 2005;66:746–50.

Multiple System Atrophy

Ryuji Sakakibara

Introduction

Multiple system atrophy (MSA) is an uncommon but well-recognized disease entity that both neurologists and urologists may encounter. The term MSA was introduced by Graham and Oppenheimer in 1969 to describe a disorder of unknown cause affecting extrapyramidal, cerebellar, and autonomic pathways [1]. MSA includes the disorders previously called striatonigral degeneration (SND) [2], sporadic olivo-pontocerebellar atrophy (OPCA) [3], and Shy–Drager syndrome [4]. The discovery in 1989 of glial cytoplasmic inclusions in the brains of patients with MSA [5] provided a pathological marker for the disorder [akin to Lewy bodies in idiopathic Parkinson's disease (IPD)] and confirmed that SND, OPCA, and Shy–Drager syndrome are the same disease with differing clinical presentations. Immunocytochemistry showed that the glial cytoplasmic inclusions of MSA are ubiquitin-, tau-, and alpha-synuclein (SNCA)-positive, possibly representing a cytoskeletal alteration in glial cells that results in neuronal degeneration [6, 7]. SNCA is a presynaptic neuronal protein encoded by the *SNCA* gene located on chromosome 4. This protein appears to play a role in dopamine and other neurotransmitter metabolism, vesicle trafficking, modification of synaptic transmission, and regulation of membrane permeability. In contrast, pathologically increased expression and abnormal conformation of SNCA are reported to reduce neurotransmitter release by inhibiting synaptic vesicle reclustering after endocytosis [6, 7]. Familial occurrence is estimated to account for 1.6% of all cases, and data on such cases are being accumulated to identify candidate genes for this disorder, including *SNCA*, *MAPT* (microtubule-associated protein tau), etc.

R. Sakakibara
Department of Neurology, Internal Medicine, Sakura Medical Center,
Toho University, Sakura, Japan
e-mail: sakakibara@sakura.med.toho-u.ac.jp

© Springer International Publishing AG, part of Springer Nature 2018
R. Dmochowski, J. Heesakkers (eds.), *Neuro-Urology*,
https://doi.org/10.1007/978-3-319-90997-4_10

Autonomic failure (postural hypotension and urinary dysfunction) is fundamental to the diagnosis of MSA: it is diagnosed when the criteria of either postural hypotension (systolic blood pressure fall >30 mmHg or diastolic >15 mmHg) or urinary dysfunction (persistent, involuntary urinary incontinence/incomplete bladder emptying) or both are fulfilled, along with poorly levodopa-responsive parkinsonism or cerebellar dysfunction being fulfilled [8]. Based on the major motor deficits, MSA can be classified as MSA-P (parkinsonism-predominant) or MSA-C (cerebellar-predominant) [1]. Clinical differential diagnosis between MSA-P, the most common clinical form, and IPD is difficult even for specialists. However, the lack of one-side dominance and resting tremor, poor response to levodopa, and rapid progression are all red flags indicating MSA. MSA-C can mostly be distinguished from hereditary spinocerebellar ataxias, although some individuals with such disorders do not have apparent heredity. Autonomic failure (AF) is almost invariably present and can be an initial manifestation (AF-MSA).[9] Autonomic failure occurs in other neurodegenerative diseases, i.e., in a subset of patients with IPD (AF-PD) as well as in pure autonomic failure (PAF), both of which are considered Lewy body diseases. This chapter reviews the current concepts of urinary dysfunction in MSA, with particular reference to urinary symptoms, (video)urodynamic assessment and sphincter electromyography (EMG), and patient management.

Urinary Symptoms

Both Overactive Bladder and Large Post-Void Residuals Occur in MSA

The second consensus statement on the diagnosis of MSA recognizes that the disease frequently begins with bladder dysfunction (although erectile dysfunction usually precedes that complaint). Patients may present with urinary incontinence, urinary retention, or a combination of incontinence and incomplete bladder emptying [8]. It is important that other common causes of poor bladder control are excluded by a urologist or urogynecologist before the disorder is attributed to the neurological condition [10]. This is presumably because the disease process of MSA might start in the brain as well as in the sacral spinal cord (Fig. 1) [10]. Patients with MSA had significantly higher prevalence of daytime frequency (45% of women, 43% of men), nighttime frequency (65%, 69%), urinary urgency (64% of men), and urgency incontinence (75%, 66%) than did the controls. Symptom of urinary urgency/frequency is also referred to as overactive bladder (OAB) [11, 12]. They also had more hesitancy of micturition (62%, 73%); prolonged, poor (71%, 81%), or intermittent stream (61%, 47%); or the need to strain to void (48%, 55%). Of particular importance is that the quality of life (QOL) index in MSA group was significantly higher (i.e., worse) in MSA patients for bladder dysfunction (70%, 76%) than that in controls. Many of them show large post-void residual urine volume >100 ml. Therefore both overactive bladder and large post-void residuals are common in MSA.

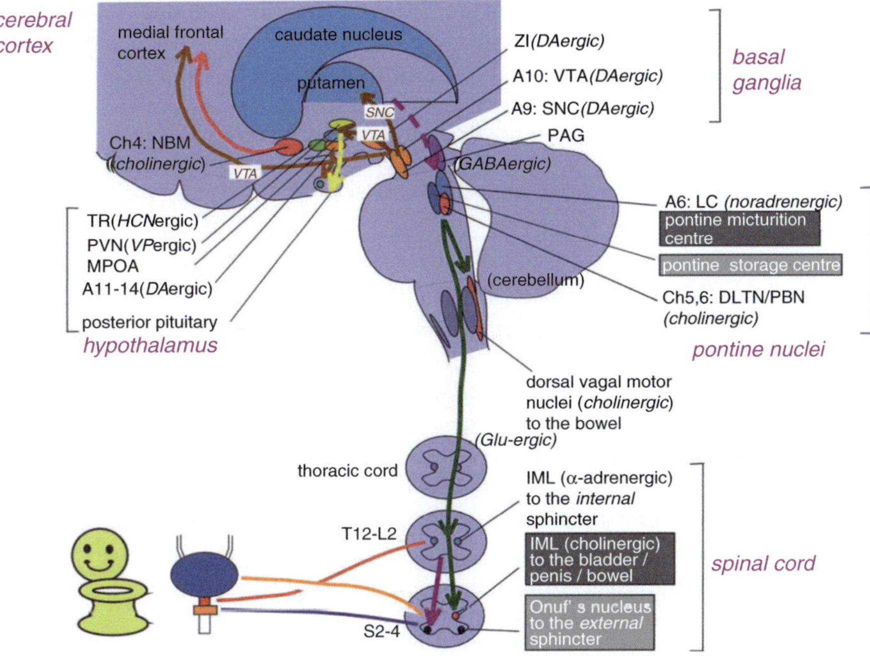

Fig. 1 Innervation of the lower urinary tract relevant to MSA. See text

Urinary Dysfunction Precedes Postural Hypotension

Of various symptoms of AF (erectile dysfunction, urinary dysfunction, postural hypotension, respiratory stridor) in patients with MSA, urinary dysfunction has attracted less attention than postural hypotension, although urinary dysfunction may result in recurrent urinary tract infection and cause morbidity. In addition, urinary incontinence results in impaired self-esteem, stress on the caregiver, and considerable financial cost. Postural hypotension was pointed out first in AF-MSA, which turned out to be a marker of autonomic involvement in this disorder. Both of the original two patients discussed by Shy and Drager had urinary frequency, incontinence, and urinary retention [4]. Other variants (MSA-P and MSA-C) rarely develop postural hypotension in their early stage. However, in the original reports, three of four patients with MSA-P showed voiding difficulty, retention, and urinary incontinence [2], and both patients with MSA-C had voiding difficulty and urinary incontinence [3]. Thus, what are the most common and earliest autonomic features of MSA?

In our previous study of 121 patients with MSA [13], urinary symptoms (96%) were more common than orthostatic symptoms (43%) ($p < 0.01$). The most frequent urinary symptom was difficulty voiding in 79% of the patients, followed by nocturnal urinary frequency in 74%. Other symptoms included sensation of urgency in 63%, urgency incontinence in 63%, diurnal urinary frequency in 45%, nocturnal enuresis in 19%, and urinary retention in 8%. The most frequent orthostatic symptom was postural faintness in 43%, followed by blurred vision in 38% and syncope in 19%. These figures are similar to those of Wenning et al. [14], who noted urinary incontinence in 71%, urinary retention in 27%, postural faintness in 53%, and syncope in 15% of 100 patients with MSA; these figures were recently confirmed by a larger study [15]. In our previous study mentioned above, among 53 patients with both urinary and orthostatic symptoms, those who had urinary symptoms first (48%) were more common than those who had orthostatic symptoms first (29%), and some patients developed both symptoms simultaneously (23%) [13].

These findings indicate that urinary dysfunction is a more common and often earlier manifestation than postural hypotension in MSA. Many factors might be involved in this phenomenon. Reports of focal lesions have shown that postural hypotension occurs in lesions below the medulla, whereas urinary dysfunction occurs in lesions at any sites in the neuraxis. MSA lesions involve the pons, the hypothalamus, and the basal ganglia, all of which might affect the lower urinary tract function as described below.

Urinary Dysfunction Also Precedes Motor Disorders

Looking at both urinary and motor disorders, we see that approximately 60% of patients with MSA develop urinary symptoms either prior to or at the time of presentation with the motor disorder [12, 13]. This indicates that many of these patients seek urological advice early in the course of their disease. Since the severity of urinary symptoms is severe enough for surgical intervention, male patients with MSA may undergo urological surgery for prostatic outflow obstruction before the correct diagnosis has been made. The results of such surgery are often transient or unfavorable because of the progressive nature of this disease. Male erectile dysfunction is often the first presentation [12, 13, 16], possibly preceding the occurrence of urinary dysfunction in MSA. The urologist confronted with a patient showing these features should be cautious about embarking on an operative approach. The neurologist encountering a patient with marked urinary symptoms might consider future investigation by brain magnetic resonance imaging (MRI) and sphincter EMG.

Since motor disorders in MSA mostly mimic those in IPD, the urogenital distinction between these two diseases is worth considering, although a number of earlier studies on "Parkinson's disease and the bladder" might inadvertently include patients with MSA. The prevalence rate of urinary dysfunction in MSA is higher than the 58–71% rate reported in IPD [13, 17–19]; similarly, that of urgency incontinence in MSA is higher than the 33% rate reported in IPD. In addition, urinary dysfunction is never the initial presentation in IPD.

Videourodynamic and Sphincter Electromyography Assessments

Since MSA is a neurodegenerative disease that affects multiple brain regions, patients with the disease may have a wide range of urodynamic abnormalities that change with progression of the illness. Videourodynamics and sphincter EMG also enable us to assess the lumbosacral cord functions, which help us distinguish MSA from other parkinsonian disorders.

Detrusor Overactivity

Filling phase abnormalities included bladder overactivity in 33–100% and uninhibited external sphincter relaxation in 33% of MSA [12, 19–21], figures similar to those reported in IPD [10, 12–16]. Bladder overactivity is urodynamically defined as an involuntary phasic increase in detrusor pressure (naïve bladder pressure—abdominal pressure) >10 cmH$_2$O during bladder filling, which is commonly associated with decreased bladder volumes at first sensation and bladder capacity. It is bladder overactivity that seems to be the major cause of urgency incontinence in patients with MSA. But when coupled with uninhibited sphincter relaxation, incontinence may worsen [22].

It is well-known that cerebral diseases can lead to a loss of the brain's inhibitory influence on the spino-bulbo-spinal micturition reflex. The information that arises from the lower urinary tract reaches the periaqueductal gray matter (PAG) and then goes down to the pontine micturition center (PMC), an area identical or just adjacent to the locus ceruleus, which then activates the descending pathway to the sacral preganglionic neurons innervating the bladder [23]. The basal ganglia are thought to be one of the higher centers for micturition, since lesions of this area lead to bladder overactivity [24–27]. Recent positron emission tomography (PET) studies have shown that the hypothalamus, PAG, midline pons, and cingulate cortex are activated during urinary filling [28, 29]. The central pathology of MSA includes neuronal loss of neuromelanin-containing cells in the locus ceruleus [30, 31] as well as in the nigrostriatal dopaminergic system ("putaminal slit sign") [6, 27] and cerebellum, and to a lesser extent in the pontomedullary raphe ("pontine cross sign") [6, 32] and the frontal cortex [33, 34]. Recent experimental studies have suggested that the raphe modulates micturition function [35]. Experimental studies have also suggested that the cerebellum controls micturition function [36]. A single-photon emission computed tomography (SPECT) study has shown that in the urinary storage and micturition phases, but not in the resting phase, activation of the cerebellar vermis was significantly lower in MSA patients than in control subjects [37]. These areas seem to be responsible for the occurrence of bladder overactivity and uninhibited sphincter relaxation in MSA patients.

Detrusor Underactivity and Detrusor-Sphincter Dyssynergia

Incomplete bladder emptying is a significant feature in MSA. In fact, 47% of patients with MSA had post-void residuals (PVR) >100 ml, whereas no patients with IPD had such levels ($p < 0.01$) [19]. The mean PVR volume was 71 ml in the first year, 129 ml in the second year (which exceeded the threshold volume for the start of clean intermittent catheterization (CIC)), and 170 ml in the fifth year from the onset of illness [38].

Factors relevant to voiding disorder in MSA include the bladder and the urethral outlet. Pressure-flow analysis refers to the simultaneous monitoring of detrusor pressure and urinary flow and to drawing the relation curve between them. Although it was originally developed for diagnosing outlet obstruction due to prostatic hypertrophy [39, 40], pressure-flow analysis is useful for evaluating neurogenic voiding difficulty [41].

Pressure-flow analysis showed that bladder underactivity (a weak detrusor contraction) during voiding is more common in MSA (71% in women and 63% in men) than in IPD (66% in women and 40% in men) [19]. The AG number represents a grade of urethral obstruction, and an AG number >40 means outflow obstruction in men [39]. The mean AG numbers were smaller in patients with MSA (12 in women and 28 in men) than in those with IPD (40 in women and 43) [19]. However, a subset of patients with MSA may have an obstructive pattern, the reason for which is unknown. Detrusor-external sphincter dyssynergia is a factor contributing to neurogenic urethral relaxation failure [41], which is noted in 47% of MSA patients [19, 42]. Therefore, it is likely that bladder underactivity accounts mostly for voiding difficulty and elevated PVR in MSA. A subset of patients with MSA has bladder overactivity during storage and underactivity during voiding (detrusor hyperactivity with impaired contractile function, DHIC) [43]. The exact mechanism of this phenomenon has yet to be ascertained. However, it has been recognized that the central mechanisms underlying bladder filling and voiding are distinct from each other; i.e., the area promoting micturition is located in the PMC and the frontal cortex, whereas that promoting urinary storage is in the pontine storage center, basal ganglia, raphe, and frontal cortex [23]. Lesions in these areas may cause various combinations of urinary filling and voiding disorders, such as DHIC.

Role of the Sympathetic System

Open Bladder Neck Suggesting Sympathetic Denervation

The bladder neck, also known as the internal (smooth) urethral sphincter, is a component in the maintenance of continence that is innervated by the sympathetic hypogastric nerve. Videourodynamic study is an established method for evaluating bladder neck function. It is a combination of visualizing the lower urinary tract simultaneously with EMG-cystometry; urethral pressure at the external urethral sphincter can be obtained with visual guidance using a radiopaque marker. In normal subjects, the bladder neck is closed throughout filling so as to avoid leaking. However, an open bladder neck is found in 46–100% of MSA patients and in 23–31% of PD patients, and an open bladder neck at the start of bladder filling, even without the accompaniment of bladder overactivity, was noted in no PD patients but in 53% of MSA patients ($p < 0.01$) [19]. Because open bladder neck is common in patients with myelodysplasia or a lower thoracic cord lesion at T12–L2 (where sympathetic thoracolumbar intermediolateral [IML] nuclei are located) and is reproduced by systemic or intraurethral application of alpha1-adrenergic blockers [44], it is likely that an open bladder neck reflects the loss of sympathetic innervation. This seems to be one of the exceptions to primary preganglionic pathology in MSA. An open bladder neck is usually considered asymptomatic but may cause incontinence and reduce bladder capacity.

Role of the Somatic System

Neurogenic Changes in Sphincter EMG Suggesting Somatic Denervation

A distinguishing pathology in MSA is neuronal cell loss in the Onuf nucleus, a group of anterior horn cells in the sacral spinal cord [6]. The first reports on neurogenic changes of external anal sphincter (EAS)-electromyography (EMG) in MSA are attributed to Sakuta et al. [45]. Since then, EAS-EMG results for over 600 MSA patients have been reported, with abnormality rates of more than 70% in many studies [46, 47]. EAS-EMG is better tolerated and yields identical results to those from EUS investigation [48]. Abnormalities have also been recorded in the bulbocavernosus muscles in MSA [49]. Figure 2a, b shows the method of sphincter EMG in clinical practice. A particular importance is not to miss the late components [50].

In our study of 84 probable MSA cases, 62% exhibited neurogenic change (Fig. 2c) [51]. The prevalence was relatively low presumably because up to 25% of our patients had a disease duration of 1 year or less. In such early cases, the diagnosis of MSA should be made with extreme caution. In addition to the clinical

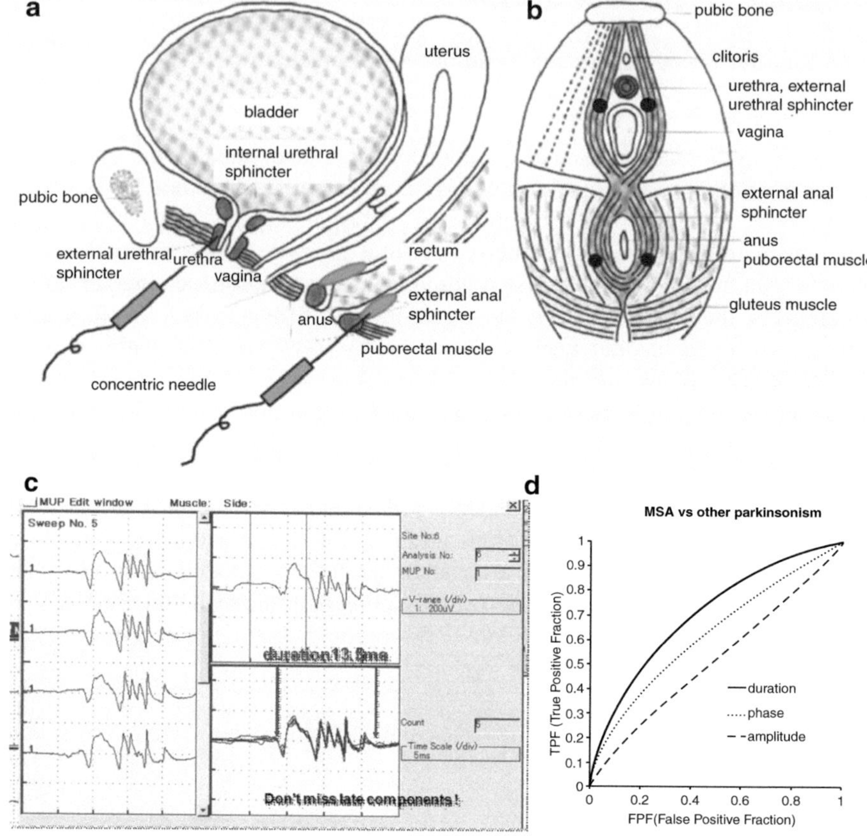

Fig. 2 External sphincter EMG in MSA. (**a**, **b**) The external anal sphincter and the external urethral sphincter. This figure illustrates where to insert concentric needles to measure external sphincter EMG. (**c**) A motor unit recorded from the anal sphincter of a patient with multiple system atrophy shows an abnormally prolonged duration (upper range of normal is <10 ms) and stable low-amplitude late components (*D* division, *EMG* electromyography, *MU* motor unit) (cited from Ref. [46]). (**d**) Receiver-operating characteristic analysis of sphincter EMG. This figure indicates high diagnostic power in terms of the duration of motor unit potentials (cited from Ref. [47])

diagnostic criteria, we usually add an imaging study, and we perform gene analysis to the extent possible. The prevalence of neurogenic change was 52% in the first year after disease onset, which increased to 83% by the fifth year ($p < 0.05$). Therefore, as expected, it is apparent that the involvement of Onuf's nucleus in MSA is time-dependent; and EAS-MUP abnormalities can distinguish MSA from idiopathic Parkinson's disease (PD) and other diseases in the first 5 years after disease onset. Receiver-operating characteristic analysis of sphincter EMG showed high diagnostic power in terms of the duration of motor unit potential (MUP) analysis (Fig. 2d) [47].

In contrast, in the early stages of illness, the prevalence of neurogenic change in MSA does not seem to be high. In only two patients who underwent repeated studies, the EAS-EMG findings tended to remain normal. We do not know whether some MSA patients never develop neurogenic change during the course of their illness. However, Wenning et al. (1994) reported three patients with normal EAS-EMG and a postmortem confirmation of MSA [14]. Therefore, a negative result cannot exclude a diagnosis of MSA. Paviour et al. (2005) reported that among 30 sets of clinical data and postmortem confirmation in MSA cases with a duration of more than 5 years, 24 (80%) had abnormal EAS-EMG, 5 (17%) had a borderline result, and only 1 had a normal EMG [52]. It has been reported that neurogenic change does not correlate directly with a clinically obvious functional deficit, although urinary incontinence was more severe in the patients with neurogenic change than in those without it ($p < 0.05$).

The prevalence of neurogenic change also increased with the severity of gait disturbance (wheelchair bound) ($p < 0.05$) in our study [51]. However, neurogenic change was not related to postural hypotension (reflecting adrenergic nerve dysfunction), erectile dysfunction in men (presumably reflecting cholinergic and nitrate oxidergic nerve dysfunction), detrusor overactivity (reflecting the central type of detrusor dysfunction), constipation (presumably reflecting both peripheral and central types of autonomic and somatic dysfunction), or gender [51]. The neurogenic change in EAS-MUP was slightly more common in those with detrusor-sphincter dyssynergia (DSD). More recently, it is suggested that not only suprasacral pathology but also sacral/peripheral lesions can produce DSD [53].

Although denervation can be found in the other skeletal muscles in MSA, it occurs much earlier in the external sphincter muscles [54]. This is in clear contrast to the case in amyotrophic lateral sclerosis, where denervation occurs in most advanced cases (respirator bound).

Changes of Bladder Patterns

Bladder Patterns Change from Central to Peripheral

The sites responsible for cardiovascular autonomic failure in MSA are mostly central, in contrast to the peripheral lesions in PAF [10]. However, 31–45% of patients with MSA also had low-compliance detrusor, defined as a maximum bladder capacity/tonic detrusor pressure increase <20 ml/cmH$_2$O [13]. Low-compliance detrusor is known to occur in patients with spina bifida or in animals with experimental cauda equina lesions, most probably reflecting neuronal loss of bladder preganglionic neurons in the sacral IML nucleus and their fibers (pelvic nerve) [55, 56]. The bethanechol test is the established method to detect lesions in the most peripheral site [57]. A minimum amount (2.5 mg) of bethanechol, a cholinergic agent, is injected subcutaneously; this amount is not sufficient to evoke bladder contraction in normal subjects. However, when the bladder is denervated, cholinergic receptor densities in the postsynaptic membrane increase, increasing abnormal detrusor pressure upon bethanechol injection. Nineteen percent of MSA patients showed denervation supersensitivity of the detrusor [13].

Repeated urodynamic studies in MSA patients showed that the cystometrogram changed from bladder overactivity to low-compliance or atonic detrusor and from negative to positive bethanechol supersensitivity [13]. In fact, as the disease progresses, symptoms may change from urinary urgency and frequency to those due to incomplete bladder emptying [12]. These findings suggest that the responsible sites of the bladder cholinergic disorder may change from the "center" (supranuclear) to the "periphery" (nuclear sacral IML and/or infranuclear) during the course of the illness. Since MSA primarily affects the preganglionic neurons in the autonomic nervous system [10], bladder findings that suggest postganglionic lesions might reflect transsynaptic degeneration of the cholinergic fibers.

Nocturnal Polyuria

Nocturnal Polyuria Also Occurs Suggesting Hypothalamic Dysfunction

Besides bladder disorders, patients with MSA may have nocturnal polyuria, which results in nocturnal urinary frequency and morning hypotension. In normal children over 7 years and adults, the circadian release of arginine vasopressin (AVP) from the posterior pituitary gland into plasma peaks at night. This leads to a nocturnal decrease in urine formation. The ratio of nighttime to daytime urine production is usually <1:2, which can be estimated by a frequency volume chart. This circadian rhythm can be impaired in cases of congestive heart failure, nephrosis, or cirrhosis with ascites. However, a postmortem study of the brains of patients with MSA revealed the degeneration of AVP neurons in the suprachiasmatic nucleus [49], leading to impairment of the circadian rhythm of the plasma AVP concentration in MSA [58, 59]. In addition, daytime postural hypotension may also cause nocturnal polyuria in patients with MSA [60]. This is probably due to a combination of factors that include compensatory supine hypertension at night, leading to increased glomerular filtration.

Management of Urinary Dysfunction

Clean, Intermittent Catheterization for Incomplete Bladder Emptying

More than half of patients with MSA have urinary dysfunction either prior to or at the time of presentation with motor disorder. Since many of these patients develop incomplete bladder emptying, they may be misdiagnosed as having prostatic hypertrophy. In fact, the results of urological surgery are rarely favorable, since bladder underactivity contributes more to voiding difficulty than does outflow obstruction. Therefore, it is important to avoid inappropriate urological surgery in patients with MSA [10]. In men with MSA, effects of transurethral resection of the prostate lasted for less than 2 years [38]. A conservative approach with medical measures to manage urinary problems can be effective.

Estimation of the PVR volume is a simple and useful test in patients with MSA; even though their urinary complaints are solely urinary urgency/frequency, they may be unaware that their bladders do not empty completely. PVR can be measured by ultrasound echography, either with specific machines (e.g., bladder manager BVI3000), abdominal echography (multiplied 3-direction diameters × 0.5), or transurethral catheterization. If the patient has a significant PVR and is symptomatic, this aspect of the problem should be managed using CIC performed by either the patient or the caregiver. However, in patients with advanced disease and severe neurological disability, a permanent indwelling catheter, either transurethral or suprapubic, or urosheath drainage may be required.

Drugs to Lessen Detrusor Overactivity

The bladder is innervated by the parasympathetic pelvic nerve and has an abundance of $M_{2/3}$ muscarinic receptors. Bladder overactivity may reflect an increased micturition reflex via either the brainstem or the sacral cord, which can be treated with anticholinergic medication such as tolterodine, oxybutynin, propiverine, or propantheline. These drugs diminish the parasympathetic tone on bladder smooth muscle and are usually tried in patients with urinary urgency and frequency. However, anticholinergic side effects, particularly dry mouth (probably mediated by M_3 receptors) and constipation ($M_2/_3$ receptors), may limit their use in a proportion of the patients. A subset of patients with MSA may develop mild cognitive decline at an advanced stage of the disease. Since the use of anticholinergic drugs carries a risk of cognitive impairment (M_1 receptors) [61], though this is much less common than the drugs' peripheral effects, we have to be careful to manage urinary dysfunction in such patients. Anticholinergic drugs do ameliorate urgency and frequency but may also reduce bladder contractility during voiding [11]. Therefore, PVR should be measured, and if it exceeds 100 ml, the medication should be withdrawn or preferably CIC should be added. If nighttime urinary urgency/frequency is the problem, a night balloon is a good alternative to drugs for patients who are performing CIC [38].

Interactions Between Drugs to Treat Bladder, Postural Hypotension, and Motor Disorder

Alpha-Adrenergic Receptors

Since incomplete bladder emptying in patients with MSA is due mostly to bladder underactivity, drugs acting on outflow obstruction are unlikely to benefit all patients. However, in some patients, alpha-adrenergic blockers may be effective in lessening

PVR volumes, due probably to detrusor-sphincter dyssynergia [62]. Uro-selective blockers such as tamsulosin and naftopidil may be of choice because they have fewer side effects such as postural hypotension. The effects of alpha-adrenergic blockers lasted for less than 2 years [38].

In contrast, the drugs most commonly used to treat postural hypotension in MSA are adrenergic agonists. However, administration of amezinium, an adrenergic drug, may increase the risk of retention and PVR volume compared to that before treatment [63]. Amezinium most probably stimulates the alpha receptors, both in the vascular wall ($alpha_{1B}$ receptors, particularly in the elderly [64]) and the proximal urethra ($alpha_{1A/D}$-adrenergic receptors).

Cholinergic Receptors

Both postural hypotension and bladder dysfunction are common clinical features in MSA. Pyridostigmine, an acetylcholinesterase inhibitor, can be effective in lessening PVR volumes, since it stimulates muscarinic acetylcholine receptors on the bladder (M2/3-muscarinic receptors) that are innervated by parasympathetic cholinergic neurons [65]. Pyridostigmine also lessens postural hypotension, presumably by enhancing nicotinic acetylcholine receptor transmission in the sympathetic ganglia [66, 67].

Dopaminergic Receptors

Whether centrally acting drugs, such as pergolide (a dopaminergic $D_{1/2}$-receptor agonist) for parkinsonism, might ameliorate urinary dysfunction in MSA has not been fully studied [68, 69]. Early untreated IPD patients with mild urgency and frequency tend to benefit from levodopa ($D_{1/2}$) treatment. However, in a 1-h time window, levodopa may augment bladder overactivity in early [70] or advanced [71] IPD patients. Since D_1 selective stimulation inhibits the micturition reflex whereas D_2 selective stimulation facilitates it, the balance of these stimulations may explain the various effects of the drugs. Levodopa ($D_{1/2}$) and its metabolites, such as norepinephrine (noradrenaline), may also contract the bladder neck by stimulating alpha1-adrenergic receptors [63].

Nocturnal Polyuria (Vasopressin Receptors)

Desmopressin is a potent analogue of AVP (hypertensive and antidiuretic effects 100 vs 100 in AVP; 0.39 vs 1200 in desmopressin, respectively), and it is used in the treatment of diabetes insipidus due to a loss of posterior pituitary AVP secretion. Mathias et al. [59] used 2–4 µg of intramuscular desmopressin in patients with autonomic failure including MSA. We also prescribed 5 µg of intranasal desmopressin once a night in MSA patients with impaired circadian rhythm of AVP and nocturnal polyuria, with benefit [72]. This small dose of desmopressin is unlikely to cause adverse effects. But hyponatremia and signs of cardiac failure should be checked for regularly. A tablet form is available and may be more convenient for patient use. Desmopressin could also ameliorate morning hypotension resulting from the abnormal loss of body fluid at night [59].

Micturition Syncope

Well-known triggers for syncope in MSA include (1) standing (postural syncope), (2) eating (postprandial syncope), and (3) exercise (post-exertional syncope) [10]. We found that syncope in patients with MSA is also triggered by (4) voiding (micturition syncope). In our patients, the systolic blood pressure increase was less pronounced during storage, whereas the systolic blood pressure decrease was significant during and after voiding as compared with control [73]. The detailed link between the bladder and the cardiovascular system is still uncertain in this condition. However, particularly in patients who experience abdominal strain upon voiding, CIC could lessen micturition syncope.

Bladder Management and Survival

Recent studies suggest that bladder management may directly, or indirectly, affect survival of MSA [74, 75]. Coon et al. suggested that while the initial onset with autonomic symptoms was not associated with shortened overall survival, early autonomic symptoms in disease course, particularly bladder symptoms and severe urinary symptoms (requiring urinary catheterization), negatively affected survival [74]. Since MSA is a progressive disease that leads to urinary retention, early differential diagnosis from Parkinson's disease is necessary in terms of catheterization [76].

Summary

Urinary dysfunction is a prominent autonomic feature in patients with MSA, and it is more common (above 90%) and occurs earlier than postural hypotension in this disorder. Since the clinical features of MSA may mimic those of IPD, a distinctive pattern of urinary dysfunction in both disorders is worth looking at. In contrast to IPD, MSA patients have more marked urinary dysfunction, which consists of both urgency incontinence and post-void residuals >100 ml. Videourodynamic and sphincter EMG analyses are important tools for understanding the extent of these dysfunctions and for determining both the diagnosis and management of the disorders. The common finding in both disorders is bladder overactivity, which accounts for urinary urgency and frequency. However, detrusor-sphincter dyssynergia, open bladder neck at the start of bladder filling (internal sphincter denervation), and neurogenic sphincter EMG (external sphincter denervation) are all characteristics of MSA. These features may reflect pathological lesions in the basal ganglia, pontine tegmentum, raphe, intermediolateral cell column, and sacral Onuf's nuclei. During the course of the disease, the pathophysiological balance shifts from central to peripheral, with bladder emptying disorder predominating.

Since MSA is a progressive disorder and impaired detrusor contractility is common, it is important to avoid inappropriate urological surgery in patients with MSA. A conservative approach with medical measures includes anticholinergics for urinary urgency and frequency, desmopressin for nocturnal polyuria, uro-selective alpha-blockers and cholinergic stimulants for voiding difficulty, and CIC for large PVR.

References

1. Graham JG, Oppenheimer DR. Orthostatic hypotension and nicotinic sensitivity in a case of multiple system atrophy. J Neurol Neurosurg Psychiatry. 1969;32:28–34.
2. Adams RD, van Bogaert L, Eecken HV. Striato–nigral degeneration. J Neuropathol Exp Neurol. 1964;23:584–608.
3. Dejerine J, Thomas A. L'atrophie olivo-ponto-cérébelleuse. Nouvelle Iconographie de la Salpêtriére. 1900;13:30–70.
4. Shy GM, Drager GA. A neurological syndrome associated with orthostatic hypotension; a clinical-pathologic study. Arch Neurol. 1960;2:511–27.
5. Papp MI, Kahn JE, Lantos PL. Glial cytoplasmic inclusions in the CNS of patients with multiple system atrophy (striatonigral degeneration, olivopontocerebellar atrophy and Shy–Drager syndrome). J Neurol Sci. 1989;94:79–100.
6. Ahmed Z, Asi YT, Sailer A, et al. The neuropathology, pathophysiology and genetics of multiple system atrophy. Neuropathol Appl Neurobiol. 2012;38:4–24.
7. Fernagut PO, Tison F. Animal models of multiple system atrophy. Neuroscience. 2012;211:77–82.
8. Gilman S, Wenning GK, Low PA, et al. Second consensus statement on the diagnosis of multiple system atrophy. Neurology. 2008;71:670–6.
9. The Consensus Committee of the American Autonomic Society and the American Academy of Neurology. Consensus statement on the definition of orthostatic hypotension, pure autonomic failure, and multiple system atrophy. Neurology. 1996;46:1470.
10. Chandiramani VA, Palace J, Fowler CJ. How to recognize patients with parkinsonism who should not have urological surgery. Br J Urol. 1997;80:100–4.
11. Yamamoto T, Sakakibara R, Uchiyama T, et al. Questionnaire-based assessment of pelvic organ dysfunction in multiple system atrophy. Mov Disord. 2009;24:972–8.
12. Abrams P, Cardozo L, Fall M, et al. The standardisation of terminology of lower urinary tract function: report from the standardisation sub-committee of the international continence society. Neurourol Urodyn. 2002;21:167–78.
13. Sakakibara R, Hattori T, Uchiyama T, et al. Urinary dysfunction and orthostatic hypotension in multiple system atrophy; which is the more common and earlier manifestation? J Neurol Neurosurg Psychiatry. 2000;68:65–9.
14. Wenning GK, Ben Shlomo Y, Magalhaes M, et al. Clinical features and natural history of multiple system atrophy: an analysis of 100 cases. Brain. 1994;117:835–45.

15. Gilman S, May SJ, Shults CW, et al. The north American multiple system atrophy study group. J Neural Transm. 2005;112:1687–94.
16. Kirchhof K, Apostolidis AN, Mathias CJ, et al. Erectile and urinary dysfunction may be the presenting features in patients with multiple system atrophy: a retrospective study. Int J Impot Res. 2003;15:293–8.
17. Christmas TJ, Chapple CR, Lees AJ, et al. Role of subcutaneous apomorphine in parkinsonian voiding dysfunction. Lancet. 1998;2:1451–3.
18. Fitzmaurice H, Fowler CJ, Richards D, et al. Micturition disturbance in Parkinson's disease. Br J Urol. 1985;57:652–6.
19. Sakakibara R, Hattori T, Uchiyama T, et al. Videourodynamic and sphincter motor unit potential analyses in Parkinson's disease and multiple system atrophy. J Neurol Neurosurg Psychiatry. 2001;71:600–6.
20. Berger Y, Salinas JM, Blaivas JG. Urodynamic differentiation of Parkinson disease and the Shy–Drager syndrome. Neurourol Urodyn. 1990;9:117–21.
21. Stocchi F, Carbone A, Inghilleri M, et al. Urodynamic and neurophysiological evaluation in Parkinson's disease and multiple system atrophy. J Neurol Neurosurg Psychiatry. 1997;62:507–11.
22. Sand PK, Bowen LW, Ostergard DR. Uninhibited urethral relaxation; an unusual cause of incontinence. Obstet Gynecol. 1986;68:645–8.
23. de Groat WC, Booth AM, Yoshimura N. Neurophysiology of micturition and its modification in animal models of human disease. In: Maggi CA, editor. The autonomic nervous system: nervous control of the urogenital system, vol. 3. London: Harwood Academic Publishers; 1993. p. 227–90.
24. Yoshimura N, Mizuta E, Kuno S, et al. The dopamine D1 receptor agonist SKF 38393 suppresses detrusor hyperreflexia in the monkey with parkinsonism induced by MPTP. Neuropharmacology. 1993;32:315–21.
25. Sakakibara R, Fowler CJ. Cerebral control of bladder, bowel, and sexual function and effects of brain disease. In: Fowler CJ, editor. Neurology of bladder, bowel, and sexual function. Boston: Butterworth-Heinemann; 1999. p. 229–43.
26. Sakakibara R, Nakazawa K, Uchiyama T, et al. Micturition-related electrophysiological properties in the substantia nigra pars compacta and the ventral tegmental area in cats. Auton Neurosci. 2002;102:30–8.
27. Yamamoto T, Sakakibara R, Hashimoto K, et al. Striatal dopamine level increases in the urinary storage phase in cats: an in vivo microdialysis study. Neuroscience. 2005;135:299–303.
28. Aswal BS, Berkley KJ, Hussain I, et al. Brain responses to changes in bladder volume and urge to void in healthy men. Brain. 2001;124:369–77.
29. Kavia RBC, Dasgupta R, Fowler CJ. Functional imaging and the central control of the bladder. J Comp Neurol. 2005;493:27–32.
30. Daniel SE. The neuropathology and neurochemistry of multiple system atrophy. In: Bannister R, Mathias CJ, editors. Autonomic failure. 3rd ed. Oxford: Oxford Medical Publications; 1992. p. 564–85.
31. Benarroch EE, Schmeichel AM. Depletion of corticotrophin-releasing factor neurons in the pontine micturition area in multiple system atrophy. Ann Neurol. 2001;50:640–5.
32. Benarroch EE, Schmeichel AM, Low PA, et al. Involvement of medullary serotonergic groups in multiple system atrophy. Ann Neurol. 2004;55:418–22.
33. Fujita T, Doi M, Ogata T, et al. Cerebral cortical pathology of sporadic olivopontocerebellar atrophy. J Neurol Sci. 1993;116:41–6.
34. Andrew J, Nathan PW. Lesions of the anterior frontal lobes and disturbances of micturition and defaecation. Brain. 1964;87:233–62.
35. Ito T, Sakakibara R, Nakazawa K, et al. Effects of electrical stimulation of the raphe area on the micturition reflex in cats. Neuroscience. 2006;142(4):1273–80. [Epub ahead of print] PMID: 16996219

36. Nishizawa O, Ebina K, Sugaya K, et al. Effect of cerebellectomy on reflex micturition in the decerebrate dog as determined by urodynamic evaluation. Urol Int. 1989;44:152–6.
37. Sakakibara R, Uchida Y, Uchiyama T, et al. Reduced cerebellar vermis activation in response to micturition in multiple system atrophy; 99mTc-labeled ECD SPECT study. Eur J Neurol. 2004;11:705–8.
38. Ito T, Sakakibara R, Yasuda K, et al. Incomplete emptying and urinary retention in multiple system atrophy: when does it occur and how do we manage it? Mov Disord. 2006;21(6):816–23. [Epub ahead of print] PMID: 16511861
39. Abrams P. Objective evaluation of bladder outlet obstruction. Br J Urol. 1995;76(Suppl 1):11–5.
40. Shäfer W. Principles and clinical application of advanced urodynamic analysis of voiding dysfunction. Urol Clin North Am. 1990;17:553–66.
41. Sakakibara R, Fowler CJ, Hattori T, et al. Pressure-flow study as an evaluating method of neurogenic urethral relaxation failure. J Auton Nerv Syst. 2000;80:85–8.
42. Blaivas JG, Sinha HP, Zayed AAH, et al. Detrusor-sphincter dyssynergia; a detailed electromyographic study. J Urol. 1981;125:545–8.
43. Yamamoto T, Sakakibara R, Uchiyama T, et al. Neurological diseases that cause detrusor hyperactivity with impaired contractile function. Neurourol Urodyn. 2006;25:356–60.
44. Yamanishi T, Yasuda K, Sakakibara R, et al. The effectiveness of terazosin, an al-blocker, on bladder neck obstruction as assessed by urodynamic hydraulic energy. BJU Int. 2000;85:249–53.
45. Sakuta M, Nakanishi T, Toyokura Y. Anal muscle electromyograms differ in amyotrophic lateral sclerosis and Shy–Drager syndrome. Neurology. 1978;28:1289–93.
46. Sakakibara R, Uchiyama T, Yamanishi T, et al. Sphincter EMG as a diagnostic tool in autonomic disorders. Clin Auton Res. 2009;19:20–31.
47. Yamamoto T, Sakakibara R, Uchiyama T, et al. Receiver operating characteristic analysis of sphincter electromyography for parkinsonian syndrome. Neurourol Urodyn. 2012;31:1128–34.
48. Beck RO, Betts CD, Fowler CJ. Genitourinary dysfunction in multiple system atrophy: clinical features and treatment in 62 cases. J Urol. 1994l;151:1336–41.
49. Ozawa T, Oyanagi K, Tanaka H, et al. Suprachiasmal nucleus in a patient with multiple system atrophy with abnormal circadian rhythm of arginine vasopressin secretion into plasma. J Neurol Sci. 1998;154:116–21.
50. Podnar S, Fowler CJ. Sphincter electromyography in diagnosis of multiple system atrophy: technical issues. Muscle Nerve. 2004;29:151–6.
51. Yamamoto T, Sakakibara R, Uchiyama T, et al. When is Onuf's nucleus involved in multiple system atrophy? A sphincter electromyography study. J Neurol Neurosurg Psychiatry. 2005;76:1645–8.
52. Paviour DC, Williams DC, Fowler CJ, et al. Is sphincter electromyography a helpful investigation in the diagnosis of multiple system atrophy? A retrospective study with pathological diagnosis. Mov Disord. 2005;20:1425–30.
53. Takahashi O, Sakakibara R, Tsunoyama K, et al. Do sacral/peripheral lesions contribute to detrusor-sphincter dyssynergia? LUTS. 2012;4:126–9.
54. Pramstaller PP, Wenning GK, Smith SJM, et al. Nerve conduction studies, skeletal muscle EMG, and sphincter EMG in multiple system atrophy. J Neurol Neurosurg Psychiatry. 1995;580:618–21.
55. Morgan C, Nadelhaft I, de Groat WC. Location of bladder preganglionic neurones within the sacral parasympathetic nucleus of the cat. Neurosci Lett. 1979;14:189–94.
56. Skehan AM, Downie JW, Awad SA. The pathophysiology of contractile activity in the chronic decentralized feline bladder. J Urol. 1993;149:1156–64.
57. Lapides J, Friend CR, Ajemian EP, et al. Denervation supersensibility as a test for neurogenic bladder. Surg Gynecol Obstet. 1962;114:241–4.
58. Ozawa T, Tanaka H, Nakano R, et al. Nocturnal decrease in vasopressin secretion into plasma in patients with multiple system atrophy. J Neurol Neurosurg Psychiatry. 1999;67:542–5.

59. Mathias CJ, Fosbraey P, DaCosta DF, et al. The effect of desmopressin on nocturnal polyuria, overnight weight loss, and morning postural hypotension in patients with autonomic failure. BMJ. 1986;293:353–6.

60. Wilcox CS, Aminoff MJ, Penn W. Basis of nocturnal polyuria in patients with autonomic failure. J Neurol Neurosurg Psychiatry. 1974;37:677.

61. Donnellan CA, Fook L, McDonald P, et al. Oxybutynin and cognitive dysfunction. BMJ. 1997;315:1363–4.

62. Sakakibara R, Hattori T, Uchiyama T, et al. Are alpha-blockers involved in lower urinary tract dysfunction in multiple system atrophy? A comparison of prazosin and moxisylyte. J Auton Nerv Syst. 2000;79:191–5.

63. Sakakibara R, Uchiyama T, Asahina M, et al. Amezinium metilsulfate, a sympathomimetic agent, may increase the risk of urinary retention in multiple system atrophy. Clin Auton Res. 2003;13(1):51–3.

64. Schwinn DA. Novel role for alpha 1-adrenergic receptor subtypes in lower urinary tract symptoms. BJU Int. 2000;86(Suppl 2):11–22.

65. Yamanishi T, Yasuda K, Kamai T, et al. Combination of a cholinergic drug and an alpha-blocker is more effective than monotherapy for the treatment of voiding difficulty in patients with underactive detrusor. Int J Urol. 2004;11:88–96.

66. Sandroni P, Opfer-Gehrking TL, Singer W, et al. Pyridostigmine for treatment of neurogenic orthostatic hypertension. A follow-up survey study. Clin Auton Res. 2005;15:51–3.

67. Yamamoto T, Sakakibara R, Yamanaka Y, et al. Pyridostigmine in autonomic failure: can we treat postural hypotension and bladder dysfunction with one drug? Clin Auton Res. 2006;16:296–8.

68. Yamamoto M. Pergolide improves neurogenic bladder in patients with Parkinson's disease. Movem Dis. 1997;12(Suppl):328.

69. Kuno S, Mizutaa E, Yamasakia S, et al. Effects of pergolide on nocturia in Parkinson's disease: three female cases selected from over 400 patients. Parkinsonism Relat Disord. 2004;10:181–7.

70. Uchiyama T, Sakakibara R, Yamanishi T, et al. Short-term effect of l-dopa on the micturitional function in patients with Parkinson's disease. Mov Disord. 2003;18:573–8.

71. Brusa L, Petta F, Pisani A, et al. Central acute D2 stimulation worsens bladder function in patients with mild Parkinson's disease. J Urol. 2006;175:202–6.

72. Sakakibara R, Matsuda S, Uchiyama T, et al. The effect of intranasal desmopressin on nocturnal waking in urination in multiple system atrophy patients with nocturnal polyuria. Clin Auton Res. 2003;13:106–8.

73. Uchiyama T, Sakakibara R, Asahina M, et al. Post-micturitional hypotension in patients with multiple system atrophy. J Neurol Neurosurg Psychiatry. 2005;76:186–90.

74. Coon EA, Sletten DM, Suarez MD, et al. Clinical features and autonomic testing predict survival in multiple system atrophy. Brain. 2015;138:3623–31.

75. Figueroa JJ, Singer W, Parsaik A, et al. Multiple system atrophy: prognostic indicators of survival. Mov Disord. 2014;29:1151–7.

76. Sakakibara R, Panicker J, Finazzi-Agro E, et al. A guideline for the management of bladder dysfunction in Parkinson's disease and other gait disorders. Neurourol Urodyn. 2015. https://doi.org/10.1002/nau.22764. [Epub ahead of print]

Part III
Diagnostics

Neuro-urological History and Clinical Examination

Hazel Ecclestone and Rizwan Hamid

Abbreviations

BMI	Body mass index
CNS	Central nervous system
EAU	European Association of Urology
MS	Multiple sclerosis
NICE	National Institute for Health and Care Excellence
QoL	Quality of life
SCI	Spinal cord injury

History Taking

As with most medical conditions, history taking is the cornerstone of evaluation of neuro-urological conditions. A thorough history should not only aim to elicit current symptomatology but should also include past history of disorders, as well as future aims and expectations of the patient. Assessment should be holistic as a variety of associated impairments will affect treatment options. Finally it is sensible to ascertain the degree of bother the patient experiences from their neuro-urological symptoms to establish whether treatment risk outweighs benefits and to track effectiveness of treatment.

Current history should include a specific urinary history along with current medication; current mobility (including ability to transfer to a toilet/commode); hand, cognitive and visual function; as well as presence or absence of bowel and sexual dysfunction. Social support including formal or informal carers should be established.

H. Ecclestone
University College London Hospitals, London, UK

R. Hamid (✉)
Department of Neurourology, Spinal Injuries Unit, Stanmore/London, UK

University College London Hospitals, London, UK

© Springer International Publishing AG, part of Springer Nature 2018 155
R. Dmochowski, J. Heesakkers (eds.), *Neuro-Urology*,
https://doi.org/10.1007/978-3-319-90997-4_11

Table 1 Examples of neurological conditions that can affect lower urinary tract function

	Congenital and perinatal conditions	Acquired stable conditions	Acquired, progressive or degenerative conditions
Brain conditions	Cerebral palsy	Stroke Head injury	Multiple sclerosis Parkinson's disease Dementia Multiple system atrophy
Suprasacral spinal cord conditions	Spinal dysraphism (such as myelomeningocoele)	Spinal cord injury	Multiple sclerosis Cervical spondylosis with myelopathy
Sacral spinal cord or peripheral nerve conditions	Spinal dysraphism Sacral agenesis Anorectal anomalies	Cauda equina syndrome Spinal cord injury Peripheral nerve injury from radical pelvic surgery	Peripheral neuropathy

Adapted from NICE guidelines on urinary incontinence in neurological disease [1]

Urinary history should include symptoms related to storage and voiding. The onset of urological symptoms is also of interest. Bladder sensation should be asked about as well as how the patient initiates micturition. The void time, flow and intermittency should be elicited as well as sensations of incomplete emptying. Presence and precipitants of incontinence should be noted. The mode of emptying (catheter/spontaneous) is also a key point.

Red flag symptoms are important to identify and include haematuria, urinary tract infection, pain or fevers. The presence of these symptoms warrants further investigation.

Past medical history. Important features in this include childhood and adolescent urological history, including a personal or family history of urolithiasis. Nature and duration of the underlying neurological condition should be assessed, including the likely clinical course of the disease. The classification of major neurological conditions that can give rise to neuro-urological symptoms is detailed in Table 1. A history of other medical co-morbidities should also be sought. In females obstetric and gynaecological history should be asked about, and fertility aims should be discussed in both sexes. A thorough past surgical history should be documented, including previous abdominal and pelvic surgery along with surgery involving the CNS or spine.

Bowel and sexual history. In patients with neuro-urological symptoms, both bowel and sexual dysfunction are common; not addressing these can lead to significant effects on patients' quality of life. It is therefore important to ask about faecal incontinence, constipation, defaecation pattern and bowel management.

It is also important to ask males about erectile function and ejaculation and both sexes about presence or absence of orgasm.

Quality of life assessment. A baseline quality of life assessment is useful, and there are a number of disease-specific quality of life validated question-

Table 2 Disease-specific patient questionnaires used to assess QoL in patients with neuro-urological complaints

Questionnaire	Underlying neurological disorder	Bladder	Bowel	Sexual function
FAMS	MS	X		X
FILMS	MS	X	X	
HAQUAMS	MS	X	X	X
IQOL	MS, SCI	X		X
MDS	MS	X	X	
MSISQ-15/MSISQ-19	MS	X	X	X
MSQLI	MS	X	X	X
MSQoL-54	MS	X	X	X
MSWDQ	MS	X	X	
NBSS	MS, SCI, congenital neurogenic bladder	X		
QoL-BM	SCI		X	
Qualiveen/ SF-Qualiveen	MS, SCI	X		X
RAYS	MS	X		X
RHSCIR	SCI	X	X	X
Fransceschini	SCI	X	X	X

Adapted from EAU guidelines on neuro-urology [2]

naires available (Table 2). These can then be repeated to assess response to treatment.

Finally it is important to elucidate what symptoms are bothersome to the patient and what their expectations for management are. It is important to gauge patients' psychological willingness to engage with medical treatment and also the acceptability of the side effects of various treatments (such as intermittent catheterisation). Without adequate adherence to a bladder management regime, many patients are at risk not only of renal deterioration but also complications such as bladder stones and urinary tract infection.

At the same time, considerable attention should be given to the social circumstance and the support network available including both family and social services for optimal planning of the management strategies.

Clinical Examination

A thorough physical examination can be very useful in determining the likely pattern of neuro-urological dysfunction. Overall a thorough examination should include a general examination, a urological examination and a neurological examination.

Physical examination should include mobility status and gait, ability to transfer as well as gross hand function. An idea of cognitive impairment is useful to ascertain, and visual function may also be impaired in some individuals. Patients should routinely have their body mass index (BMI) measured, as BMI can have an impact on treatment options and success. Patients with impaired sensation are also at risk of pressure sores, and a careful examination of the sacrum and ischial tuberosities as well as any other pressure-bearing areas is useful. Some neurological conditions, such as high spinal cord injury, are associated with a marked drop in blood pressure with changes in posture, and a baseline lying and sitting blood pressure can be useful in deciding on safe bladder management options.

Urological examination. Urologically it is prudent to examine the abdomen and external genitalia as well as performing vaginal or rectal examination.

When examining the abdomen, it is useful to note presence of obesity, previous surgical scars or abdominal distension. Palpation aims to identify abdominal masses, especially an enlarged bladder or kidneys, as well as eliciting tenderness.

The presence of indwelling catheters should be noted. If indwelling catheters are inserted urethrally, it is important to look for urethral trauma and erosion (traumatic hypospadias in males and patulous urethra in females).

Digital rectal examination is useful to assess anal tone but has the advantage in males of also allowing assessment of the prostate gland.

In females a focused pelvic examination should be performed looking for stress urinary incontinence and quantifying pelvic floor tone (Table 3 describes the ICS grading system of pelvic floor muscle tone). Furthermore females with neurological conditions are at risk of pelvic organ prolapse that should be assessed as this may be responsible for symptoms and also has important implications for future management.

Neurological examination includes the above points (mobility, hand function, cognition, visual acuity) as well as presence or absence of limb weakness or paralysis, with or without spasticity, all of which can affect ability to transfer on and off a toilet or perform self-catheterisation without assistance. Neurological examination should also document sensation, especially in S2–S5 dermatomes (light touch and pinprick), reflexes (sacral, knee and ankle jerk), muscle tone (anal sphincter) and strength of muscle contraction of the anal sphincter and pelvic floor.

A focused neuro-urological examination primarily concentrates on lumbar and sacral segment function, looking both at sensory and motor components. Figure 1 details lumbosacral dermatomes, cutaneous nerves and reflexes.

Table 3 Pelvic floor muscle tone assessment

Grade	Description
Absent	No contraction palpated or present
Weak	Weak contraction palpated
Normal	Normal contraction palpated
Strong	Strong contraction palpated

Adapted from the International Continence Society grading [3]

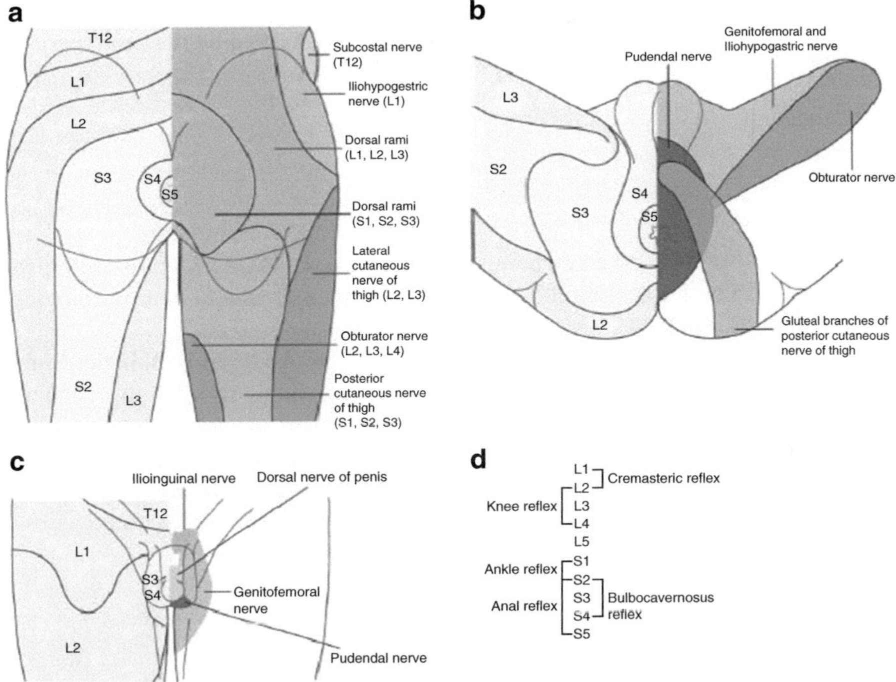

Fig. 1 Lumbosacral dermatomes, cutaneous nerves and reflexes [2]

Sacral Reflexes

Sacral reflexes are motor responses evoked following sensory stimulation of the perineum. Stimulation can be elicited physically or electrically. The three most commonly used in clinical practice are detailed below, with the sacral segments they assess in parentheses.

- *Bulbospongiosus/bulbocavernosus (S2/S3)*—the dorsal nerve of the penis is stimulated, e.g. by squeezing the glans penis, and a motor response in the bulbo-spongiosus muscle is observed for. This muscle is located between the scrotum and anal sphincter. The sensitivity of this test is not fully known and its clinical utility is therefore uncertain.
- *Bulboanal (S3/S4)*—again this reflex uses stimulation of the dorsal nerve of the penis but looks at the motor response of the anal sphincter. This is technically easier to perform clinically and therefore is more widely utilised clinically.
- *Anal wink (S4/S5)* stimulation of the S5 dermatome—by stroking the skin adjacent to the anus, it causes a reflex contraction. This reflex tests the lowest nerve roots of the sacral segment.

Absence of sacral reflexes indicates damage to the sacral nerves or sacral spinal cord and can predict the type of bladder dysfunction likely to be present (suprasacral or infrasacral bladder).

Summary

Table 4 below highlights the key points to consider when taking a neuro-urological history, with Table 5 detailing the key points to remember about neuro-urological examination.

In summary a full neuro-urological assessment should be truly holistic. Many neurological conditions affect multiple organ systems, and these will impact on possible treatment options. The social situation and support of the patient is equally important. Most important is to establish a good relationship with the patient, as without their investment and compliance, the outcome is likely to be unsatisfactory for all involved. Key to developing a good long-term relationship is a careful assessment of an individual's future aims and expectations.

Table 4 Key points in history

Past history	Childhood/adolescent history
	Neurological history
	Nature and course of disease
	Obstetric history (female)
	Surgical history (CNS, abdominal, pelvic)
Current history	Mobility, hand/visual/cognitive function
	Medication
	QoL
	Social situation
Neurological history	Underlying condition
	Acquired or congenital
	Stable or progressive
	Spasticity
Urological history	Voiding method (use of catheter)
	Bladder sensation
	Initiation of micturition, interruption to void
	Frequency, voided volume
	Incontinence/enuresis
	Incomplete emptying
	Red flags (haematuria, UTI, pain)
Bowel history	Bowel management regime
	Initiation of defaecation
	Rectal sensation
	Faecal incontinence/urgency
Sexual history	Genital sensation
	Male—erectile, ejaculatory and orgasm
	Female—dyspareunia, orgasm

Table 5 Key points in examination

Neurological	Sensation	Pinprick/light touch S2–S5—present/absent/altered
	Reflexes	Knee jerk (L3/L4) Ankle jerk (S1/S2) Sacral reflexes (S2/S5)
	Motor function	Anal sphincter tone Voluntary contraction anal sphincter/levator ani
Urological	External	Abdominal—palpable bladder/kidney Abdominal mass, tenderness, distension, scar Presence of catheter External genital examination
	Internal	Male—prostate examination Female—pelvic organ prolapse

Conclusion

The neuro-urologist primarily strives to prevent deterioration of the upper urinary tract, as well as instigating management that is both safe and acceptable to the patient. The difficulty comes when patient and physician expectations do not meet. Holistic assessment is the cornerstone in evaluating neuro-urology patients. A thorough history and examination allows the neuro-urologist to assess what is feasible in terms of management options, as well as evaluating patients' desires and wishes.

References

1. NICE guideline panel 2012. Urinary incontinence in neurological disease: assessment and management, available from https://www.nice.org.uk/guidance/cg148/resources/urinary-incontinence-in-neurological-disease-assessment-and-management-pdf-35109577553605. Accessed 1 Nov 2017.
2. Blok B, Pannek P, Castro-Diaz D, et al. European Association of Urology (EAU) guidelines on neuro-urology. Presented at the EAU Annual Congress London; 2017. 978-90-79754-91-5. Arnhem, The Netherlands: EAU Guidelines Office.
3. Messelink B, Benson T, Berghmans B, et al. Standardization of terminology of pelvic floor muscle function and dysfunction: report from the pelvic floor clinical assessment group of the International Continence Society. Neurourol Urodyn. 2005;24(4):374.

Practice of Urodynamics in Patients with Neurogenic Lower Urinary Tract Dysfunction

Peter F. W. M. Rosier

Introduction

Neurological diseases affect the nervous system, however, with consequences for the organs or structures that the affected nerve(s) innervate. Nerve damage may not only cause loss of sensation and/or paralysis and/or autonomic dysfunction but also pain and spasticity.

The lower urinary tract is innervated by the somatosensory system and also by the autonomic nervous system. As is explained in other chapters, urinary storage and voiding are autonomic reflexes that are modulated (or 'overruled') by the sensory and somatic nervous system. This modulation of an autonomic reflex is not unique for the lower urinary tract because (autonomic) reflexes like coughing or eye-blinking can be inhibited by (somatosensory) will to a certain extent as well.

If a neurological lesion occurs in one or more of the nerves from and to the lower urinary tract, both functions of the bladder and its outlet may be altered. Pure autonomic failure will affect (sympathetic bladder neck/sphincter) closure and continence function and also (parasympathetic detrusor dome) volume increase adaptation and voiding function. Somatosensory dysfunction shall affect the voluntary inhibition of the voiding reflex as well as the sustained continuous relaxation of the striated pelvic floor muscle outlet to initiate or continue the micturition reflex. Furthermore, bladder filling, muscle stretch sensation (detrusor muscle spindle—proprioceptis) as well as urinary passage sensation may be lost or be diminished. Needless to mention that also sexual dysfunction or lower bowel (anal) dysfunction may be present with any disease that affects the lower urinary tract. Discussion of sexual or bowel dysfunction is however outside the scope of this chapter.

P. F. W. M. Rosier
Department of Urology C.04.236, University Medical Center Utrecht, Utrecht, The Netherlands
e-mail: p.f.w.m.rosier@umcutrecht.nl

© Springer International Publishing AG, part of Springer Nature 2018
R. Dmochowski, J. Heesakkers (eds.), *Neuro-Urology*,
https://doi.org/10.1007/978-3-319-90997-4_12

Almost all neurological diseases can have an effect on the lower urinary tract; very local neurology as, e.g. carpal tunnel syndrome, thoracic outlet syndrome or trigeminal neuralgia, is some of the exceptions. Central neurological diseases affect 'higher centres of control' for the lower urinary tract and shall usually also affect mobility. Frontal, periaqueductal and pontine centres are well known in relation to lower urinary tract function and last but not least the spinal nucleus of Onuf in the medullary cone. Peripheral nerves to the lower urinary tract may be damaged, most frequently by trauma or surgery in the lower abdomen, which will result in dysfunction.

The most prevalent neurological abnormality that is congenital is meningomyelocele. If meningomyelocele is the case, the innervation to the lower urinary tract is disturbed already before birth, with obvious potential consequences for the prenatal development of the bladder as well as the ureterovesical junction, the bladder outlet and the pelvic floor muscles, partially determining the dysfunction in later life.

Traumatic spinal cord lesion, or other (e.g. surgical) lesion of the cord, is a prevalent cause of acquired neurological disease, and multiple sclerosis and Parkinson's disease are also well known for their association with lower urinary tract dysfunction. Some patients have a history of lower urinary tract dysfunction or symptoms, before the onset of the neurological disease and unravelling of the primary dysfunction and the effect of the neurological disease may be difficult or impossible in those.

Urodynamic investigation and tests may be used for the objective diagnosis of dysfunction when a neurological diagnosis—deemed to be relevant for lower urinary tract dysfunction—is established. Especially when sensory loss is one of the signs of the disease and/or dysfunction, the symptoms may not be very reliable. Specific scores that measure the burden of disease of patients with neurogenic dysfunction of the lower urinary tract, which may have some relevance in outcome research, are available. However it is never precisely established whether signs or symptoms of the lower urinary tract, in combination with the neurological diagnosis, are more or less reliable towards the dysfunction diagnosis in patients with neurogenic dysfunction than in patients without neurogenic dysfunction.

Urodynamic Investigation

Spinal Cord Injury

Without exception, the clinical practice guidelines recommend (invasive) urodynamic investigation for the diagnosis of lower urinary tract function, for every patient with spinal cord injury (SCI). Especially relatively unnoticed or asymptomatic, long periods of high intravesical pressure pose a risk to the upper urinary tract. Urodynamic investigation, more precisely cystometry, is not only relevant for initial diagnosis after the injury but also in the follow-up. Urodynamic investigation is recommended to optimise management with regard to the prevention of upper urinary tract damage and to aid with management advices with regard to (in-) continence and bladder emptying. There is however no unanimity on how frequently urodynamic control should be performed in the follow-up, and further discussion of this is not in the scope of this chapter.

Multiple Sclerosis

Almost all patients that have multiple sclerosis (or other demyelinating disease) will have lower urinary tract dysfunction at a certain stage. Sensation, voiding reflex inhibition and low-pressure storage as well as synergic and effective voiding are all prone to alterations as the consequence of the nerve damage. Urodynamic investigation may also uncover unnoticed post-voiding residual (e.g. as a cause of frequent and/or urgent voiding).

Parkinson's Disease

Parkinson's disease (and variants) is one of the central neurological diseases that has also more or less influence on the autonomic nervous system. The lower urinary dysfunction may be caused by this autonomic dysfunction and/or by the somatosensory dysfunction. However because Parkinson's disease affects older persons, the other diseases of advanced life such as benign prostatic obstruction or stress urinary incontinence may alone or in combination play a role. Signs and symptoms may be unable to unravel the precise cause of the dysfunction in this situation, but also the results of urodynamic investigation should be precisely interpreted and combined with the results of clinical examination as, e.g. prostate size and/or pelvic floor muscle tone.

Some specific practice elements of urodynamic investigation for persons with a neurological disease and signs and/or symptoms of lower urinary tract dysfunction are provided here below, without discussing indications and/or follow-up interval of urodynamic investigation and other exams. Here it is emphasised that urodynamic investigation should be performed only after appropriate indication, clinical exam, laboratory exam and voiding diary, and further refer to the clinical practice guidelines and/or the other chapters of this book for this.

Preparation

The patient should be properly informed about the test while this is ordered. It is advisable that the patient carries extra continence material and/or (condom) catheters, if relevant, to the urodynamics lab. The person performing urodynamics should be informed about the 'usual' emptied bladder volumes or 'capacity' on the basis of a diary that includes catheterisation and/or voiding or incontinence frequency and volumes, as well as volumes of fluid intake. These volumes should give a basis for the anticipation of cystometry volume. The values are however also relevant to estimate a total amount of high intravesical pressure. (An example is: cystometry can show that intravesical pressure rises to high levels beginning at 60% of the usual catheterisation volume; it can thus be concluded that in an estimated 40% of the daily lifetime of that person, the pressure is high.)

The patient should also be instructed on the continuation of the usual medication. LUT dysfunction is chronic, and whereas the urodynamic investigation should allow estimation on upper tract risk, it is preferable to take all medication as usual, to optimally replicate the 'daily life situation' during the urodynamic investigation and make an adequate risk estimation as was mentioned here above.

Usually no prophylaxis is needed for invasive urodynamic investigation especially since the predominance of the patients already performs clean intermittent catheterisation—or may have an indwelling catheter; sterile catheterisation for urodynamic investigation will not put a patient at extra risk for UTI in this regard. Patients should also be specifically instructed for the use of antibiotics; patients on antibiotic prophylaxis can usually continue this. Patients should also be instructed to use laxatives as usual or empty their bowel as usual. The specific prescription of laxatives before urodynamic investigation, in a patient not accustomed to this, will give extra bowel irritation and will interfere with the representativeness (and also the readability) of the urodynamic investigation.

The equipment for tests will be standard urodynamic machinery, with at least two pressure channels and a pressure subtraction channel. Furthermore a filling pump and a flowmeter are useful. The value and applicability of pelvic muscle surface EMG for urodynamic investigation and diagnosis of patients with neurological abnormalities are not very well documented, but the feature will be available on most of the machines.

Many patients with neurogenic dysfunction will not be able to void by will (in daily life), and it might be considered to perform urodynamic investigation while the patient is on a normal bed or on a comfortably upholstered chair. This may be advantageous over using a urodynamic chair, both for patient transfer from wheelchair to urodynamic position and prevention of pressure sores. Furthermore many urodynamic chairs do not offer the necessary stability for patients with motoric dysfunction. If the patient is able to void or when there is a necessity to document the urine leakage on a flowmeter (channel), the flow chair should nevertheless also be selected or built to minimise pressure sore risk and maximise comfort. A patient lift may be helpful for transfers. In any case the urodynamics lab should be spacious enough for the demands of these patients, and also an adequate dressing room and wheelchair-accessible toilet are a necessity. Certainly these preventive measures should also be available in a video-urodynamics laboratory (see below).

Last but not least, the patient should be supported by experienced personnel and adequate equipment and material, for (un)dressing, cleaning, redressing and retransfer after the test. The personnel there above should be professional in the handling and specific care of persons with sensory and mobility problems.

Basic Pathophysiology Relevant to Urodynamic Investigation in Persons with SCI

The myelum lesion of patients with SCI determines the dysfunction. Complete transection above the spinal micturition centre in the medullary cone results in an upper motor neuron lesion (spastic paralysis) after some latency (spinal shock phase), and a lesion below or through this micturition centre will result in a lower motor neuron disease.

In the spinal shock phase of a lesion above the spinal micturition centre and also when a lower motor neuron lesion exists, a flaccid (high compliance, acontractile) detrusor can be expected together with a paralysed (non-contracted/non-contractile) pelvic floor muscles. When an upper motor neuron lesion exists a few months, the detrusor becomes overactive with high pressures as a result of the also 'overactive' (dyssynergic) bladder outlet and pelvic floor muscles. This new situation is a result of the lack of inhibition and coordination of the spinal Onuf's nucleus. This neuronal centre initiates reflex voiding again as was existing before potty training, however, without the pontine coordination of the autonomic with the somatosensory system. This results in reflex detrusor contraction as a reaction on muscle stretch (due to filling) at low volume and reactive bladder outlet and pelvic contraction as a consequence of an uninhibited guarding reflex/pelvic floor muscle spasm.

These two archetypes of dysfunction are however frequently imperfect. The clinical/orthopaedic lesion (the level of the lesioned vertebrum) is not perfectly predicting the (N)LUTD because the medullary lesion can be incomplete at that level or can extend below the upper margin of the vertebral and clinical lesion. Furthermore, in the follow-up it may become relevant that, e.g. indwelling catheters or chronic high intravesical pressure can result in structural changes of the bladder or urethra. The results of the urodynamic investigation should always be interpreted with the lesion in mind; apart from the fact that an upper motor neuron lesion requires some time (months) to fully develop, the potential consequences of the management that has been initiated or maintained should also be kept in mind.

Basic Pathophysiology Relevant to Urodynamic Investigation in Persons with Meningomyelocele

Both archetypical lesions as mentioned here above are also the basis for the dysfunction in patients with meningomyelocele. However because the dysfunction is already present before birth, the end organs may never have had a chance to develop properly. Muscular structures have very likely not been able to develop normally during prenatal development when innervation is lacking, which frequently can be visible in the legs of children affected with meningomyelocele but which may—less visible—also be present in the pelvic floor muscles or in the detrusor muscle. There is however not a precise association of leg anatomy and/or leg function with lower urinary tract function and continence function. Frequently there exists a (underdevelopment) dysfunction of the entire pelvic floor muscle system, and therefore urinary incontinence may be associated with faecal incontinence with consequence for the management of both of these symptoms. In the situation of an underdeveloped detrusor, a flaccid or a stiff (fibrotic) bladder may result. A flaccid bladder has a usually good volume adaptation at low pressures without the ability to contract (for voiding) and with usually no typical sensation of filling. A stiff detrusor/bladder has a continuous pressure increment, while the fill volume increases as a sign of lacking volume adaptation. Frequently a low-compliance bladder is also unable to contract, and also here the usually incremental (normal) sensation of bladder filling may be underdeveloped. Depending on the sphincter/pelvic floor function, urinary incontinence will occur at a certain amount of bladder filling in both situations but usually at lesser intravesical volumes and higher pressures in low compliance bladders. Depending on the level of the spinal defects, pelvic floor muscle sensation can be present, while normal bladder filling sensation is absent, and sensation of leakage (or urine entering the bladder neck/striated sphincter area) can be perceived. In the situation that the bladder has maintained some muscle structure, detrusor overactivity may occur, with or without sensation and with or without urinary incontinence.

The hampered development and the abnormal intravesical pressures during prenatal development can also have consequences for the vesicoureteral valve system, and persons with meningomyelocele have a higher incidence of vesicoureteral reflux than persons who have acquired—in later life—neurological disease.

Technique and Interpretation

Patients are asked to arrive at the urodynamics lab with a bladder that is as 'full as usual at the time of voiding or catheterisation' when that is possible without excessive effort or discomfort. After positioning of the patient, the emptying of the bladder will give an extra—or first—impression of the usual volume at the time of 'subjectively full bladder'. As indicated here above, the position of the patient may depend on whether a flowmetry (or leakage detection on the flow channel of the measurement) is deemed relevant. In all patients the risk of pressure sores should be balanced against the necessary positioning.

After emptying the bladder, the urodynamic investigation is performed in the ICS standard manner, medium fill rate and room temperature, via a double-lumen 6–8F transurethral catheter. Fill rate may be further selected to be 10% of the estimated predicted individual's maximal bladder capacity per minute. For intrarectal (abdominal) pressure, a fluid-filled catheter with a punctured and flaccid balloon is used, as also per ICS standard.

Bladder filling should continue until the usual capacity or more when the pressure remains low and safe (as a rule of thumb <40 cmH$_2$O). If the pressure rises continuously (reduced compliance) and/or phasic (detrusor contraction), the diagnosis of filling phase is established accordingly. It will be relevant to continue filling until leakage or dyssynergic voiding if that is deemed necessary on the basis of history, signs and symptoms. On the other hand, if high pressures are observed at low volume whether or not the volume is representative, it may be considered to end the cystometry since further filling would not change the diagnosis.

If visible leakage occurs, this should be adequately marked, and the detrusor pressure at leakage (DLPP) will be noted. There is no evidence that the leakage pressure should be determined very precisely and that video is especially needed for this. Leakage pressure estimation in units of $10cmH_2O$ is sufficient to establish management, also because the aim of any management is to reduce vesical pressure in the first place. Dyssynergic voiding or leakage can be recognised by the pattern of detrusor pressure increment simultaneous with the flowrate significantly reducing or stopping.

Sensation during filling, whether or not specific, should be recorded in ICS standard terms. When no sensation and no pressure event or incontinence has occurred and 800 mL has been filled, the cystometry may be stopped. In patients with lower motor neuron disease and pelvic floor muscle weakness, stress urinary incontinence may be observed and/or tested as usual by coughing. When the abdominal muscles are too weak, external pressure on the abdomen by the hand of the investigator may be helpful or movements like the patient self-lifting from the urodynamic chair. On the other hand, if stress leak point pressure is very low (and fill volume cannot increase), it might be necessary to fill the bladder with a closed urethra, e.g. with indwelling balloon catheter or penile compression, to evaluate the reserve capacity of the detrusor, especially when anti-incontinence procedures are considered.

Persons with autonomic dysreflexia will usually be aware of this, but signs and symptoms indicative for this should always be asked for during testing. If such symptoms arise, filling should be stopped instantaneously and the bladder emptied. Some experts advise continuous blood pressure monitoring; however, the symptoms usually precede the blood pressure rise, and symptoms are easily recognisable. Nevertheless it is recommendable to have blood pressure-reducing medication (as per local protocol) available in the urodynamic testing room.

Video-Urodynamic Testing

The addition of roentgen monitoring to standard urodynamic testing, video-urodynamic testing, can be of auxiliary value and is a recommended test, when primary or secondary anatomical abnormalities of the LUT are to be expected or are known to be present and possibly relevant for the basis of treatment or management decisions in the individual patient.

Abnormalities in the LUT are common in patients with meningomyelocele as the sequelae of abnormal development. Secondary abnormalities can be expected in patients with spinal cord lesions or other neurological lesions of the LUT. Vesicoureteral reflux or ureteroceles are anatomical LUT abnormalities that are associated with LUT dysfunction, especially in children. Video urodynamics is recommended in the diagnosis and follow-up of patients with neurogenic LUT dysfunction, however, with a frequency that is not precisely defined on the basis of evidence. Video-urodynamic testing is also recommended in the routine follow-up after surgical interventions, such as augmentation cystoplasties, or after failed (e.g. anti-incontinence) surgery.

Despite the fact that video-urodynamic testing has been known for many years, standardisation of the video technique is lacking. Video-urodynamic technique is not mentioned in the ICS Good Urodynamic Practices reports, and there is probably a wide variation in clinical practice. The number of images to be acquired and/or the timing and length of the video recording are yet undetermined.

Many studies have reported the use of video with urodynamics without any description of the roentgen technique used nor of number of pictures taken. The results of what has been observed or how have not been standardised. In short, good evidence is lacking, with regard to the reproducibility, the sensitivity, the specificity and the predictive value of the observations done during video urodynamics. Only very few reports, most of them non(gynaeco-)-urologic, have discussed radiation exposure, dose, field of view or fluoroscopy time. In radiology the ALARA (as low (radiation dose) as reasonably achievable) -principle is commonly accepted. For example, technical improvements have made pulsed fluoroscopy available. Pulsed fluoroscopy with 7.5 frames or even 3.75 frames per second has been demonstrated to be demonstrated to perform equivalent to continuous fluoroscopy. One urologic handbook suggests that a radiation time of <1 min is possible to do a video-urodynamic investigation.

With this in mind, a video-urodynamic study should be performed in adult patients with neurogenic lower urinary tract dysfunction when relevant anatomical abnormalities related with the lower urinary tract dysfunction are suspected. Video urodynamics can be done with pulsed fluoroscopy with a frame rate of 3.75/s without loss of clinical relevant information.

During the storage (filling) phase of the test, some 'snapshots <1 sec' can usually provide relevant information: one snapshot at first sensation of filling, one during detrusor (over-) activity and one at strong desire to void/catheterise, the end of filling or urodynamic capacity. During storage phase a stress test can be performed with fluoroscopic monitoring during 1 or 2 s (if deemed clinically relevant, usually at or just before strong desire to void).

During voiding phase a short fluoroscopic monitoring (1 s) can be done at the initiation of the voiding (detrusor pressure starts to rise) and a snapshot at (just after) maximum detrusor pressure if deemed relevant. The field of view can usually be close around the bladder neck, to prevent (male) gonadal radiation dose as much as possible, but especially for patients with neurogenic lower urinary tract dysfunction, one wider-view (abdominal) snapshot (<1 s) at the start of the investigation may provide relevant information. Certainly another snapshot at maximum contraction (at 'leak point') can usually demonstrate vesicoureteral reflux.

Concluding the Urodynamic Test(s) and Consequences

During and directly after the test, a diagnosis of the LUT dysfunction can be made and discussed with the patient. For the patient it is important whether the sensations that arise are meaningful or what the 'safe volume' is. The 'safe volume' may be considered as the volume at pressures considered low enough to ensure continence and also low enough to preserve the kidney function. The safe volume may guide catheterisation frequency and may also direct or provide arguments for the necessity of alterations of the management.

Figures and Clinical Scenarios

Five clinical cases are presented with this chapter for teaching purposes (see Figs. 1, 2, 3, 4, 5, 6).

Conclusion

This chapter has explained the theory and practice of performing, interpreting and evaluating urodynamics in patients with neurogenic dysfunction of the lower urinary tract.

Case 1

Man, 19 years old, meningomyelocele, CIC every 3–4 h (not during night-time) with volumes around 300 mL, usually with some sensation of fullness. He never voids and has very low frequency of symptomatic urinary tract infections (less than once a year without prophylaxis). He is using antimuscarinics now after long-term anticholinergics at childhood. He infrequently experiences urinary incontinence which is not bothersome for him. Recently slight dilatation was observed of the right kidney during ultrasound, not present 2 years earlier (refer to Fig. 1).

Urodynamics (Cystometry)

Urodynamic diagnosis: (Neurogenic) detrusor overactivity with reduced capacity until unsafe pressure and preserved filling sensation. *Clinical conclusion* may be that the capacity until unsafe pressure is not very large and that although the patient has occasional urine incontinence, he is content with his quality of life. The slight and new onset of upper tract dilatation and the, although not bothersome, incontinence may be a reason to discuss the upgrading of the medical management with him and/or to increase the neuro-urological monitoring frequency.

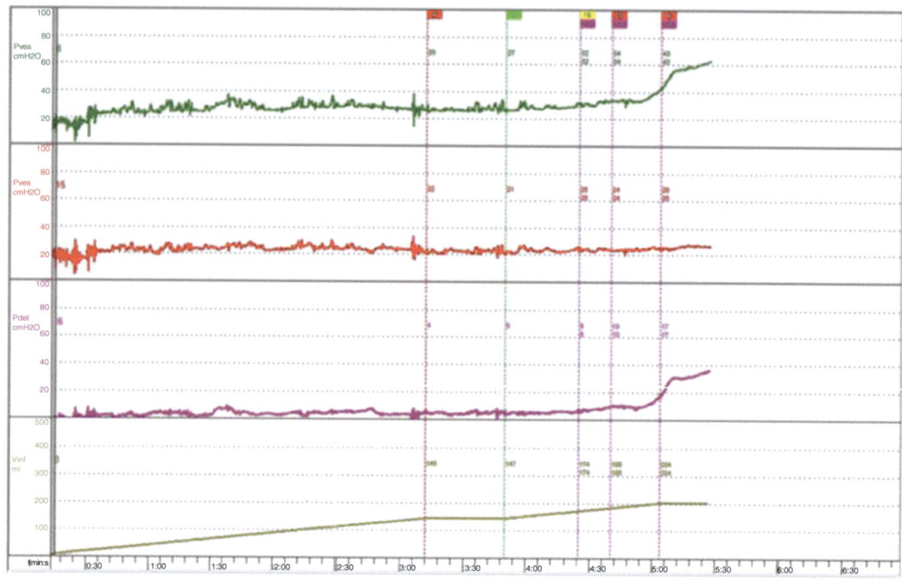

Fig. 1 Cystometry: At 90 mL filling (after 1 min and 30 s), a phasic pressure increment of 10 cm H_2O is visible and later at a volume of ±200 mL again. Following on to that, the pressure increment is steeper until a pressure of nearly 40 cmH_2O. Urodynamic filling is stopped, but pressure rise continues. The first sensation of filling occurred at the start of the detrusor pressure rise at 174 mL, and normal desire to void that similar to 'the need to catheterize' in this patient was seen at 200 mL. After emptying the bladder, it was observed that almost 50 mL of diuresis had been added to the measured capacity. Therefore his urodynamic capacity until unsafe pressure is ±250 mL

Case 2

Man, 46 years and 8 months old after thoracic transverse myelitis. Walking has recovered and he is ambulant with a cane. He has urinary incontinence and is not able to void voluntarily. He senses the urine leakage, but he reports his bladder sensation to be less or absent. He also reports that it is difficult to perceive whether the rectum is filled, but he is continent after using a laxative in the morning. His urinary incontinence is managed with a condom sheath catheter, and he does self-catheterisation before the night. He had two urinary tract infections in the last 3 months (refer to Fig. 2).

Urodynamics (Cystometry)

Urodynamic diagnosis: Neurogenic detrusor overactivity with high pressure and detrusor activity incontinence with ineffective dyssynergic emptying (and inability to void with intent). Chronic residual urine or 'chronic ineffective emptying/overactivity urinary incontinence'. *Clinical conclusion*: The patient considers the spurts of

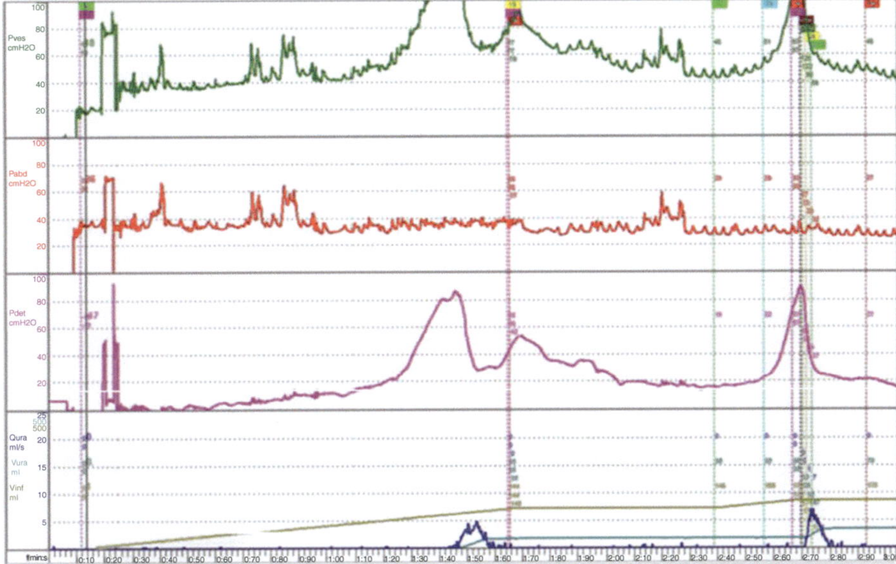

Fig. 2 Cystometry demonstrates detrusor contraction, starting from ±70 to 80 mL incrementing to a high detrusor pressure of 90 cmH$_2$O when 110 mL are filled, when the 'guarding reflex' gives way and when a spurt of urine is seen. Further filling after a pause, while the (after-) contraction fades away (but not entirely to baseline zero), shows an almost immediate new contraction and a new spurt of voiding again. Both spurts empty about 30% of the bladder content. He was unable to voluntarily empty the rest of the intravesical volume (not shown on this trace). (Detrusor) Leak point pressure is around 35 cmH$_2$O

leakage a sign of 'recovery of the voiding function', which he very much hopes for to further improve. He is very frustrated about the need for self-catheterisation. The periods of elevated pressure and the chronic residual urine are however a long-term risk; moreover he already had a few symptomatic UTIs. The management should balance the risks of the contemporary situation with the hopes and wishes of the patient and the chance of further recovery as well as the disadvantageous and longer-term consequences of initiating antimuscarinic management and more frequent self-catheterisation.

Case 3

Man, 55 years old, cervical lesion since 5 years. Catheterisation volumes of ±500 mL 4 times a day, with the help of a caregiver. Early morning volumes are sometimes ±600 mL. He has no sensation of filling and no signs of autonomic dysreflexia. He experiences no urinary incontinence and has had less than 1 UTI/year. Last urodynamic investigation was 3 years ago. He uses antimuscarinics and spasmolytics for his leg spasms (refer to Fig. 3).

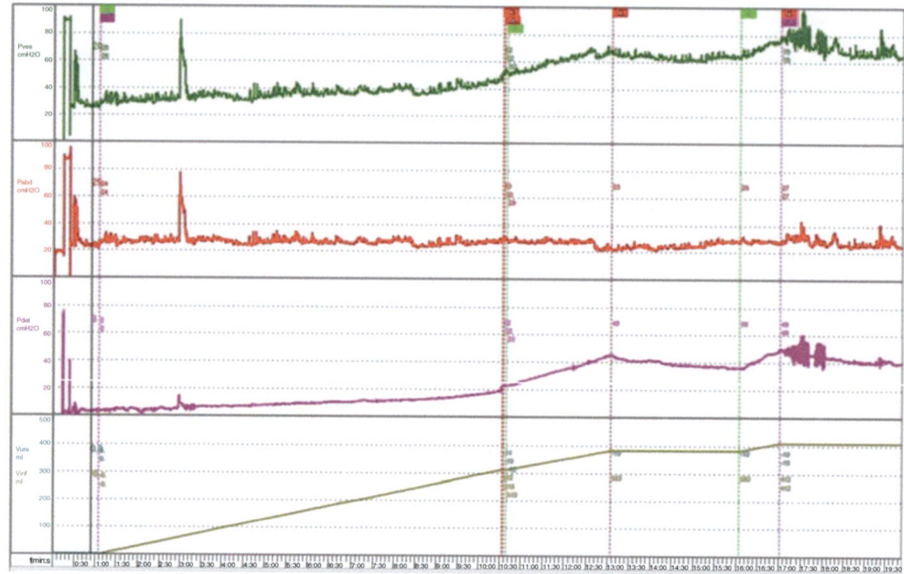

Fig. 3 Filling was continued until 380 mL, and from ±250 mL, compliance is lacking; pressure is rising until 40 cmH₂O. Filling was stopped and pressure slightly diminished. When filling was switched on again, an immediate pressure rise was seen

Urodynamics (Cystometry)

Urodynamic diagnosis: Reduced compliance with little amount of detrusor contraction dynamics. Capacity until 40 cmH₂O is ±400 mL. *Clinical conclusion*: Although the patient has no symptoms, the pressure at his usual capacity is not optimal. Because increase of the catheterisation frequency (by caregiver) would have a lot of practical consequences, he was treated with intra-detrusor botulinum toxin (refer to Fig. 4).

Case 3 Repeated Urodynamics After 3 Months

Urodynamic conclusion: Reduced compliance but—relatively—safe pressure until his usual catheterisation volume. *Clinical conclusion*: it is considered likely that the new initiated management results in reduced risk for upper tract deterioration although the compliance has not significantly altered/improved.

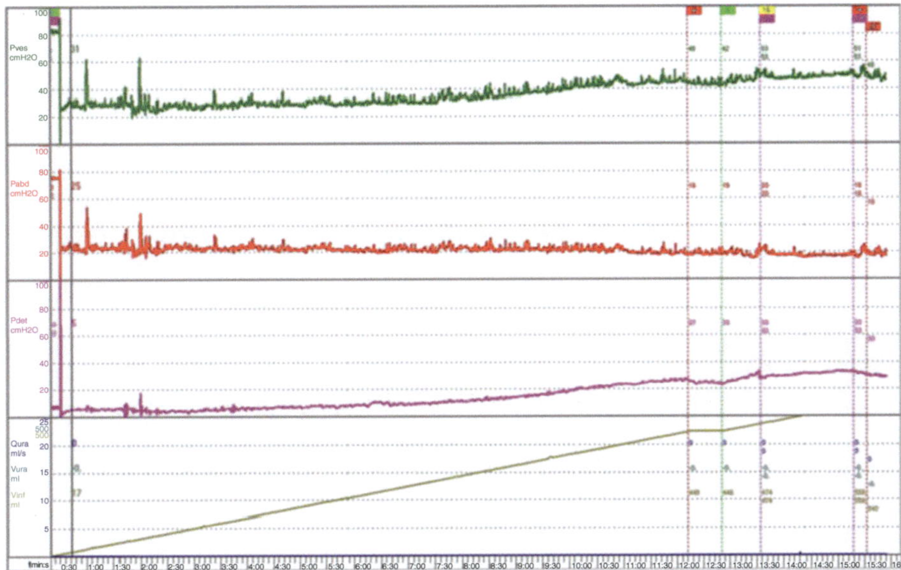

Fig. 4 Filling was continued until 550 mL now, and he experienced some sensation of 'abdominal fullness' at 480 mL. Compliance was slightly better than before, and pressure at a somewhat larger capacity was 35 cmH₂O. Obvious detrusor contraction effects were not observed any more

Case 4

Woman, 46 years old, spinal arteriovenous malformation and partial lesion and lumbar lesion after haemorrhage and surgery. Six months after the lesion, she was able to walk some steps but predominantly wheelchair bound. Urinary incontinence and frequent voiding small volumes, voiding diary 12 times ±90–120 mL during daytime hours and 2 times during the night. Perineal sensation was recovered, and anal closure was normal. She had no urinary tract infections and no urinary tract dysfunction symptoms before the onset of neurological symptoms (refer to Fig. 5).

Urodynamics (Cystometry)

Urodynamic diagnosis: Neurogenic detrusor overactivity with sensation and reduced capacity until an imperative need to void. Ineffective voiding as a consequence of unsustained detrusor voiding contraction and ineffective abdominal straining. *Clinical conclusion*: Spontaneous recovery and/or improvement is not

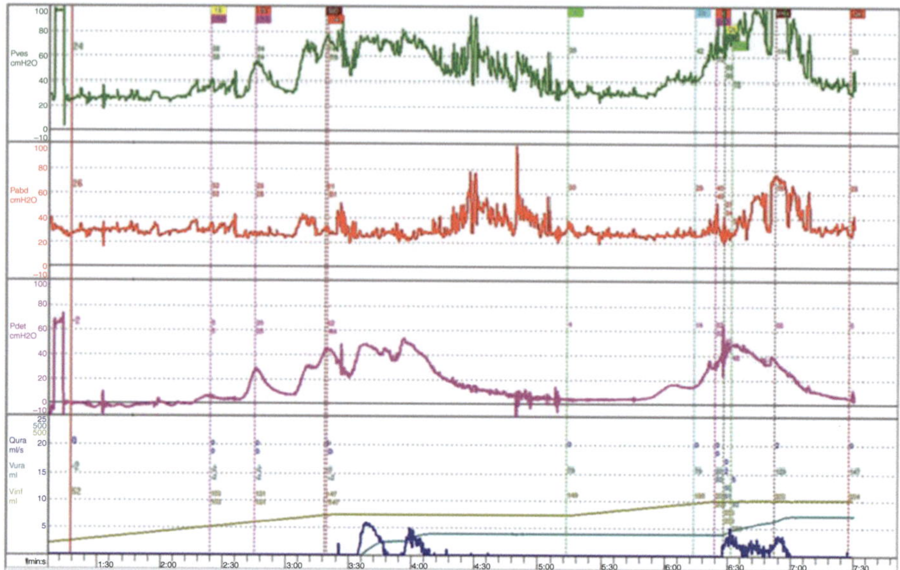

Fig. 5 (Start of the filling not on figure) First sensation of filling is at 100 mL, and a detrusor pressure rise is visible. Normal desire to void was at 120 mL and strong desire with fear of leakage at 150 mL. Pressure increments were seen up to 45 cmH$_2$O. Permission to void was given, and with two portions 80 mL was emptied. There was a sensation of residual volume. When detrusor pressure was at baseline level again, filling was resumed, and contractions were seen again. Permission was followed by another ineffective—and not continuous—voiding of 70 mL. Now ending with an ineffective attempt to improve the emptying with abdominal straining (also straining is visible after the first voiding)

impossible and may be expected in the months to follow. She produces a normal volume of fluid per 24 h. Symptoms—frequent voiding and nocturia—may be alleviated with antimuscarinics. Pelvic muscle training, especially to improve relaxation during voiding, may be added. Potentially her straining increases her chance to become stress urinary incontinent. However there is little chance of recovery of the lower urinary tract and pelvic floor muscles when the general neurological situation (walking) does not improve. In her perspective the advantages and disadvantages of clean intermittent self-catheterisation should also be discussed, especially when good bladder storage volumes can be achieved with conservative measures. An indwelling catheter will certainly *not* be a good option.

Case 5

Man, 55 years old, secondary-progressive multiple sclerosis, EDSS 6.5 nearing 7 (wheelchair needed, but able to stand supported). He uses anticholinergics prescribed by his neurologist since 16 months. He voids nine times during the day

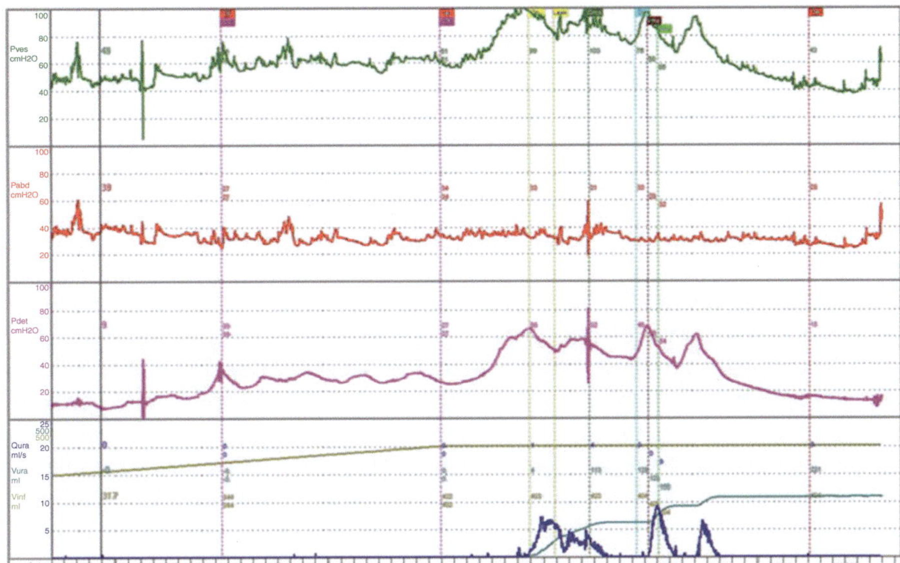

Fig. 6 Patient had a very strong urge to void when he arrived at the urodynamics lab. Seated on the flowmeter, he voided 120 mL with a maximum flow of 11 mL/s. Post-void residual was 420 mL. He drank 500 mL of water just before the test 'to fill his bladder'

(usually 2–300 mL) and three times at night, which is the most bothersome for him because of his mobility problems but also because he never feels that the bladder is empty. Sometimes he loses a few drops of urine, and he always has a urinary bottle with him, but he wears no incontinence material. Defecation is cumbersome, and he uses laxatives but sometimes needs digital evacuation. He reports that postponing the voiding and sitting result in subjectively lesser good voiding. He had no urinary tract infections and no previous history of urinary tract problems.

Based on questioning, his leg propriocepsis was significantly reduced. Clinical exam revealed little or no loss of saddle region sensation and normal anal tone. Both cremasteric and anal reflex were very lively. While catheters were inserted (after initial voiding and after pressure flow, to empty the bladder, and with urodynamic double lumen catheter for cystometry), pelvic muscular contraction (pelvic floor defence) and leg adductor muscle spasms were noted. On rectal exam his prostate was estimated to be not enlarged (refer to Fig. 6).

Urodynamics

Cystometry is shown from a 350 mL of pump filling and shows phasic detrusor pressure rises. There was strong desire to void at 400 mL of filling. Patient was in a standing position (from ±200 mL) during cystometry, with good arm and hand support, close to the flowmeter which was adjusted to his height. After permission to void (12:25), a new—now voluntarily initiated—detrusor contraction was seen with a latency (hesitancy) of almost 30 s before flow started. In three spurts 220 mL was emptied, and no further detrusor activity could be elicited. After the test 300 mL was evacuated, and it was concluded that 120 mL diuresis was added to the cystometry.

Urodynamic diagnosis: Neurogenic detrusor overactivity and dyssynergic and chronically ineffective voiding and reduced functional capacity. (Of note not shown, standard ICS pressure flow plot shows no (BPH, static) bladder outlet obstruction.) The detrusor sphincter dyssynergy is diagnosed on the basis of the typical pressure flow pattern; flowrate and detrusor increment are asynchronous; flowrate reduces when detrusor pressure increases and vice versa. *Clinical conclusion*: It can be advisable to discuss the likelihood of disease progression and his life expectancy with the treating neurologist. There is not much danger for the upper tract, as long as he does not need an indwelling (suprapubic) catheter (which is however certainly a valuable option when his EDSS increases to 8 or more). The lower urinary tract dysfunction may be managed with a variety of alternative (other than anticholinergics) medication to reduce detrusor overactivity and/or bladder neck overactivity. Continence material advice and (occupational or physiotherapeutic) methods to support him to be able to void in standing position should certainly be discussed. (Better) Measures to support defecation as also clean intermittent self-catheterisation and (medical) night-time fluid management (since this is his most important/bothersome problem) should be considered. The management must be based on quality of life and patient preference and practical consequences.

Suggested Readings

Abrams P, Cardozo L, Fall M, Griffiths D, Rosier P, Ulmsten U, Van Kerrebroeck P, Victor A, Wein A, Standardisation Sub-Committee of the International Continence Society. The standardisation of terminology in lower urinary tract function: report from the standardisation sub-committee of the international continence society. Urology. 2003;61(1):37–49. Review

Nijeholt GJ, van Walderveen MA, Castelijns JA, van Waesberghe JH, Polman C, Scheltens P, Rosier PF, Jongen PJ, Barkhof F. Brain and spinal cord abnormalities in multiple sclerosis. Correlation between MRI parameters, clinical subtypes and symptoms. Brain. 1998;121(Pt 4):687–97.

Rosier PF, Szabó L, Capewell A, Gajewski JB, Sand PK, Hosker GL, International Consultation on Incontinence 2008 Committee on Dynamic Testing. Executive summary: the international consultation on incontinence 2008 – committee on: "dynamic testing"; for urinary or fecal incontinence. Part 2: urodynamic testing in male patients with symptoms of urinary incontinence, in patients with relevant neurological abnormalities, and in children and in frail elderly with symptoms of urinary incontinence. Neurourol Urodyn. 2010;29(1):146–52. https://doi.org/10.1002/nau.20763. Review

Rosier PFWM, Schaefer W, Lose G, Goldman HB, Guralnick M, Eustice S, Dickinson T, Hashim H. International continence society good urodynamic practices and terms 2016: urodynamics, uroflowmetry, cystometry, and pressure-flow study. Neurourol Urodyn. 2017;36(5):1243–60. https://doi.org/10.1002/nau.23124. Epub 2016 Dec 5. Review

Sakakibara R, Panicker J, Finazzi-Agro E, Iacovelli V, Bruschini H, Parkinson's Disease Subcomitee, The Neurourology Promotion Committee in The International Continence

Society. A guideline for the management of bladder dysfunction in Parkinson's disease and other gait disorders. Neurourol Urodyn. 2016;35(5):551–63. https://doi.org/10.1002/nau.22764. Epub 2015 Mar 25. Review

Schurch B, Iacovelli V, Averbeck MA, Stefano C, Altaweel W, Finazzi AE. Urodynamics in patients with spinal cord injury: a clinical review and best practice paper by a working group of the international continence society urodynamics committee. Neurourol Urodyn. 2017. https://doi.org/10.1002/nau.23369. [Epub ahead of print] Review. PubMed PMID: 28762566

Clinical Neuro-urophysiological Investigations

Hazel Ecclestone and Rizwan Hamid

Abbreviations

BCR	Bulbocavernosus reflex
CT	Computerised tomography
DSD	Detrusor sphincter dyssynergia
EMG	Electromyography
MRI	Magnetic resonance imaging
SEP	Somatosensory potential

Introduction

Although urodynamics remain a fundamental part of the assessment of neuro-urological patients, there are a number of other investigations that can be performed to help give an insight into neuro-urological dysfunction. The type and timing of investigation will largely depend on the underlying neurological pathology and may also be guided by changes in symptoms.

The predominant aim of a neuro-urologist is to protect the upper urinary tract from deterioration. Secondary aims include improving continence and sexual function and reducing the impact of urological symptoms on patients' quality of life.

The nervous system responsible for the control of micturition is split into the central (brain and spinal cord) and peripheral nervous systems. The peripheral ner-

H. Ecclestone
University College London Hospitals, London, UK

R. Hamid (✉)
Department of Neurourology, Spinal Injuries Unit, Stanmore/London, UK

University College London Hospitals, London, UK

© Springer International Publishing AG, part of Springer Nature 2018
R. Dmochowski, J. Heesakkers (eds.), *Neuro-Urology*,
https://doi.org/10.1007/978-3-319-90997-4_13

vous system has both somatic and autonomic functions. Damage to any of the branches of the nervous system can have significant impact on micturition. Conventional imaging such as MRI and CT may not show up the location and degree of nerve damage, and so specialised uro-neurophysiological tests can be employed to improve diagnostic accuracy.

Common reasons for requiring these specialist uro-neurophysiological tests in the neuro-urology population include urinary incontinence or voiding dysfunction, faecal incontinence, urological symptoms with suspected underlying neurological condition and patients with Parkinson's-type symptoms to differentiate from the diagnosis of multisystem atrophy.

Uro-neurophysiological Tests (Electrodiagnostics)

There are a number of specialised neurophysiological tests that can be performed if there is diagnostic uncertainty with a neuro-urology patient [1]. The difficulty, especially in polyneuropathies, is that the somatic and autonomic nervous systems can both be affected to varying degrees, and therefore the following neurophysiological tests may be of benefit to define the degree and location of impairment.

Classification of Uro-neurophysiological Tests

These tests are an extension of the clinical examination. The nervous system is divided into somatic and autonomic nervous systems. Both systems have central pathways and peripheral nerves.

Hence, the uro-electrophysiological tests can be divided into:

1. Somatic motor system tests

    (a) Electromyography (EMG)
    (b) Nerve conduction tests
    (c) Motor evoked potentials

2. Somatosensory

    (a) Sensory neurography
    (b) Somatosensory evoked potentials

3. Reflexes
4. Autonomic nervous system tests

    (a) For sympathetic or parasympathetic fibres

Electromyography (EMG)

This looks at the neuromuscular electrical activity of muscle using recording electrodes inserted into or placed on the surface of a muscle. Bioelectric signals are recorded, filtered and amplified during muscle depolarisation, and the results are translated graphically and via an oscilloscope for auditory analysis. EMGs are commonly performed on the striated muscles of the pelvic floor, urethral sphincter and/or anal sphincter. Needle electrode recording, intra-vaginal/anal probes with surface detectors as well as skin surface electrodes can be used. The kinesiological EMG studies using surface electrodes can be performed at the same time as urodynamic studies to gain extra insight into lower urinary tract function. Of particular interest is the behaviour of the pelvic floor and urethral sphincter during voiding. The advantage of these surface electrodes is that they are simple to use and are tolerated well by patients by virtue of their noninvasive nature; however, they are very sensitive and thus can pick up signals from other muscles causing artefacts.

ICS guidelines on urodynamic standardisation suggest placement of two signal electrodes as close as possible to the muscle of interest (usually the anal sphincter) with a third (reference) electrode, attached ideally over a bony prominence (see Fig. 1). ICS also suggest efforts are made to obtain good electrical contact with the skin by ensuring good mechanical adherence with skin preparation if necessary [2].

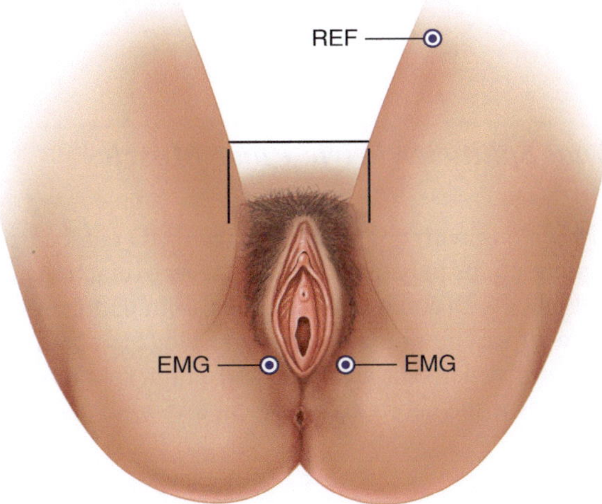

Fig. 1 shows surface electrode placement for EMG, as used during urodynamic evaluation—REF, reference/ground electrode [3]

The utility of EMG of both the anal and urethral sphincters is still debated, with some authors arguing the results are highly unreliable in neuro-urology patients [4], whereas others feel anal sphincter EMG is the optimal diagnostic test in cases of sacral nerve lesions [1]. A number of authors also agree that EMG is of great benefit in atypical cases of Parkinson disease, where a diagnosis of multisystem atrophy is potentially differential [1, 5].

EMG of the Urethral Sphincter

Urinary sphincter EMG has been used for some time in the diagnosis of NLUTD, but the practical value still has not been adequately quantified. Additionally, it is still debated if needle or surface electrodes should be used though needle electrodes were found to be superior for evaluating relaxation of muscle during voiding [6]. It is suggested that sphincter EMG is the most sensitive test for focal sacral lesions and atypical Parkinson. Fowler [7] evaluated the sphincter motor units with needle electrodes and showed this to be helpful in evaluating patients with disorders of micturition. It is now considered to be the diagnostic test for Fowler's syndrome [8]. It has also been shown that sphincter EMG is valuable in differentiating patients between Parkinsonism and multiple system atrophy [9]. The sphincter EMG can be used in conjunction with video images during simultaneous video urodynamics to diagnose detrusor sphincter dyssynergia (DSD). DSD is particularly important to identify in neurological patients, as it is an independent risk factor for upper tract deterioration [10].

EMG of the Anal Sphincter/Pelvic Floor Muscles

Anal sphincter EMG along with urethral sphincter EMG can be used to detect the onset of detrusor contractions in patients with detrusor overactivity. This can lead to development of therapies with continuous electrical stimulation of sensory nerves to control neurogenic overactivity of the detrusor muscle [11, 12]. It has been demonstrated that in patients with detrusor areflexia, and a high spinal cord lesion EMG of the pelvic floor muscles is the neurophysiological test which best predicts detrusor contractility [13].

EMG of the Detrusor Muscle

Although EMG of detrusor muscle is technically possible, it has not been adequately studied and remains an area for future research. It is therefore not part of standard neurophysiological workup [14, 15].

Nerve Conduction Studies

These look at the resistance along a nerve as it transmits an action potential. A reduced nerve conduction speed is indicative of nerve damage, be that due to axonal loss or demyelination. The pudendal and levator ani nerves can both be studied. The St Marks disposable electrode is most frequently used to study the pudendal nerve (Fig. 2). Despite nerve conduction studies being a routine part of standard diagnostic neurophysiology workup, their use in the pelvis is not widely practiced, and as such, no 'norms' exist to aid with interpretation. Furthermore, the autonomic nerve supply to the pelvis is unmyelinated, and therefore nerve conduction studies in this situation are unhelpful. For these reasons, some authors do not recommend the routine use of nerve conduction studies in the pelvis, especially as there is no correlation between the results and the outcomes for surgery [16]. If there is a suspicion of a polyneuropathy or pathology of the lumbosacral plexus or nerve roots, then standard lower limb nerve conduction studies may be of added benefit.

The nerve conduction velocities are decreased in patients with diabetes mellitus with a delayed response to electrical stimulation of the penis, bladder neck and anus [17, 18].

Motor Evoked Potentials (MEP)

Motor evoked potentials have been used to assess neurogenic lesions affecting the urethral compressive musculature with simultaneous recording of evoked pressure curves. MEP recording is an accurate and easily applicable test for the diagnosis of

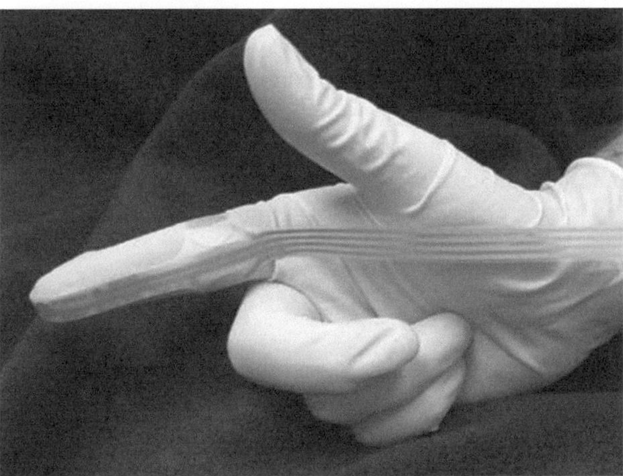

Fig. 2 Disposable St Marks electrode, stimulating anode/cathode at the fingertip; with the recording electrode at the base of the index finger (Adapted from GLOWM [19])

lumbosacral spinal cord lesions [20]. It is possible to depolarise the motor cortex and record a response from the pelvic floor by either magnetic or electric stimulation. Magnetic cortical stimulation is better tolerated. The stimulation is performed at two sites: the brain and spinal roots. One can get three conduction times; a total time, a peripheral time and a central time. The total conduction time is from the brain to the muscle with the peripheral time from sacral roots to the muscle. The central conduction time is obtained by subtracting the two. A central conduction time of 15–16 ms without and 13–14 ms with facilitation is obtained for pelvic floor and sphincter muscles [21, 22].

It has been shown that there are significantly longer central conduction times in patients with multiple sclerosis and spinal cord lesions as compared to healthy controls [22, 23]. Hence, MEPs may be useful in patients with unclear localisation of spinal lesions [22]. Theoretically, MEP may help to differentiate between involvement of motor and sensory pathways. However, the clinical utility of these measurements is not established.

Somatosensory Evoked Potentials (SSEP)

The SSEP are electric waveforms of biological origin provoked by stimulation of a sensory nerve. The most commonly performed tests in the urogenitoanal region are pudendal SSEP. These assess conduction in large fibre pathways between the site of nerve stimulation and the parietal sensory cortex. The technique of recording evoked potentials in humans secondary to stimulation was described by Badr [24]. Later on, Galloway [25] described a method to measure the integrity and function of the lower sacral segments by stimulation at the urethral and anal sphincters. The pudendal SSEP can be elicited by electrical stimulation of penile or clitoral perineal nerve. This has have been advocated in patients with neurogenic bladder dysfunction, e.g. in multiple sclerosis and spinal cord injury. The presence of NLUTD is closely correlated with relatively slow evoked spinal cord potentials (ESCP) velocity. Curt [26] demonstrated a good significance of SSEP recordings in predicting the recovery of bladder function in acute traumatic spinal cord injury. There was good correlation with the recovery of the external urethral sphincter function.

Bulbocavernosus Reflex (BCR)

Reflex latency measurement uses electrical/magnetic or mechanical stimulation to elicit BCR and anal reflex arcs described in chapter "Neuroanatomy Relevant for the Urologist" of this section. Recording electrodes are then placed within the anal sphincter or bulbocavernosus muscle [27]. The results indicate that an enhanced BCR is a contributing factor to increased urethral resistance during micturition.

The evoked potential of the BCR (BCR-EP) can be recorded with a concentric needle electrode at the periurethral striated muscle. This has been found to be suppressed during voluntary voiding in normal subjects, but it was insufficiently suppressed in the neurogenic patients [28]. It is thought that the measurement of BCR-EP could distinguish involuntary voiding caused by pathological urethral sphincter relaxation from voluntary voiding. It has also been shown that the sacral reflex activity was accelerated by bladder filling in SCI patients [29]. This information may be useful to evaluate the continuity of sacral segment and supraspinal micturition centre.

This is a more accurate way of registering and quantifying the presence of sacral reflexes and can have important implications for bladder management. Niu [30, 31] demonstrated in cauda equina syndrome sufferers up to 95% of patients had abnormal bulbocavernosus reflex latency results, compared to only 8% of those with spinal cord injury. Despite this relatively promising study, the routine use of BCR latency is not currently a routine part of practice.

Autonomic Function Tests

The autonomic function can be assessed by looking at sensations in the bladder, rectum and urethra. Urodynamics also give an indication of autonomic bladder function. Anal manometry may also be useful to fully assess autonomic dysfunction.

Summary

Electrodiagnostics are widely used by neurophysiologists in settings outside the pelvis. The utility of electrodiagnostics in the evaluation of lower urinary tract dysfunction in neurogenic patients is not yet fully established. The most widely used electrodiagnostic test in this setting is EMG, often performed alongside urodynamics. The primary use of EMG in the neuro-urology population is to aid in the diagnosis of DSD. Nerve conduction studies can be useful in the further differentiation of the nerve deficits in cases of neurologic pathology of the bladder as can the SSEP be of use in evaluation of neurological conditions affecting lower urinary tract. The other uro-neurophysiological tests including detrusor EMG, BCR-EP and MEP are techniques of experimental interest, but with insufficient basis for use as standard clinical diagnostic tests.

Hence, these tests still remain potentially promising investigations in the armamentarium of a neuro-urologist, and much more research is needed before these tests can be incorporated in the routine clinical practice.

References

1. Podner S, et al. Lower urinary tract dysfunction in patients with peripheral nervous system lesions. Handb Clin Neurol. 2015;130:203–24.
2. Homma Y, Batista J, Bauer S, et al. Urodynamics. Incontinence: international consultation on incontinence. Plymouth: Health Publication Ltd.; 2002. p. 317.
3. Padilla-Fernandez B, Batista J, Bauer S, et al. Urodynamics. Incontinence: international consultation on incontinence. Plymouth: Health Publication Ltd.; 2002. p. 317.
4. Nordling J, Meyhoff HH. Dissociation of urethral and anal sphincter activity in neurogenic bladder dysfunction. J Urol. 1979;122:352–6.
5. Palace J, Chandiramani VA, Fowler CJ. Value of sphincter electromyography in the diagnosis of multiple system atrophy. Muscle Nerve. 1997;20:1396–403.
6. Mahajan ST, Fitzgerald MP, Kenton K, Shott S, Brubaker L. Concentric needle electrodes are superior to perineal surface-patch electrodes for electromyographic documentation of urethral sphincter relaxation during voiding. BJU Int. 2006;97:117–20.
7. Fowler CJ, Kirby RS, Harrison MJ, Milroy EJ, Turner-Warwick R. Individual motor unit analysis in the diagnosis of disorders of urethral sphincter innervation. J Neurol Neurosurg Psychiatry. 1984;47:637–41.
8. Kavia RB, Datta SN, Dasgupta R, Elneil S, Fowler CJ. Urinary retention in women: its causes and management. BJU Int. 2006;97(2):281–7.
9. Fowler CJ. Investigational techniques. Eur Urol. 1998;34(Suppl 1):10–2.
10. Mundy AR, Borzyskowski M, Saxton HM. Videourodynamics evaluation of neuropathic vesicourethral dysfunction in children. BJU Int. 1982;54:645–9.
11. Wenzel BJ, Boggs JW, Gustafson KJ, Creasey GH, Grill WM. Detection of neurogenic detrusor contractions from the activity of the external anal sphincter in cat and human. Neurourol Urodyn. 2006;25:140–7.
12. Hansen J, Borau A, Rodríguez A, Vidal J, Sinkjaer T, Rijkhoff NJ. Urethral sphincter EMG as event detector for neurogenic detrusor overactivity. IEEE Trans Biomed Eng. 2007;54:1212–9.
13. Light JK, Faganel J, Beric A. Detrusor areflexia in suprasacral spinal cord injuries. J Urol. 1985;134:295–7.
14. La Joie WJ, Cosgrove MD, Jones WG. Electromyographic evaluation of human detrusor muscle activity in relation to abdominal muscle activity. Arch Phys Med Rehabil. 1976;57:382–6.
15. Kinder M, Gommer E, Janknegt R, van Waalwijk van Doorn E. Recording the detrusor electromyogram is still a difficult and controversial enterprise. Neurourol Urodyn. 1998;17:571–3.
16. Kjolhede P, Lindehammar H. Pelvic floor neuropathy in relation to the outcome of Burch colposuspension. Int Urogynecol J Pelvic Floor Dysfunct. 1997;8:61–5.
17. Andersen JT, Bradley WE. Abnormalities of bladder innervation in diabetes mellitus. Urology. 1976;7:442–8.
18. Vereecken RL, De Meirsman J, Puers B, Van Mulders J. Electrophysiological exploration of the sacral conus. J Neurol. 1982;227:135–44.
19. GLOWM- global library of women medicine. http://www.glowm.com/section_view/heading/Neurophysiologistesting. Accessed 1 Nov 2017.
20. Di Lazzaro V, Pilato F, Oliviero A, Saturno E, Dileone M, Tonali PA. Role of motor evoked potentials in diagnosis of cauda equina and lumbosacral cord lesions. Neurology. 2004;63:2266–71.
21. Brostrom S. Motor evoked potentials from the pelvic floor. Neurourol Urodyn. 2003;22:620–37.
22. Schmid DM, Curt A, Hauri D, Schurch B. Motor evoked potentials (MEP) and evoked pressure curves (EPC) from the urethral compressive musculature (UCM) by functional magnetic stimulation in healthy volunteers and patients with neurogenic incontinence. Neurourol Urodyn. 2005;24:117–27.
23. Eardley I, Nagendran K, Lecky B, Chapple CR, Kirby RS, Fowler CJ. Neurophysiology of the striated urethral sphincter in multiple sclerosis. Br J Urol. 1991;68:81–8.

24. Badr G, Carlsson CA, Fall M, Friberg S, Lindström L, Ohlsson B. Cortical evoked potentials following stimulation of the urinary bladder in man. Electroencephalogr Clin Neurophysiol. 1982;54:494–8.
25. Galloway NT, Chisholm GD, McInnes A. Patterns and significance of the sacral evoked response (the urologist's knee jerk). Br J Urol. 1985;57:145–7.
26. Curt A, Rodic B, Schurch B, Dietz V. Recovery of bladder function in patients with acute spinal cord injury: significance of ASIA scores and somatosensory evoked potentials. Spinal Cord. 1997;35:368–73.
27. Fowler CJ, Benson JT, Craggs MD, et al. Clinical neurophysiology in 2nd international consultation on incontinence. Plymouth: Health Publication Ltd.; 2002. p. 391–424.
28. Kaiho Y, Namima T, Uchi K, Nakagawa H, Aizawa M, Orikasa S. Electromyographic study of the striated urethral sphincter by using the bulbocavernosus reflex: study of the normal voluntary voiding and the involuntary sphincter relaxation. Nippon Hinyokika Gakkai Zasshi. 1999;90:893–900.
29. Kaiho Y, Namima T, Uchi K, et al. Electromyographic study of the striated urethral sphincter by using the bulbocavernosus reflex: study of the normal voluntary voiding and the involuntary sphincter relaxation. Nippon Hinyokika Gakkai Zasshi. 2000;91:715–22.
30. Niu X, Shao B, Ni P, Wang X, Chen X, Zhu B, Wang Z, Teng H, Jin K. Bulbocavernosus reflex and pudendal nerve somatosensory-evoked potentials responses in female patients with nerve system diseases. J Clin Neurophysiol. 2010;27:207–11.
31. Niu X, Wang X, Ni P, Huang H, Zhang Y, Lin Y, Chen X, Teng H, Shao B. Bulbocavernosus reflex and pudendal nerve somatosensory evoked potential are valuable for the diagnosis of cauda equina syndrome in male patients. Int J Clin Exp Med. 2015;8:1162.

Part IV
Clinical Entities: Urinary Problems

Incontinence

Riyad Taher Al-Mousa and Hashim Hashim

Overview

Normal micturition is a complex process that is controlled by the neural integration between the central and peripheral nervous systems [1] to coordinate sympathetic, parasympathetic, and somatic nervous system activity to allow for normal micturition and urinary continence.

Any neurological or mechanical abnormalities in this circuit may result in lower urinary tract dysfunction (LUTD). Various neurological diseases can cause neurogenic lower urinary tract dysfunction (NLUTD). The degree of dysfunction and severity of symptoms are highly dependent on the nature, location, and extent of the neurological disease. This variation also affects the prevalence of the NLUTD among this group of patients. The variation in prevalence is also related to low levels of evidence and smaller sample sizes in most published data when it comes to treatment [2].

NLUTD has been found in 40–90% of patients with multiple sclerosis (MS), 37–72% of patients with Parkinsonism, and 15% of patients with stroke [3, 4].

Many other conditions like spina bifida, diabetes mellitus, pelvic surgeries, and cauda equina syndrome resulting from lumbar spine pathology are associated with varying degrees of lower urinary tract symptoms (LUTS) [3, 5].

Spinal cord injuries (SCI) often cause NLUTD [6]. 70–84% of patients with SCI have at least some degree of bladder dysfunction [3, 7].

R. T. Al-Mousa
Department of Urology, King Fahad Specialist Hospital,
Dammam, Saudi Arabia

H. Hashim (✉)
Bristol Urological Institute, Southmead Hospital, Bristol, UK

© Springer International Publishing AG, part of Springer Nature 2018
R. Dmochowski, J. Heesakkers (eds.), *Neuro-Urology*,
https://doi.org/10.1007/978-3-319-90997-4_14

In addition to the psychological, social, economic, and quality of life negative impact of NLUTD in this group of patients, NLUTD may cause a higher risk of upper urinary tract damage and renal function impairment compared to idiopathic causes of voiding dysfunction [3, 7, 8].

Lower urinary tract symptoms (LUTS) are classified by the International Continence Society (ICS) into storage, voiding, and post-micturition symptoms. Urinary incontinence is one of the common manifestations of NLUTD.

Urinary incontinence (UI), the involuntary loss of urine, is a term that can describe a symptom (patient's complaint), a sign (objective demonstration), or a condition of LUTS (the underlying cause). UI may occur with any patient with NLUTD. The mechanism of action is similar to that of idiopathic UI, but it carries more risk of upper urinary tract damage due to the comorbidities of such patients [8].

Process of Micturition

The bladder works as a reservoir to store urine at low pressure and empty when it is convenient and appropriate. This function is controlled by complex processes at all levels of the nervous system [3, 9].

There are three voiding centers that control micturition [9, 10] which are:

- The sacral micturition center
- The pontine micturition center
- The cerebral cortex

In general, urine storage is a function of the sympathetic nervous system through the hypogastric nerve (through signals from the spinal cord at levels T10–L2), whereas micturition is a function of the parasympathetic nervous system through the pelvic nerve (and these signals originate from the spinal cord levels at S2–S4). While both are autonomic functions in nature, the somatic nervous system is responsible for the control of the external urinary sphincter, allowing for volitional continence through the pudendal nerve [11]. Therefore, the lower urinary tract is unique organ in the body, having triple innervation.

Parasympathetic activity inhibition causes relaxation of the detrusor muscle. A competent urethral sphincter is mediated by the sympathetic and pudendal nerves (and pelvic nerve to a lesser degree) to prevent leakage during filling [12].

During voiding, the detrusor muscle contracts and the pelvic floor muscles and urethral sphincter relax by inhibition of sympathetic activity and the pudendal nerve [12] (details about the neuroanatomy can be found in Part I).

As mentioned before, a disruption to this triple innervation can cause LUTD.

Definition

Urinary incontinence (UI): complaint of any involuntary loss of urine [13].

Types of UI [13, 14]

UI can be divided into six general types:

1. **Total continuous UI:** continuous involuntary loss of urine without normal voiding.
   Causes: major sphincteric abnormalities (e.g., exstrophy of the bladder, epispadias), ectopic ureteral orifices, or vesicovaginal fistula
2. **Urgency UI:** involuntary loss of urine associated with urgency. It's usually as a result of an involuntary detrusor muscle contraction that leads to a rise in intravesical pressure that overcomes the outlet resistance.
3. **Stress UI:** involuntary loss of urine on effort or physical exertion and not caused by a bladder contraction (e.g., loss of urine during sneezing, coughing, laughing, lifting, and exercise).
   Causes: could be due to weak pelvic floor muscles (e.g., following multiple vaginal deliveries in females) or could be due to iatrogenic injuries to the external urethral sphincter post-surgery (e.g., post-prostatectomy)
4. **Mixed UI:** complaint of involuntary loss of urine associated with urgency and also with effort or physical exertion or on sneezing or coughing.
5. **Enuresis:** complaint of involuntary loss of urine which occurs during sleep.
6. **Incontinence associated with chronic retention** of urine and failure of the bladder to empty. It is commonly known as **overflow incontinence**, but this is no longer recommended by the ICS. This type of UI is dangerous in neurogenic patients due to risk of autonomic dysreflexia in patients with spinal cord injuries above T10.
7. **Other Less Common Types of UI**

   (a) Postural urinary incontinence: Complaint of involuntary loss of urine associated with change of body position, for example, rising from a seated or lying position.
   (b) Insensible urinary incontinence: Complaint of urinary incontinence where the individual is unaware of how it occurred.
   (c) Coital incontinence (for women only): Complaint of involuntary loss of urine with coitus. This symptom can be further divided into that occurring with penetration, suggestive of stress urinary incontinence, and that occurring at orgasm, suggestive of detrusor overactivity.

(d) Functional incontinence: Involuntary loss of urine that results from an inability to reach the toilet due to cognitive, functional, or mobility impairments in the presence of an intact lower urinary tract system, as can happen in frail elderly or disabled patients.

(e) Multifactorial incontinence: Involuntary loss of urine related to multiple interacting risk factors like comorbidity, medication, age-related physiological changes, and other environmental factors.

Causes and Risk Factors for UI [15–21]

The level of the injury can sometimes help predict the type of incontinence that a patient may suffer. In suprapontine lesions, patients are unaware of bladder filling and can't initiate a void at social times and therefore can suffer with enuresis. In infra-pontine/supra-sacral injuries, the patient may get detrusor sphincter dyssynergia and/or neurogenic detrusor overactivity. In sub-sacral lesions, there may be detrusor areflexia (acontractility), SUI, and potentially poor compliance. Finally in peripheral lesions, there can be areflexia and overflow UI or SUI.

The non-neurological causes can also affect neurological patients and may be an extra factor as to why patients with NLUTD are incontinent (Table 1).

Also, the term **DIAPPERS** can be used to help remember the functional and multifactorial contributors to incontinence, especially in the frail elderly [22]:

D: Delirium
I: Infection, urinary
A: Atrophic urethritis or vaginitis
P: Pharmacologic agents
P: Psychiatric illness

Table 1 Causes and risk factors for urgency and stress urinary incontinence

Urgency urinary incontinence (UUI)	Stress urinary incontinence (SUI)
• Diabetes mellitus and other metabolic conditions	• Obesity
• Heavy occupational work	• Chronic cough
• Neuropsychiatric disorders	• Chronic obstructive pulmonary disease (COPD)
• Smoking	• Heavy occupational work
• Previous pelvic surgery	• Smoking
• Constipation	• Previous pelvic surgery
• Radiotherapy	• Connective tissue disorders
• Congestive heart failure	• Postmenopausal hypoestrogenism
• Connective tissue disorders	• CNS or spinal cord disorders
• CNS or spinal cord disorders	• Cancer of pelvic organs
• Chronic UTIs	
• Urinary tract stones	
• Benign prostatic enlargement/obstruction	
• Cancer of pelvic organs	

E: Endocrine disorders
R: Reduced mobility or dexterity
S: Stool impaction

Assessment (See Part III for Further Details)

Patient with UI should undergo a basic evaluation that starts with a detailed history, physical examination, basic laboratory investigations, and specific diagnostic tests [13, 23] (Fig. 1).

- *History*

  - Nature of the neurological disease
  - Congenital abnormalities
  - Urological symptoms and complications (type of UI, frequency, severity, precipitating factors, other associated urological symptoms)
  - Effect on hygiene
  - Quality of life
  - The measures used to contain the leakage
  - Previous surgeries and treatments
  - Medications
  - Bowel, sexual obstetric, and family history
  - Social history like work, smoking, and alcohol
  - Presence of caregiver

- *Physical examination* [24, 25]

  - General physical examination should be done in all those patients.
  - Special attention shall be directed toward:

    Degree of mobility
    Sensation
    Spasticity
    Mental orientation
    Lower abdomen
    Pelvic floor
    External genitalia and perineal skin
    Neurological examination, especially of the lower limbs, including gait, power, tone, and reflexes
    Rectal examination feeling for anal tone, sensation, and strength of pelvic squeeze

- *Diagnostic tests*

  - Bladder diary is helpful to record voiding pattern, incontinence episodes, pad usage, and other information related to fluid intake [26].

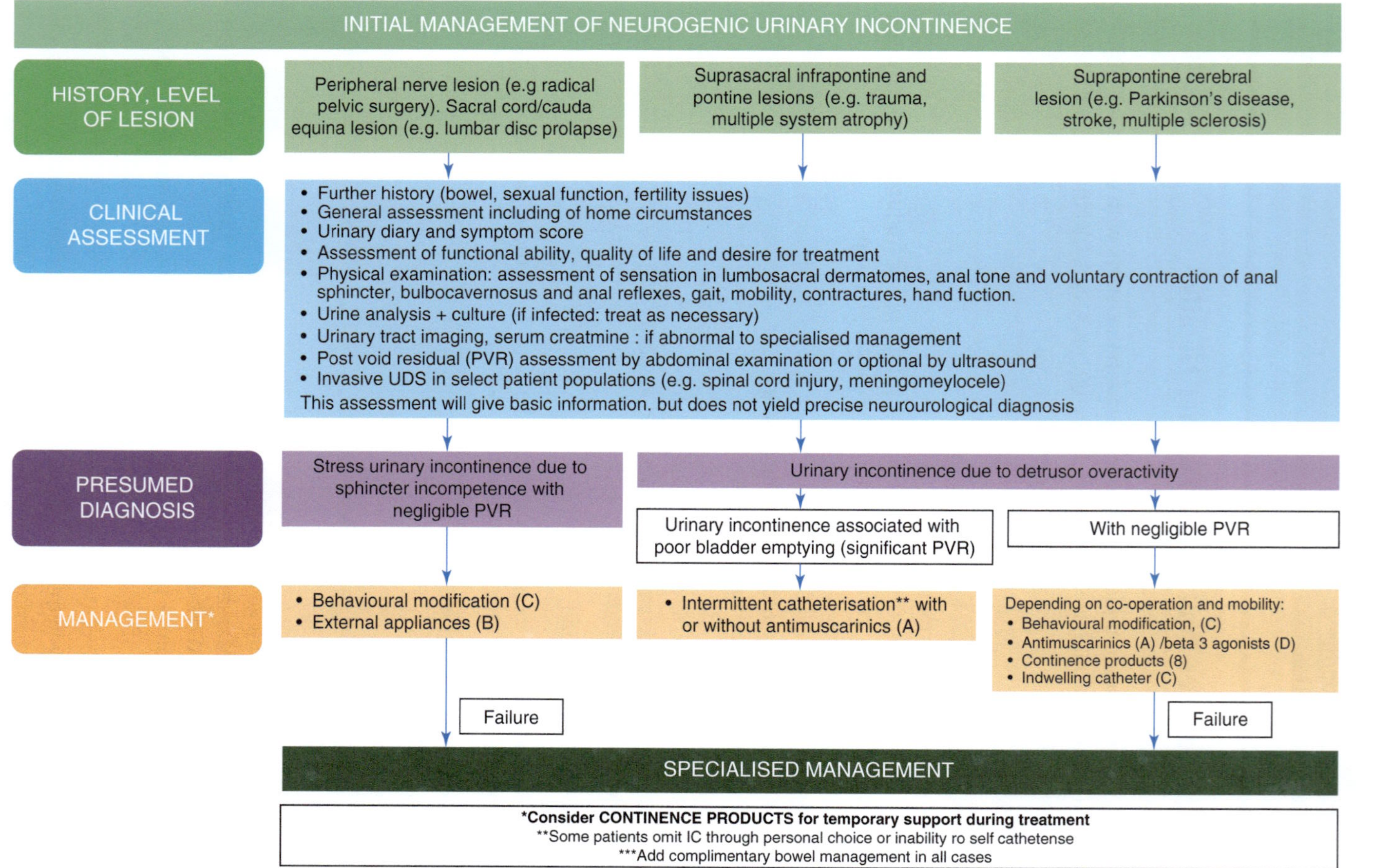

Fig. 1 Initial management of neurogenic UI (Incontinence, 6th edition 2017)

- Laboratory tests: Urine dipstick is mandatory, and if there are signs or symptoms of infection, then the urine should be sent for microscopy, culture, and sensitivity. If the patient is self-catheterizing, then there may be leucocytes and nitrites in the urine dipstick.
- Renal function test is indicated if the residual is high or the patient has other medical conditions such as diabetes [27, 28].
- Flow rate and post-void residual volume are important in patients who are voiding to assess the pattern of flow.
- Radiological tests: Ultrasound is helpful to assess the upper urinary tracts and check post-void residual volume. X-ray or CT KUB or further tests are indicated if there is a suspicion of stones [29].
- Urodynamic studies: Mainly in patients with spinal cord injuries, patients who did not respond to conservative and medical treatment and those who are planning to undergo any surgical intervention [30, 31].
- Cystoscopy: In selected patients like patients with hematuria or suspected urethral stricture or bladder outlet obstruction [32, 33].

Management (See Part IV for Further Details)

In order to have a successful treatment of urinary incontinence, a tailored management toward the specific type of incontinence and its related cause (in order to treat the underlying cause) must be followed [34].

The options of treatment depend on the underlying cause that may lead to the specific type of NLUTD and UI.

Neurogenic detrusor overactivity (NDO) leads to urgency incontinence, while detrusor acontractility might cause retention and overflow incontinence. SUI can be due to an incompetent urethral sphincter in such patients.

The aim of treatment is to preserve upper urinary tract, control continence, and improve quality of life. Treatment options include conservative, pharmacotherapy, minimally invasive procedures, and major surgery (see Fig. 2).

- *Conservative*

Conservative therapy is considered to be the initial line of treatment. It includes timed voiding, fluid manipulation, and hygiene care. These measures can be applied to all types of incontinence. Pelvic floor muscle training is another example of conservative measure that is more applicable in patients with SUI [35]. Bladder expression can be used in patients with low pressure bladders and should be avoided in patients with high-pressure "dangerous" bladders due to risk of upper tract damage.

Drainage using clean intermittent catheterization (CIC) by the person or a caregiver, condom sheath catheter, indwelling catheter (urethral or suprapubic), can be considered in persistence of UI [35–37]. It is important to try to avoid prolonged indwelling urethral catheters as they may cause a traumatic hypospadias

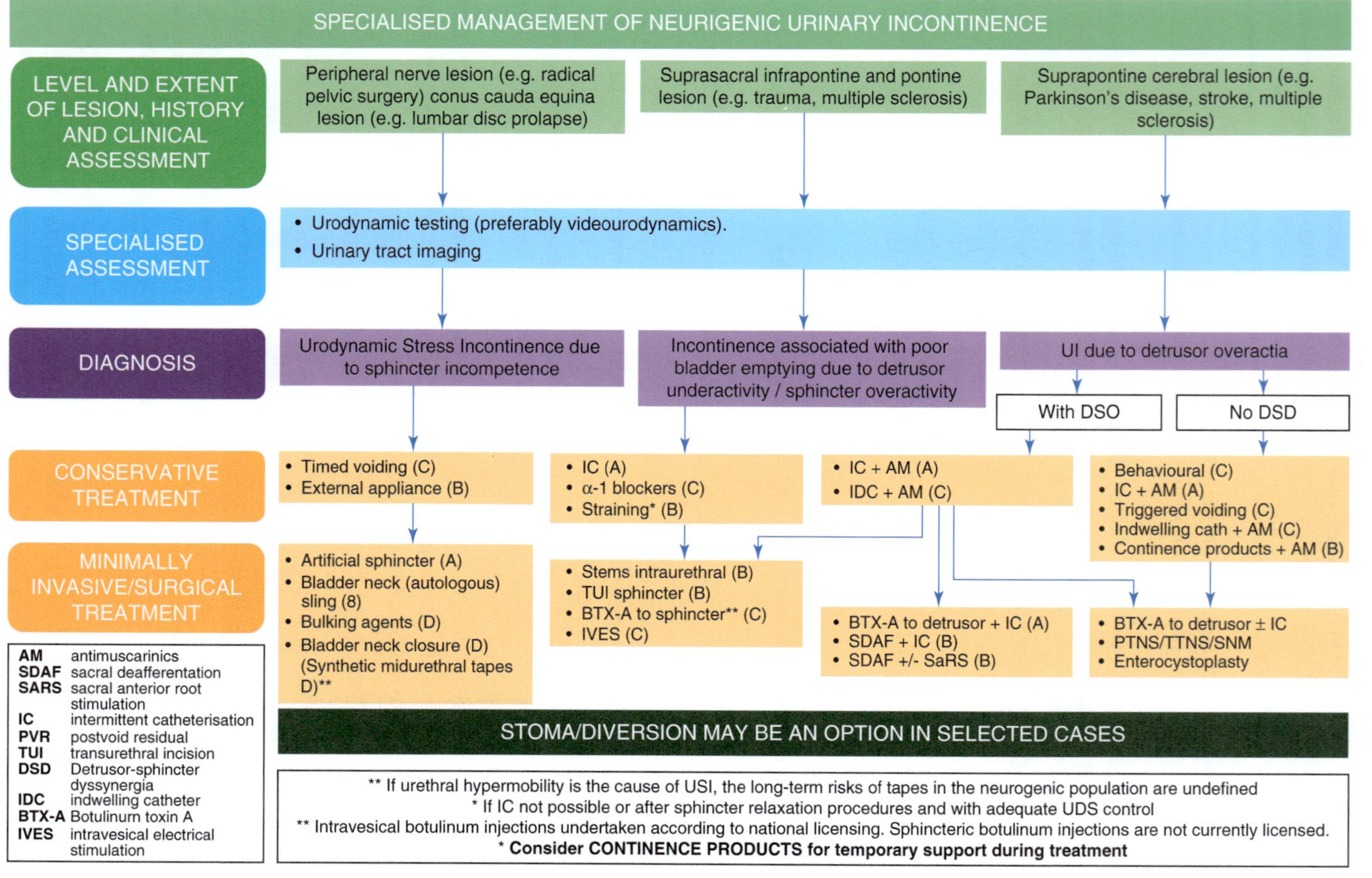

Fig. 2 Specialized management of neurogenic UI (Incontinence, 6th edition 2017)

and in patients with very high-pressure bladders could lead to the expulsion of the catheter with an intact balloon which would traumatize the urethra.
CIC is the preferred method if can be used by the patient or his caregiver [37, 38].

- *Medications*

  Drugs can be used as a single-line therapy, in combination with multiple drugs or in combination with other therapeutic measures (conservative or surgical).

  1. Drugs that are used to increase bladder capacity and decrease detrusor overactivity (DO):

     (a) Anticholinergic/antimuscarinic medications: Although considered to be the mainstay of pharmacotherapy in treating patients with idiopathic urgency UI [39], the efficacy of anticholinergic medications in neurogenic bladder patients has been documented in many studies [40–44]. On the other hand, there are recent data that shows that their efficacy is limited [45].

     (b) Beta3 agonists: Relatively new approved drug with studies showed significant improvement in bladder capacity, frequency, and incontinence episodes in neurogenic bladder patients, but more studies are needed to support its efficacy [46].

  2. Drugs that are used for urethral sphincter competency:

     (a) To increase sphincter resistance: Many drugs have been tried in the past such as alpha-agonist, estrogens, beta adrenergic agonists, tricyclic antidepressant, and duloxetine with no proven benefits.

     (b) To decrease outlet resistance: Alpha-blockers are widely used in men with benign prostatic obstruction, but studies have shown that they can improve bladder emptying [47, 48] in some male and female neurological patients.

- *Surgery*

  1. Minimally invasive surgeries for neurogenic UUI:

     (a) Botulinum neurotoxin type A (BoNT/A) injection: It is a relatively new approved treatment modality for patients with neurogenic UI with numerous literatures that support the efficacy and safety of BoNT/A [49–56], with reported failure rate in some cases of up to 30% [51]. BoNT/A also showed relative efficacy in treating detrusor sphincter dyssynergia (DSD) by sphincter injection [57, 58] (chemical sphincterotomy); however, this is an unlicensed use. Onabotulinum toxin A (Botox®) at a dose of 200 units in 30 mls and 30 injections is currently the only licensed formulation for neurogenic detrusor overactivity. Trials are ongoing with other formulations of BoNT/A.

(b) Electrical stimulation: It varies from simple local stimulation like anogenital stimulation, posterior tibial nerve stimulation, or pudendal nerve stimulation to more advanced procedures like sacral neuromodulation (SNM) or deep brain stimulation. In urgency-frequency syndrome, idiopathic UUI, and non-obstructed urinary retention, the efficacy of SNM has been well studied and proven [59]. The efficacy of electrical stimulation in neurogenic cases is controversial with available data that support the use of SNM in patients with incomplete spinal cord or incomplete medullary lesions [60–64] and stable multiple sclerosis.

2. Surgeries for SUI:

    (a) Artificial urinary sphincter [65]
    (b) Bulking agents [66, 67]
    (c) Autologous sling [68]
    (d) Bladder neck closure and continent urinary diversion [69]

3. Other surgical procedures: More invasive surgical procedures are considered to be the last resort in case of failure of all previous measures. Examples of these procedures include:

    (a) Denervation procedures for treatment of UUI due DO [70, 71]
    (b) Surgeries for DSD: endoscopic sphincterotomy or prosthetic sphincterotomy (stent) [72, 73]
    (c) Surgeries to increase detrusor strength: like latissimus dorsi myoplasty on the bladder which is a promising technique but still needs further validation [74]
    (d) Bladder augmentation and diversion [75–77]

Conclusion

Neurogenic lower urinary tract dysfunction and urinary incontinence negatively affect the quality of life of neurogenic patients. UI can result from disruption of the nerve supply to the lower urinary tract, and depending on the level of the injury, different types of urinary incontinence can be experienced. Treatment is aimed at protecting the upper urinary tracts and improving quality of life and should follow a pathway starting with conservative and medical therapy and then progressing to minimally invasive surgery with major surgery left as a last resort. The main thing is treatment of NLUTD should be individualized and tailored to the needs of the patient.

References

1. Del Popolo G, Panariello G, Del Croso F, et al. Diagnosis and therapy for neurogenic bladder dysfunctions in multiple sclerosis patients. Neurol Sci. 2008;29(suppl 4):S352–5. https://doi.org/10.1007/s10072-008-1042-y.
2. Kaplan SA, Chancellor MB, Blaivas JG. Bladder and sphincter behavior in patients with spinal cord lesions. J Urol. 1991;146:113–7.
3. Dorsher PT, McIntosh PM. Neurogenic bladder [published online February 8, 2012]. Adv Urol. 2012;2012:816274. https://doi.org/10.1155/2012/816274.
4. Lansang RS, Krouskop AC. Bladder management. In: Massagli TL, et al., editors. eMedicine; 2004.
5. Verhoef M, Lurvink M, Barf HA, et al. High prevalence of incontinence among young adults with spina bifida: description, prediction and problem perception. Spinal Cord. 2005;43:331–40.
6. Blok B, Pannek J, Castro-Diaz D et al. EAU Guidelines on Neuro-Urology. 2015. http://uroweb.org/guideline/neuro-urology. Accessed Mar 2015.
7. Manack A, Mostko SP, Haag-Molkenteller, et al. Epidemiology and healthcare utilization of neurogenic bladder patients in a US claims database. NeurourolUrodyn. 2011;30:395–401.
8. Linsenmeyer TA, Culkin D. APS recommendations for the urological evaluation of patients with spinal cord injury. J Spinal Cord Med. 1999;22:139–42.
9. Griffiths D, Derbyshire S, Stenger A, Resnick N. Brain control of normal and overactive bladder. J Urol. 2005;174(5):1862–7.
10. Panicker JN, de Seze M, Fowler CJ, et al. Rehabilitation in practice: neurogenic lower urinary tract dysfunction and its management. Clin Rehabil. 2010;24:579–89.
11. Fowler CJ, Griffiths D, de Groat WC. The neural control of micturition. Nat Rev Neurosci. 2008;9:453–66.
12. Ouslander JG. Management of overactive bladder. N Engl J Med. 2004;350(8):786–99.
13. Al-Shukri SA. Neurogenic bladder-assessment, investigation, and treatment. Eur Urol Rev. 2012;7:55–60.
14. Abrams P, Cardozo L, Fall M, Griffiths D, Rosier P, Ulmsten U, et al. The standardisation of terminology of lower urinary tract function: report from the standardisation sub-committee of the inter-national continence society. NeurourolUrodyn. 2002;21(2):167–78.
15. Haylen BT, de Ridder D, Freeman RM, Swift SE, Berghmans B, Lee J, et al. An International Urogynecological Association (IUGA)/International Continence Society (ICS) joint report on the terminology for female pelvic floor dysfunction. NeurourolUrodyn. 2010;29(1):4–20.
16. Dursun M, Otunctemur A, Ozbek E, Sahin S, Besiroglu H, Koklu I. Stress urinary incontinence and visceral adipose index: a new risk parameter. Int Urol Nephrol. 2014;46(12):2297–300.
17. Vissers D, Neels H, Vermandel A, De Wachter S, Tjalma WA, Wyndaele JJ, et al. The effect of non-surgical weight loss interventions on urinary incontinence in overweight women: a systematic review and meta-analysis. Obes Rev. 2014;15(7):610–7.
18. Lenherr SM, Clemens JQ, Braffett BH, Dunn RL, Cleary PA, Kim C, et al. Glycaemic control and risk of incident urinary incontinence in women with type 1 diabetes: results from the Diabetes Control and Complications Trial and Epidemiology of Diabetes Interventions and Complications study (DCCT/EDIC). Diabet Med. 2016;33(11):1528–35.
19. Ahn KS, Hong HP, Kweon HJ, Ahn AL, Oh EJ, Choi JK, et al. Correlation between overactive bladder syndrome and obsessive compulsive disorder in women. Korean J Fam Med. 2016;37(1):25–30.
20. Walid MS. Prevalence of urinary incontinence in female residents of American nursing homes and association with neuropsychiatric disorders. J Clin Med Res. 2009;1(1):37–9.
21. Nygaard IE, Shaw JM, Bardsley T, Egger MJ. Lifetime physical activity and female stress urinary incontinence. Am J Obstet Gynecol. 2015;213(1):40.e1–10.

22. Sheyn D, James RL, Taylor AK, Sam-marco AG, Benchek P, Mahajan ST. Tobacco use as a risk factor for reoperation in patients with stress urinary incontinence: a multi-institutional electronic medical record database analysis. Int Urogynecol J. 2015;26(9):1379–84.
23. DuBeau CE. The continuum of urinary incontinence in an aging population. Geriatrics. 2002;57(Suppl 1):S12–7.
24. Jensen JK, Nielsen FR Jr, Ostergard DR. The role of patient history in the diagnosis of urinary incontinence. Obstet Gynecol. 1994;83(5 Pt 2):904–10.
25. Schurch B, Schmid DM, Karsenty G, Reitz A. Can neurologic examination predict type of detrusor sphincter-dyssynergia in patients with spinal cord injury? Urology. 2005;65:243–6.
26. Abrams P, Agarwal M, Drake M, et al. A proposed guideline for the urological management of patients with spinal cord injury. BJU Int. 2008;101:989–94.
27. Wyndaele JJ, De Sy WA. Correlation between the findings of a clinical neurological examination and the urodynamic dysfunction in children with myelodysplasia. J Urol. 1985;133:638–40.
28. Hill TC, Baverstock R, Carlson KV, Estey EP, Gray GJ, Hill DC, Ho C, McGinnis RH, Moore K, Parmar R. Best practices for the treatment and prevention of urinary tract infection in the spinal cord injured population: the Alberta context. Can Urol Assoc J. 2013;7(3- 4):122–30.
29. Drake MJ. Re: influences on renal function in chronic spinal cord injured patients. J Urol. 2001;165(6 Pt 1):2006.
30. Bright E, Cotterill N, Drake M, Abrams P. Developing and validating the international consultation on incontinence questionnaire bladder diary. Eur Urol. 2014;66:294–300.
31. Wyndaele JJ. A critical review of urodynamic investigations in spinal cord injury patients. Paraplegia. 1984;22:138–44.
32. Nitti VW, Adler H, Combs AJ. The role of urodynamics in the evaluation of voiding dysfunction in men after cerebrovascular accident. J Urol. 1996;155:263–6.
33. Hamid R, Bycroft J, Arya M, Shah PJ. Screening cystoscopy and biopsy in patients with neuropathic bladder and chronic suprapubic indwelling catheters: is it valid? J Urol. 2003;170:425–7.
34. Sammer U, Walter M, Knüpfer SC, Mehnert U, Bode-Lesniewska B, Kessler TM. Do we need surveillance Urethro-cystoscopy in patients with neurogenic lower urinary tract dysfunction? PLoS One. 2015;10(10):e0140970.
35. Lucas MG, Bosch RJ, Burkhard FC, Cruz F, Madden TB, Nambiar AK, et al. EAU guidelines on assessment and nonsurgical management of urinary incontinence. Eur Urol. 2012;62(6):1130–42. Erratum in: Eur Urol. 2013;64(1):e20
36. Bothig R, Hirschfeld S, Thietje R. Quality of life and urological morbidity in tetraplegics with artificial ventilation managed with suprapubic or intermittent catheterisation. Spinal Cord. 2012;50:247–51.
37. Cameron AP, Wallner LP, Forchheimer MB, et al. Medical and psychosocial complications associated with method of bladder management after traumatic spinal cord injury. Arch Phys Med Rehabil. 2011;92:449–56.
38. Di Benedetto P. Clean intermittent self-catheterization in neuro-urology. Eur J Phys Rehabil Med. 2011;47:651–9.
39. Kochakarn W, Ratana-Olarn K, Lertsithichai P, Roongreungsilp U. Follow-up of long-term treatment with clean intermittent catheterization for neurogenic bladder in children. Asian J Surg. 2004;27:134–6.
40. Gajewski JB, Awad SA. Oxybutynin versus propantheline in patients with multiple sclerosis and detrusor hyperreflexia. J Urol. 1986;135:966–8.
41. Lee JH, Kim KR, Lee YS, Han SW, Kim KS, Song SH, Baek M, Park K. Efficacy, tolerability, and safety of oxybutynin chloride in pediatricneurogenic bladder with spinal dysraphism: a retrospective, multicenter, observational study. Korean J Urol. 2014;55(12):828–33.
42. Mazo EB, Krivoborodov GG, Shkol'nikov ME, Babanina GA, Kozyrev SV, Korshunov ES. Trospium chloride in the treatment of idiopathic and neurogenic detrusor overactivity. Urologiia. 2005:56–9.
43. Mazo EB, Babanina GA. Trospium chloride (spasmex) in the treatment of lower urinary tract symptoms in patients with neurogenic hyperactive urinary bladder caused by vertebrogenic lesions. Urologiia. 2007:15–9.

44. van Rey F, Heesakkers J. Solifenacin in multiple sclerosis patients with overactive bladder: a prospective study. Adv Urol. 2011;2011:834753.
45. Krebs J, Pannek J. Effects of Solifenacin in patients with neurogenic detrusor overactivity as a result of spinal cord lesion. Spinal Cord. 2013;51:306–9.
46. Nicholas RS, Friede T, Hollis S, Young CA. Anticholinergics for urinary symptoms in multiple sclerosis. Cochrane Database Syst Rev. 2009;(1):CD004193.
47. Wöllner J, Pannek J. Initial experience with the treatment of neurogenic detrusor overactivity with a new beta-3 agonist (Mirabegron) in patients with spinal cord injury. Spinal Cord. 2016;54(1):78–82.
48. Stankovich E, Borisov VV, Demina TL. Tamsulosin in the treatment of detrusor sphincter dyssynergia of the urinary bladder in patients with multiple sclerosis. Urologia. 2004:48–51.
49. Abrams P, Amarenco G, Bakke A, Buczynski A, Castro-Diaz D, Harrison S, et al. Tamsulosin: efficacy and safety in patients with neurogenic lower urinary tract dysfunction due to suprasacral spinal cord injury. J Urol. 2003;170:1242–51.
50. Karsenty G, Denys P, et al. Botulinum toxin A (Botox) intradetrusor injections in adults with neurogenic detrusor overactivity/neurogenic overactive bladder: a systematic literature review. Eur Urol. 2008;53(2):275–7.
51. Apostolidis A, Dasgupta P, Denys P, Elneil S, Fowler CJ, Giannantoni A, et al. Recommendations on the use of botulinum toxin in the treatment of lower urinary tract disorders and pelvic floor dysfunctions: a European consensus panel report. Eur Urol 2009;55:100-120.
52. Mangera A, Andersson KE, Apostolidis A, Chapple C, Dasgupta P, Giannantoni A, et al. Contemporary management of lower urinary tract disease with botulinum toxin A: a systematic review of botox (onabotulinumtoxinA) and dysport (abobotulinumtoxinA). Eur Urol. 2011;60(4):784–95.
53. Duthie JB, Vincent M, Herbison GP, Wilson DI, Wilson D. Botulinum toxin injections for adults with overactive bladder syndrome. Cochrane Database Syst Rev. 2011;12:CD005493.
54. Mangera A, Apostolidis A, Andersson KE, Dasgupta P, Giannantoni A, Roehrborn C, et al. An updated systematic review and statistical comparison of standardised mean outcomes for the use of botulinum toxin in the management of lower urinary tract disorders. Eur Urol. 2014;65(5):981–90.
55. Zhang R, Xu Y, Yang S, Liang H, Zhang Y, Liu Y. OnabotulinumtoxinA for neurogenic detrusor overactivity and dose differences: a systematic review. Int Braz J Urol. 2015;41(2):207–19.
56. Schurch B, de Seze M, Denys P, Chartier- Kastler E, Haab F, Everaert K, et al. Botulinum toxin type a is a safe and effective treatment for neurogenic urinary incontinence: results of a single treatment, randomized, placebo controlled 6-month study. J Urol. 2005;174(1):196–200.
57. Giannantoni A, Di Stasi SM, Stephen RL, Bini V, Konstantini E, Porena M. Intravesical resiniferatoxin versus botulinum-A toxin injections for neurogenic detrusor overactivity: a prospective randomized study. J Urol. 2004;172(1):240–3.
58. de Seze M, Petit H, Gallien P, de Seze MP, Joseph PA, Mazaux JM, et al. Botulinum a toxin and detrusor sphincter dyssynergia: a double blind lidocaine-controlled study in 13 patients with spinal cord disease. Eur Urol. 2002;42(1):56–62.
59. Gallien P, Reymann JM, Amarenco G, Nicolas B, de Seze M, Bellissant E. Placebo controlled, randomised, double blind study of the effects of botulinum A toxin on detrusor sphincter dyssynergia in multiple sclerosis patients. J Neurol Neurosurg Psychiatry. 2005;76(12):1670–6.
60. van Kerrebroeck PE, van Voskuilen AC, Heesakkers JP, Lycklama a Nijholt AA, Siegel S, Jonas U, et al. Results of sacral neuromodulation therapy for urinary voiding dysfunction: outcomes of a prospective, worldwide clinical study. J Urol. 2007;178:2029–34.
61. de Seze M, Raibaut P, Gallien P, et al. Transcutaneous posterior tibial nerve stimulation for treatment of the overactive bladder syndrome in multiple sclerosis: results of a multicenter prospective study. NeurourolUrodyn. 2011;30:306–11.
62. Hagerty JA, Richards I, Kaplan WE. Intravesical electrotherapy for neurogenic bladder dysfunction: a 22-year experience. J Urol. 2007;178:1680–3.
63. Vodusek DB, Light JK, Libby JM. Detrusor inhibition induced by stimulation of pudendal nerve afferents. NeurourolUrodyn. 1986;5:381–90.

64. Chartier-Kastler EJ, Ruud Bosch JL, Perrigot M, Chancellor MB, Richard F, Denys P. Long term results of sacral nerve stimulation (S3) for the treatment of neurogenic refractory urge incontinence related to detrusor hyperreflexia. J Urol. 2000;164:1476–80.
65. Bosch RJL, Groen J. Neuromodulation: urodynamic effects of sacral (S3) spinal nerve stimulation in patients with detrusor instability or detrusor hyperflexia. Behav Brain Res. 1998;92:141–50.
66. Zvara P, Sahi S, Hassouna MM. An animal model for the neuromodulation of neurogenic bladder dysfunction. Br J Urol. 1998;82:267–71.
67. Kessler TM, Burkhard FC, Z'Brun S, Stibal A, Studer UE, Hess CW, et al. Effect of thalamic deep brain stimulation on lower urinary tract function. Eur Urol. 2008;53:607–12.
68. Blok BF, Groen J, Bosch JL, Veltman DJ, Lammertsma AA. Different brain effects during chronic and acute sacral neuromodulation in urge incontinent patients with implanted neurostimulators. BJU Int. 2006;98:1238–43.
69. Colli J, Lloyd LK. Bladder neck closure and suprapubic catheter placement as definitive management of neurogenic bladder. J Spinal Cord Med. 2011;34(3):273–7.
70. Westney OL, Lee JT, McGuire EJ, Palmer JL, Cespedes RD, Amundsen CL. Long-term results of Ingelman-Sundberg denervation procedure for urge incontinence refractory to medical therapy. J Urol. 2002;168:1044–7.
71. Cespedes RD, Cross CA, McGuire EJ. Modified Ingelman-Sundberg bladder denervation procedure for intractable urge incontinence. J Urol. 1996;156:1744–7.
72. Ross JC, Damanski M, Giddons N. Resection of the external urethral sphincter in the paraplegic- preliminary report. J Urol. 1958;79:742–6.
73. Chancellor MB, Gajewski J, Ackman CF, Appell RA, Bennett J, Binard J, et al. Long-term follow up of the North American multicenter UroLume trial for the treatment of external detrusor- sphincter dyssynergia. J Urol. 1999;161:1545–50.
74. Ninkovic M, Stenzl A, Schwabegger A, Bartsch G, Prosser R, Ninkovic M. Free neurovascular transfer of latissimus dorsi muscle for the treatment of bladder acontractility: II. Clinical results. J Urol. 2003;169:1379–83.
75. Gundeti MS, Acharya SS, Zagaja GP, Shalhav AL. Paediatric robotic-assisted laparoscopic augmentation ileocystoplasty and Mitrofanoff appendicovesicostomy (RALIMA): feasibility of and initial experience with the University of Chicago technique. BJU Int. 2011;107:962–9.
76. Ehrlich RM, Gershman A. Laparoscopic seromyotomy (auto-augmentation) for non-neurogenic neurogenic bladder in a child: initial case report. Urology. 1993;42:175–8.
77. Mollard P, Gauriau L, Bonnet JP, Mure PY. Continent cystostomy (Mitrofanoff's procedure) for neurogenic bladder in children and adolescent (56 cases: long-term results). Eur J Pediatr Surg. 1997;7:34–7.

Urinary Retention and Voiding Dysfunction

Dominique Malacarne Pape and Victor W. Nitti

Introduction

Normal voluntary micturition in adults involves a delicate balance of various components of the autonomic and somatic nervous systems and coordination of the brain and spinal cord. Disruption of this symbiosis, whether functional or anatomic, can lead to significant dysfunction of the lower urinary tract and ultimately both lower and upper tract decompensation. At rest, the sympathetic and somatic nervous systems work to store urine; this is mediated by the buildup of cyclic adenosine monophosphate (AMP) leading to relaxation of bladder smooth muscle (beta-3 receptors) and the simultaneous contraction of urethral smooth muscle via the hypogastric nerve (alpha-1 receptors). The parasympathetic system is activated with sufficient bladder filling to reflexively inhibit this storage mode, resulting in release of acetylcholine to induce outlet relaxation and detrusor contraction via M3 receptor stimulation [1]. Voluntary urination subsequently ensues in the appropriate social setting. With disturbance of this system comes disrupted voiding patterns and ultimately the inability to execute complete bladder emptying. Proper bladder emptying requires generation of a detrusor contraction that will overcome bladder outlet resistance [2]. When there is a lack of coordination between these two processes, dysfunction can result. That dysfunction can lie with the bladder or the outlet or a combination of both. Thus one must consider the possibility of detrusor underactivity, increased resistance of the bladder outlet, or a component of both. To adequately diagnose and treat voiding dysfunction,

D. Malacarne Pape (✉) · V. W. Nitti
Department of Urology, Female Pelvic Medicine and Reconstructive Surgery,
NYU Langone Medical Center, New York, NY, USA
e-mail: malacd01@nyumc.org; Victor.Nitti@nyumc.org

© Springer International Publishing AG, part of Springer Nature 2018
R. Dmochowski, J. Heesakkers (eds.), *Neuro-Urology*,
https://doi.org/10.1007/978-3-319-90997-4_15

it is imperative to understand the different neurologic, endocrine, cognitive, and musculoskeletal factors that can plague normal voiding. This chapter aims to review the pathophysiology of urinary retention and potential etiologies of voiding dysfunction in men and women. Additionally, the focus of accurate diagnosis and various treatment modalities for both bladder dysfunction and outlet dysfunction will be emphasized. In this chapter we use the term "voiding dysfunction" to describe problems with the voiding phase of the micturition cycle, independent of the storage phase.

Prevalence and Pathophysiology of Voiding Dysfunction

Approximately 50% of all elderly patients experience some form of voiding dysfunction. The EPIC trial revealed that both men and women $\geq$60 years old experience some type of voiding symptom, ranging from slow urinary stream, intermittency, terminal dribbling, to straining (37.2% and 27.6% of women and men, respectively) [3, 4]. While more commonly found in our ageing population, voiding dysfunction and incomplete bladder emptying can affect patients of all ages and can result from physiologic or anatomic insults. In a more recent trial surveying the USA, the UK, and Sweden, the prevalence of voiding and storage LUTS was examined using ICS definitions. The prevalence of at least one LUTS at least "sometimes" was 72.3% for men and 76.3% for women. The average age of participants was 56.6 years (40–99) [5]. The reported LUTS in men and women over the age of 40 years old appears higher than previously understood and is demonstrated similarly in men and women. When looking at different racial and ethnic groups, one recent study found significant differences in type of LUTS when comparing white, African-American (AA), and Hispanic groups of both men and women. Differences in nine categories of LUTS were identified among different racial/ethnic groups in men, and Hispanic men were more likely to suffer from perception of urinary frequency, urgency with fear of leak, straining, split stream, and hesitancy ($p < 0.05$). When looking at women only, split stream (11.8%), nocturia (37.6%), and urgency urinary incontinence (UUI) (19.3%) were highest among AA women, while stress urinary incontinence (SUI) (40.1%) and leak for no reason (5.9%) were highest among white women. AA and Hispanic men and women tended to have higher prevalence of LUTS despite reporting fewer comorbid conditions and LUTS risk factors [6]. This epidemiologic information is invaluable for understanding patient risk factors for voiding dysfunction and incomplete bladder-emptying symptoms.

The biological process of micturition constitutes transition from the storage phase of the cycle to the voiding phase. This process begins with the desire to urinate and/or the anticipation of an inability to void (lack of socially appropriate accessibility to a toilet). Multiple centers of the central nervous system (CNS) coordinate to initiate this process. In storage mode, the bladder neck is contracted, and the detrusor muscle is relaxed through control of the sympathetic nervous system (SNS). Conversely, the urinary sphincter, controlled by Onuf's nucleus, is contracted at baseline. During transition to voiding mode, the parasympathetic nucleus is activated to generate detrusor contraction, which reflexively inhibits the SNS and somatic systems. This results in relaxation of the urinary sphincter and bladder neck and expulsion of urine ensues [7, 8]. When emptying is complete, or when voiding needs to be unexpectedly terminated, the neuromuscular processes of the micturition complex allow for restoration of storage mode. Various pharmacologic factors are also responsible for normal voiding processes. Loss of excitatory motor innervation results in dysfunction of this complex matrix. This can occur with neurogenic insult, bladder outlet obstruction, or human ageing, and careful workup is imperative to arrive at an accurate etiology of voiding dysfunction [9].

The physiologic effects of bladder outlet obstruction are well understood. Bladder outlet obstruction can be fixed (anatomical) or functional, and it is recognized that with reversal of obstruction, the bladder has an amazing ability to recover as early as 14 days following reversal of the inciting event [10]. It is known that chronic outlet obstruction, whether fixed or functional, causes changes in the extracellular matrix and smooth muscle enzymatic complex of the bladder. This leads to an increase in collagenous deposits and a subsequent decrease in myosin deposition leading to a loss of contractility of the muscle matrix and a decrease in the force of the detrusor contraction. The viscoelastic properties of the bladder are thought to be compromised due to ischemic changes that are a secondary result of obstruction [11, 12]. The severity of bladder muscle dysfunction has been continually found to correlate more with degree of collagen deposition, calcium dysregulation, and tissue hypertrophy and less with duration of obstruction [13, 14]. Histologic studies reveal connective tissue found in between smooth muscle cells and bundles, blocking muscle contraction [15]. Even with smooth muscle cell recovery, collagen distribution inhibits the ability for organized and sustained contractions, thereby resulting in significant bladder decompensation.

The pathophysiology of bladder dysfunction without identifiable obstruction is less clear; however we do know there are various neurogenic, pharmacologic, and myogenic entities that can be involved. Structural changes that accompany normal ageing include decreased ratios of detrusor muscle to collagen deposition and widespread detrusor myocyte disruption and axonal degeneration, much like those changes related to BOO. There is also a decline in autonomic nerve innervation in normal human bladders correlating directly with age [16, 17]. These factors are thought to contribute to insufficient contraction and subsequent voiding dysfunction. Apart from myogenic etiologies, there can also be dysfunction of the central neural control of the voiding reflex. Various animal studies have revealed that neurons of the pontine micturition center (PMC) that fire during reflex bladder contraction pass through the lumbosacral spinal cord. The trajectory of these direct neurons is found to be similar in humans [18, 19]. Diseases with direct neuronal injury, such as multisystem atrophy, Parkinson's disease, and multiple sclerosis, are likely associated with disruption in the efferent nerves, resulting in likely reduced neuromuscular activation and subsequent poor detrusor contractility. Disruption to the afferent system can cause detrusor underactivity by reducing or prematurely ending the micturition reflex. In various diseases such as diabetic cystopathy, this system is disrupted. Subsequently, sensory input is dulled and detrusor smooth muscle matrix is compromised [20–21]. This results in inefficient voiding due to the inability to accurately monitor storage volumes and the magnitude of smooth muscle contraction. More initiatives are needed to understand these physiologic mechanisms of myogenic and neuropathic compromise.

While it is clear there are molecular changes associated with urinary retention and voiding dysfunction, it is less clear as to what leads to the development of bothersome symptoms for some individuals. A number of theories exist, including the makeup of the detrusor muscle itself. It has been suggested that the detrusor is comprised of circumscribed modules controlled by a peripheral myovesical plexus, intramural ganglia, and interstitial cells. The reduction of blood flow that results with BOO then leads to ischemic insult leading to denervation of many of these modules. There is a reflexive excitation that ensues in the affected muscle modules, and eventually denervation progresses giving way to detrusor decompensation [22]. This postulation can explain why resolution of symptoms is not always reached with treatment. Other studies have focused on smooth muscle proteins. Increased fluid pressure from urinary retention has been found to cause a four- to fivefold increase in certain gap junction proteins, particularly Connexin 26 and Connexin 43, thought to cause irritative (storage) symptoms. Other studies have focused on alpha-1 adrenergic receptor subtypes as having a marked role in the development of symptomatology associated with urinary retention and voiding dysfunction [23, 24].

Voiding Dysfunction Terminology and Etiologies

There is a vital importance of a common understanding of the terminology, for purposes of reporting results and developing guidelines for treatment of bladder-emptying disorders. The International Continence Society (ICS) originally established terminology guidelines in 1998 for a variety of lower urinary tract symptoms (LUTS) and diagnoses. LUTS now serves as a global term that refers to symptoms representative of any bladder, urinary outlet, musculoskeletal, or neurologic abnormalities related to voiding and storage of urine. A terminology consensus has been most recently updated in 2002 with additions in 2016, and a terminology report for adult neurogenic lower urinary tract dysfunction (ANLUTD) has been added in 2017 [25–27]. Table 1 reviews definitions from these reports as they pertain to urinary retention and disorders of voiding dysfunction.

Various etiologies can contribute to incomplete bladder emptying, and it is important to classify these causes appropriately in order to arrive at optimal diagnostic and treatment modalities for a specific condition. We have found the functional classification system proposed by Wein et al. to be the most practical [28]. In simple anatomic terms voiding, dysfunction is categorized as dysfunction of the bladder, dysfunction of the bladder outlet, or both (Fig. 1). The subsequent consequences of these problems can then be classified as failure to store urine, failure to empty urine, and failure to store and empty urine. While insight into the functional and structural causes of voiding dysfunction is important, this should be understood in conjunction with the ability to distinguish neurogenic from non-neurogenic

Table 1 ICS definitions of LUTS as they pertain to urinary retention and bladder-emptying disorders

Terminology	Definition
Normal detrusor function	A voluntarily initiated continuous detrusor contraction that leads to complete bladder emptying within a normal time span and in the absence of obstruction For a given detrusor contraction, the magnitude of the recorded pressure rise will depend on the degree of outlet resistance
Lower urinary tract symptoms (LUTS)	The subjective indicator of a disease or condition as perceived by the patient, caregiver, or partner that may lead him/her to seek help from healthcare professionals *Storage symptoms: Frequency, nocturia, urgency, urinary incontinence* *Voiding symptoms: Slow stream, splitting or spraying, intermittency, hesitancy, straining, terminal dribble* *Post-micturition symptoms: Feeling of incomplete emptying, post-micturition dribble*
Underactive bladder	Slow urinary stream, hesitancy, and straining to void, with or without a feeling of incomplete bladder emptying and dribbling, often with storage symptoms "Occurs in association with diverse pathologies and based on current knowledge there is no single distinguishing symptom" "Storage symptoms in UAB are varied and may be highly prevalent, including nocturia, increased daytime frequency, reduced sensation of filling, and incontinence" "Underlying mechanisms of storage symptoms are diverse and are often related to a significant post voiding residual urine volume"
Detrusor underactivity	A contraction of reduced strength and/or duration, resulting in prolonged bladder emptying and/or a failure to achieve complete bladder emptying within a normal time span
Acontractile detrusor	One that cannot be demonstrated to contract during urodynamic studies
Neurogenic detrusor underactivity	A contraction of reduced strength and/or duration, resulting in prolonged bladder emptying and/or a failure to achieve complete bladder emptying within a normal time span in the setting of a clinically relevant neurologic disorder
Neurogenic acontractile detrusor	One that cannot be demonstrated to contract during urodynamic studies in the setting of a clinically relevant neurologic lesion
Bladder outlet obstruction	The generic term for obstruction during voiding and is characterized by increased detrusor pressure and reduced urine flow rate. It is usually diagnosed by studying the synchronous values of flowrate and detrusor pressure *Further stated that bladder outlet dysfunction has been defined for men but, as yet, not adequately in women and children*
Dysfunctional voiding	Voiding characterized by an intermittent and/or fluctuating flow rate due to involuntary intermittent contractions of the peri-urethral striated muscle during voiding in neurologically normal individuals *It has also be termed non-neurogenic neurogenic bladder, idiopathic detrusor sphincter dyssynergia, or sphincter overactivity voiding dysfunction*
Detrusor sphincter dyssynergia	A detrusor contraction concurrent with an involuntary contraction of the urethral and/or peri-urethral striated muscle. Occasionally, flow may be prevented altogether *Occurs in patients with a supra-sacral lesion and is uncommon in lesions of the lower cord*

(continued)

Table 1 (continued)

Terminology	Definition
Non-relaxing urethral sphincter obstruction	Usually occurs in individuals with a neurological lesion and is characterized by a non-relaxing, obstructing urethra resulting in reduced urine flow *Found in sacral and infra-sacral lesions. This term replaces isolated distal sphincter obstruction*
Delayed relaxation of the urethral sphincter	Impaired and hindered relaxation of the sphincter during voiding attempt resulting in delay of urine flow
Acute retention of urine	A painful, palpable, or percussible bladder, when the patient is unable to pass any urine *In certain circumstances pain may not be a presenting feature (herniated vertebral disc, postanesthesia,* postpartum*)*
Chronic retention of urine	A non-painful bladder, which remains palpable or percussible after the patient has passed urine. Such patients may be incontinent *Implies a significant residual urine (a minimum figure of 300 mL has been previously mentioned in men)*
Complete urinary retention	Inability to empty any amount of bladder volume (or the requirement for use of a catheter, consciously or unconsciously due to anatomical or functional bladder outlet obstruction, detrusor underactivity, or both)
Incomplete urinary retention	Impaired bladder emptying due to anatomical or functional bladder outlet obstruction, detrusor underactivity, or both, when the voided volume is smaller than post-void residual
Benign prostatic obstruction	A form of *bladder outlet obstruction* and may be diagnosed when the cause of outlet obstruction is known to be benign prostatic enlargement, due to histologic benign prostatic hyperplasia

International Continence Society Sub-Committee Standardization of Terminology in Lower Urinary Tract Function and report on terminology for Adult Neurogenic Lower Urinary Tract Dysfunction (ANLUTD)

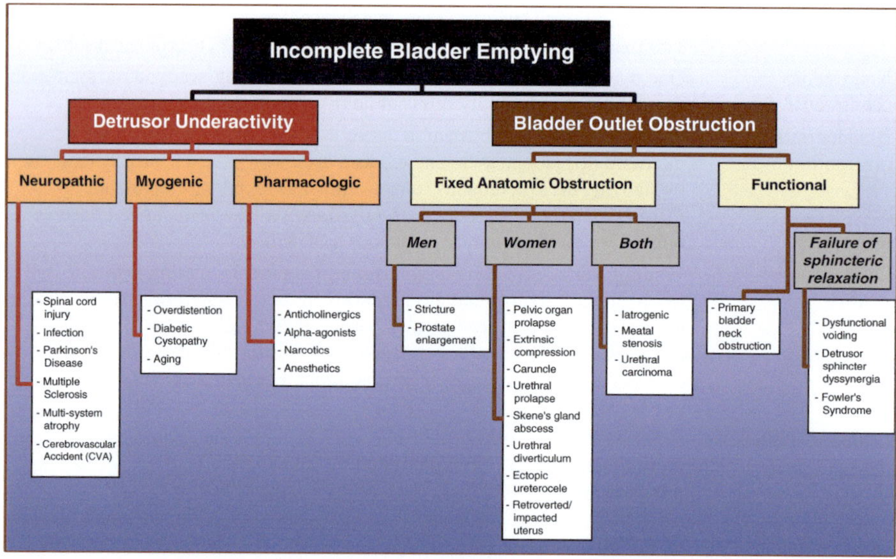

Fig. 1 Causes of voiding dysfunction and urinary retention

causes of voiding dysfunction. With neurogenic voiding dysfunction, it is important to discern the different innervation levels, and pathologic processes at each of these levels should be considered. Newly defined clinical diagnoses have been established depending on which part(s) of the nervous system is affected [27]. When diagnosing and treating these conditions, it is crucial to recognize that neurologic processes can affect both bladder and outlet dysfunction (Fig. 2).

Detrusor Underactivity

Detrusor underactivity (DU) is a fairly common cause of LUTS and is thought to occur in about 9–48% of men and 12–45% of women undergoing urodynamic evaluation [29]. It is important to recognize that these estimates may be skewed, as voiding under testing conditions may be influenced by anxiety and the voiding reflex may be blunted and detrusor contraction inhibited. It is important to recognize this in evaluating the comprehensive clinical scenario of incomplete bladder emptying and make sure to consider subjective symptoms and objective findings in combination. ICS recently published a review on urodynamic practices and terms and suggests "situational inability to void" when attempted voiding is not representative of a usual situation. This document also suggests further characterization using terms "unsustained contraction" when waxing and waning or "fading contraction" to describe certain patterns during a urodynamic evaluation [30]. When evaluating patients with concern for detrusor underactivity, these terms may assist with characterizing urodynamic findings and arriving at appropriate diagnoses. Additionally, in order to decrease ambiguity and confusion, it is important to always consider underlying etiologies and note that neurogenic and non-neurogenic causes may present similarly yet come with varying treatment modalities.

Neurogenic Causes

Various medical conditions are known to cause impaired detrusor function as a secondary sequela of neurological insult. Infectious sources such as HIV, herpes simplex virus, tertiary syphilis, or post-infectious polyneuritis causing Guillain-Barre syndrome have been linked to impaired detrusor function in certain cohorts [31, 32]. These should be considered in patients with risk factors or prior infectious history. Various suprapontine lesions are associated with voiding dysfunction, as they cause a loss of inhibitory input to the PMC; however sphincter reflexes are not affected, leading to uninhibited bladder contractions or neurogenic detrusor overactivity (NDO). Parkinson's disease is routinely found to cause NDO but has been demonstrated to present with detrusor underactivity or acontractility as well. Studies reveal a prevalence of DU ranging from 16% to 53% of Parkinson's patients tested [32]. This can be due to either pseudodyssynergia of the external urethral sphincter during detrusor overactivity or bradykinesia of the external urethral sphincter during volitional voiding [33]. Similar symptoms are

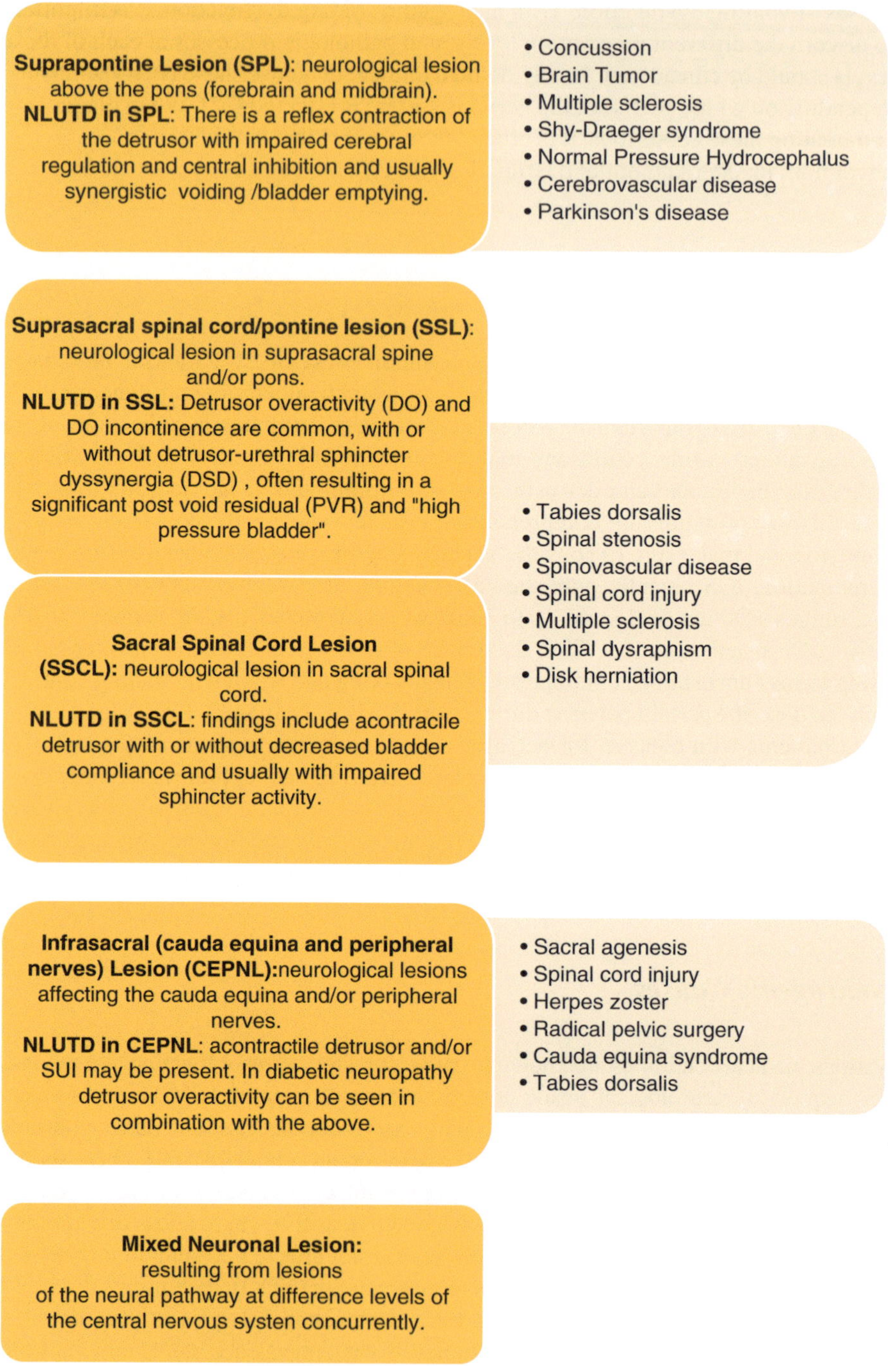

Suprapontine Lesion (SPL): neurological lesion above the pons (forebrain and midbrain).
NLUTD in SPL: There is a reflex contraction of the detrusor with impaired cerebral regulation and central inhibition and usually synergistic voiding /bladder emptying.

- Concussion
- Brain Tumor
- Multiple sclerosis
- Shy-Draeger syndrome
- Normal Pressure Hydrocephalus
- Cerebrovascular disease
- Parkinson's disease

Suprasacral spinal cord/pontine lesion (SSL): neurological lesion in suprasacral spine and/or pons.
NLUTD in SSL: Detrusor overactivity (DO) and DO incontinence are common, with or without detrusor-urethral sphincter dyssynergia (DSD) , often resulting in a significant post void residual (PVR) and "high pressure bladder".

- Tabies dorsalis
- Spinal stenosis
- Spinovascular disease
- Spinal cord injury
- Multiple sclerosis
- Spinal dysraphism
- Disk herniation

Sacral Spinal Cord Lesion (SSCL): neurological lesion in sacral spinal cord.
NLUTD in SSCL: findings include acontracile detrusor with or without decreased bladder compliance and usually with impaired sphincter activity.

Infrasacral (cauda equina and peripheral nerves) Lesion (CEPNL):neurological lesions affecting the cauda equina and/or peripheral nerves.
NLUTD in CEPNL: acontractile detrusor and/or SUI may be present. In diabetic neuropathy detrusor overactivity can be seen in combination with the above.

- Sacral agenesis
- Spinal cord injury
- Herpes zoster
- Radical pelvic surgery
- Cauda equina syndrome
- Tabies dorsalis

Mixed Neuronal Lesion:
resulting from lesions of the neural pathway at difference levels of the central nervous systen concurrently.

Fig. 2 ICS terminology of neural lesions found in common neurogenic voiding dysfunction

often reported following cerebrovascular accident (CVA) or stroke. In the acute phase of the incident, up to 50% of patients can experience urinary retention. In these cases, upper motor neuron damage is the underlying cause of detrusor areflexia, particularly with hemorrhagic or cerebellar infarcts [34]. The majority of the time, the detrusor dysfunction is transient, and symptoms resolve; however patients suffering these injuries often also have other comorbidities such as diabetes that may contribute to their prolonged bladder dysfunction. Damage to lower motor neurons exiting from the lumbosacral vertebrae or sub-sacral lesions may also result in impaired detrusor contractility or poor urethral sphincter function. This can be due to spinal cord injury, multiple sclerosis, or traumatic brain injury, among other etiologies.

Symptoms related to voiding dysfunction are of the leading causes of hospitalizations in spinal cord injury patients [35]. The exact type of bladder impairment is based upon the level of spinal cord lesion; however in most instances while the parasympathetic and spinal sensory centers are preserved, there is a breakdown in communication between the PMC and sacral cord [36]. NDO usually results primarily; however, with any supracervical spinal cord lesion, there can also be loss of coordination between external urethral relaxation and detrusor contraction leading to detrusor-external sphincter dyssynergia (DESD). DESD inherently lends itself to high bladder storage pressures (as the bladder attempts to empty against a close or partially closed sphincter) and incomplete bladder emptying. DU resultantly ensues and upper tract deterioration is a risk in these patients. Sacral spinal injury can also lead to damage of both the sacral parasympathetic and Onuf's nuclei. With destruction of these nuclei, there is impaired compliance and loss of sensation [36]. While these patients are less at risk for upper tract damage, compliance can be altered due to neurologic decentralization, and periodic urodynamic assessment is crucial in these patients. Lower thoracic cord lesions lend themselves to lack of internal sphincter coordination, termed detrusor internal sphincter dyssynergia (DISD).

In multiple sclerosis (MS), focal demyelination and plaque formation can be found throughout the brain and spinal cord, and so pathology can be found from the suprapontine to sacral regions. Voiding and/or storage can be affected depending on where the lesions occur. Roughly 10% of MS diagnoses are made when patients present for urologic evaluation. While NDO is the more likely presenting bladder symptom, both DU and DESD can be found in MS patients, and these findings are mostly associated with cervical cord or pontine lesions [37]. Although these are the most common neurogenic causes of detrusor underactivity, consideration should also be given to the possibility of disc herniation, spinal stenosis, myelodysplasia, and cranial or spinal arteriovenous malformations as possible contributors.

Myogenic Causes

The myogenic basis for detrusor underactivity assumes that there is an intact nervous system and surrounds two postulations, one that ischemia leads to detrusor denervation, subsequently affecting the entire myovesical plexus. Alternatively, this detrusor dysfunction could be due to inability for myocytes to generate intrinsic contractile activity regardless of external stimuli [29, 38]. It is unclear whether these changes are representative of cause or effect.

As previously discussed, normal ageing has been directly linked to morphological changes in detrusor muscle cell matrix. There has been an objective loss of bladder contractility and voiding efficacy when looking at urodynamic studies in an ageing population and a direct correlation with elevation in PVR [39]. When analyzing the visceral sensation brain center, MRI findings of the brain reveal there is a diminished response to bladder filling in neurologically intact ageing humans [40]. While the myogenic hypothesis hones in on peripheral dysfunction, or the initial defect in the muscle leading to a resultant inefficient detrusor contraction, it should be recognized that this might not be truly distinct from the neurogenic hypothesis or the thought that the primary defect is in afferent innervation effecting efferent outflow [41, 42]. These two theories likely have some overlap, and reasons for detrusor underactivity caused by myogenic deterioration can also be influenced by neurogenic or even functional factors. Women can also exhibit detrusor underactivity as a secondary component of menopause, whether natural or surgical, as in vivo studies have shown that oophorectomy is affiliated with axonal degeneration and loss of detrusor muscle cells [43]. Although ageing and factors that are associated with this process are contributing factors for DU in some patients, it is clear that not all ageing individuals have voiding dysfunction, and DU should not be minimalized to simply a natural progression of the ageing process.

Urinary complications related to diabetic cystopathy are becoming more prevalent, and symptoms range from "sensory urgency" without findings of measurable detrusor overactivity to detrusor underactivity (impaired bladder contractility) and incomplete bladder emptying. There are multiple causes of diabetic cystopathy, ranging from neuronal to urothelial dysfunction as well as altered detrusor physiology. Chronic hyperglycemia also contributes to nerve damage through increased free radical production and decreased levels of nerve growth factor (NGF) [20, 44]. While diabetic cystopathy is categorized by some as a myogenic cause of DU and others deem it a neurogenic cause, the underlying pathogenesis is likely multifactorial.

Overdistention of the urinary bladder is known to result in cellular changes and alteration of smooth muscle contractile function, which results in subsequent DU. This can be caused by various entities causing effects on the vascular supply or detrusor muscle itself and described as acute or chronic. Acute prolonged bladder overdistention (ApBO) is defined as a bladder-filling volume at the time of diagnosis of at least 120% of a normal bladder capacity, which has lasted at least 24 h. This is more often associated with pelvic or orthopedic surgical procedures, and most patients are not immediately aware of an inability to empty the bladder completely [45]. This differs from acute retention secondary to obstructive causes, where significant symptoms arise. A recent review quoted postoperative urinary retention incidence to vary from 4% to 29% with hernia repair procedures, arthroplasties of the knee, and hip and gynecologic procedures having the highest rates associated [46]. Factors predictive of postoperative urinary retention include age greater than 50, intraoperative fluids greater than 750 mL, bladder volume greater than 270 mL on entry to PACU [28], male gender, obstructive preoperative symptoms, spinal/epidural anesthesia, prolonged postoperative analgesia [29], and anesthesia time greater than 2 h [47]. Childbirth has also been associated with overdistention and possible overdistention injury. A study evaluating 8000 consecutive births found a 0.05% incidence of prolonged voiding dysfunction [48]. It has also been suggested that labor exceeding 700 min increases the risk for postpartum voiding dysfunction [49].

Pharmacologic Causes

Various medications can also contribute to detrusor underactivity, the most common of these being antimuscarinics, anesthetics, and analgesics including narcotics, neuroleptics, and alpha-agonists (phenylephrine, pseudoephedrine, clonidine). Nonsteroidal anti-inflammatory drugs (NSAIDs) have been correlated with urinary retention, and it is theorized that this is due to inhibition of prostaglandin-mediated detrusor contraction [50]. Other studies reveal there may be modifiable anesthetic risk factors associated with perioperative care of patients. Mayo et al. found that 20% of patients develop urinary retention after routine lumbar spine surgery, and increasing doses of neostigmine and phenylephrine were strongly associated with retention incidence ($p < 0.05$) [51]. Further research is needed to identify specific anesthetic risk factors of urinary retention and alter practices to improve patient outcomes and reduce costs related to urinary retention in the postoperative period. Narcotics have also been held responsible for diminishing detrusor function. Many of these associations are found with postoperative use of narcotic analgesia. Research demonstrates, however, that preoperative use of narcotics and anti-inflammatory medications actually is associated with lower rates of urinary retention [52]. This could be due to lower narcotic requirement postoperatively with preemptive use of analgesic medications.

Bladder Outlet Obstruction (BOO)

Anatomic Obstruction (Fixed)

There are various causes of anatomic obstruction that can occur, and while some affect men and women alike, such as meatal stenosis, urethral malignancy, iatrogenic causes (catheterization, transurethral surgery), dysfunctional voiding, DESD, and primary bladder neck obstruction, most etiologies are sex-specific. While urethral strictures can occur in men and women, they are much more prevalent in males. They are often associated with trauma, urethral pathology, urethral instrumentation, or infection. Other iatrogenic causes of obstruction in men include artificial urinary sphincter placement (AUS). In a study of 117 patients, transcorporal AUS placement was associated with a significantly higher rate of urinary retention when compared with traditional AUS (27% vs. 2%). Larger cuff size was also associated with higher retention rates. Overall retention rate was significant at 15%, and postoperative catheterization ranged from days to 6 weeks in duration [53]. The most common cause of bladder outlet obstruction in the male patient is benign prostatic hyperplasia (BPH), and this is well studied. This phenomenon includes both smooth muscle hyperplasia and prostatic enlargement leading to bladder dysfunction and outlet obstruction, resulting most commonly in significant LUTS, which are the most common clinical manifestations of BPH. It is important to recognize that the natural history of BPH is highly variable, and while both prostate volume and PSA correlate with urinary retention rates, other factors should also be acknowledged.

Functional Obstruction

Outlet dysfunction in the absence of obstruction is a result of poor muscle relaxation, either at the level of the bladder neck and urethra or pelvic floor. Primary bladder neck obstruction (PBNO) is defined as a failure of the bladder neck to open adequately during micturition. In addition there can be no identifiable anatomic obstruction and no increase in striated sphincter activity [54]. We have further categorized PBNO into three distinct types: (1) classic high-pressure, low-flow voiding; (2) normal-pressure, low-flow voiding with narrowing at the bladder neck; and (3) delayed opening of the bladder neck [55]. While PBNO was initially thought to be a diagnosis mostly commonly found in the male patient, substantial evidence of this condition in females has emerged, and urodynamic series have uncovered a prevalence of 9–16% of women with urinary retention and obstructive symptoms [56, 57]. Some have proposed this condition is due to failure of dissolution of mesenchymal elements with additional connective tissue and smooth muscle hypertrophy [58]. Other hypotheses revolve around underlying neurologic pathology that is responsible for this obstruction [59]. The symptomatology can vary in this condition and can be very similar to other "functional" disorders.

A second type of functional outlet obstruction surrounds conditions where there is failure of sphincteric relaxation. This can be a result of three separate disorders. Dysfunctional voiding is characterized by habitual variable contractions at the time of micturition that prevent normal bladder emptying. These are likely in response to pelvic floor pain or discomfort (can be due to constipation, IBS symptoms, lower extremity injury such as hip or knee damage, reflex due to prior abuse or sexual assault) or can be a response to urinary symptoms such as urinary urgency. Many adults present with a multitude of voiding symptoms. These are likely the resulting compensatory response of a reflexive urethral sphincter contraction as a reaction to primary detrusor instability. This habitual routine becomes very bothersome to patients causing them to seek medication treatment. As touched on previously, patients with underlying neurologic conditions that also have this same cluster of symptoms will often be diagnosed with detrusor sphincter dyssynergia (DSD), and dysfunction can occur with the external or internal sphincters, or there can be coexistence of the conditions. While dysfunctional voiding is learned and can therefore at times be unlearned, the latter is due to interruption of a neural pathway connection to the PMC, and the resultant lack of coordination is a permanent sequelae.

The third condition of inhibited sphincteric relaxation is Fowler's syndrome. This disorder differs from dysfunctional voiding and DSD as patients are asymptomatic and are often in retention at time of diagnosis [60]. It is a rare condition found most commonly in young women, typically postmenarche, and in the second and third decades of life, with long-standing detrusor inhibition from a chronically non-relaxing external urethral sphincter. The original paper describing Fowler's syndrome in 1988 made an association to polycystic ovaries because 14 of the 22 patients with abnormal EMG activity had the condition, which thereby postulated a hormonal cause [61]. There is conflicting evidence about the relationship between this cause and effect relationship. More research is needed to confirm this correlation, as polycystic ovaries tend to be common in this age group and could be a confounder. The major difference between Fowler's syndrome and dysfunctional voiding or DSD is that with the latter two, the bladder actually contracts, while in Fowler's syndrome it does not.

Evaluation and Diagnostic Workup

Thorough evaluation of the patient is imperative when dealing with disorders of bladder emptying, and it is important to identify patient risk factors, provide appropriate and timely treatment modalities, and avoid superfluous testing and procedures. Regardless of the underlying cause of urinary retention, symptoms can be very disruptive to patients even when objective findings are minimal. Conversely, urinary retention can be found incidentally. The primary objective should be to arrive at a judicious diagnosis and initiate proper treatment and provide surveillance for those at higher risk for long-term complications.

Medical History

When taking a patient's history, emphasis should be placed on eliciting the nature, acuity, and duration of the urinary symptoms. It is crucial to differentiate between storage symptoms (frequency, nocturia, urgency, or incontinence) and voiding symptoms (slow stream, splitting of spraying of the stream, intermittency, hesitancy, straining, or terminal dribbling) or post-void symptoms (a sensation of incomplete emptying or post-void dribbling). Past medical history should be obtained, and patients should be asked specifically about diabetes, stroke, infection, trauma, prior surgeries, prolonged anesthesia or childbirth, or abdominal or pelvic radiation. It is also important to ask specifically about prior treatments requiring catheterization and symptomatic episodes of an inability to void within the last 6 months. If prior incontinence or prolapse surgeries were performed, obtaining past operative reports is essential. Abnormal childhood voiding patterns, urinary tract infection history, and bowel symptoms such as constipation and accidental bowel leakage should also be assessed. Sexual history is an important part of the medical record and sexual orientation; history of sexually transmitted infections and history of sexual abuse should be elicited. In female patients a thorough obstetrical and gynecological history should be taken, and symptoms of sexual dysfunction or prolapse symptoms should be obtained. Finally, it is important to understand the patient's living situation and overall functional status, as this may impact your treatment choices.

In patients where upper tract deterioration is not a concern, the degree of bother is the driving force for evaluation and management. Using one of the validated urinary questionnaires, in addition to obtaining a medical history, can elucidate the impact of LUTS on a patient's quality of life. A number of validated questionnaires are available for initial assessment but can also be useful throughout the course of management to assess for improvement or worsening of symptoms. Lepor et al. evaluated the American Urological Association Symptom Index (AUASI) survey results in both men and women and found that ageing men and women have similar rates of bothersome symptoms, thereby suggesting that the AUASI can be used for assessment of LUTS regardless of sex [62]. This tool also has been found to be helpful in assessing lower urinary tract symptoms in women independent of incontinence [63, 64].

Physical Exam

Particular attention should be paid to certain aspects of the physical examination. The bladder should be assessed, and a palpable or percussible bladder during the abdominal exam is a pertinent finding. The patient's back should be thoroughly examined for any scars or vertebral pathology, as well as costovertebral angle tenderness. During digital rectal examination, rectal tone should be assessed, and hard stools, fecal impaction, or any palpable masses should be documented. The urethral meatus should be evaluated for any abnormalities. A neurological assessment is crucial, especially in patients with neurological complaints of numbness or weakness or urinary symptoms occurring simultaneously with a surgery or trauma. In women, the physician should assess for pelvic organ and rectal prolapse, pain during palpation of the levator or obturator complex, or urethral or vaginal masses. Masses should be assessed for firmness and fluctuance to better categorize and triage these findings. In men, the penis should be examined for plaques or masses, and the prostate should be examined to ascertain size and presence of tenderness.

Diagnostics

There are a number of procedures and studies that can be used to assess for etiology of urinary retention and voiding complaints. Information that is obtained through a comprehensive history and physical should guide the provider to what studies to proceed with, in order to avoid a potentially costly and invasive workup. In all patients risk assessment of upper tract deterioration or development of urinary tract infections should also help to guide the evaluation process.

Post-void Residual (PVR)

A post-void residual is a simple and very valuable test that can be performed with a bedside bladder scan or ultrasound or catheterization. Both techniques are comparable; however reverting to catheterization may be necessary if a sonographic finding seems inaccurate [65]. It is important to note that especially in women, elevated PVR findings on bedside bladder scans can also be due to gynecological pathology. While a range of PVR values have been proposed to correlate with incomplete bladder emptying, there is no consensus on the value cutoff to define an abnormal residual. The more recent guidelines from the UK National Institute for Health and Clinical Excellence proposed using a PVR of greater than 1 L, while the Italian Association of Urology Guidelines for BPH define a pathological PVR "more than one-third of total bladder capacity" [66, 67]. Negro and colleagues suggest using a PVR of >300 mL in those who can void and a PVR of >1000 mL in those who are unable to void [66], and this seems reasonable. However absolute values are less important than interpreting a PVR volume in conjunction with the clinical scenario. Thus, it is critically important to interpret post-void residual data in the context of the patients symptoms and, when available, urodynamic findings. For example, an "elevated" post-void residual in a patient with poor or decreased compliance likely has more clinical significance than the same PVR in a patient with a compliant bladder.

Uroflowmetry

A uroflow measurement is helpful for understanding a patient's time to void and flow rate and can also uncover the presence of straining with urination. This is often used in unison with a PVR to assess bladder capacity; however it may not be accurate if patient is not at capacity when these measurements are obtained. The maximum flow rate is also a helpful measurement and will be discussed in more detail with the urodynamic evaluation.

Labs

The most readily available lab test in the office setting is the urine dipstick. In patients that exhibit findings of a urine infection, either because of the dipstick findings or symptoms, a urine sample should be sent for urinalysis and/or culture. Patients that have concern for upper tract dysfunction should have a basic metabolic panel in order to check serum creatinine, electrolytes, and glomerular filtration rate (GFR).

Imaging

With elevated PVR or any concern for upper tract pathology, urinary imaging is important. Renal and bladder ultrasound can be used to detect hydronephrosis, renal stones, or parenchymal thinning of the kidney. Ureteral jet and PVR measurements can also be taken. A contrast CT will not provide additional information in regard to incomplete emptying and should not be performed in those with renal dysfunction. An MRI is helpful in cases of concern for urethral diverticulum. In a patient who does not exhibit a degree of prolapse that coincides with symptomatology, a dynamic MRI may help to assess this, but it should be used with caution, as it is an expensive study that may not provide any additional information about bladder emptying. Gadolinium should be avoided in patients on dialysis due to the risk of nephrogenic systemic fibrosis.

Cystourethroscopy

Cystourethroscopy alone is not adequate in diagnosis of bladder outlet obstruction; however it can help with uncovering etiology or any abnormal urethral or bladder anatomy. Indications for this procedure include evaluation for masses or lesions that may be the source of voiding symptoms, especially in those at elevated risk for genitourinary malignancy. The urethra can be appropriately evaluated as well in patients where there is concern for urethral stricture. Urethral angle, distention ability, presence of diverticula, or any foreign body can also be assessed. The prostate can also be assessed for contour, and any prominent or obstructing lobes can be identified.

Urodynamics

When evaluating a patient for the underlying cause of incomplete bladder emptying, the definitive study to assist in diagnosis is urodynamics (UDS) [68]. While this test is very helpful in assessing bladder compliance and capacity, as well as presence of involuntary detrusor contractions, detrusor pressures, storage pressures, flow rates, and PVR, care should be taken to only utilize this procedure when necessary, as it is somewhat invasive and can cause discomfort and/or anxiety that could falsely alter findings. For evaluation of detrusor contractility and pressure-flow analysis, and degree of obstruction, UDS is the gold standard. Videourodynamics can be immensely helpful in the identification of obstruction and further classification of exact level of the blockage, especially in female patients. This is particularly helpful when trying to differentiate between the various functional causes of bladder outlet obstruction. In primary bladder neck obstruction, the obstruction is at the bladder neck, versus in dysfunctional voiding or detrusor external sphincter dyssynergia, the obstruction is at the level of the external sphincter and may reveal a "spinning-top" urethra. Independent of maximum flow rate and detrusor pressures, we have found fluoroscopy to be the best identifier of obstruction, and for assessment of this etiology, we use it routinely when there is high suspicion [56]. Fluoroscopy can also be very helpful in identifying vesicoureteral reflux and any structural abnormalities, such as diverticulum, trabeculations, filling defects, or urethral stricture. When multichannel urodynamics is not needed, a voiding cystourethrogram can be used to identify the structural etiologies above. EMG can also be a useful component of urodynamics; however it should be utilized in conjunction with the full clinical picture. When there is concern for DSD, an increase in EMG activity at the time of increase in detrusor pressure can help to make the diagnosis and further help to classify DESD based on specific type. We have found VUD to be superior to EMG alone in differentiating between DV and PBNO, although it is helpful to have the parameter as part of the complete urodynamic picture [69].

Nomograms

Various nomograms have been constructed over the last decade to help with defining obstruction; however these largely apply only to male patients. The bladder outlet obstruction index (BOOI) from the Abrams-Griffiths nomogram is measured by the equation BOOI = Pdet @ $Q_{max} - 2(Q_{max})$ [70]. With this nomogram men are divided into three separate categories: (1) obstructed if BOOI >40, (2) equivocal if BOOI 20–40, and (3) unobstructed if BOOI <20. More recently a retrospective study turned attention to the presence of abdominal strain on intravesical pressure and the resultant underestimation of BOOI. They suggested a modified BOOI to more accurately correlate with endoscopically proven obstruction [71]. The bladder contractility index (BCI) is derived from the Schaefer nomogram and is calculated by the formula BCI = PdetQ_{max} +5(Q_{max}) and defines contractility as strong if >150, normal if 100–150, and weak if <100 [72]. This is helpful in men with bladder outlet obstruction; however thresholds to distinguish normal contractility and DU remain a subject of debate. Recently Oelke and colleagues set out to construct a nomogram using detrusor contractility scores and BOO grades as continuous variables in order to better classify patients. They correlated BOO grades with detrusor contraction power (W_{max}) and determined specific percentiles using linear interpolation. They propose a diagnosis of DU for patients that fall below the 25th percentile in this nomogram. These men were found to be older and had higher cystometric capacity and PVR and significantly lower voiding efficiency when compared to men in higher percentile groups [73]. More research is needed in this area to confirm this classification of DU; however it is a helpful tool when evaluating men with LUTS.

We do not have clearly defined urodynamic criteria that may be indicative of obstruction in female patients, likely because the prevalence and causes of obstruction are quite different. Although a consensus of an objective definition of BOO in females is lacking, the condition has received more attention recently in connection with voiding dysfunction, and it likely requires a combination of pressure/flow data, imaging, and EMG [74].

Variable criteria have been suggested for women, including peak flows of less than 12 mL/s to15mL/s, as well as values for detrusor pressure at peak flows of greater than 20cmH20 to greater than 50cmH20 [75, 76]. The Blaivas-Groutz nomogram defines obstruction as a maximum flow rate less than 12 mL/s, with or without radiographic evidence of obstruction, in the presence of a sustained detrusor contraction greater than 20 cmH20, and/or an inability to void [77]. In practice, these criteria can overestimate BOO in certain instances. Choi et al. utilized variants of this nomogram to evaluate LUTS in women and defined "voiding difficulty" at a Qmax less than or equal to 15 mL/s. Those with detrusor pressure at peak flow >20 cmH20 were subclassified as having bladder outlet obstruction, and those with <20 cmH20 were diagnosed with detrusor underactivity [78]. A new nomogram has been recently published to assist with diagnosing BOO in females. Cluster analysis revealed the equation Pdet.Q_{max} = 2*Qmax to best differentiate between those who were obstructed versus unobstructed, and this SG nomogram demonstrated both high sensitivity and specificity [79]. We have found that pressure-flow patterns in obstructed women are quite variable and the diagnosis requires an individualized approach.

Treatment of Urinary Retention and Voiding Dysfunction

Two main factors should drive the treatment of patients with voiding dysfunction: degree of symptom bother and risk for upper tract deterioration or debilitating infection. Any patient categorized as high risk should be strongly advised to undergo some treatment to maintain decompression of the bladder. Those without risk can be stratified by degree of bother and offered treatment based on the cause of their incomplete emptying. It is also imperative to categorize chronic urinary retention (CUR) as neurogenic or non-neurogenic. Figure 3 lists recommendations for treatment of patients with non-neurogenic CUR as defined by the AUA CUR workgroup [80].

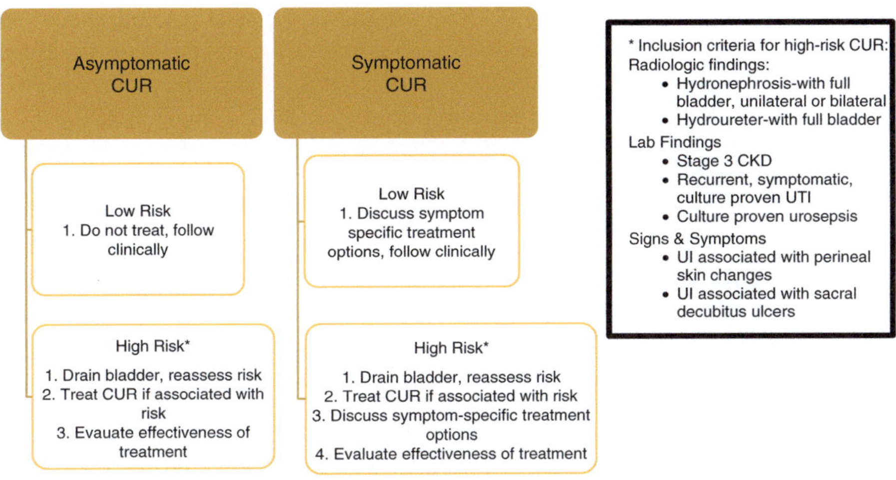

Fig. 3 AUA recommendations for treatment of non-neurogenic CUR

Detrusor Underactivity

The majority of causes of detrusor underactivity are irreversible, particularly neuropathic and myogenic causes. Early intervention and optimal management of neurological disorders may help to delay detrusor dysfunction, but ultimately it may be inevitable. It is important to emphasize active management of comorbid conditions such as diabetes, and judicious restriction of fluid intake may assist in halting the deterioration of bladder contractility. Modifiable pharmacologic contributions should be discontinued if at all possible. The patient should be treated with conservative therapies and catheterization if needed, with frequent assessment of improvement in detrusor function. Various oral therapies such as alpha-adrenergic antagonists, muscarinic receptor agonists (e.g., bethanechol), and prostaglandin E have been derived to stimulate contractility of the detrusor, but these come with very limited efficacy [31]. Sacral neuromodulation has been aggressively studied in animal models showing promising results that there is stimulation of sacral efferents and modulation of the micturition reflex; however more studies are needed in humans. In the current studies of human subjects, there have been reductions in mean urinary volume per catheterization and mean urinary catheterization number per day [9]. A number of investigative studies around gene therapies have been published, particularly involving NGF. It has been extensively studied in animal models and has been found to have a protective effect on diabetic rodent bladders. Studies replacing NGF and other neuroprotective agents such as alpha-lipoic acid have revealed a potential therapeutic intervention for DU [80, 81]. Animal models of stem cell injection have shown improved bladder contraction and decreased PVR urine volumes; however more work is needed in this particular area [82, 83]. Oftentimes with cases of detrusor underactivity, there can also be concomitant outlet obstruction. With objective DU findings, these particular patients should be extensively counseled regarding any outlet procedure, and risks should be discussed including persistence of voiding dysfunction symptoms, as the outlet reduction procedure will not be addressing one probably etiology of their bladder symptoms. In patients with chronic long-standing obstruction, it is valuable to discuss the potential of irrecoverable detrusor function.

Bladder Outlet Dysfunction

Fixed Anatomic Obstruction

With this type of obstruction, there is high likelihood return to normal bladder emptying with removal of the obstruction. In men with bothersome prostatic enlargement, management with medications is usually first in line. In those who are refractory to medical procedures to reduce obstruction to the outlet can be performed. These may be performed abdominally (prostatectomy) or transurethrally (transurethral resection of the prostate (TURP), greenlight vaporization, holmium laser enucleation). A large systematic review by Lourenco et al. compared minimally invasive BPH management to traditional TURP and found that patients undergoing minimally invasive types of management had less blood loss, lower stricture rate, and lower incontinence rates and were less likely to have loss of ejaculation. Laser coagulation, although shorter than TURP, had higher urinary retention rates and postop UTI in comparison with other modalities. Minimally invasive procedures however did have a higher need for reoperation [81].

Treatment of strictures may include dilation if short; however recurrent or long strictures will likely require a urethroplasty. At times grafts from the buccal mucosa may be harvested to promote procedural success; however patients should be carefully selected for these procedures as these grafts can incur higher procedural costs [82]. Meatoplasty can be performed in those with meatal stenosis. Patients with urethral carcinoma should be referred to a urologic oncologist and managed per oncologic guidelines based on grading and depth of invasion of the tumor, as well as other patient risk factors.

Anatomic abnormalities in women (urethral caruncle, diverticulum, pelvic organ prolapse, Skene's gland abscess, or vaginal cysts) may require surgical intervention. Urinary retention after incontinence surgery should always be considered in those with voiding difficulties after this type of procedure. Revision of slings, either made from autologous fascia or synthetically derived, may be necessary for relief of bladder outlet obstruction in the female patient. A recent study revealed a 30% incidence of sling lysis with autologous sling and 42% risk of long-term catheterization [83]. Loosening or cutting of transvaginal tapes (TVTs) has shown excellent results with marked improvement in storage and voiding symptoms; however risk of recurrent SUI after sling lysis is thought to reach nearly 60% [84, 85]. These statistics should be discussed with patients preoperatively as part of a shared decision-making process.

Functional Obstruction

Once a patient has been found to have a functional cause of obstruction, it is imperative to identify which type of functional obstruction is at play, as treatments are different for each. In patients that have failure of the sphincter to relax, those with dysfunctional voiding may benefit from physical therapy (PT) and biofeedback in order to "relearn" how to void with proper coordination, and standardized protocols have been published [86]. For those who have a history of sexual abuse or trauma, psychotherapy could also be helpful in conjunction with PT. Other therapies that have been implemented include Botox injections into the external urethral sphincter, sacroneuromodulation, and muscle relaxants.

In patients with a neurological cause that prevents their sphincter from relaxing (DSD), botulinum toxin injections into the external urinary sphincter can be attempted. Other options include sphincterotomy; however, one major risk of this includes high-grade urinary incontinence, and this may increase overall morbidity for these patients. For some individuals, the optimal treatment may intermittent catheterization, or in those with functional impairment, indwelling catheter (either transurethral or suprapubic), or a urinary diversion. A continent diversion may be considered in those that have good dexterity of their upper extremities and hands. In patients diagnosed with Fowler's syndrome, the treatment of choice is sacral neuromodulation. Its postulated mechanism of action is retraining of the nerve input to the pelvic floor. Lastly, in those with primary bladder neck obstruction, alpha-blocker therapy can be tried. It may act as both a diagnostic and therapeutic modality prior to proceeding with a transurethral incision of the bladder neck, which would be the next step in these patients.

Discussion

Disorders of voiding dysfunction and urinary retention should be categorized as either a failure of either the detrusor (detrusor underactivity) or of the outlet (bladder outlet obstruction). Regardless of categorization, however, symptoms can be quite debilitating in large population of patients and can contribute to recurrent urinary tract infections and/or upper tract function decline. Modifiable risk factors should be identified and reduced if at all possible. The diagnostic tests and treatment modalities are numerous and vary based on etiology. For this reason it is important to educate patients regarding the roles for different procedures and interventions. The gold standard study to determine the cause of incomplete bladder emptying is urodynamics and should be utilized when there is not a clear etiology. Addition of fluoroscopy can be a pertinent factor in uncovering cause of bladder dysfunction, and this should be sought out when necessary. Treatments for bladder outlet obstruction are numerous and should be offered only after meticulous and well-thought out assessment. While the therapies for detrusor underactivity are limited, there is promising research concerning a variety of investigational therapies, and hopefully this will continue to evolve.

References

1. Fowler CJ, Griffiths D, deGroat WC. The neural control of micturition. Nat Rev Neurosci. 2008;9(6):453–66.
2. Brucker BM, Nitti VW. Evaluation of urinary retention in women: pelvic floor dysfunction or primary bladder neck obstruction. Curr Bladder Dysfunct Rep. 2012;7:222–9.
3. Nassau D, Gerber J, Weiss J. The prevalence and treatment of voiding dysfunction in the elderly. Curr Geriatr Rep. 2014;3:33–41.
4. Irwin DE, et al. Population-based survey of urinary incontinence, overactive bladder, and other urinary tract symptoms in five countries: results of the EPIC study. Eur Urol. 2006;50:1306–15.
5. Coyne K, Sexton C, Thompson C, et al. The prevalence of lower urinary tract symptoms (LUTS) in the USA, the UK and Sweden: results from the Epidemiology of LUTS (EpiLUTS) study. BJU. 2009;104(3):352–60.
6. Coyne KS, Sexton CC, Bell JA, Thompson CL, Dmochowski R, Bavendam T, Chen CI, Quentin Clemens J. The prevalence of lower urinary tract symptoms (LUTS) and overactive bladder (OAB) by racial/ethnic group and age: results from OAB-POLL. Neurourol Urodyn. 2013;32:230–7. https://doi.org/10.1002/nau.22295.
7. Sadananda P, Vahabi B, Drake MJ. Bladder outlet physiology in the context of lower urinary tract dysfunction. Neurourol Urodyn. 2011;30:708–13.
8. De Groat WC, Wickens C. Organization of the neural switching circuitry underlying reflex micturition. Acta Physiol (Oxf). 2013;207:66–84.
9. Drake MJ, et al. Voiding dysfunction due to detrusor underactivity: an overview. Nat Rev Urol. 2014;11:454–64.
10. Elbadawi A, Meyer S, Regnier CH. Role of ischemia in structural changes in the rabbit detrusor following partial bladder outlet obstruction: a working hypothesis and a biomechanical/structural model proposal. NeurourolUrodyn. 1989;8:151–62.
11. Malmqvist U, Arner A, Uvelius B. Contractile and cytoskeletal proteins in smooth muscle during hypertrophy and its reversal. Am J Physiol. 1991;63:86–93.
12. Sjuve R, Haase H, Morano I, et al. Contraction kinetics and myosin isoform composition in smooth muscle from hypertrophied rat urinary bladder. J Cell Biochem. 1996;63:86–93.
13. Wolffenbuttel KP, de Jong BW, Scheepe JR, Kok DJ. Potential for recovery in bladder function after removing a urethral obstruction. NeurourolUrodyn. 2008;27:782–8.
14. Jock M, Leggett RE, Schuler C, et al. Effect of partial bladder outlet obstruction and reversal on rabbit bladder physiology and biochemistry: duration of recovery period and severity of function. BJU Int. 2014;114:946–54.
15. Levin RM, Reed TP, Whitbeck C, Chichester P, Damaser M. Effect of strip length on the contractile dysfunction of bladder smooth muscle after partial outlet obstruction. Urology. 2005;66:659–64.
16. Gilpin SA, Gilpin CJ, Dixon JS, et al. The effect of age on the autonomic innervation of the urinary bladder. Br J Urol. 1986;58:378–81.
17. Elbadawi A, Yalla SV, Resnick NM. Structural basis of geriatric voiding dysfunction. III Detrusor overactivity. J Urol. 1993;150:1681–95.
18. Sugaya K, et al. Ascending and descending brainstem neuronal activity during cystometry in decerebrate cats. Neurourol Urodyn. 2003;22:343–50.
19. Blok BF, Willesmsen AT, Holstege G. A PET study on brain control of micturition in humans. Brain. 1997;120:111–21.
20. Yoshimura N, Chancellor MB, Andersson KE, Christ GJ. Recent advances in understanding the biology of diabetes-associated bladder complications and novel therapy. BJU Int. 2005;95:733–8.
21. Suskind AM, Smith PP. A new look at detrusor underactivity: impaired contractility versus afferent dysfunction. Curr Urol Rep. 2009;10:347–51.
22. Drake MJ, Mills IW, Gillespie JI. Model of peripheral autonomous modules and a myovesical plexus in normal and overactive bladder function. Lancet. 2001;358:401–3.

23. Haefliger JA, Tissieres P, Tawadros T, et al. Connexins 43 and 26 are differentially increased after rat bladder outlet obstruction. Exp Cell Res. 2002;274:216–25.
24. Hampel C, Dolber PC, Smith MP, et al. Modulation of bladder alpha-1 adrenergic receptor subtype expression by bladder outlet obstruction. J Urol. 2002;167:1513–21.
25. Abrams P, Cardozo L, Fall M, Griffiths D, Rosier P, Ulmsten U, van Kerrebroeck P, Victor A, Wein A. The standardization of terminology of lower urinary tract function: report from the standardisation sub-committee of the international continence society. NeurourolUrodyn. 2002;21:167–78.
26. Wein A, Chapple C. Introduction and terminology. In: Chapple C, Wein A, Osman N, editors. Underactive bladder. Switzerland: Springer; 2017. p. ix–xiii.
27. Gajewski JB, Schurch B, Hamid R, et al. An International Continence Society (ICS) report on the terminology for adult neurogenic lower urinary tract dysfunction (ANLUTD). Neurourol Urodyn. 2018;37(3):1152–61.
28. Wein AJ. Classification of neurogenic voiding dysfunction. J Urol. 1981;125:605.
29. Osman N, et al. Detrusor underactivity and the underactive bladder: a new clinical entitity? A review of current terminology, definitions, epidemiology, aetiology and diagnosis. Eur Urol. 2014;65:389–98.
30. Rosier P, Schaefer W, Lose G, et al. International continence society good urodynamic practices and terms 2016: urodynamics, uroflowmetry, cystometry, and pressure-flow study. NeurourolUrodyn. 2016;9999:1–18.
31. Araki I, Kitahara M, Oida T, Kuno S. Voiding dysfunction and Parkinson's disease: urodynamic abnormalities and urinary symptoms. J Urol. 2000;164:1640–3.
32. Campeau L, Soler R, Andersson KE. Bladder dysfunction and Parkinsonism: current pathophysiological understanding and management strategies. Curr Urol Rep. 2011;12:396–403.
33. Burney TL, Senapati M, Desai S, et al. Acute cerebrovascular accident and lower urinary tract dysfunction: a prospective correlation of the site of brain injury with urodynamic findings. J Urol. 1996;156:1748–50.
34. Manack A, Motsko SP, Haag-Molkenteller C, et al. Epidemiology and healthcare utilization of neurogenic bladder patients in a us claims database. NeurourolUrodyn. 2011;30:395–401.
35. Cruz CD, Coelho A, Antunes-Lopes T, et al. Biomarkers of spinal cord injury and ensuing bladder dysfunction. Adv Drug Deliv Rev. 2015;82–83:153–9.
36. Litwiller SE, Frohman EM, Zimmern PE. Multiple sclerosis and the urologist. J Urol. 1999;161:743–57.
37. Andersson KE, Arner A. Urinary bladder contraction and relaxation: physiology and pathophysiology. Physiol Rev. 2004;84:935–86.
38. Madersbacher S, Pycha A, Schatzl G, et al. The aging lower urinary tract: a comparative urodynamic study of men and women. Urology. 1998;51:206–12.
39. Griffiths D, Tadic SD, Schaefer W, Resnick NM. Cerebral control of the bladder in normal and urge-incontinent women. Neuroimage. 2007;37:1–7.
40. Tyagi P, Smith PP, Kuchel GA, et al. Pathophysiology and animal modeling of underactive bladder. Int Urol Nephrol. 2014;46:S11–21.
41. Smith PP, Birder LA, Abrams P, Wein AJ, Chapple CR. Detrusor underactivity and the underactive bladder: symptoms, function, cause-what do we mean? ICI-RS think tank 2014. NeurourolUrodyn. 2016;35(2):312–7. https://doi.org/10.1002/nau.22807. Review
42. Zhu Q, et al. Role of ovarian hormones in the parthogenesis of impaired detrusor contractility: evidence in ovariectomized rodents. J Urol. 2001;166:1136–41.
43. Sasaki K, Chancellor MB, Goins WF, et al. Gene therapy using replication-defective herpes simplex virus vectors expressing nerve growth factor in a rat model of diabetic cystopathy. Diabetes. 2004;53:2723–30.
44. Madersbacher H, Cardozo L, Chapple C, Abrams P, Toozs-Hobson P, Young JS, Wyndaele JJ, deWachter S, Campeau L, Gajewski JB. What are the causes and consequences of bladder overdistention?:ICI-RS 2011. Neurourol Urodyn. 2012;31:317–21.
45. Darrah DM, Griebling TL, Silverstein JH. Postoperative urinary retention. Anesthesiol Clin. 2009;27:465–84.

46. Sivasankaran MV, Pham T, Divino CM. Incidence and risk factors for urinary retention following laparoscopic inguinal hernia repair. Am J Surg. 2014;2017:288–92.
47. Yip SK, Sahota D, Pang MW, et al. Screening test model using duration of labor for the detection of postpartum urinary retention. NeurourolUrodyn. 2005;24:248–53.
48. Groutz A, Gordon D, Woman I, et al. Persistent postpartum urinary retention in contemporary obstetric practice. Definition, prevalence, and clinical implications. J Reprod Med. 2001;46:44–8.
49. Verhamme KM, Dieleman JP, Van Wijk MA, et al. Nonsteroidal anti-inflammatory drugs and increased risk of acute urinary retention. Arch Intern Med. 2005;165(13):1547–51.
50. Mayo BC, Louie PK, Bohl DD, et al. Effects of intraoperative anesthetic medications on postoperative urinary retention after single-level lumber fusion. Spine. 2016;41(18):1441–6.
51. Boulis NM, Mian FS, Rodriguez D, et al. Urinary retention following routine neurosurgical spine procedures. Surg Neurol. 2001;55(1):23–7; discussion: 27–8
52. Smith PJ, Hudak SJ, Scott F, Zhao LC, Morey A. Transcorporal artificial urinary sphincter cuff placement is associated with a higher risk of postoperative urinary retention. Can J Urol. 2013;20(3):6773–7.
53. Padmanabhan P, Nitti VW. Primary bladder neck obstruction in men, women, and children. Curr Urol Rep. 2007;8:379–84.
54. Nitti VW, Lefkowitz G, Ficazzola M, Dixon CM. Lower urinary tract symptoms in young men: videourodynamic findings and correlation with noninvasive measures. J Urol. 2002;168(1):135–8.
55. Nitti VW, Ru LM, Gitlin J. Diagnosing bladder outlet obstruction in women. J Urol. 1999;161(5):1535–40.
56. Kuo HC. Videourodynamic characteristics and lower urinary tract symptoms of female bladder outlet obstruction. Urology. 2005;66(5):1005–9.
57. Leadbetter GW, Leadbetter WF. Diagnosis and treatment of congenital bladder neck obstruction in children. N Engl J Med. 1959;260(13):633–7.
58. Awad SA, Downie JW, Lywood DW, Young RA, Jarzylo SV. Sympathetic activity in the proximal urethra in patients with urinary obstruction. J Urol. 1976;115(5):545–7.
59. Osman N, Chapple C. Fowler's syndrome- a cause of unexplained urinary retention in young women? Nat Rev Urol. 2014;11:87–98.
60. Fowler CJ, et al. Abnormal electromyographic activity of the urethral sphincter, voiding dysfunction, and polycystic ovaries: a new syndrome? BMJ. 1988;297:1436–8.
61. Lepor H, Machi G. Comparison of AUA symptom index in unselected males and females between fifty-five and seventy-nine years of age. Urology. 1993;42:36–41.
62. Hsiao SM, Lin HH, Kuo HC. International prostate symptom score for assessing lower urinary tract dysfunction in women. Int Urogynecol J. 2013;24:263–7.
63. Scarpero HM, Fiske J, Xue X, Nitti VW. American urological association symptom index for lower urinary tract symptoms in women: correlation with degree of bother and impact on quality of life. Urology. 2003;61(6):1118–22.
64. Huang YH, Bih LI, Chen SL, et al. The accuracy of ultrasonic estimation of bladder volume: a comparison of portable and stationary equipment. Arch Phys Med Rehabil. 2004;85:138–41.
65. Negro CL, Muir GH. Chronic urinary retention in men: how we define it, and how does it affect treatment outcome. BJU Int. 2012;110:1590–4.
66. Spatafora S, Conti G, Perachino M, Casarico A, Mazzi G, Pappagallo GL, AURO. it BPH Guidelines Committee. Evidence-based guidelines for the management of lower urinary tract symptoms related to uncomplicated benign prostatic hyperplasia in Italy: updated summary. Curr Med Res Opin. 2007;23:1715–32.
67. Nitti VW. Pressure flow urodynamic studies: the gold standard for diagnosing bladder outlet obstruction. Rev Urol. 2005;7(Suppl 6):S14–21.
68. Griffiths D, Hofner K, van Mastrigt R, Rollema HR, Spangberg A, Gleason D. Standardization of terminology of lower urinary tract function: pressure-flow studies of voiding, urethral resistance, and urethral obstruction. Neurourol Urodyn. 1997;16:1–18.

69. Brucker B, Fong E, Shah S, Kelly C, Rosenblum N, Nitti V. Urodynamic differences between dysfunctional voiding and primary bladder neck obstruction in women. Urology. 2012;80:55–60.
70. Han JH, Yu HS, Lee JY, et al. Simple modification of the bladder outlet obstruction index for better prediction of endoscopically-proven prostatic obstruction: a preliminary study. PLoS One. 2015;10:e0141745.
71. Abrams P. Bladder outlet obstruction index, bladder contractility index and bladder voiding efficiency: three simple indices to define bladder voiding function. BJU Int. 1999;84:14–5.
72. Oelke M, Rademakers K, van Koeveringe GA. Unraveling detrusor underactivity: development of a bladder outlet resistance-bladder contractility nomogram for adult male patients with lower urinary tract symptoms. NeurourolUrodyn. 2016;35:980–6.
73. Meier K, Padmanabhan P. Female bladder outlet obstruction: an update on diagnosis and management. Curr Opin Urol. 2016;26(4):334–41.
74. Defreitas GA, Zimmern PE, Lemack GE, Shariat SF. Refining diagnosis of anatomic female bladder outlet obstruction: comparison of pressure-flow study parameters in clinically obstructed women with those of normal controls. Urology. 2004;64:675–9.
75. Gammie A, Kaper M, Dorrepaal C, Kos T, Abrams P. Signs and symptoms of detrusor underactivity: an analysis of clinical presentation and urodynamic tests from a large group of patients undergoing pressure flow studies. Eur Urol. 2016;69(2):361–9.
76. Blaivas JG, Groutz A. Bladder outlet obstruction nomogram for women with lower urinary tract symptomatology. NeurourolUrodyn. 2000;19:553–64.
77. Choi YS, Kim JC, Lee KS, Seo JT, Kim HJ, Yoo TK, Lee JB, Choo MS, Lee JG, Lee JY. Analysis of female voiding dysfunction: a prospective, multi-center study. Int Urol Nephrol. 2013,45:989–94.
78. Stoffel JT, Peterson AC, Sandhu JS, Suskind AM, Wei JT, LIghtner DJ. AUA white paper: non-neurogenic chronic urinary retention: consensus definition, treatment algorithm and outcome endpoints. J Urol. 2017;198(1):153–60.
79. Apfel SC. Nerve growth factor administration protects against experimental diabetic sensory neuropathy. Brain Res. 1994;634:7–12.
80. Garrett NE. Alpha-lipoic acid corrects neuropeptide deficits in diabetic rats via induction of trophic support. Neurosci Lett. 1997;222:191–4.
81. Lourenco T, Pickard R, Vale L, Grant A, Fraser C, MacLennan G, N'Dow J. Minimally invasive treatments for benign prostatic enlargement: systematic review of randomized controlled trials. BMJ. 2008;337(a1662):1–8.
82. Harris C, et al. National variation in urethroplasty cost and predictors of extreme cost: a cost analysis with policy implications. Urology. 2016;94:246–54.
83. Gomelsky A, Scapero HM, Dmochowski RR. Sling surgery for stress urinary incontinence in the female: what surgery, which material? AUA Update Ser. 2003;22(34):266–76.
84. Rardin CR, Rosenblatt PL, Kohli N, Miklos JR, Heit M, Lucente VR. Release of tension-free vaginal tape for the treatment of refractory post-operative voiding dysfunction. Obstet Gynecol. 2002;100:898–902.
85. Viereck V, Rautenberg O, Kociszeski J, et al. Midurethral sling incision: indications and outcomes. Int Urogynecol J. 2013;24(4):645–53.
86. Pedraza R, Nieto J, Ibarra S, Haas E. Pelvic muscle rehabilitation: a standardized protocol for pelvic floor dysfunction. Adv Urol. 2014;2014:487436. https://doi.org/10.1155/2014/487436.

Upper Urinary Tract Function (Reflux, Obstruction, and Kidney Function)

Paul W. Veenboer and J. L. H. Ruud Bosch

Abbreviations

^{99m}Tc-DSMA	Technetium-99m dimercaptosuccinic acid
^{99m}Tc-DTPA	Technetium-99m diethylenetriamine pentaacetic acid
^{99m}Tc-MAG3	Technetium-99m mercaptoacetyl triglycine
BUO	Bilateral ureteric obstruction
EAU	European Association of Urology
eGFR	Estimated glomerular filtration rate
GFR	Glomerular filtration rate
RBF	Renal blood flow
RVR	Renal vascular resistance
SCI	Spinal cord injury
T½	Half-life time
UPJ	Ureteropelvic junction
UUO	Unilateral ureteric obstruction
VUJ	Vesicoureteric junction

Normal Pyelo-ureteral Urodynamics [Function]

Normal and Abnormal Pyelo-ureteral Fluid Dynamics

In physical terms, i.e., in terms of fluid mechanics, the ureter can be seen as a collapsible tube with peristalsis. The peristaltic waves originate from pacemaker cells in the pyelocaliceal system, also known as Cajal cells. There are several pacemaker cells in the pyelocaliceal system, but not all action potentials originating from these cells "cross" the ureteropelvic junction (UPJ). The propagation of the

P. W. Veenboer · J. L. H. Ruud Bosch (✉)
Department of Urology, University Medical Center Utrecht, Utrecht, The Netherlands
e-mail: p.w.veenboer-2@umcutrecht.nl; j.l.h.r.bosch@umcutrecht.nl

© Springer International Publishing AG, part of Springer Nature 2018
R. Dmochowski, J. Heesakkers (eds.), *Neuro-Urology*,
https://doi.org/10.1007/978-3-319-90997-4_16

"

action potentials is possible because of excitation-contraction coupling via gap junctions between the smooth muscle cells in the pyelocaliceal system and the ureteral wall. Action potentials can be blocked when they arrive at smooth muscle cells that are in their refractory period; the refractory period of these muscle cells is several seconds long. Conduction can also be blocked at the UPJ when the incoming signals are not synchronized. So, normally, not every action potential leads to propagation of smooth muscle activity/contraction beyond the UPJ. Therefore the UPJ is a functional (and may be an anatomical) checkpoint in the fluid transport mechanism. Griffiths and Notschaele have given a detailed description of the physical aspects of ureteral urine transport [1]. A schematic representation of their description of these mechanisms is shown in Fig. 1: contraction waves originating from the most proximal part of the ureter move down the ureter and propagate boluses of urine toward the bladder. So, contraction of ureteral smooth muscle cells leads to increased intraluminal pressure and propagation of peristaltic waves down the ureter. Intraluminal manometry has shown that the ureter basically acts as a peristaltic pump that increases the intraluminal pressure and in this way delivers boluses of urine in the bladder. A peristaltic wave

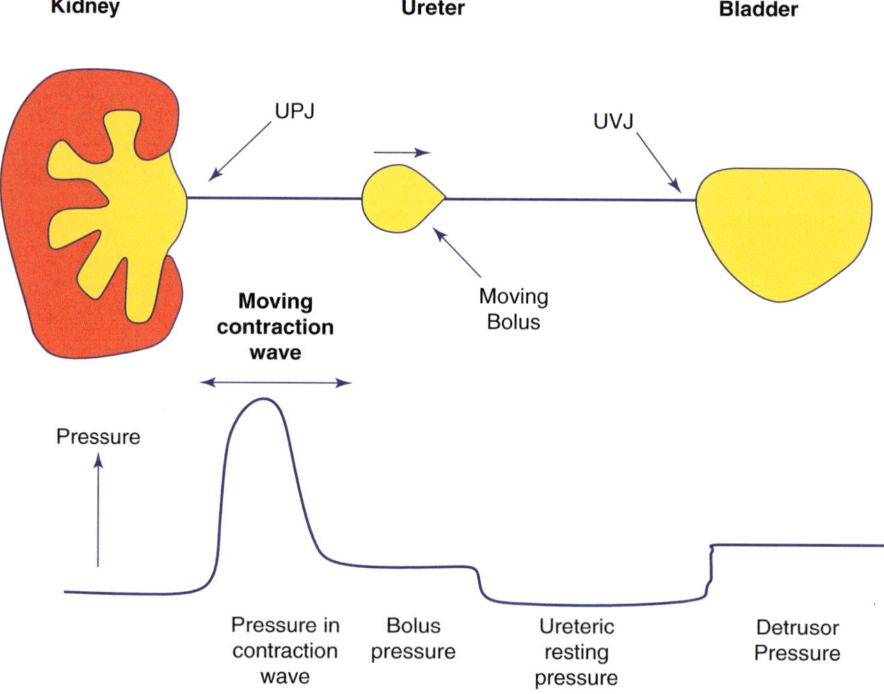

Fig. 1 Schematic representation of the physical aspects of ureteral urine transport including distribution of pressure in the pyelocaliceal system, ureter, and bladder. Contraction waves originating from the most proximal part of the ureter, indicated in the figure by UPJ, move down the ureter and propagate boluses of urine toward the bladder

lasts about 6 s and has a velocity of about 2 cm/s [2]. These peristaltic waves "catch" separate urine boluses that are propagated toward the bladder. Because this peristaltic activity creates separate urine boluses, the kidney with its pyelocaliceal system is effectively isolated from the bladder and the high pressures that can sometimes be generated in this organ. The frequency or periodicity of the peristaltic contractions is not strictly fixed; it is dependent on the rate of diuresis. When the ureter relaxes between two peristaltic boluses, urine can "leak" from the bolus, thus creating extra-peristaltic flow; this can occur particularly at low rates of diuresis. The peristaltic transport capacity of the ureter has an upper limit of a certain volume of urine per time unit (mL/min). Above this limit, boluses that follow upon each other cannot be separated anymore. Normally, increasing diuresis (urine flow) leads to a higher frequency of peristaltic waves up to the point where the upper limit of peristaltic transport capacity is reached. The higher frequency of peristaltic waves in case of a high rate of diuresis serves to maintain the isolation of the bladder from the upper tract. When the maximal peristaltic transport capacity is reached, the ureter becomes an "open" tube. Although an open tube can transport more urine per time unit, particularly when the subject is in the upright position, it may also lead to a harmful translation of high bladder pressures to the upper tract and kidney.

From its course down from the pyclo-ureteral junction, which is a functional checkpoint, there are two additional anatomical holdups in the ureter. The first is situated at the point where the ureter crosses the iliac blood vessels and the second where the ureter enters the bladder through its muscular wall before it courses submucosally for a few centimeters. The thicker the bladder wall, the more relevant the holdup. In neurogenic bladder disease, a thick bladder wall regularly acts as the obstructive locus. The submucosal tunnel serves as an additional obstructive area during times when detrusor pressure is high or when the bladder is full; that is when the capacity is (nearly) reached. Short-lasting periods of high pressure typically occur during an (neurogenic or non-neurogenic) overactive detrusor contraction or during voiding. Long-lasting periods of high pressure occur when the bladder is poorly compliant. Poor compliance can have an active neuromuscular or a passive origin due to bladder wall fibrosis; sometimes both factors play a significant role. The two anatomic checkpoints are particularly important with extra-peristaltic flow at low rates.

There is a clear intraluminal pressure gradient from the upper ureter toward the submucosal tunnel. At the ureterovesical junction, the ureter can freely slide in its tunnel through the bladder wall. It can shorten its length thus decreasing the length of the tunnel, but it is not able to actively decrease its diameter [2]. When the urine bolus arrives at the junction of the ureter with the bladder, it is delivered into the bladder by an active retraction or shortening of the ureteric wall over the urine bolus. Distal spreading of a ureteric contraction wave into the superficial trigone increases the submucosal ureteric length, thus passively preventing reflux. Thickening of the contracted portion of the ureter in its transmural tunnel contributes to the prevention of reflux.

When the ureter is acutely obstructed, the frequency of peristaltic waves increases. When the ureter is chronically dilated, interestingly, the frequency of ureteric peristaltic waves decreases.

In a chronically instrumented animal model, administration of atropine or carbachol neither changed the force of the contraction nor the frequency of the peristaltic waves [2]. This seems to be at variance with the notion that atropine and pethidine are effective in the treatment of collicy pain from a passing ureteral stone. Adrenergic stimulation of alpha-1 and beta-adrenoceptors leads to an increase of peristaltic pressure and a decrease of peristaltic frequency [2]. An inhibition of the alpha-1 and beta-adrenoceptors diminishes the contractile force but does not affect the frequency; this seems to be in line with clinical studies that do not show a significant effect of tamsulosin over placebo in the expulsion of ureteral stones [3].

Diagnostic Urodynamics and Functional Imaging of the Upper Tract

Nuclear Renography

For the evaluation of obstruction and renal function, several i.v. injectable agents are available. Gamma scintillation cameras can measure the radiation that is emitted by the injected radioisotope. The measured data are processed into perfusion (renal blood flow) images and perfusion time-activity curves. The agents most often used in urology are technetium-99m diethylenetriamine pentaacetic acid (^{99m}Tc-DTPA), technetium 99m-dimercaptosuccinic acid (^{99m}Tc-DSMA), and technetium-99m mercaptoacetyl triglycine (^{99m}Tc-MAG3).

^{99m}Tc-DTPA is primarily a glomerular filtration agent. Since it is excreted through the kidney and depends on the kidney function/the glomerular filtration rate, it is less useful in the evaluation of the collecting system and ureters in patients with impaired glomerular filtration rate (GFR).

^{99m}Tc-DSMA is very useful for the evaluation of the renal cortex. Renal clearance is by glomerular filtration and secretion; the agent mainly accumulates in the renal cortex and is therefore ideal for the detection of renal cortical defects and ectopic kidneys.

^{99m}Tc-MAG3 is mainly cleared through tubular secretion and has a 6-h half-life ($T_{1/2}$). It is an excellent agent for the evaluation of ureteral obstruction even in patients with renal insufficiency. With ^{99m}Tc-MAG3, differential renal function and clearance time of the left and right kidney can be assessed.

An example of a ^{99m}Tc-MAG3 renogram is shown in Fig. 2. In the first phase of the examination, the flow phase (about 3 min) renal uptake occurs showing background clearance, vascular abnormalities, and bleeding. In the second phase, called the renal phase (about 30 min), renal (dys)function is assessed. In the first 2 min of this phase, the time-to-peak uptake is measured. At the onset of the third phase, the transit phase, a diuretic (usually furosemide) is injected when the visualized collect-

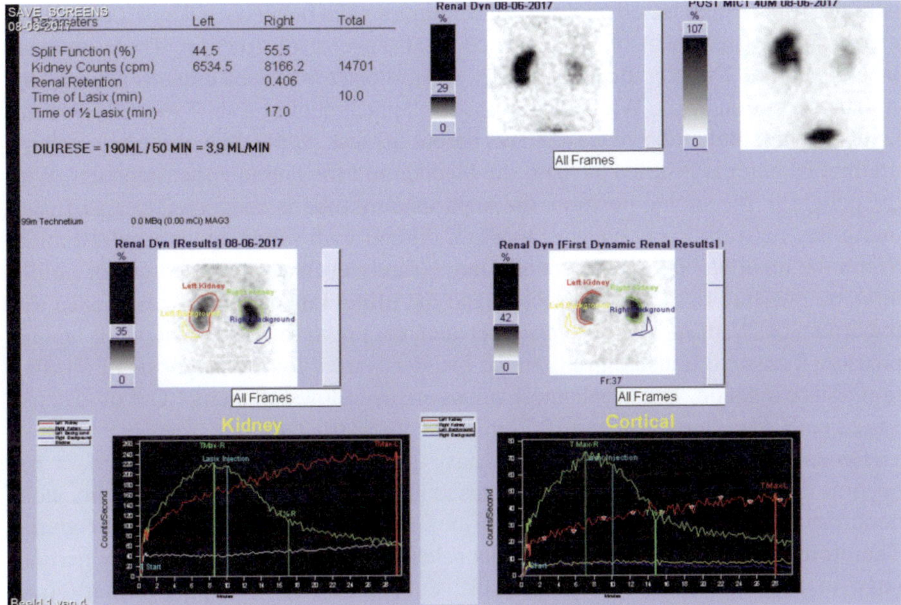

Fig. 2 MAG3 renogram. This examination shows the case of a 66-year-old woman with a total obstruction of the left kidney. In this case, both kidneys take up an approximately similar amount of radioisotope (with a split renal function of 44.5% vs. 55.5%). After injection of a diuretic (in this case, furosemide or Lasix® i.v.), the green curve (=the right kidney) descents steeply, showing that urine transport from the left kidney is unobstructed. However, the red curve does not show any sign of descent, corresponding with a total lack of runoff from the obstructed left system

ing system activity is at its maximum. It is crucial that the technician who executes the examination identifies the moment of maximum activity correctly and not too late or too early. The time it takes from the injection of the diuretic, for the collecting system activity to decrease 50%, is called $T_{1/2}$. When the $T_{1/2}$ is less than 10 min, this indicates that the system is not obstructed. A transit time of 10–20 min represents a moderate delay and may be consistent with obstruction, whereas a $T_{1/2}$ that is longer than 20 min indicates clear obstruction. Often the level of obstruction can be visualized. These examinations are noninvasive.

Whitaker Test

In 1973, Whitaker introduced a method for the urodynamic assessment of the upper urinary tract: the perfusion pressure-flow (PPF) test, thereafter known as the Whitaker test [4, 5]. The test has not been widely accepted because of its invasiveness and perceived unphysiological approach. Early analyses of its use have pointed out that its ability to predict the functional outcome of reconstructive surgery for obstructive hydronephrosis is inconsistent [6]. Around the time of its introduction, other noninvasive methods based on imaging techniques were being considered more convenient for the assessment of the presence or absence of obstruction. These methods include diuretic Doppler ultrasonography and radioisotope-based diuresis renography.

The execution of the Whitaker test involves placement of a (6–7 *French*) percutaneous nephrostomy tube, at least 3 days before the test. At the time of the test, a transurethral catheter is inserted to drain the bladder and for pressure measurement. With the patient in the supine position, the nephrostomy tube is connected to a perfusion pump that delivers X-ray contrast medium diluted with saline, at a rate of 10 mL/s. When the renal pelvis is exceptionally large (rarely even several hundreds of milliliters), no pressure rise will be detected, and the filling rate can then be increased to a maximum of 20 mL/s. The difference between the pressure in the renal pelvis and the pressure measured transurethrally in the bladder is used for the diagnosis of obstruction or its exclusion. The usual cutoff values are as follows: >22 cmH_2O = obstructed, 15–22 cmH_2O = equivocal, and <15 cmH_2O = unobstructed.

Recently, Lupton and George [7] have pointed out that its invasiveness has become less important with the increased use of renal access via percutaneous nephrostomy and the popularity of various minimally invasive renal procedures. Therefore, the Whitaker test still has its role in modern urological surgery particularly in the evaluation of the difficult, equivocal case of upper urinary tract dilatation.

In their report on the 35-year experience with this test [7], Lupton and George found that in patients with idiopathic hydronephrosis, there was agreement between the results of the perfusion pressure-flow studies and diuresis renography in 72%. The test determined or contributed to the clinical management in 84% of the cases studied. It was accurate in its prediction of outcome in 77% of cases where obstruction was diagnosed and in 77% of unobstructive cases. They concluded that the Whitaker test should be reserved for assessing potential upper urinary tract obstruction in the following circumstances: equivocal results from less invasive tests, suspected obstruction with poor kidney function, loin pain with a negative diuresis renogram, suspected intermittent obstruction, and gross dilatation with a positive diuresis renogram.

Cystometry and Pressure-Flow Study in Neuro-urology: Effects on the Upper Tract

A full (video)urodynamic study that includes cystometry to evaluate bladder function and a pressure-flow study to evaluate the outflow tract are often less easy to perform in patients with neurologic defects than in neurologically intact patients. Nevertheless, important aspects of the examination that might indicate the presence of a "hostile" bladder can most often be assessed adequately. The term hostile bladder indicates the high pressures in the bladder may lead to hydroureteronephrosis allowing transmission of the high pressures to the kidney. It is most important to evaluate the compliance of the bladder and the presence of neurogenic detrusor overactivity. During X-ray screening (video), active (during contraction) or passive vesicoureteral reflux can be detected. Detrusor-sphincter dyssynergia can also be detected during the voiding phase when using video urodynamics. Wang and McGuire [8] have reported that spina bifida patients with a poor compliance leading to a detrusor leak point pressure (DLPP) of more than 40 cmH$_2$O have a 81% chance of developing kidney damage whereas those with a DLPP of less than 40 cmH$_2$O developed kidney damage in only 10% of the cases.

Normal and Abnormal Renal Function

Assessment of Renal Function

In clinical practice, GFR is often used to measure global renal function. GFR has been defined as the clearance for any substance which is freely filtered and is neither absorbed, secreted, nor metabolized by the kidney [9]. The gold standard for determining GFR is a 24-h inulin clearance. However, there are some drawbacks to this method, especially the fact that it is labor-intensive and has limited availability and intravenous access will be needed.

The same practical limitations hamper the widespread use of radioactive isotopes such as ^{51}Cr-EDTA and DTPA. Another method to determine GFR is using 24-h creatinine clearance, which does not have the drawbacks of needing intravenous access and (expensive) isotopes. However, 24-h urine collection is still rather labor-intensive for the patient and especially difficult in patients with urinary incontinence (in whom the entire 24-h portion cannot be collected). In patients with one- or two-sided percutaneous nephrostomy tube drainage of urine in addition to spontaneous voiding, it is clear that all urine must be collected. Therefore, most clinicians will determine the "estimated" GFR (eGFR) in everyday practice.

eGFR is usually based on a single serum measurement of a marker. In healthy individuals, creatinine is usually used for this purpose. Using a single serum creatinine, eGFR can be calculated using a range of formulas, e.g., Cockroft-Gault, CKD-EPI, and MDRD. In everyday practice, the CKD-EPI formula is recommended for the general population [10].

It is known that creatinine has some drawbacks, especially its dependence on muscle mass. In patients with neurological diseases, muscle atrophy causes the normal creatinine value to be lower than in the healthy population. In some (stable) neuromuscular disease, especially congenital diseases like spinal dysraphism, the course of serum creatinine could be followed over time to see if any deterioration takes place. However, in neurodegenerative diseases such as amyotrophic lateral sclerosis and multiple sclerosis, loss of muscle mass may take place over time, and a deteriorating GFR might not be detected.

Several markers have been proposed to overcome this problem. The first one of interest is cystatin C, a cysteine protease inhibitor. This small molecule has some interesting features which make it a possible marker for GFR, especially the fact that it is independent of muscle mass (being produced by every nucleated cell in the body) and that it is filtered by the glomerulus without being reabsorbed. Despite what was formerly claimed, serum levels of cystatin C are influenced by higher lean body mass, fat mass, diabetes, markers of inflammation, age, and thyroid malfunctioning [10].

Formulas estimating GFR using cystatin C have been developed, as well as a formula combining serum creatinine and serum cystatin C [11]. The combined formula turned out to be more reliable in estimating eGFR than creatinine alone in one very large study with 5352 individuals.

Hemodynamic Changes with Obstruction

Glomerular Filtration Rate (GFR)

As a result of obstruction of the upper urinary tract, GFR can be impaired. The volume of filtrated blood directly depends on three factors: glomerular hydrostatic pressure, glomerular colloid osmotic (oncotic) pressure, and the pressure in Bowman's capsule [12]. As described in more detail below, the hydrostatic pressure and pressure in Bowman's capsule are affected by obstruction of the urinary tract, thus eventually reducing GFR.

Renal Blood Flow (RBF)

The kidneys receive about 25% of the cardiac output; this is controlled by an autoregulation system, meaning that approximately 1 L of blood per minute is filtrated in physiologic circumstances. RBF has been defined as the pressure difference between the renal artery and renal vein divided by the renal vascular resistance [9].

Regulation of the RBF takes place via vasoconstriction of arterioles as a response to increased blood pressure as well as tubuloglomerular feedback via the juxtaglomerular apparatus. Apart from autoregulation mechanisms, paracrine and endocrine mechanisms are also involved in regulating RBF. Under normal circumstances, renal blood flow remains remarkably constant when blood pressure ranges between 80 and 180 mmHg.

Renal Vascular Resistance (RVR)

As discussed in the section above, vascular resistance in the kidney is regulated tightly thanks to autoregulation mechanisms. RVR is mainly regulated by the cortical radial arteries and especially by afferent arterioles [13]. Normally, the resistance is determined by the preglomerular segment (afferent arteriole and the interlobular artery) and the postglomerular segment (efferent vessel). In case of obstruction the total vascular resistance may be influenced by the peritubular capillary network [14].

The effects of ureteral obstruction are mainly known from animal studies and focus primarily on acute occlusion.

Unilateral Ureteral Obstruction

Unilateral ureteral obstruction (UUO) will be more often caused by non-neurogenic than neurogenic causes. Neurogenic obstruction is usually caused by functional or anatomical changes in the lower urinary tract, i.e., the bladder or the vesicoureteric junction, and therefore will most often lead to a bilateral problem.

The effects of unilateral ureteral obstructions have been studied in animal experiments [15]. UUO causes subacute renal injury due to tubular cell injury, interstitial inflammation, and fibrosis. After acute unilateral obstruction, a triphasic change in renal blood flow occurs [16].

After 0–90 min, there is an increase in both RBF and ureteral pressure; after 90–300 min, RBF decreases while ureteral pressure continues to rise. After 300 min, both ureteral pressure and RBF decrease. Prostaglandin E2 and nitric oxide are the most important mediators responsible for dilation of the afferent arteriole; they enhance RBF in the first hours after acute obstruction [17].

In another study, conducted in young lambs by Kim et al., the initial phase of increase of RBF was not observed; during a follow-up period of 5 days, RBF decreased with 29%, and after an initial rise in ureteral pressure from 9 to 37 mmHg, this declined very slowly during the following days [18].

Vasoconstriction of the afferent arteriole in the later phases of acute obstruction is primarily mediated by angiotensin II. Apart from global changes in kidney perfusion, some parts of the kidney are better perfused than others: the superficial cortex receives relatively less blood than the juxtaglomerular part of the kidney.

The effects of treatment of unilateral ureteral obstruction have also been studied in dogs. Leahy et al. have studied a group of 21 dogs in which unilateral obstruction had been applied [19]. Obstruction was relieved by stenting after 14, 28, and 60 days. In the first group, recovery of renal function was 100%, whereas in the other two groups, only 31% and 8% recovered full function, respectively. Microscopic studies revealed arteriolar constriction in the second group, suggesting that renal damage after ureteral constriction is in fact a vascular disease.

Bilateral Ureteral Obstruction

In bilateral ureteral obstruction (BUO), the changes in renal blood flow are different from those in unilateral obstruction. In bilateral ureteral obstruction (or in obstruction of a solitary kidney), there is only a minor increase in RBF after occlusion, lasting for about 90 min. However, RBF will soon drop due to postglomerular vasoconstriction. Another change with BUO is that the blood flow is directed to the outer part of the kidney (the cortex) instead of the central part, which is exactly the opposite in UUO [17].

Postobstructive polyuria is often encountered after alleviating BUO, and this is thought to be a response to the accumulation of fluid and solute. The incidence varies between 0.5% and 52.0% [20]. After UUO, postobstructive polyuria is much rarer because of compensatory mechanisms from the contralateral kidney (with the logical exception of the patient with a solitary kidney).

There are several theories to explain the pathophysiology of postobstructive polyuria—the exact cause is probably multifactorial [21]. One of these is a progressive reduction in the medullary concentration gradient secondary to vascular washout and downregulation of sodium transporters in the thick ascending loop of Henle. Another theory states that ischemia of the tubular structures will occur due to reduced renal blood flow and hence dysregulation of the juxtaglomerular apparatus. Furthermore, due to renal damage, the effects of antidiuretic hormone on the kidney may also be reduced, thus triggering a large diuresis.

Effect of Obstruction on Tubular Function

Despite the emphasis on renal blood flow and GFR, these processes only take place in small part of the kidney. In fact, 80% of the renal volume is occupied by the tubulo-interstitium. Much about the effects of ureteral obstruction is known from animal experiments [15]. Ureteral obstruction causes subacute renal injury due to tubular cell injury, interstitial inflammation, and fibrosis. In acute obstruction, it is known that urinary production may continue, sometimes leading to calyceal blowout. In chronic settings (as in neurogenic cases), fluid will often exit through the renal venous system again, and a blowout will not occur.

However, due to the reduction in renal blood flow, a state of local ischemia will start in the tubulo-interstitium. Damaged cells will release cytokines attracting macrophages and T-lymphocytes, initiating a vicious circle of inflammation and fibrosis. Apart from the local ischemia, mediators released by the activation of the renin-angiotensin system like angiotensin II will stimulate the influx of cytokines promoting interstitial fibrosis. The most important mediator of this process seems to be tumor growth factor-bèta. Apart from stimulation of fibrosis, TGF-bèta also degrades nitric oxide which normally prevents macrophages from entering the kidney [12]. Unfortunately, reversal of kidney obstruction will not immediately stop these processes: it may in fact take weeks before inflammation resides [22].

Effect of Reflux on Renal Function

Vesicoureteral reflux (VUR) in neurogenic bladder can be both active and passive; the mechanisms are described below in more detail.

Reflux can cause renal damage by scarring. One study showed an 18-fold increase in renal scarring in patients with high-grade reflux [23]. After urine reaches the kidney due to reflux, intrarenal reflux is prevented by the shape of the papillae. Most of the (healthy) kidney is composed of so-called convex papillae, comprising about 2/3 of all papillae. These papillae, also called "simple papillae," have slit-like orifices which close automatically during raised intrarenal pressure. However, 1/3 of the kidney, predominantly the upper and lower pole regions, is comprised of "compound" papillae. The latter have much larger orifices which will not close, allowing intrarenal reflux to take place. Since intrarenal reflux will first take place in these papillae, renal scarring is initially observed in the lower and upper poles of the kidney. It has been observed that the scarring leads to distortion of architecture and causes neighboring simple papillae to change into compound papillae, thus enhancing the process of intrarenal reflux. This mechanism also explains why scarring in nuclear studies is often detected first in the upper and lower poles of the kidneys.

In any case, if reflux occurs intrarenally, renal scarring can occur. This especially happens when urine infected with bacterial products (most importantly, lipopolysaccharides) enters the renal parenchyma and triggers an immune response. However, in high-pressure obstructed systems such as in neurogenic bladder disease, scarring can also occur when the urine is sterile [24].

Ureteropelvic Junction (UPJ) Stenosis

In physiologic situations, the UPJ has a physiological "blockage" meaning the frequency of contraction at the level of the calyces and renal pelvis is higher than that of the UPJ [25]. This has already been discussed in more detail above. Only when enough urine has accumulated in the renal pelvis, urinary propulsion down the ureter will start.

UPJ obstruction is frequently encountered as a stand-alone problem without any relation to neurogenic dysfunction. The estimated incidence of this entity is about 1:1000 and is the single most common cause of antenatal hydronephrosis. Intrinsic and extrinsic forms of UPJ stenosis can be distinguished, the first form being caused by disturbances in the muscular fibers of the UPJ and thus compromising motility of the UPJ [9]. A lack of interstitial cells of Cajal (the pacemaker cells) can also contribute to impaired peristalsis [26]. The treatment of choice for this entity is a pyeloplasty, with very high success rates.

UPJ obstruction in neurogenic disease is likely to be caused by disturbances in motility of the ureter. Peristalsis in the pelvis and proximal ureter is regulated by the interstitial cells of Cajal and seems to respond to the amount of urine flowing through, which means that the number and intensity of contractions are regulated by the volume of urine passing. Interestingly, this process seems to take place in an entirely autonomic fashion—contractions of the upper tract continue to take place after denervation of the kidney and after transplantation [27]. In the case of neurogenic lower urinary tract dysfunction, it is likely that high bladder pressures will eventually cause the peristalsis of the entire ureter and pyelocalyceal system to cease, a pathophysiological phenomenon which is described in more detail below.

Although there might be a regulatory role for the autonomic nerve system, studies concerning this regulation are conflicting and fall outside the scope of this chapter.

Obstruction Between UPJ and Vesicoureteral Junction (VUJ)

This concerns the midsection of the ureter. Normally, the ureter propulses urine to the bladder when intravesical pressures are below 40 cmH$_2$O; above this point, pressure in the ureter causes dilation and termination of propulsion [28]. In the normal resting state, intra-ureteric pressure is ca. 0–5 cmH$_2$O, and the ureter is completely collapsed. In case of high intravesical pressure, it is known that ureteric dilatation can occur, thereby compromising the possibility of proper ureteric contraction, eventually ceasing entirely.

In case of acute obstruction, it has been observed that the inter-ureteric pressure rises. At the same time, the frequency and amplitude of ureteric contractions increase [29]. After a couple of hours, the resting pressure as well as the amplitude and frequency of contractions decrease, whereas the diameter of the ureter will continue to increase if obstruction is not alleviated. After a period of weeks, muscular hypertrophy of the ureters occurs leading to a marked increase in contractile capability of these ureters. However, due to the ever-increasing ureteral luminal radius, the ureter is not able to generate a proper bolus propulsion [30]. This is explained by Laplace's law, in which pressure is the resultant of "stress" times "wall thickness" divided by the "radius" of the ureter.

Apart from the abovementioned, it should be noted that infection of the ureter (i.e., by stasis of infected urine) can further decrease ureteral motility.

Vesicoureteral Reflux in Neuro-urology

Passive Reflux

This is also called primary reflux. Passive VUR has been defined as reflux occurring due to failure of the passive anti-reflux mechanism. It occurs at relatively low bladder pressures. This mechanism is based on compression of the intramural portion of the distal ureter and depends on the length of the intramural (or more specifically intra-detrusor) tunnel and the diameter of the ureter [31].

Pacquin et al. have reported back in 1959 that the ideal tunnel-length-to-ureteral diameter should be 3:1, whereas in refluxing ureters, this ratio is only 1.4:1 [32]. Essentially, this type of reflux requires no other treatment and follow-up than that of reflux in otherwise healthy individuals.

Active Reflux

In neurogenic bladder disease, reflux is often secondary to overactivity and high bladder pressures. This form of VUR occurs when there is a (pathologic) bladder contraction; it has also been called secondary reflux. The active mechanism preventing VUR is based upon contraction of muscles in the trigone. Treatment relies on lowering intravesical pressures rather than surgical reconstruction of the intravesical ureteric tract. As stated above, the critical pressure limit in the neurogenic bladder has been defined at 40 cmH$_2$O. According to the European Association of Urology (EAU) Guidelines on Neuro-urology, video urodynamics are recommended if urodynamic studies are conducted in patients with a neurogenic bladder, because fluoroscopy can show reflux and record whether this takes place during a detrusor contraction or not [33].

There is some literature on active reflux in patients with spinal cord injury (SCI). Reflux can be present particularly in those patients with a high-pressure bladder (often due to suprasacral lesions). In 1965, Hackler reported that 60% of patients with SCI who died from renal failure had VUR [34]. In one recent series with a very long follow-up (median 45 years), 33% developed VUR during follow-up [35]. Treatment should be directed toward converting the lower urinary tract into a low-pressure reservoir and should be individually tailored, comprising medication (e.g., anticholinergics) and self-catheterization. The EAU Guidelines point out that procedures to treat sphincteric incontinence are only suitable if no significant ureteral reflux is present [33]. If these modalities fail, neuromodulation, sphincterotomy, or augmentation cystoplasty can be considered. Long-term treatment with an indwelling catheter is not recommended because of the risk of bladder shrinkage and bladder wall fibrosis as well as chronic infection, further decreasing bladder compliance.

Another neuro-urologic entity in which VUR is observed is spinal dysraphism. This is usually seen in the children with detrusor-sphincter dyssynergia [36]. Although the incidence at birth is only 3–5%, this increases to 30–40% if the impaired bladder function is left untreated. In one series in which 159 children were followed up between 1972 and 1992, reflux eventually occurred in almost 60%. In the same series, cortical scarring was seen significantly more often in children with VUR than those without VUR ($p < 0.05$) [37]. In children with spinal dysraphism, treatment of the neurogenic bladder is the mainstay in treating VUR; treatment modalities used are comparable to those in SCI.

Specific Clinical Neuro-urologic Entities with Effects on the Upper Tract

Neurogenic bladder dysfunction can lead to difficulties with urine transport from the pyelocaliceal system down the ureter and into the bladder, possibly resulting in hydroureteronephrosis and kidney failure. Detrusor pressure is high during short-lasting periods of (neurogenic or non-neurogenic) overactive detrusor contraction or during a normal voiding contraction. The more detrimental long-lasting periods of high pressure typically occur when the bladder is poorly compliant. Poor compliance can have an active neuromuscular basis or a passive basis due to bladder wall fibrosis; sometimes both factors play a significant role. Both upper and lower motor neuron diseases can lead to neurogenic bladder dysfunction.

In somewhat simple terms, the micturition reflex can be described as a modulated spinobulbospinal (spinal cord-brainstem-spinal cord) reflex. This reflex is under voluntarily cortical cerebral control. The pontine micturition center is an important center integrating signals from various higher cerebral nuclei and the cortex and controlling an on-off switch in the brainstem. When this switch is in the on-mode, the pontine micturition center sends coordinated signals down to the sacral micturition center leading to the onset of bladder contraction and sphincter relaxation. The sacral micturition center is located in the conus medullaris; here, fine-tuning of the lower urinary tract function occurs. For example, incoming neural traffic from a full rectum inhibits the micturition reflex. Basically, and somewhat simplified, the reflex pathways can be damaged between the pontine and the sacral micturition center or peripherally from the sacral micturition center; the former situation leads to upper motor neuron disease and the latter to lower motor neuron disease. In chronic neurogenic bladder, the bladder wall thickens leading to additional obstruction to the ureteric urine flow.

Upper Motor Neuron Disease

When the neural pathways between the pontine and sacral micturition center are completely severed as in a complete spinal cord lesion, a normal reflex is not possible anymore leading to an acontractile bladder in the acute spinal shock phase. Weeks to months later, a new spinal reflex emerges. In patients with chronic spinal cord injury, this spinal reflex is not under control of the higher centers anymore, leading to hyperreflexia and detrusor-sphincter dyssynergia. The urodynamic pattern seen in a complete upper motor lesion, therefore, is characterized by neurogenic detrusor overactivity, involving involuntary hyperreflexive phasic detrusor contractions at a generally low bladder volume. During these contractions, micturition is not initiated or incomplete because of detrusor-sphincter dyssynergia, further increasing the deleterious pressures in the bladder. In patients with partial spinal cord lesions, the urodynamic picture can be mitigated. The most typical example of upper motor neuron disease is a complete spinal cord injury. In multiple sclerosis, plaques in the cervical spinal cord lead to an incomplete spinal cord lesion.

Lower Motor Neuron Disease

When the neural pathways are completely severed at or below the sacral micturition center, as can be the case in a conus medullaris lesion or a complete lesion of the cauda equina or the pelvic plexus, a normal reflex is not possible anymore; this results in an acontractile bladder. A new spinal reflex cannot emerge since no connection with the sacral micturition center is left. The bladder is not only acontractile but due to local axon reflexes also develops a state of poor compliance. So, the hostile bladder in lower motor neuron disease is characterized urodynamically by an acontractile bladder with a poor compliance and a nonfunctioning sphincter. Lower motor neuron disease typically occurs in patients with myelomeningocele (spina bifida) or in patients with a pelvic plexus lesion as can be seen after extensive ablative rectal surgery or radical hysterectomy.

So, in summary, in upper as well as lower motor neuron disease, the bladder pressures can become deleteriously high during prolonged periods of time, leading to impaired urine transport down the ureter and to hydroureteronephrosis.

References

1. Griffiths DJ, Notschaele C. The mechanics of urine transport in the upper urinary tract: 1. The dynamics of the isolated bolus. NeurourolUrodyn. 1983;2(2):155–66.
2. Roshani H. Dynamics and modulation of ureteric peristalsis. Amsterdam: Academic thesis, University of Amsterdam; 2003.
3. Pickard R, Starr K, MacLennan G, Lam T, Thomas R, Burr J, et al. Medical expulsive therapy in adults with ureteric colic: a multicentre, randomised, placebo-controlled trial. Lancet. 2015;386(9991):341–9.
4. Whitaker RH. Methods of assessing obstruction in dilated ureters. Br J Urol. 1973;45(1):15–22.
5. Whitaker RH. The Whitaker test. Urol Clin North Am. 1979;6(3):529–39.
6. Djurhuus JC, Sorensen SS, Jorgensen TM, Taagehoj-Jensen F. Predictive value of pressure flow studies for the functional outcome of reconstructive surgery for hydronephrosis. Br J Urol. 1985;57(1):6–9.
7. Lupton EW, George NJ. The Whitaker test: 35 years on. BJU Int. 2010;105(1):94–100.
8. Wang SC, McGuire EJ, Bloom DA. A bladder pressure management system for myelodysplasia—clinical outcome. J Urol. 1988;140(6):1499–502.
9. Reynard J, Brewster S, Biers S, editors. Oxford handbook of urology. 3rd ed. Oxford: Oxford University Press; 2013.
10. Inker LA, Perrone RD. Assessment of kidney function. 2017. https://www.uptodate.com/contents/assessment-of-kidney-function?source=search_result&search=renal%20function&selectedTitle=1~150#H23. Accessed 12 Apr 2017.
11. Inker LA, Schmid CH, Tighiouart H, Eckfeldt JH, Feldman HI, Greene T, et al. Estimating glomerular filtration rate from serum creatinine and cystatin C. N Engl J Med. 2012;367(1):20–9.
12. Nayyar R, Anil KS, Kaza R, Anand VJ. Review article- the obstructed kidney. Indian J Surg. 2005;67:1.
13. Carlstrom M, Wilcox CS, Arendshorst WJ. Renal autoregulation in health and disease. Physiol Rev. 2015;95(2):405–511.
14. Wright FS. Effects of urinary tract obstruction on glomerular filtration rate and renal blood flow. Semin Nephrol. 2017;2(1):5–16.
15. Ucero AC, Benito-Martin A, Izquierdo MC, Sanchez-Nino MD, Sanz AB, Ramos AM, et al. Unilateral ureteral obstruction: beyond obstruction. Int Urol Nephrol. 2014;46(4):765–76.
16. Moody TE, Vaughn ED Jr, Gillenwater JY. Relationship between renal blood flow and ureteral pressure during 18 hours of total unilateral ureteral occlusion. Implications for changing sites of increased renal resistance. Invest Urol. 1975;13(3):246–51.
17. Singh I, Standhoy JW, Assimos DG. Pathophysiology of urinary tract obstruction. In: Wein AJ, editor. Campbell-Walsh urology. 10th ed. Philadelphia, PA: Elsevier Saunders; 2012. p. 1091.

18. Kim KM, Bogaert GA, Nguyen HT, Borirakchanyavat S, Kogan BA. Hemodynamic changes after complete unilateral ureteral obstruction in the young lamb. J Urol. 1997;158(3 Pt 2):1090–3.
19. Leahy AL, Ryan PC, McEntee GM, Nelson AC, Fitzpatrick JM. Renal injury and recovery in partial ureteric obstruction. J Urol. 1989;142(1):199–203.
20. Nyman MA, Schwenk NM, Silverstein MD. Management of urinary retention: rapid versus gradual decompression and risk of complications. Mayo Clin Proc. 1997;72(10):951–6.
21. Halbgewachs C, Domes T. Postobstructive diuresis: pay close attention to urinary retention. Can Fam Physician. 2015;61(2):137–42.
22. Vaughan ED Jr, Gillenwater JY. Recovery following complete chronic unilateral ureteral occlusion: functional, radiographic and pathologic alterations. J Urol. 1971;106(1):27–35.
23. Tepmongkol S, Chotipanich C, Sirisalipoch S, Chaiwatanarat T, Vilaichon AO, Wattana D. Relationship between vesicoureteral reflux and renal cortical scar development in Thai children: the significance of renal cortical scintigraphy and direct radionuclide cystography. J Med Assoc Thai. 2002;85(Suppl 1):S203–9.
24. Smellie JM, Normand C. Reflux nephropathy in childhood. In: Hodson CJ, Kincaid-Smith P, editors. Reflux nephropathy. New York: Masson Publishing; 1979. p. 14–20.
25. Morita T, Ishizuka G, Tsuchida S. Initiation and propagation of stimulus from the renal pelvic pacemaker in pig kidney. Invest Urol. 1981;19(3):157–60.
26. Solari V, Piotrowska AP, Puri P. Altered expression of interstitial cells of Cajal in congenital ureteropelvic junction obstruction. J Urol. 2003;170(6 Pt 1):2420–2.
27. Lang RJ, Davidson ME, Exintaris B. Pyeloureteral motility and ureteral peristalsis: essential role of sensory nerves and endogenous prostaglandins. Exp Physiol. 2002;87(2):129–46.
28. McGuire EJ, Woodside JR, Borden TA, Weiss RM. Prognostic value of urodynamic testing in myelodysplastic patients. J Urol. 1981;126(2):205–9.
29. Rose JG, Gillenwater JY. Effects of obstruction on ureteral function. Urology. 1978;12(2):139–45.
30. Biancani P, Hausman M, Weiss RM. Effect of obstruction on ureteral circumferential force-length relations. Am J Physiol. 1982;243(2):F204–10.
31. Arena S, Iacona R, Impellizzeri P, Russo T, Marseglia L, Gitto E, et al. Physiopathology of vesico-ureteral reflux. Ital J Pediatr. 2016;42(1):103.
32. Paquin AJ Jr. Ureterovesical anastomosis: the description and evaluation of a technique. J Urol. 1959;82:573–83.
33. Groen J, Pannek J, Castro Diaz D, Del Popolo G, Gross T, Hamid R, et al. Summary of European Association of Urology (EAU) Guidelines on Neuro-Urology. Eur Urol. 2016;69(2):324–33.
34. Hackler RH, Dalton JJ Jr, Bunts RC. Changing concepts in the preservation of renal function in the paraplegic. J Urol. 1965;94:107–11.
35. Gao Y, Danforth T, Ginsberg DA. Urologic management and complications in spinal cord injury patients: a 40- to 50-year follow-up study. Urology. 2017;104:52–8.
36. Seki N, Akazawa K, Senoh K, Kubo S, Tsunoda T, Kimoto Y, et al. An analysis of risk factors for upper urinary tract deterioration in patients with myelodysplasia. BJU Int. 1999;84(6):679–82.
37. Filler G, Gharib M, Casier S, Lodige P, Ehrich JH, Dave S. Prevention of chronic kidney disease in spina bifida. Int Urol Nephrol. 2012;44(3):817–27.

Infections in Neuro-urology

Muhammad Rasheed and Arndt van Ophoven

Abbreviations

ACSS	Acute cystitis symptom score
ACTH	Adrenocorticotrophic hormone
AUC	Acute urinary cystitis
BPH	Benign prostatic hyperplasia
CA	Catheter associated
CA-AB	Catheter-associated bacteriuria
CA-AB	Catheter-associated asymptomatic bacteriuria
CA-UTI	Catheter-associated urinary tract infection
CAUTI	Community-associated UTI
CFU	Colony forming unit
CIC	Clean intermittent catheterization
DSD	Detrusor sphincter dyssynergia
DSD	Detrusor sphincter dyssynergia
ESBL	Extended-spectrum beta-lactamase
GAG	Glycosaminoglycan
HAUTI	Healthcare-associated urinary tract infection
IC	Indwelling catheter
IDSA	Infectious Disease Society of America
IL	Interleukin
MDR	Multidrug-resistant
MRSA	Methicillin-resistant Staphylococcus aureus
MS	Multiple sclerosis
NAUTI	Nosocomial urinary tract infections

M. Rasheed (✉) · A. van Ophoven
Department of Neuro-Urology, Marien Hospital Herne, University Clinic Bochum,
The Ruhr University Bochum, Herne, Germany
e-mail: muhammad.rasheed@ruhr-uni-bochum.de; neuro-urologie@marienhospital-herne.de

© Springer International Publishing AG, part of Springer Nature 2018
R. Dmochowski, J. Heesakkers (eds.), *Neuro-Urology*,
https://doi.org/10.1007/978-3-319-90997-4_17

NB	Neurogenic bladder
NDO	Neurogenic detrusor overactivity
NF-kB	Nuclear factor kappa-light-chain-enhancer of activated B cells
qSOFA	Quick sequential (sepsis-related) organ failure assessment
SCI	Spinal cord injury
S-IgA	Secretory immunoglobulin-A
SOFA	Sequential (sepsis-related) organ failure assessment
SPC	Supra pubic catheterization
TLR	Toll-like receptors
TMP-SMX	Trimethoprim-sulfamethoxazole
TNF	Tumor necrosis factor
UDS	Urodynamics
UTI	Urinary tract infection
VUDS	Video urodynamics
VUR	Vesicoureteral reflux

Urinary Tract Infection in Neurogenic Bladder Dysfunction

Introduction

Congenital abnormalities like meningomyelocele and damage of the central, peripheral, or autonomic nerve system can cause neurogenic bladder dysfunction. Inadequate bladder management can result in recurrent urinary tract infection that can cause progressive renal damage and urinary incontinence. Infection means the presence of microorganisms in a normally sterile site that is usually accompanied by an inflammatory host response. The clinical symptoms suggestive of urinary tract infection and evidence of bacteriuria or pyuria in urine are called urinary tract infections (UTIs). Infection can occur in all parts of the urinary system such as urethra, urethritis; urinary bladder, cystitis; and kidney infection, pyelonephritis. Most infections involve the lower urogenital tract, urinary bladder, and urethra. Women are at greater risk of developing infection in the urinary bladder than men. The infection in the bladder can be painful and irritating. Not everyone with UTI has symptoms, but common symptoms include urgency, frequency, and pain or burning when urinating. Physical obstruction such as formation of stones and cysts within the urinary tract leads to severe urinary tract infection. Inappropriate treatment of urinary tract infection can damage the renal function due to reflex pyelonephritis and vesicoureteral reflux. The patients with neurogenic bladder may suffer with lower urinary tract dysfunction with neurologic disorder range from 12% to 19% after stroke and up to 90% suffering from multiple sclerosis (MS).

Neurogenic bladder dysfunctions have high incidence of UTI in patients with spinal cord injuries and neurological conditions like multiple sclerosis, Parkinson's disease, cerebral palsy, and spina bifida. Inappropriate bladder management may not only cause kidney damage but also incontinence, vesicoureteral reflux infection, and lethal urosepsis. Modern medical science along with advanced technologies and better understanding of pathophysiology of functional urology has reduced the occurrence of many of these complications. However, infections in neuro-urology remain as challenging to diagnose, treat, and prevent in patients with neurological disorder. The management of neurogenic bladder consists of behavioral modification, clean intermittent catheterization, pharmacotherapy, intravesical botulinum toxin-A injections, or major reconstructive surgery including bladder augmentation and urinary diversion. Neuromodulation is a well-known treatment method for the patients with non-neurogenic overactive bladder and urinary retention who have previously failed more conservative therapies.

Global Epidemiology of Urinary Tract Infection

The prevalence of community-associated urinary tract infection (CAUTI) is 0.7% with main risk factors, i.e., age, sexual activity, and diabetes mellitus [1]. The most common pathogen is *Escherichia coli*, and its resistance rate to antibiotics depends on the geographical location. The incidence of UTI is higher in patients with neurogenic bladder dysfunction than normal community. Approximately 20–30% of female have a dysuria episode per year. In a retrospective study of 46,271, neurogenic bladder patients in the United States reported that more than one third (36.4%) of patients were diagnosed with a lower urinary tract infection.

In neurogenic bladder the UTI episodes are frequently treated during the acute exacerbation of multiple sclerosis. The prospective studies depict that the viral infections are common triggers of infection with the pathogenic mechanism involving T cells and cytokines. Furthermore, the retrospective data also support the bacterial infection as an important MS exacerbation trigger that significantly impacts neurogenic bladder management. A prospective study of spinal cord injury showed 16% of patients with neurogenic bladder are diagnosed with urinary tract infection. This ratio is much higher as compared to the non-neurogenic population.

Risk Factors in Healthcare-Associated Urinary Tract Infection (HAUTI)

An infection occurs due to the imbalance between the host defense mechanisms and micro pathogens. The influencing factors contributing in the context of healthcare-associated infections are related to the patient (host defense), pathogen virulence, healthcare intervention, and environment. Indwelling urinary catheters are considered as one of the most important factors in developing HAUTIs [2, 3]. The other risk factors like prolonged hospital stay, female gender, neurological disease, limited mobility prior to admission, and bone fracture have also been postulated as risk factors. In addition to the patient characteristics or the medical setting, the following available resources also play a vital role in the frequency of healthcare-associated infections [4]:

• Poor infrastructure	• Understaffing
• Insufficient equipment	• Overcrowding
• Poor knowledge and application of basic infection measures	• Lack of procedure
• Inadequate environmental hygienic conditions and waste disposal	• Absence of local and national guidelines and policies

Etiology

The most common isolated organism in neurogenic bladder is the *Enterobacteriaceae* family. Within this family, *E. coli* and *Klebsiella* species dominate with a *E. coli* comprising 50% of all strains isolated in two large studies [5, 6]. The frequency of *E. coli* and *Klebsiella* infections are lower in non-neurogenic patients. The incidence of the following bacteria in the neurogenic population is *Pseudomonas* 8.7–15%, *Acinetobacter* 6–15%, and *Enterococcus* 6–12% [7, 8]. The neurogenic bladder patients have increased risk of nosocomial organisms and to fungal infections which have been found to be associated with recent antibiotic use and indwelling catheterization. In prospective study of spinal cord injury patients, the incidence of candiduria was found to be 17%. The patients with indwelling catheterization and suprapubic catheter were ten times more likely to develop candiduria compared to the patients who used clean intermittent catheterization [9].

Figure 1 illustrates the urinary tract infection among women is extremely common; approximately 13% of women between the ages of 18 and 90 years will have an annual incidence of urinary tract infection. Based on the 2010 US census data, an estimated 15 million women will have a UTI annually in the United States. Percentages are proportional to the area of circles.

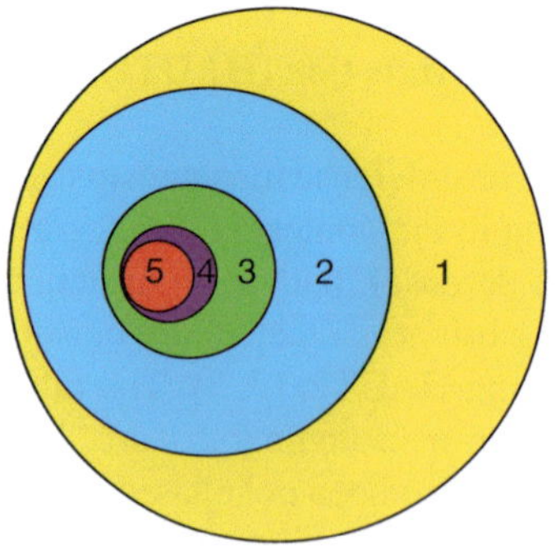

1. All Women.

2. 50% of all women will have a UTI in their lifetime.

3. Nearly 20% of women who have one UTI will have another.

4. 30% of those will have yet another UTI (recurrent).

5. 80% of those, 2.4% of all women, will have very frequent UTI.

Fig. 1 Percentage of infected women anually by Urinary tract infection [10]

Classification of Urinary Tract Infections

UTIs are classified into uncomplicated, complicated, recurrent, catheter-associated UTIs and urosepsis according to clinical symptoms, anatomical structure, severity level, risk factors, laboratory data, and microbiological findings.

Uncomplicated UTI: Asymptomatic bacteriuria with or without leucocytes and absence of clinical symptoms are called uncomplicated urinary tract infection. It refers to the invasion of microorganism but without structural and functional abnormalities. For example, asymptomatic cystitis, uncomplicated pyelonephritis limited to nonpregnant and premenopausal women.

Complicated UTI: Symptomatic urinary infection means the presence of pathogen bacteria in urine along with clinical signs that are evaluated by physician is called complicated urinary tract infection. The complication chances are increased in pregnant women, patients with immune suppressive diseases, and anatomical or functional abnormalities of the urinary tract.

Recurrent UTIs: Urinary infections that occur at least three episodes/year or two episodes in the last 6 months are called as recurrent urinary tract infection.

Catheter-associated UTIs: Urinary infection occurring in patients whose urinary tract is catheterized currently or within the past 48 h is called CA-UTI.

Urosepsis: Infection followed by signs of systemic inflammation, presence of symptoms of organ dysfunction, and persistent hypotension associated with tissue anoxia is called urosepsis.

Figure 2 illustrates the epidemiology of urinary tract infections that is caused by a wide range of pathogens, including Gram-negative and Gram-positive bacteria, as well as fungi. Uncomplicated UTIs typically affect women, children, and elderly patients who are otherwise healthy. Complicated UTIs are usually associated with

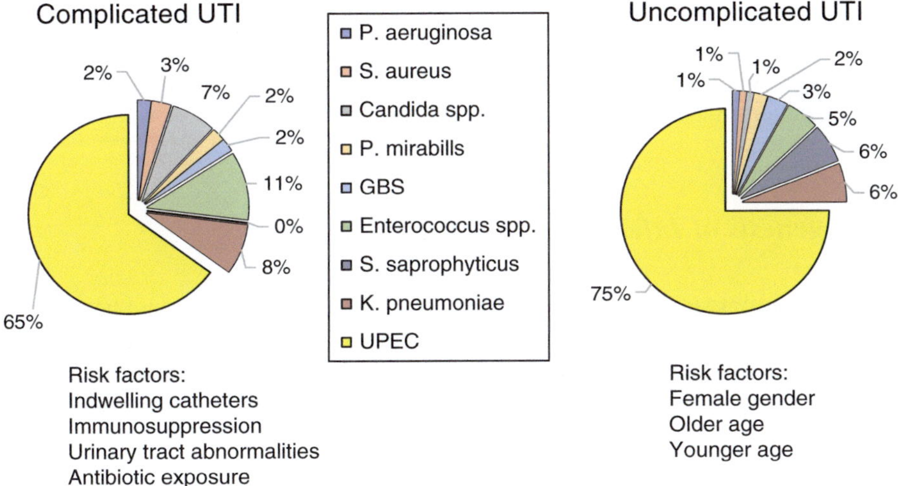

Fig. 2 Comparative epidemiology of urinary tract infection [11]

indwelling catheters, urinary tract abnormalities, immunosuppression, or exposure to antibiotics. The most common causative agent for both uncomplicated and complicated UTIs is uropathogenic *Escherichia coli* (UPEC). For uncomplicated UTIs, other causative agents are (in order of prevalence) *Klebsiella pneumoniae*, *Staphylococcus saprophyticus*, *Enterococcus faecalis*, group B *Streptococcus* (GBS), *Proteus mirabilis*, *Pseudomonas aeruginosa*, *Staphylococcus aureus*, and *Candida* spp. For complicated UTIs, the other causative agents are (in order of prevalence) *Enterococcus* spp., *K. pneumoniae*, *Candida* spp., *S. aureus*, *P. mirabilis*, *P. aeruginosa*, and GBS.

Figure 2 Comparative epidemiology of urinary tract infection [11] in neurogenic bladder patients. In general, complicated urinary infections are associated with biomedical devices, storage and voiding dysfunction, upper tract abnormalities, and immunosuppression, whereas uncomplicated infections occur in healthy patients, usually in females, children, and the elderly. *Escherichia coli* accounts for the most of infections in both groups of patients; however, there is a shift in the prevalence of pathogens toward nosocomial organisms in the complicated group of patients

Host Risk Factors in Urinary Tract Infection

According to ORENUC, host risk factors in UTI are describes as explained in Table 1

Acute cystitis is a common diagnosis in women. The incidence ratio of cystitis in middle-aged women to men is 30:1. The incidence and prevalence of acute cystitis vary, in different reports depending on the criteria used for urine analysis vs. urine culture. The National Health and Nutrition Survey reports the incident for UTIs: 13,320 per 100 thousand adult women per year. Among 25% of young women with cystitis, the infection recurs within 6 months after the first episode. Acute cystitis symptom scores may help to reduce recurrent urinary tract infections, vesicoureteral reflux, and assessment of everyday activity and quality of life in neurogenic bladder patients that is not yet validated in neuro-urology.

Pathogenesis of Infection in Neurogenic Bladder

Usually, microorganisms enter the urinary tract through lymphatic and hematogenous pathway, but some clinical and experimental evidences demonstrated that the ascent of microorganisms from the urethra is the most common passage that leads to UTI, especially bacteria from the gut (e.g., *E. coli* and other *Enterobacteriaceae*). This provides a logical explanation for the higher frequency of cystitis in women than in men due to their small size of urethra in female. Insertion of one-time catheter into the urinary bladder can cause infection in 1–2% among ambulatory patients. Bacteriuria found in almost 100% cases within 2–3 days of indwelling catheters with open-drainage systems. The use of closed-drainage system, including a valve

Table 1 Host risk factors in UTI according to ORENUC [12]

Type	Category of risk factor	Examples of risk factors
O	**NO** known/associated RF	– Healthy premenopausal women
R	**R**ecurrent UTI RF, but no risk of severe outcome	– Sexual behavior and contraceptive devices – Hormonal deficiency in post menopause – Secretory type of certain blood groups – Controlled diabetes mellitus
E	**E**xtra-urogenital RF, with risk of more severe outcome	– Pregnancy – Male gender – Badly controlled diabetes mellitus – Relevant immunosuppression* – Connective tissue diseases* – Prematurity, newborn
N	**N**ephropathic disease, with risk of more severe outcome	– Relevant renal insufficiency* – Polycystic nephropathy
U	**U**rological RF, with risk of more severe outcome, which can be resolved during therapy	– Ureteral obstruction (i.e., stone, stricture) – Transient short-term urinary tract catheter – Asymptomatic bacteriuria** – Controlled neurogenic bladder dysfunction urological surgery
C	Permanent urinary **c**atheter and non-resolvable urological RF, with risk of more severe outcome	– Long-term urinary tract catheter treatment – Non-resolvable urinary obstruction – Badly controlled neurogenic bladder

RF = risk factor; * = not well defined; ** = usually in combination with other RF (i.e. pregnancy, urological internvention)

to prevent retrograde flow, delays the onset of infection, but ultimately does not prevent it. It is assumed that bacteria migrate within the mucopurulent space between the urethra and catheter and that results in development of bacteriuria in almost all patients within ~4 weeks.

Mechanism of Infection Manifestation in Neurogenic Bladder

The early stage of acute cystitis shows hyperemia of bladder wall, edema, and infiltration of neutrophil granulocytes. The uropathogenic bacteria could adhere to, and often internalize into, the apical urothelial cells in the urinary tracts. Through pathogen-host interactions such as film-h/uroplakin-1a and LPS/toll-like receptor binding, a local immune and resultant inflammatory response occurs [11]. The mucosa membrane damages and replaces with granulation tissue. The bladder ischemia resulting from increased intravesical pressure and over distention is believed to predispose to infection from tissue hypoperfusion and decreased deliver of inflammatory cells and antibiotics. In some parts of the mucosa, ulceration with exudate can occur. Normally the lamina muscularis will not involve with the inflammation. In later stage the inflammation can cause hemorrhage and necrosis without adequate therapy. Bladder overdistention or urinary stasis similarly contribute to risk of infection by eliminating one of the most important nature protective mechanism: voiding [13]. Voiding dysfunction can result from problems with the detrusor muscle or sphincter dysfunction, i.e., detrusor sphincter dyssynergia (DSD). In a study of spinal cord injury patients, a residual volume <50 cc was associated with a 5% rate of UTI compared to 24% patients with a residual >251 cc [14]. DSD leads to high intravesical and proximal ureteral pressure that can result in chronic dilatation of the posterior urethra and bladder neck. Patients with DSD classically show ballooning of the posterior urethra/bladder neck [15]. Elevated intravesical pressure can similarly predispose to vesicoureteral reflux (VUR) which has been shown to significantly increase the risk of UTI in neurogenic patients. Prospective study of 128 spinal cord injury patients demonstrated that patients with VUR had a 23-fold risk for the development of repeat infection [8].

Innate Immunity

The protective microbiological architecture of the perineum and in female vagina is disrupted in neurogenic bladder patient. Approximately 74.1% of spinal cord injury patients that represents with significant bacteriuria had at least one urinary infection. The bacterial species present in the urine also present in the perianal or urethral cultures [16]. The glycosaminoglycan (GAG) layer lining the urothelium serves as a protective barrier preventing bacteria binding. Thus the innovation and medical research play an important role in prevention of urinary tract infection [17]. Disruption of the GAG layer has been shown to increase the infection. This layer in neurogenic bladder patient is continually subject to chronic inflammation and infection that lead to disruption and impending regeneration [13, 15, 18]. Secretory immunoglobulin-A (S-IgA) that is secreted onto mucosal surfaces plays a very important role in the innate immunity of the bladder. High concentration of S-IgA exists in the epical cells of the urothelium, and it functions primarily by agglutinating bacteria and preventing their adherence to the urothelium [19]. UTI is more common and vulnerable in the neuro-urology due to deficiency of immunoglobulin in neurogenic bladder patients. Biopsies taken from non-neurogenic bladder patients demonstrated strong immunostaining for S-IgA in 100% of samples. In the neurogenic bladder population, however, <50% of samples demonstrated strong or moderate immunostaining [20].

Adaptive Immunity

Mast cells play an important role in the inflammatory process due to releasing mediators that induce inflammation from storage granules histamine and heparin into the local microenvironment. The adaptive response to infection is initiated by the manifestation of microphages and mast cells [21]. A failure to activate this system is likely related to the dysregulated innate response. Bone marrow aspirates in both quadriplegic and paraplegic patients demonstrated that both lymphocytic-mediated non-specific (NK cell) and adaptive (B and T cells) immunity were significantly impaired and had no correlation with the time since injury [22].

Diagnosis

Appropriate specimen collection is the most important and needs to be standardized for all patients so that the results accurately reflect microbial environment of the neurogenic bladder. Accurate diagnosis of symptomatic UTI in patients with neuro-urological disease is clouded by the high rate of lower urinary tract colonization. There is no standard definition for the bacteria in patients who are catheterized or have a neurogenic bladder [23]. The Infectious Disease Society of America recommended as follows:

1. Catheter-associated urinary tract infection (CA-UTI) in patients with indwelling urethral, indwelling suprapubic, or intermittent catheterization is defined by the presence of symptoms and identified source with 10^3 CFU/mL of ≥ 1 bacteria species in single catheter urine specimen and also in a midstream voided urine from a patient whose urethral, suprapubic, or condom catheter has been removed within 48 h [23].
2. The IDSA is very strict in defining CA-AB (catheter-associated asymptomatic bacteriuria) reporting a cutoff $\geq 10^5$ with the absence of symptoms compatible with a UTI. A higher cutoff increased the specificity and underscores their motivation to prevent antimicrobial overuse [23].
3. IDSA argues against the interpretation of pyuria for defining a catheter-associated urinary tract infection and serving as threshold for antimicrobial treatment. The sensitivity of pyuria is reported among three articles of ranging quality to be 70–83% [24].

A retrospective study of 89 spinal cord injury patients with different bladder management methods evaluated the incidence of asymptomatic bacteriuria and correlated this with urine analysis [25]. They found that 45% of patients with positive nitrites and that 100% of patients with positive nitrites had culture positive asymptomatic bacteriuria. In patients with negative nitrites, 55% had asymptomatic bacteriuria.

Flexible or Rigid Cystoscopy in Neurogenic Bladder

Neurogenic bladder patients need more invasive diagnostic evaluation with cystoscopy in the cases of recurrent infection and recurrent catheter blockage. Retrospective study of 262 SCI patients managed with either an IC or SPC underwent total of 419 cystoscopies and were divided into symptomatic and asymptomatic group. The most common indications in both the IC and SPC groups were UTI and recurrent blockage, although 31% of patients that were in the IC group also underwent cystoscopy for the insertion of the SPC. No significance difference was seen in the incidence of finding between the two groups. However, 69% of SPC and 36% of IC patients in the symptomatic group were identified to have either significant proteinaceous debris or bladder calculi on cystoscopy [26]. Therefore, cystoscopy should be considered as part of the workup in NB patients with recurrent infections or catheter blockage especially if they are managed with a SPC.

Urodynamic and Video Urodynamic (UDS and VUDS)

Urodynamic investigations play a very important role in the evaluation and diagnostic of a neurogenic bladder patient with recurrent urinary tract infections. It is well established that elevated bladder pressure predisposes to infection as well as VUR and upper tract deterioration. Therefore, recognizing can allow for targeted therapy, e.g., anticholinergic medications or intravesical Botox injections [27]. The use of ultrasound is also recommended according to results of systematic reviews because of its cost effectiveness and noninvasive nature. Ultrasound has good sensitivity for the detection of urinary tract stones and hydro nephrosis which can significantly impact on treatment or urodynamic [24].

Clinical Features of Urinary Tract Infection

The patients with an intact central nervous system have different symptoms as compared to neurogenic bladder patients. International spinal cord injury patients with UTI show following signs [28]:

• Fever	• Spasticity
• Malaise/discomfort	• Lethargy or sense of unease
• Cloudy urine	• Malodorous urine
• Back pain	• Bladder pain
• Dysuria	• Autonomic dysreflexia
• Urinary incontinence/failure of control or leaking around catheter	• Urinary frequency/ Pollakisuria

The spinal cord injury patients with symptomatic UTI and performing CIC (clean intermittent catheterization) are defined according to American Paraplegia Society as $\geq 10^2$ CFU/mL with at least one sign or symptom. The total of 381 episodes of symptomatic UTI were recorded. The frequent clinical symptoms were cloudy and malodourous urine (51.4%), urinary incontinence (51.2%) and fatigue are sense of unease (41.7%), then fever (30.7%) and increased spasticity

(30.2%). The different signs occurred in many different permutations; however, one third of patients experienced an isolated sign, one third experienced two signs, and one third experienced three signs. Increased spasticity, autonomic dysreflexia, and fatigue or sense of unease occurred very rarely in isolation. In patients presenting with an isolated sign, there was no significant difference in white blood cell count and colony-forming units per millimeter compared to the asymptomatic group [29].

Treatment

Acute Bacterial UTI

The IDSA-recommended antimicrobial treatments in addition to basic primary care for the neurogenic bladder patients with symptomatic UTI are as follows:

1. Any catheter that has been in place for over 2 weeks should be immediately removed and then replaced, and the urine specimen should be obtained from the new catheter before the initiation of antimicrobial therapy.
2. Urine cultures should always be obtained prior to antimicrobial therapy because of increased risk of nosocomial organisms [23].
3. UTI often represents an overarching term for many complicated infections including prostatitis, pyelonephritis, bacteremia, and simple cystitis. Therefore, patients should be clinically assessed carefully to determine the optimal route, spectrum of coverage, and duration of antibiotics.

Antibiotic Stewardship in NB UTI and IDSA Recommendation

- The patients must be treated with narrow-spectrum antibiotics, when possible, for the shortest duration.
- A 7-day course of antibiotics for patients with quick clinical response. Patients with significant infection or a delayed response should have the duration of treatment extended to 10–14 days [30].
- A 5-day regimen of levofloxacin is a suitable therapy in patients with CA-UTI that are not significantly ill.
- The patients carrying MRSA (methicillin-resistant *Staphylococcus aureus*) should be treated with vancomycin as first-line therapy if very serious infection is found.
- Out patient management with MRSA UTI should be treated with trimethoprim-sulfamethoxazole.
- Nitrofurantoin is recommended with mild UTI and ideal because it does not change bowl or vaginal flora.

- Patients with *Pseudomonas* and *Proteus* tend to be highly resistant; therefore, antibiotics should be prescribed according to antibiograms.
- Fosfomycin tromethamine administrated as a single 3 g dose for the treatment of uncomplicated UTIs in females; however, it helps to reduce recurrent infection in neurogenic patients. Fosfomycin interferes with cell wall synthesis by inhabiting the formation of peptidoglycan and act against biofilms in the neurogenic patients [31, 32]
- MRSA and extended-spectrum beta-lactamase (ESBL) as well as typical urinary Gram-negative organisms should be treated effectively as a 7–10-day course in accordance with local antibiogram [31]. The safety profile of Fosfomycin is excellent and it is very well tolerated and safe during pregnancy. The oral dosage does not need to be adjusted in the setting of hepatic and renal failure [31]

Prevention of UTI in Neurogenic Bladder

Closed Catheter Drainage

- Close catheter drainage system remains one of the most important prevention measures against infection and for the prevention of CA-UTI in patients with IC and SPC [23].
- Some studies support its role in the prevention of infection with 95% incidence of catheter-associated bacteriuria after 96 h in patients without closed drainage [33].
- Frequent violation of the close drainage junction has been shown to significantly increase the risk of catheter-associated bacteriuria [23, 34, 35].
- The location of urinary drainage bag is of equal importance, and catheter-associated bacteriuria follows contamination of the urinary bag. Therefore, the drainage bag and tubing should always be situated below the level of bladder [36, 37]

Routine Catheter Changes

A 4–6 weeks catheter change interval is generally recommended for neurogenic bladder patients with IC and SPC. Because of the tendency for catheters to develop biofilms and incrustation, it seems plausible that routine changes with fresh catheters maintain the microbial burden manageable by removing established intra- and extra luminal biofilms. Comparison of urine culture results in patients with long-term catheters, and those immediately following catheter replacement demonstrates both a qualitative and quantitative reduction in bacterial species [23, 38, 39].

Intravesical Botulinum Toxin A and Reduction of UTI in Neuro-urology

Botulinum toxin A injected intravesical for the treatment of neurogenic detrusor overactivity caused by spinal cord injury or multiple sclerosis (MS). Botulinum toxin therapy provides significant improvement in UDS parameters, continence, and quality of life [40]. Additionally, it may impart protection against infection in a subset of NB patient [27]. It is possible that elevated bladder pressures predispose to vesicoureteral reflux, bladder ischemia, and stasis, all of which are significant risk factors for UTI in NB patients [15]. Intravesical botulinum toxin-A injections are an attractive option for the prevention of UTI in neurogenic bladder dysfunction.

Peri-interventional Antibiotic Prophylaxis During Botulinum Toxin A

Antibiotic prophylaxis may not be necessary in patients with asymptomatic bacteriuria undergoing intravesical botulinum toxin-A injections for neurogenic detrusor overactivity [41]. According to EAU Guidelines on urological infections, peri-interventional antibiotic prophylaxis is not generally recommended during cystoscopy and fulguration of small bladder tumors. Asymptomatic bacteriuria in patients undergoing intravesical botulinum toxin-A injections for neurogenic detrusor overactivity did not affect safety and efficacy outcomes. Thus, antibiotic prophylaxis is not justified and needs to be critically reconsidered, especially considering the alarming antibiotic resistance worldwide.

Sacral Neuromodulation and Prevention of UTI

Bladder pacemaker or sacral neuromodulation is a treatment used to help patients with detrusor overactivity or urge incontinence, underactive bladder, fecal incontinence, erectile function, and nonobstructive urinary retention. Sacral neuromodulation therapies improve urodynamic parameter and are helpful to prevent UTIs in patients with neurogenic bladder dysfunction [27]. Normally, the brain controls the bladder by sending electrical signals down nerve pathways that run from the brain to the spinal cord and through the lower back called sacral area. These sacral nerves control the muscles in the pelvic floor, the bladder, and those needed for urinary control bladder sensation or also relayed via these nerves to brain. Sacral neuromodulation helps to correct inappropriate, unwanted, or even erroneous messages sent along these nerve pathways. It is also known as Interstim-II therapy. A cross-sectional study of SCI patient with NDO who previously underwent implantation of a Brindley sacral stimulator reported improved quality of life, continence, and infrequent UTIs compared to control group of NDO patients managed by alternative methods. The patient with sacral neuromodulation had a mean of 0.5 UTIs/year compared to 3.8 in the control group [42].

Bacterial Interference

Bacterial interference is characterized by intentional bladder colonization with a bacterial strain of low virulence. This leads to prevention of uropathogenic bacterial binding, internalization, and consecutive infection of neurogenic bladder. The average number of episodes of UTI/patient-year was significantly lower in experimental group (0.50) compared to control group (1.68) after successful bladder colonization and protection against infection [43].

Figure 3 illustrates the pathogenesis of urinary tract infections. (**a**) Uncomplicated urinary tract infections (UTIs) begin when uropathogens that reside in the gut contaminate the periurethral area (step 1) and are able to colonize the urethra. Subsequent migration to the bladder (step 2) and expression of pili and adhesins results in colonization and invasion of the superficial umbrella cells (step 3). Host inflammatory responses, including neutrophil infiltration (step 4), begin to clear extracellular bacteria. Some bacteria evade the immune system, either through host cell invasion or through morphological changes that result in resistance to neutrophils, and these bacteria undergo multiplication (step 5) and biofilm formation (step 6). These bacteria produce toxins and proteases that induce host cell damage (step 7), releasing essential nutrients that promote bacterial survival and ascension to the kidneys (step 8). Kidney colonization (step 9) results in bacterial toxin production and host tissue damage (step 10). If left untreated, UTIs can ultimately progress to bacteremia if the pathogen crosses the tubular epithelial barrier in the kidneys (step 11). (**b**) Uropathogens that cause complicated UTIs follow the same initial steps as those described for uncomplicated infections, including periurethral colonization (step 1), progression to the urethra, and migration to the bladder (step 2). However, in order for the pathogens to cause infection, the bladder must be compromised. The most common cause of a compromised bladder is catheterization. Owing to the robust immune response induced by catheterization (step 3), fibrinogen accumulates on the catheter, providing an ideal environment for the attachment of uropathogens that express fibrinogen-binding proteins. Infection induces neutrophil infiltration (step 4), but after their initial attachment to the fibrinogen-coated catheters, the bacteria multiply (step 5), form biofilms (step 6), promote epithelial damage (step 7), and can seed infection of the kidneys (steps 8 and 9), where toxin production induces tissue damage (step 10). If left untreated, uropathogens that cause complicated UTIs can also progress to bacteremia by crossing the tubular epithelial cell barrier (step 11).

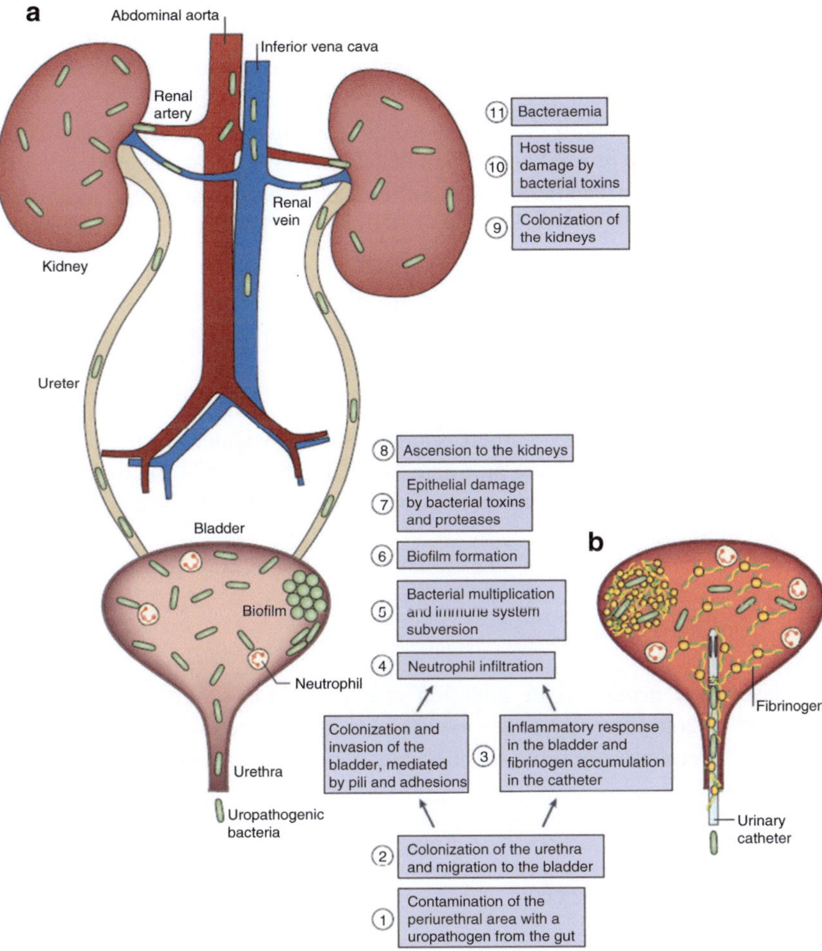

Fig. 3 Pathogenesis of urinary tract infections [11]

Nonsurgical Bladder Management Methods in Neuro-urology

The following factors must be considered for bladder management in patients with neurogenic bladder dysfunction including status of lower urinary tract, duration of catheterization, degree of mobility sensation and dexterity, and access to healthcare personnel and patients' preferences [23]. Clean intermittent catheterization is associated with reduced infections, fewer stone formation, and complications compared to the other commonly used methods like suprapubic catheterization. Condom catheter drainage provides a less painful and more comfortable alternative in neurogenic bladder patients [23]. Although noninvasive, bacteriuria is still a problem and studies have shown that condom catheters are significantly associated with *Pseudomonas* and *Klebsiella bacteriuria* [44, 45]. However the incidence of condom catheter-associated bacteriuria is less than indwelling catheter, and the incidence of CA-UTI appears to be comparable to that of clean intermittent catheterization [8, 23, 30]. Significantly increased incidences of UTIs were seen in the Crede/reflex voiding and IC groups compared with the normal voiding groups. This difference was not appreciated between the normal voiding and CIC group [46]. Current evidence supports intermittent catheterization as the optimal bladder management method in neurogenic bladder patients to reduce CA-AB and CA-UTI. And this is also recommended by IDSA [23].

Impregnated Catheters

The antibiotic and silver-coated catheters have been investigated for the prevention of UTIs. Both catheter types have an impact on bacteriuria and infection for short term of time [27, 47]. But for long term of usage, antibiotics resistance and silver toxicity increased [27, 48].

Catheter-Associated UTIs

Catheter-associated urinary tract infection refers to UTIs occurring in a person whose urinary tract is currently catheterized or has been catheterized within the past 48 h. The EAU recommendations for the management of catheter-associated UTI are described in Table 2.

Antimicrobial Prophylaxis

Antibiotic Prophylaxis in General

The IDSA recommended against the prophylactic use of antibiotics for the reduction of catheter-associated infections because of increased antimicrobial resistance. Thus, antibiotic prophylaxis is not recommended for the prevention of UTI in neurogenic bladder patients. With regard to antibiotic prophylaxis at the time of catheter replacement, no studies currently exist and the IDSA recommends against this as well as pre-replacement bladder irrigation to prevent CA-AB and CA-UTI [23].

The patients with refractory NDO (neurogenic detrusor overactivity) got intravesical botulinum toxin-A injections without antibiotic prophylaxis; safety and efficacy of the therapy could be ensured, even if asymptomatic bacteriuria was present. Within 6 weeks after treatment, UTI occurred in 5% of the patients with asymptomatic bacteriuria pretreatment and in 7% of those with a sterile urine culture. The efficacy rate of 70%, i.e., appropriate clinical and urodynamic effect, was without any association between asymptomatic bacteriuria and therapy failure [41].

Table 2 EAU recommendation for the management of catheter-associated UTI [49]

EAU recommendations for diagnostic evaluation of catheter-associated UTIs	LE	GR
Do not carry out routine urine culture in asymptomatic catheterized patients	1a	A
Do not use pyuria as an indicator for catheter-associated UTI	2	A
Do not use the presence, absence, or degree of pyuria to differentiate catheter-associated asymptomatic bacteriuria from catheter-associated UTI	2	A
Do not use the presence or absence of odorous or cloudy urine alone to differentiate catheter-associated asymptomatic bacteriuria from catheter-associated UTI	3	C
EAU recommendations for disease management and prevention of catheter-associated UTIs	**LE**	**GR**
Take a urine culture prior to initiating antimicrobial therapy in catheterized patients in whom the catheter has been removed	3	A[a]
Do not treat catheter-associated asymptomatic bacteriuria in general	1a	A
Treat catheter-associated asymptomatic bacteriuria prior to traumatic urinary tract interventions (e.g., transurethral resection of the prostate)	1a	A
Replace or remove the indwelling catheter before starting antimicrobial therapy	4	B[a]
Do not apply topical antiseptics or antimicrobials to the catheter, urethra, or meatus	1a	A
Do not use prophylactic antimicrobials to prevent catheter-associated UTIs	1a	A
The duration of catheterization should be minimal	2a	B
Remove an indwelling catheter after non-urological operation within the same day	1b	B
Change long-term indwelling catheters at intervals adapted to the individual patient	3	C

[a]Upgraded based on panel consensus

Cranberry Prophylaxis

The literature does not support the use of cranberry for the prevention of UTI in NB population [23, 50]. Only a single study has demonstrated a significant reduction in the incidence of UTI with cranberry prophylaxis in the NB population. The frequency of UTI was reduced to 0.3 UTI per year vs. 1.0 UTI per year while receiving placebo. However, this study has been criticized for its small sample size and for the fact that 74% of patients were managed with condom catheter [51].

Methenamine Salt Prophylaxis

In urine, methenamine salts hydrolyze into ammonia and formaldehyde. The antimicrobial activity of these agents is correlated with the urinary concentration of formaldehyde which is dependent on urinary methenamine concentration, pH, and dwell time [23]. For these reasons its use has been limited in the NB population that is largely catheterized, thereby shortening the dwell tie significantly. A meta-analysis failed to show a significant effect for methenamine for preventing in NB patients when the results for specific agents were pooled [52]. Therefore, at this time methenamine salt is not recommended for the prevention of a catheter-associated UTI and catheter-associated bacteriuria [23].

Antibiotic Resistance in Patients with Nosocomial Infection

Urinary tract infection is one of the most frequently occurring nosocomial infections and is correlated with increasing antimicrobial resistance. To present the worldwide antibiotic resistance rates of uropathogens reported in nosocomial urinary tract infections (NAUTI) during the period of 2003–2010. The global prevalence of infections in urology study is an Internet-based surveillance study carried out at annually since 2003, specifically evaluating bacterial spectrum and antimicrobial resistance in urological patients with NAUTIs [1]. Geographic differences were assessed according to four regions (North Europe, South Europe, Asia, Africa + South America). Antimicrobial susceptibility of the following pathogens was recorded: *Escherichia coli*, *Klebsiella* spp., *Proteus* spp., *Citrobacter* spp., *Enterobacter* spp., *Pseudomonas aeruginosa*, *Enterococcus* spp., coagulase-negative *Staphylococcus*, and *S. aureus*.

The resistance rates against the following antibiotics were analyzed: aminopenicillin (ampicillin or amoxicillin) in combination with beta-lactamase inhibitor, piperacillin in combination with tazobactam as beta-lactamase inhibitor, trimethoprim in combination with sulfamethoxazole (TMP-SMX), ciprofloxacin, cefuroxime, cefotaxime, ceftazidime, gentamicin, and imipenem. In general, the lowest resistance rates were seen in north Europe, while the highest resistance rates against most of the antibiotics tested were seen in Asia.

Asia exhibited the highest rates in general. The only antibiotics tested with an overall resistance rate below 10% was imipenem, representing the carbapenems. All other antibiotics have much higher overall resistance rates including so-called broad-spectrum antibiotics such as piperacillin/tazobactam, ciprofloxacin, and gentamicin. Knowledge of regional and local resistance data and prudent use of antibiotics are necessary to optimize antibiotic therapy in urological patients with NAUTI. The evidence of uropathogen spectrum and resistance is gathered from complicated UTI reports [53, 54] and local surveillance data [55]. At that time, ceftazidime and levofloxacin were one of the recommended first-line treatments in the urosepsis [56]. It is not appropriate to use the pathogen spectrum and resistance of other clinical diagnosis of HAUTIs as representative of urosepsis [57].

Asymptomatic Bacteriuria and Treatment Recommendation

The antibiotic treatment is recommended during pregnancy and prior to damage of mucus membrane during urinary tract intervention. Antimicrobial therapy is not required in asymptomatic bacteriuria if the patients are nonpregnant women, elderly with indwelling catheters, and female with diabetes mellitus.

Figure 4 illustrate the global and regional resistance rates of all pathogens and Fig. 5 illustrates the global and regional resistance rates of *E. coli*. This showed the resistance patterns of nosocomial urinary tract infections in a study of the global prevalence of infections in urology.

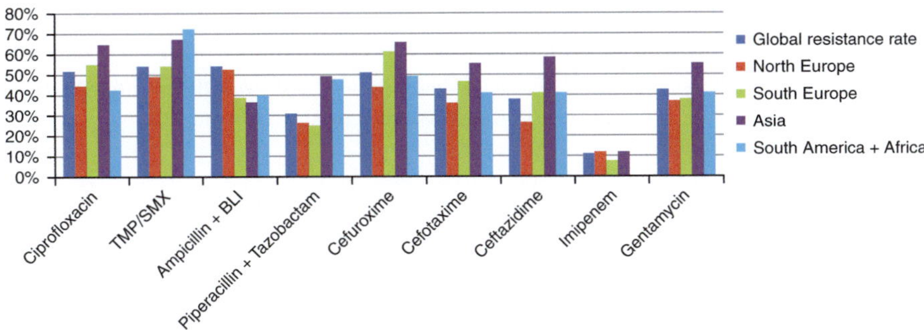

Fig. 4 Global and regional resistance rates of all pathogen [58]

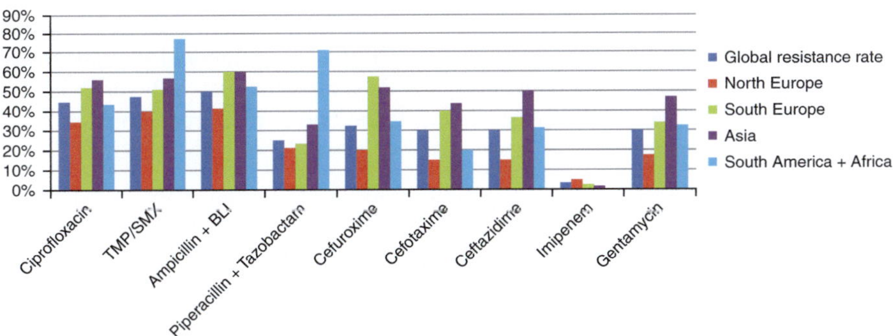

Fig. 5 Global and regional resistance rates of *E. coli* [58]

Acute Pyelonephritis

The local and systemic manifestations of microorganisms in renal parenchyma are associated with flank pain, nausea, vomiting, fever (>38° C), and elevation of leucocytes.

Etiology and Pathogenesis

The common causes of acute pyelonephritis are stones and structures in the urogenital tract, prostatic obstruction urinary catheters, neurogenic bladder, polycystic kidney disease, immune suppression, pregnancy, and post-renal transplant. These are the following main causative microorganisms: Gram positives like *Enterococcus faecalis* and *S. aureus* or either Gram negatives like *E. coli*, *Klebsiella*, *Proteus*, *Pseudomonas*, and *Enterobacter*. *E.* coli-induced pyelonephritis was shown that epithelial signaling produced an increase in cellular oxygen consumption and affected microvascular flow by clotting, causing localized ischemia. The subsequent ischemic damage led to actin rearrangement and epithelial sloughing, leading to paracellular bacterial movement. A denuded tubular-basement membrane was able to hinder immediate dissemination of bacteria, giving the host time to isolate the infection by clotting. Interestingly, suppression of clotting by heparin treatment caused fatal urosepsis [59].

Clinical Symptoms

Pyelonephritis is a non-specific infection without inflammatory process in which the collecting systems and renal parenchyma are involved. The severity of pyelonephritis depends on the interstitial edema of the kidney tissue. Women suffer five times more than men with pyelonephritis. In 90% of cases, the cause of disease is penetration of Gram-negative bacteria. The microorganisms penetrate into the kidney through hematogenous and urinogenous. Clinical symptoms of pyelonephritis are unilateral or bilateral flank pain and systemic symptoms such as fever (>38° C), chills, and malaise. The focal nephritis is limited to one or more renal lobules, comparable to lobular pneumonia.

Diagnostic Recommendations

For the diagnosis and differential diagnosis of obstructive and nonobstructive pyelonephritis, the following procedures are necessary:

1. Urinary dipstick and urine culture.
2. Blood tests mostly indicate leukocytosis and left shift.
3. Ultrasounds of abdomen and pelvic showed the lesion with interrupted echoes, which break through the normal cortex-medulla organization.
4. The imaging indicated if suspicious of complicated pyelonephritis or symptom donors improve with 48–72 h of treatment. The CT scan shows typical wedge-shaped, poorly limited areas of diminished sonographic density. As differential diagnosis, renal abscess, tumor, and a renal infarction must be considered. Emphysematous pyelonephritis shows gas formation in the renal parenchyma and perirenal space [60].
5. DMSA scan can be used to help secure the diagnosis, e.g., a photogenic defect indicates active infection or scar in nuclear medicine investigations.

Treatment

1. Hemodynamically stable patient:
   Outpatient oral antibiotic therapy like ciprofloxacin and third generation of cephalosporin or trimethoprim TMP-SMX.

2. Severe or non-resolving patient:
   These patients must be admitted in the hospital for intravenous antibiotics and volume substitution.
3. Emphysematous pyelonephritis:
   These patients required temporary nephrostomy tubes and some patients receive nephrectomy after intravenous antibiotic treatment.
4. Renal obstruction:
   Patient with renal obstruction admitted in hospitals for percutaneous nephrostomy tube or double-J ureteral stent.

For the treatment of uncomplicated urinary tract infection, the resistance percentages of causative microorganisms must be <20% to consider an agent suitable for empirical treatment of a lower UTI and must be <10% for the treatment of an upper UTI. Considering the current resistance percentages of amoxicillin, co-amoxiclav, trimethoprim, and trimethoprim-sulfamethoxazole, it can be concluded that these agents are not suitable for the empirical treatment of pyelonephritis in a normal host and, therefore, also not for treatment of UTIs [61]. The same applies to ciprofloxacin and other fluoroquinolones in urological patients [61].

The current recommendations for the antibiotic treatment of urinary tract infections and urosepsis are described in Table 3.

Multidrug-Resistant (MDR) Bacteria in a Patient with Neurogenic Bladder and New Combination Therapy

The US Food and Drug Administration approved a new antimicrobial drug combining a cephalosporin and β-lactamase inhibitor (ceftolozane/tazobactam) especially for spinal cord injury patients. Due to multidrug resistance phenotype and the nephrotoxicity of colistin and amikacin, the antibiotic therapy was switched to ceftolozane/tazobactam at 1 g per 500 mg TID for 7 days. Ceftolozane shows potent activity against *Pseudomonas aeruginosa* compared to ceftazidime and cefepime [62]. This combination therapy is newly recommended for febrile UTI due to multidrug resistance *Pseudomonas aeruginosa* in patients with neurogenic bladder.

Sepsis/Urosepsis

There are new sepsis definitions focusing on severity of sepsis as described below:
Urosepsis: A very severe infection in the urogenital tract that leads to life-threatening organ dysfunction caused by a dysregulated host response to pathogen organism is called urosepsis.
Bacteremia: The presence of bacteria or pathogen organism in blood stream as confirmed by culture is called bacteremia.

Table 3 Antibiotics recommended for the treatment of urinary tract infections [60]

Antibiotic group	Substance	Dosage	
		Oral	IV[a]
Aminopenicillin + BLI[b]	Ampicillin/ sulbactam	0.750 g twice daily	0.75–3 g 3 times daily
	Amoxicillin/ clavulanic acid	1 g twice daily or 0.625 g 3 times daily	1.2–2.2 g 3 times daily
Acyl ureidopenicillin + BLI	Piperacillin/ tazobactam	–	2.5–4.5 g 3 times daily
	Piperacillin/ combactam	–	5 g 3 times daily
Cephalosporin Gr. 1	Cephalexin	Prophylaxis only	–
Cephalosporin Gr. 2	Cefuroxime axetil	500 mg twice daily	–
	Cefuroxime	–	0.75–1.5 g 3 times daily
	Cefotiam	–	1–2 g 2–3 times daily
Cephalosporin Gr. 3	Cefpodoxime proxetil	200 mg twice daily	–
	Ceftibuten	200–400 mg daily	–
Cephalosporin Gr. 3a	Cefotaxime	–	1–2 g 2–3 times daily
	Ceftriaxone	–	1–2 g daily
Cephalosporin Gr. 3b	Ceftazidime	–	1–2 g 2–3 times daily
Cephalosporin Gr. 4	Cefepime	–	2 g twice daily
Carbapenem Gr. 1	Imipenem	–	0.5–1 g q 6–8 h
	Meropenem	–	0.5–1 g 3 times daily
	Doripenem	–	0.5 g 3 times daily
Carbapenem Gr. 2	Ertapenem	–	1 g daily
Fluoroquinolone Gr. 2	Ciprofloxacin Ciprofloxacin XR	500–750 mg twice daily 1000 mg daily	400 mg twice daily –
Fluoroquinolone Gr. 3	Levofloxacin	500–750 mg daily	500 mg daily
Antimycotic group			
Azole derivatives	Fluconazole Voriconazole	400–800 mg daily 4–6 mg/kg BW[c] daily	400–800 mg daily 4–6 mg/kg BW daily
Pyrimidine analog Echinocandin	Flucytosine Caspofungin		100–150 mg/kg BW 4 times daily 50–70 mg daily

[a]*IV* intravenous
[b]*BLI* β-lactamase inhibitor
[c]*BW* body weight

Systemic inflammatory response syndrome (SIRS): An inflammatory state affecting the whole body, frequently a response of immune system to infection or noninfectious etiology (e.g., burns pancreatitis). The system response in manifested by two or more of the following conditions:

- Temperature $\geq 38°$ C or $\leq 36°$ C
- Heart rate ≥ 90 beats/min
- Respiratory rate ≥ 20/min or $Paco_2$ ≤ 32 mmHg (4.3 kPa)
- WBC $\geq 12,000$ cells/mm^3 or ≤ 4000 cells/mm^3 or $\geq 10\%$ immature bands

Sepsis: Activation of the inflammatory process due to infections that leads to life-threatening organ dysfunction caused by dysregulated host response. Commonly it can be defined as, SIRS with presumed or proved infection.

Septic shock: Sepsis with hypotension (i.e., a systolic blood pressure of <90 mmHg or a reduction of >40 mmHg from base line in the absence of other causes) despite adequate fluid resuscitation along with the pressure of perfusion abnormalities that may include, but are not limited to, lactic acidosis, oliguria, or an acute alteration in mental status. Patients who are on inotropic or vasopressor agents may not be hypotensive at the time that perfusion abnormalities are measured.

Refractory septic shock: Septic shock that lasts for more than 1 h and does not respond to fluid administration or pharmacological intervention.

The third international consensus definition for sepsis and septic shock task force recently introduced a new clinical score termed quick sequential (sepsis-related) organ failure assessment (qSOFA) for the identification of patients at risk of sepsis outside the intensive care unit. A comparison of qSOFA and SIRS is done for predicting adverse outcomes of patients with suspicion of sepsis in intensive care unit. The results suggest that qSOFA is more accurate than SIRS for predicting in-hospital mortality and ICU-free days, but not ventilator-free days, any organ dysfunction-free days, or renal dysfunction-free days [63].

Epidemiology of Urosepsis

In approximately 30% of all septic patients, the infectious focus is localized in the urogenital tract and arises from infection of the parenchymatous urogenital organs, e.g., kidneys, prostrate, or testicles [60]. This can be due to subvesicular obstruction like urethra stricture and ureteral stones or stenosis in urogenital tract.

Classification of Sepsis

The sepsis is classified and differentiated according to severity levels:

- Severe sepsis is defined as sepsis associated with organ dysfunction; the term severe sepsis is now obsolete.
- Septic shock is persistence of hyper perfusion or hypotension despite fluid resuscitation and signs of organ damage.
- Refractory septic shock is defined by an absence of response to therapy.

Pathophysiology of Urosepsis

Mostly pathogen organisms reach the urinary tract by way of the intraluminal-ascending route. Inflammation is the physiologic response of the body to infections and is mediated by the release of soluble substances by cells of the immune system. Urosepsis is established when pathogen organisms reach the blood stream from urinary tract. An initially overwhelming proinflammatory reaction, activated by mediators such as bacterial toxin, is accompanied by a counter-regulatory anti-inflammatory response syndrome. Complete bacteria and components of bacterial cell walls act as exogenous pyrogens on eukaryotic target cells of patients. These include lipopolysaccharides, especially the endotoxin of the outer membrane of Gram-negative bacteria; the peptidoglycan; lipoteichoic acid of Gram-positive bacteria; and toxins like toxic-shock syndrome toxin 1 and *Staphylococcus aureus* toxin A. Many of these factors bind two cellular receptors and co-receptors of the innate immune system (e.g., CD 14, "Toll-like receptors," TLR2 and TLR4, CD 18, and selectin) on the surface of macrophages, neutrophils, and endothelial cells [60]. Intracellular molecule such as nuclear factor kappa-light-chain-enhancer of activated B cells (NF-kB) or protein-kinase C is activated, which induces transcription of mediator genes and thus the synthesis of numerous endogenous mediators, such as cytokines.

Cytokines as Markers of the Septic Response

Cytokines are produced with different kinetics and are classified into anti-inflammatory and proinflammatory cytokines. Tumor necrosis factor (TNF)-α and interleukin (IL)-1 are the most important proinflammatory cytokines. They influence the temperature-regulatory centers in the hypothalamus, which results in fever. They also have an effect on *formatio reticularis* in the brain stem that renders the patients somnolent and comatose. Release of adrenocorticotrophic hormone (ACTH) in the pituitary gland is increased, which stimulates the adrenal gland [60].

New Approaches in Diagnosis and Management of Sepsis

Sepsis patients require less invasive but equally an effective approach to access organ perfusion and oxygenation for better treatment.

Lactates

Lactate elevation reflects the pathophysiological changes of sepsis (hypotension, tissue hypoperfusion, and organ dysfunction); it defines the diagnosis and prognosis of septic patients.

Procalcitonin

Procalcitonin is the marker related to the presence of bacterial infection, the concentration of which is correlated to the severity of the infection. Monitoring procalcitonin level could be helpful in evaluating the efficacy and even in the decision to stop antibiotic therapy. If PCT dropped 50% or more from baseline at day 4, no change in antibiotic treatment was advised. The antimicrobial therapy can stop if PCT was 1.0 ng/mL or less at day 7 or dropped 50% more from day 4 [64].

Beta-D Glucan and Anti-mannan Antibodies

Blood cultures are essential to rule out invasive fungal infections. Fungal biomarkers and metabolites could be assessed in plasmatic samples to anticipate the diagnosis. The combined detection of mannan and anti-mannan antibodies represents a specific method for the diagnosis of candidemia (80% sensitivity, 85% specificity, >85% negative predictive value) with ammine anticipation of 6 days prior to blood cultures positivization. Galactomannan does not represent to detect candidiasis, but it is useful for the diagnosis of aspergillus infections [65]. Real-time PCR represents an alternative method for the diagnosis of fungal and bacterial infections, with high sensitivity and specificity.

Sequential [Sepsis-Related] Organ Failure Assessment Score (SOFA)

The application of sequential organ failure assessment score in intensive care unit reduces the high economic burden of the society while achieving sufficient reduction in morbidity and mortality of patients. The SOFA score is helpful to assess the severity of patients in intensive care units.

The baseline sequential [sepsis-related] organ failure assessment (SOFA) score should be assumed to be zero unless the patient is known to have preexisting (acute or chronic) organ dysfunction before the onset of infection. qSOFA indicates quick SOFA; MAP (mean arterial pressure) [63].

Table 4 illustrates the SOFA score for the assessment of organ failure.

Figure 6 explains about the qSOFA and clinical criteria of patients. The baseline sequential [sepsis-related] organ failure assessment (SOFA) score should be assumed to be zero unless the patient is known to have preexisting (acute or chronic) organ dysfunction before the onset of infection. qSOFA indicates quick SOFA; MAP (mean arterial pressure)

Table 4 Sequential [sepsis-related] organ failure assessment score [63]

System	Score				
	0	1	2	3	4
Respiration					
PaO_2/FIO_2, mm Hg (kPa)	≥400 (53.3)	<400 (53.3)	<300 (40)	<200 (26.7) with respiratory support	<100 (13.3) with respiratory support
Coagulation					
Platelets, $×10^3$/ μL	≥150	<150	<100	<50	<20
Liver					
Bilirubin, mg/ dL (μmol/L)	<1.2 (20)	1.2–1.9 (20–32)	2.0–5.9 (33–101)	6.0–11.9 (102–204)	>12.0 (204)
Cardiovascular	MAP ≥70 mm Hg	MAP <70 mm Hg	Dopamine <5 or dobutamine (any dose)[a]	Dopamine 5.1–15 or epinephrine ≤0.1 or norepinephrine ≤0.1[a]	Dopamine >15 or epinephrine >0.1 or norepinephrine >0.1[a]
Central nervous system					
Glasgow coma scale score[b]	15	13–14	12-Oct	9-Jun	<6
Renal					
Creatinine, mg/ dL (μmol/L)	<1.2 (110)	1.2–1.9 (110–170)	2.0–3.4 (171–299)	3.5–4.9 (300–440)	>5.0 (440)
Urine output, mL/d				<500	<200

Abbreviations: *FIO₂* fraction of inspired oxygen, *MAP* mean arterial pressure, *PaO₂* partial pressure of oxygen

Adapted from Vincent et al. [27]

[a]Catecholamine doses are given as μg/kg/min for at least 1 h

[b]Glasgow Coma Scale scores range from 3 to 15; higher score indicates better neurological function

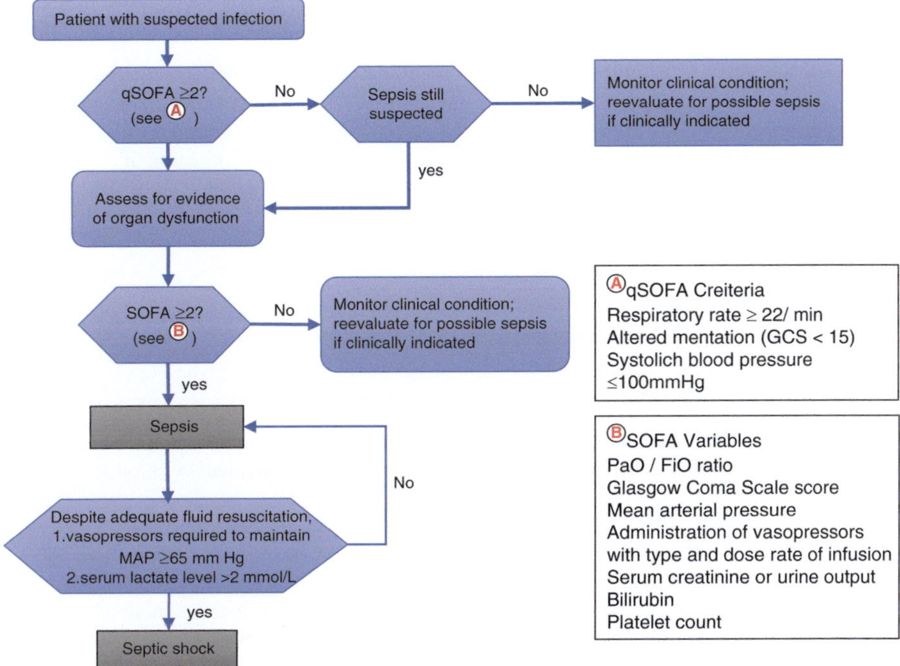

Fig. 6 Operationalization of clinical criteria identifying patients with sepsis and septic shock [63]

Antimicrobial Treatment of Sepsis

The recommendation for application of IV antimicrobial treatment after the recognition and is initiated within 1 h for both sepsis and septic shock [66].

Table 5 illustrates the recommendation for the treatment of urosepsis as below.

Table 6 illustrates the important terminologies for antimicrobial recommendations.

Table 7 illustrates the EAU recommendation for parental antimicrobial therapy of urosepsis.

Detection of Bacteriuria Prior to Urological Procedures

Identification of bacteria in urine prior to diagnostic and therapeutic procedures is recommended to reduce the risk of infectious complications by controlling any pre-operative detected bacteriuria and to streamline the antimicrobial coverage in conjunction with the procedure,

Table 8 illustrates the EAU recommendation detection of bacteriuria prior to urological procedures.

Table 5 Antibiotics recommended for the treatment of urosepsis [60]

Most frequent pathogens/species	Initial, empirical antimicrobial therapy	Therapy duration
E. coli other enterobacteria	Cephalosporin (group 3a/b) Fluoroquinolone[a]	3–5 days after defervescence or control/ elimination of complicating factor
After urological interventions multiresistant pathogens		
Pseudomonas spp., *Proteus* spp., *Serratia* spp., *Enterobacter* spp.	Anti-pseudomonas active acylaminopenicillin/BLI carbapenem ± aminoglycoside	

[a]Only in regions where fluoroquinolone resistance is below 10%

Table 6 Important terminology for antimicrobial recommendations [66]

Empiric therapy	Initial therapy started in the absence of definitive microbiologic pathogen identification. Empiric therapy may be mono, combination, or broad-spectrum, and/or multidrug in nature
Targeted/ definitive therapy	Therapy targeted to a specific pathogen (usually after microbiologic identification). Targeted/definitive therapy may be mono or combination, but is not intended to be broad-spectrum
Broad-spectrum therapy	The use of one or more antimicrobial agents with the specific intent of broadening the range of potential pathogens covered, usually during empiric therapy (e.g., piperacillin/tazobactam, vancomycin, and anidulafungin; each is used to cover a different group of pathogens) broad-spectrum therapy is typically empiric since the usual purpose is to ensure antimicrobial coverage with at least one drug when there is uncertainty about the possible pathogen. On occasion, broad-spectrum therapy may be continued into the targeted/definitive therapy phase if multiple pathogens are isolated
Multidrug therapy	Therapy with multiple antimicrobials to deliver broad-spectrum therapy (i.e., to broaden coverage) for empiric therapy (i.e., where pathogen is unknown) or to potentially accelerate pathogen clearance (combination therapy) with respect to a specific pathogen(s) where the pathogen(s) is known or suspected (i.e., for both targeted or empiric therapy). This term therefore includes combination therapy
Combination therapy	The use of multiple antibiotics (usually of different mechanistic classes) with the specific intent of covering the known or suspected pathogen(s) with more than one antibiotic (e.g., piperacillin/tazobactam and an aminoglycoside or fluoroquinolone for Gram-negative pathogens) to accelerate pathogen clearance rather than to broaden antimicrobial coverage. Other proposed applications of combination therapy include inhibition of bacterial toxin production (e.g., clindamycin with β-lactams for streptococcal toxic shock) or potential immune modulatory effects (macrolides with a β-lactam for pneumococcal pneumonia)

Perioperative Antibacterial Prophylaxis in Urology

The purpose of antimicrobial prophylaxis in urology is to prevent infectious complications resulting from diagnostic and therapeutic procedures. However, evidence for the best choice of antimicrobials and regimens is limited.

Table 9 illustrates the EAU recommendation for perioperative antibacterial prophylaxis in urology.

Table 7 EAU recommendation for parenteral antimicrobial therapy of urosepsis [49]

EAU recommendations				
Antimicrobials	Daily dose	LE	GR	Comments
Cefotaxime	2 g t.i.d	2	A[a]	Not studied as monotherapy in acute uncomplicated pyelonephritis
Ceftazidime	1–2 g t.i.d	2	A[a]	
Ceftriaxone	1-2 g q.d	1b	A[a]	Lower dose studied but higher dose recommended. Same protocol for acute uncomplicated pyelonephritis and complicated UTI (stratification not always possible)
Cefepime	1–2 g b.i.d	1b	B	
Piperacillin/ tazobactam	2.5– 4.5 g t.i.d	1b	A[a]	
Ceftolozane/ tazobactam	1.5 g t.i.d	1b	B	
Ceftazidime/ avibactam	2.5 g t.i.d	1b	B	
Gentamicin	5 mg/kg q.d	1b	B	Not studied as monotherapy in acute uncomplicated pyelonephritis
Amikacin	15 mg/kg q.d	1b	B	
Ertapenem	1 g q.d	1b	B	Same protocol for acute uncomplicated pyelonephritis and complicated UTI (stratification not always possible)
Imipenem/ cilastatin	0.5/0.5 g t.i.d	1b	B	
Meropenem	1 g t.i.d	2	B	
Doripenem	0.5 g t.i.d	1b	B	

b.i.d twice daily, *t.i.d* three times daily, *q.d* every day
[a]Upgraded based on panel consensus

Table 8 EAU recommendation detection of bacteriuria prior to urological procedures [49]

EAU recommendation	LE	GR
Laboratory urine culture is the recommended method to determine the presence or absence of clinically significant bacteriuria in patients prior to undergoing urological interventions	3	B

Table 9 EAU recommendations for perioperative antibacterial prophylaxis in urology [49]

Procedure	Comments	Antimicrobial prophylaxis	LE	GR
Diagnostic procedures				
Cystoscopy	Individual risk factors for UTI (i.e., asymptomatic bacteriuria, history of febrile UTI)	Not recommended	1b	A
Urodynamic study	Low frequency of infections Consider individual risk factors for UTI (i.e., asymptomatic bacteriuria, history of febrile UTI)	Not recommended	1a	A
Diagnostic ureteroscopy	No available studies	Optional	4	C
Fulguration of small bladder tumors	Low frequency of infections	Optional	2b	C

References

1. Tandogdu Z, Wagenlehner FM. Global epidemiology of urinary tract infections. Curr Opin Infect Dis. 2016;29(1):73–9. https://doi.org/10.1097/QCO.0000000000000228.
2. Gardner A, Mitchell B, Beckingham W, Fasugba O. A point prevalence cross-sectional study of healthcare-associated urinary tract infections in six Australian hospitals. BMJ Open. 2014;4(7):e005099. https://doi.org/10.1136/bmjopen-2014-005099.
3. Graves N, Tong E, Morton AP, Halton K, Curtis M, Lairson D, et al. Factors associated with health care-acquired urinary tract infection. Am J Infect Control. 2007;35(6):387–92. https://doi.org/10.1016/j.ajic.2006.09.006.
4. World health organization: Health care-associated infections fact sheet, http://www.who.int/gpsc/country_work/gpsc_ccisc_fact_sheet_en.pdf. Accessed 7 Oct 2015.
5. Togan T, Azap OK, Durukan E, Arslan H. The prevalence, etiologic agents and risk factors for urinary tract infection among spinal cord injury patients. Jundishapur J Microbiol. 2014;7(1):e8905. https://doi.org/10.5812/jjm.8905.
6. Martins CF, Bronzatto E, Neto JM, Magalhaes GS, D'Anconna CA, Cliquet A Jr. Urinary tract infection analysis in a spinal cord injured population undergoing rehabilitation—how to treat? Spinal Cord. 2013;51(3):193–5. https://doi.org/10.1038/sc.2012.104.
7. Yoon SB, Lee BS, Lee KD, Hwang SI, Lee HJ, Han ZA. Comparison of bacterial strains and antibiotic susceptibilities in urinary isolates of spinal cord injury patients from the community and hospital. Spinal Cord. 2014;52(4):298–301. https://doi.org/10.1038/sc.2014.10.
8. Esclarin De Ruz A, Garcia Leoni E, Herruzo Cabrera R. Epidemiology and risk factors for urinary tract infection in patients with spinal cord injury. J Urol. 2000;164(4):1285–9.
9. Vigil HR, Hickling DR. Urinary tract infection in the neurogenic bladder. Transl Androl Urol. 2016;5(1):72–87. https://doi.org/10.3978/j.issn.2223-4683.2016.01.06.
10. Brumbaugh AR, Mobley HL. Preventing urinary tract infection: progress toward an effective Escherichia coli vaccine. Expert Rev Vaccines. 2012;11(6):663–76. https://doi.org/10.1586/erv.12.36.
11. Flores-Mireles AL, Walker JN, Caparon M, Hultgren SJ. Urinary tract infections: epidemiology, mechanisms of infection and treatment options. Nat Rev Microbiol. 2015;13(5):269–84. https://doi.org/10.1038/nrmicro3432.
12. Grabe M, Bartoletti R, Bjerklund Johansen TE, Cai T, Çek M, Köves B, Naber KG, Pickard RS, Tenke P, Wagenlehner F, Wullt B. Guidelines on Urological Infections. European Association of Urology. 2015.
13. Neal DE Jr. Host defense mechanisms in urinary tract infections. Urol Clin North Am. 1999;26(4):677–86. vii
14. Merritt JL. Residual urine volume: correlate of urinary tract infection in patients with spinal cord injury. Arch Phys Med Rehabil. 1981;62(11):558–61.
15. Vasudeva P, Madersbacher H. Factors implicated in pathogenesis of urinary tract infections in neurogenic bladders: some revered, few forgotten, others ignored. NeurourolUrodyn. 2014;33(1):95–100. https://doi.org/10.1002/nau.22378.
16. Waites KB, Canupp KC, DeVivo MJ. Microbiology of the urethra and perineum and its relationship to bacteriuria in community-residing men with spinal cord injury. J Spinal Cord Med. 2004;27(5):448–52.
17. Parsons CL, Greenspan C, Moore SW, Mulholland SG. Role of surface mucin in primary antibacterial defense of bladder. Urology. 1977;9(1):48–52.
18. Parsons CL, Shrom SH, Hanno PM, Mulholland SG. Bladder surface mucin. Examination of possible mechanisms for its antibacterial effect. Invest Urol. 1978;16(3):196–200.
19. Wold AE, Mestecky J, Tomana M, Kobata A, Ohbayashi H, Endo T, et al. Secretory immunoglobulin A carries oligosaccharide receptors for Escherichia coli type 1 fimbrial lectin. Infect Immun. 1990;58(9):3073–7.

20. Vaidyanathan S, McDicken IW, Soni BM, Singh G, Sett P, Husin NM. Secretory immunoglobulin A in the vesical urothelium of patients with neuropathic bladder—an immunohistochemical study. Spinal Cord. 2000;38(6):378–81.

21. Chaudhry R, Madden-Fuentes RJ, Ortiz TK, Balsara Z, Tang Y, Nseyo U, et al. Inflammatory response to Escherichia coli urinary tract infection in the neurogenic bladder of the spinal cord injured host. J Urol. 2014;191(5):1454–61. https://doi.org/10.1016/j.juro.2013.12.013.

22. Iversen PO, Hjeltnes N, Holm B, Flatebo T, Strom-Gundersen I, Ronning W, et al. Depressed immunity and impaired proliferation of hematopoietic progenitor cells in patients with complete spinal cord injury. Blood. 2000;96(6):2081–3.

23. Hooton TM, Bradley SF, Cardenas DD, Colgan R, Geerlings SE, Rice JC, et al. Diagnosis, prevention, and treatment of catheter-associated urinary tract infection in adults: 2009 International Clinical Practice Guidelines from the Infectious Diseases Society of America. Clin Infect Dis. 2010;50(5):625–63.

24. Cameron AP, Rodriguez GM, Schomer KG. Systematic review of urological followup after spinal cord injury. J Urol. 2012;187(2):391–7. https://doi.org/10.1016/j.juro.2011.10.020.

25. Jayawardena V, Midha M. Significance of bacteriuria in neurogenic bladder. J Spinal Cord Med. 2004;27(2):102–5.

26. El Masri y WS, Patil S, Prasanna KV, Chowdhury JR. To cystoscope or not to cystoscope patients with traumatic spinal cord injuries managed with indwelling urethral or suprapubic catheters? That is the question! Spinal Cord. 2014;52(1):49–53. https://doi.org/10.1038/sc.2013.119.

27. Salameh A, Al Mohajer M, Darouiche RO. Prevention of urinary tract infections in patients with spinal cord injury. CMAJ. 2015;187(11):807–11. https://doi.org/10.1503/cmaj.141044.

28. Goetz LL, Cardenas DD, Kennelly M, Bonne Lee BS, Linsenmeyer T, Moser C, et al. International spinal cord injury urinary tract infection basic data set. Spinal Cord. 2013;51(9):700–4. https://doi.org/10.1038/sc.2013.72.

29. Ronco E, Denys P, Bernede-Bauduin C, Laffont I, Martel P, Salomon J, et al. Diagnostic criteria of urinary tract infection in male patients with spinal cord injury. Neurorehabil Neural Repair. 2011;25(4):351–8. https://doi.org/10.1177/1545968310383432.

30. Siroky MB. Pathogenesis of bacteriuria and infection in the spinal cord injured patient. Am J Med. 2002;113(Suppl 1A):67s–79s.

31. Michalopoulos AS, Livaditis IG, Gougoutas V. The revival of fosfomycin. Int J Infect Dis. 2011;15(11):e732–9. https://doi.org/10.1016/j.ijid.2011.07.007.

32. Kahan FM, Kahan JS, Cassidy PJ, Kropp H. The mechanism of action of fosfomycin (phosphonomycin). Ann N Y Acad Sci. 1974;235:364–86.

33. Kass EH. Asymptomatic infections of the urinary tract. Trans Assoc Am Physicians. 1956;69:56–64.

34. Warren JW, Platt R, Thomas RJ, Rosner B, Kass EH. Antibiotic irrigation and catheter-associated urinary-tract infections. N Engl J Med. 1978;299(11):570–3. https://doi.org/10.1056/nejm197809142991103.

35. Platt R, Polk BF, Murdock B, Rosner B. Reduction of mortality associated with nosocomial urinary tract infection. Lancet. 1983;1(8330):893–7.

36. Garibaldi RA, Burke JP, Dickman ML, Smith CB. Factors predisposing to bacteriuria during indwelling urethral catheterization. N Engl J Med. 1974;291(5):215–9. https://doi.org/10.1056/nejm197408012910501.

37. Hartstein AI, Garber SB, Ward TT, Jones SR, Morthland VH. Nosocomial urinary tract infection: a prospective evaluation of 108 catheterized patients. Infect Control. 1981;2(5):380–6.

38. Tenney JH, Warren JW. Bacteriuria in women with long-term catheters: paired comparison of indwelling and replacement catheters. J Infect Dis. 1988;157(1):199–202.

39. Grahn D, Norman DC, White ML, Cantrell M, Yoshikawa TT. Validity of urinary catheter specimen for diagnosis of urinary tract infection in the elderly. Arch Intern Med. 1985;145(10):1858–60.

40. Cruz F, Nitti V. Chapter 5: clinical data in neurogenic detrusor overactivity (NDO) and overactive bladder (OAB). NeurourolUrodyn. 2014;33(Suppl 3):S26–31. https://doi.org/10.1002/nau.22630.
41. Leitner L, Sammer U, Walter M, Knupfer SC, Schneider MP, Seifert B, et al. Antibiotic prophylaxis may not be necessary in patients with asymptomatic bacteriuria undergoing intradetrusor onabotulinumtoxinA injections for neurogenic detrusor overactivity. Sci Rep. 2016;6:33197. https://doi.org/10.1038/srep33197.
42. Sievert KD, Amend B, Gakis G, Toomey P, Badke A, Kaps HP, et al. Early sacral neuromodulation prevents urinary incontinence after complete spinal cord injury. Ann Neurol. 2010;67(1):74–84. https://doi.org/10.1002/ana.21814.
43. Darouiche RO, Green BG, Donovan WH, Chen D, Schwartz M, Merritt J, et al. Multicenter randomized controlled trial of bacterial interference for prevention of urinary tract infection in patients with neurogenic bladder. Urology. 2011;78(2):341–6. https://doi.org/10.1016/j.urology.2011.03.062.
44. Montgomerie JZ, Morrow JW. Long-term Pseudomonas colonization in spinal cord injury patients. Am J Epidemiol. 1980;112(4):508–17.
45. Montgomerie JZ, Gilmore DS, Graham IE, Schick DG, Ashley MA, Morrow JW, et al. Klebsiella pneumoniae colonization in patients with spinal cord injury. Diagn Microbiol Infect Dis. 1987;7(4):229–35.
46. Shen L, Zheng X, Zhang C, Zeng B, Hou C. Influence of different urination methods on the urinary systems of patients with spinal cord injury. J Int Med Res. 2012;40(5):1949–57. https://doi.org/10.1177/030006051204000536.
47. Prieto J, Murphy CL, Moore KN, Fader M. Intermittent catheterisation for long-term bladder management. Cochrane Database Syst Rev. 2014;(9):Cd006008. https://doi.org/10.1002/14651858.CD006008.pub3.
48. Siddiq DM, Darouiche RO. New strategies to prevent catheter-associated urinary tract infections. Nat Rev Urol. 2012;9(6):305–14. https://doi.org/10.1038/nrurol.2012.68.
49. EAU. http://uroweb.org/guideline/urological-infections/.
50. Opperman EA. Cranberry is not effective for the prevention or treatment of urinary tract infections in individuals with spinal cord injury. Spinal Cord. 2010;48(6):451–6. https://doi.org/10.1038/sc.2009.159.
51. Hess MJ, Hess PE, Sullivan MR, Nee M, Yalla SV. Evaluation of cranberry tablets for the prevention of urinary tract infections in spinal cord injured patients with neurogenic bladder. Spinal Cord. 2008;46(9):622–6. https://doi.org/10.1038/sc.2008.25.
52. Morton SC, Shekelle PG, Adams JL, Bennett C, Dobkin BH, Montgomerie J, et al. Antimicrobial prophylaxis for urinary tract infection in persons with spinal cord dysfunction. Arch Phys Med Rehabil. 2002;83(1):129–38.
53. Bouza E, San Juan R, Munoz P, Voss A, Kluytmans J. A European perspective on nosocomial urinary tract infections I. Report on the microbiology workload, etiology and antimicrobial susceptibility (ESGNI-003 study). European Study Group on Nosocomial Infections. Clin Microbiol Infect. 2001;7(10):523–31.
54. Gordon KA, Jones RN. Susceptibility patterns of orally administered antimicrobials among urinary tract infection pathogens from hospitalized patients in North America: comparison report to Europe and Latin America. Results from the SENTRY Antimicrobial Surveillance Program (2000). Diagn Microbiol Infect Dis. 2003;45(4):295–301.
55. DasGupta R, Sullivan R, French G, O'Brien T. Evidence-based prescription of antibiotics in urology: a 5-year review of microbiology. BJU Int. 2009;104(6):760–4. https://doi.org/10.1111/j.1464-410X.2009.08779.x.
56. Bone RC, Balk RA, Cerra FB, Dellinger RP, Fein AM, Knaus WA, et al. Definitions for sepsis and organ failure and guidelines for the use of innovative therapies in sepsis. The ACCP/SCCM Consensus Conference Committee. American College of Chest Physicians/Society of Critical Care Medicine. Chest. 1992;101(6):1644–55.

57. Tandogdu Z, Bartoletti R, Cai T, Cek M, Grabe M, Kulchavenya E, et al. Antimicrobial resistance in urosepsis: outcomes from the multinational, multicenter global prevalence of infections in urology (GPIU) study 2003-2013. World J Urol. 2016;34(8):1193–200. https://doi.org/10.1007/s00345-015-1722-1.
58. Tandogdu Z, Cek M, Wagenlehner F, Naber K, Tenke P, van Ostrum E, et al. Resistance patterns of nosocomial urinary tract infections in urology departments: 8-year results of the global prevalence of infections in urology study. World J Urol. 2014;32(3):791–801. https://doi.org/10.1007/s00345-013-1154-8.
59. Melican K, Boekel J, Mansson LE, Sandoval RM, Tanner GA, Kallskog O, et al. Bacterial infection-mediated mucosal signalling induces local renal ischaemia as a defence against sepsis. Cell Microbiol. 2008;10(10):1987–98. https://doi.org/10.1111/j.1462-5822.2008.01182.x.
60. Wagenlehner FM, Pilatz A, Weidner W, Naber KG. Urosepsis: overview of the diagnostic and treatment challenges. Microbiol Spectr. 2015;3(5). https://doi.org/10.1128/microbiolspec.UTI-0003-2012.
61. Wagenlehner F, Tandogdu Z, Bartoletti R, Cai T, Cek M, Kulchavenya E, et al. The global prevalence of infections in urology study: a long-term, worldwide surveillance study on urological infections. Pathogens. 2016;5(1):E10. https://doi.org/10.3390/pathogens5010010.
62. Dinh A, Davido B, Calin R, Paquereau J, Duran C, Bouchand F, et al. Ceftolozane/tazobactam for febrile UTI due to multidrug-resistant Pseudomonas aeruginosa in a patient with neurogenic bladder. Spinal cord Ser Cases. 2017;3:17019. https://doi.org/10.1038/scsandc2017.19.
63. Singer M, Deutschman CS, Seymour CW, Shankar-Hari M, Annane D, Bauer M, et al. The third international consensus definitions for sepsis and septic shock (Sepsis-3). JAMA. 2016;315(8):801–10. https://doi.org/10.1001/jama.2016.0287.
64. Bloos F, Trips E, Nicrhaus A, Briegel J, Heyland DK, Jaschinski U, et al. Effect of sodium selenite administration and procalcitonin-guided therapy on mortality in patients with severe sepsis or septic shock: a randomized clinical trial. JAMA Intern Med. 2016;176(9):1266–76. https://doi.org/10.1001/jamainternmed.2016.2514.
65. Zaccone V, Tosoni A, Passaro G, Vallone C, Impagnatiello M, Li Puma DD, et al. Sepsis in internal medicine wards: current knowledge, uncertainties and new approaches for management optimization. Ann Med. 2017:1–26. https://doi.org/10.1080/07853890.2017.1332776.
66. Rhodes A, Evans LE, Alhazzani W, Levy MM, Antonelli M, Ferrer R, et al. Surviving sepsis campaign: international guidelines for management of sepsis and septic shock: 2016. Intensive Care Med. 2017;43(3):304–77. https://doi.org/10.1007/s00134-017-4683-6.

Part V
Clinical Entities: Bowel Disorders

Neurogenic Bowel Dysfunction

Herjan van der Steeg, André J. A. Bremers, and Ivo de Blaauw

Introduction

Individuals suffering from a central neurological condition such as spinal cord injury (SCI), spina bifida, multiple sclerosis (MS), Alzheimer's disease, Parkinson's disease, and transverse myelitis often experience severely debilitating lower urinary and bowel dysfunction in addition to physical disabilities. These dysfunctions often have a severe impact on the quality of life. Despite its high prevalence in neurologically affected individuals, neurogenic bowel dysfunction (NBD) has received much less attention by the medical providers compared to bladder dysfunction [1, 2]. This chapter will provide the reader with an insight in the prevalence, treatment, and impact of NBD, whether of post-traumatic, congenital, degenerative, ischemic, or neoplastic origin.

Gut Motility

Several physiological factors play an important role in fecal continence. Normal propulsive activity of the bowel wall, rectal wall compliance, an adequate resting tone of the anal sphincters, contractility of the smooth and striated anal sphincters, intact anal canal sensation, and afferent nervous information from the rectal wall all have a decisive influence on physiological defecation and fecal continence.

H. van der Steeg (✉) · I. de Blaauw
Department of Surgery-Pediatric Surgery, Radboudumc-Amalia
Children's Hospital, Nijmegen, The Netherlands
e-mail: herjan.vandersteeg@radboudumc.nl

A. J. A. Bremers
Department of Surgery, Radboudumc, Nijmegen, The Netherlands

© Springer International Publishing AG, part of Springer Nature 2018
R. Dmochowski, J. Heesakkers (eds.), *Neuro-Urology*,
https://doi.org/10.1007/978-3-319-90997-4_18

The internal anal sphincter (IAS), which is the thickening of the inner circular muscle layer of the bowel wall at the level of the anal canal, is composed of smooth muscle fibers. It is responsible for 70–80% of the anorectal resting pressure and is under reflex control by the autonomous nervous system; even in the absence of normal external innervation, the internal anal sphincter will have some tone and contractility.

The striated muscle fibers of the external anal sphincter (EAS) have a small additional effect on the resting pressure but are easily exhausted. Therefore, the EAS can never fully compensate for an IAS dysfunction. The EAS muscle fibers are under both reflex and voluntary control via somatic lower motor neurons in the pudendal nerve from the sacral cord. In the absence of normal external innervation, the EAS will be areflexic, hypotonic, and atrophic [3].

The intrinsic or enteric nervous system is embedded in the gut wall as two plexuses, the submucosal plexus of Meissner and the mucosal plexus of Auerbach. This enteric nervous system coordinates gut secretion, blood flow, and muscular activity. It coordinates peristalsis, the wavelike flow of contraction that pushes the stool in stages toward the anus.

The extrinsic neurological input to the gut is via the autonomic nervous system. Parasympathetic input increases motility in the gut and relaxes sphincters, preparing the body for involuntary defecation. Parasympathetic fibers to the ascending and part of the transverse colon originate for the vagus nerve. The remainder of the colon, rectum, and anal canal receives its parasympathetic input via sacral roots S2–S4 through the pelvic nerves. Sympathetic innervation comes from T6–L2 nerve roots and decreases motility and tone of the colon but stimulates contraction of the IAS, preventing defecation. This autonomic nervous system influences the activity of the enteric nervous system and in itself is modulated by centers in the spinal cord and brain (hypothalamus).

Bowel contents enter the colon through the ileocecal valve and are propulsed through the colon via peristalsis. The innate rhythmicity within the smooth muscle fibers of the gut arises from the cells of Cajal which generate slow waves which persist in the absence of other neural input, e.g., after complete spinal cord transection [3]. Almost constant mixing movements, called haustral churning, ensure the frequent presentation and representation of stool to colonic mucosa, thus facilitating absorption of water and electrolytes. Occasional "mass" movements propulse the stool through the colon and occur two to three times a day. The gastrocolic reflex is responsible for the association between food ingestion and colonic mass movements [4].

Mechanism of Defecation

Filling of the rectum, which ultimately leads to urge of defecation, is evoked by various reflexes, such as the gastrocolic and ileocolic reflex (contraction of the colon by filling of the stomach and ileum, respectively) as well as voluntary contraction of the abdominal wall musculature. When the volume of the rectal fecal contents increases, intrarectal pressure will rise. The strain in the rectal wall causes a relaxation of the IAS by a reflex of the autonomous nervous system known as the rectalanal inhibitory reflex, at the same time stimulating the peristalsis in the descending and sigmoid colon. Proprioceptive receptors in the puborectalis muscle and parapuborectal tissues ultimately lead to the conscious feeling of an urge to defecate. Feces hereby reach the upper anal canal, where hypersensitive mucosa is able to distinguish flatus from liquid or solid stool. The reflex or voluntary contraction of the EAS and puborectalis muscle will produce an aboral-oral pressure gradient, preventing expulsion of flatus or stool, and thus inhibits defecation. If evacuation of stool at that time would be appropriate, the EAS is then voluntarily relaxed.

An intrarectal pressure of 25–30 mmHg will stimulate a reflex which inhibits the anorectal sphincters and puborectalis muscle. Voluntary contraction of the abdominal wall musculature and diaphragm will also cause a reciprocal inhibition of the striated muscles of the pelvic floor, diminishing the anorectal angle by straightening the rectum whereby defecation commences. Additionally, the contraction of the abdominal muscles and diaphragm will increase the intra-abdominal pressure, triggering peristalsis in the colon and rectum. Relaxation of smooth muscle fibers causes dilatation of the anal canal, starting at the upper part, continuing down, allowing stool to pass [5, 6]. This complex process relies upon the existence of intact reflex arcs between the colon, rectum and anal canal and spinal cord and intact voluntary pathways between the anorectum and hypothalamus. These reflexes can be easily witnessed in clinical examination: in physiological circumstances a pinprick to the perianal skin causes the external anal sphincter to contract and introduction of the finger in the anal canal on a digital examination causes the external anal sphincter to relax within seconds.

Neurogenic Bowel Dysfunction (NBD)

"Neurogenic bowel dysfunction" is the term used to describe dysfunction of the colon, rectum, and anus, resulting in constipation, fecal incontinence, and disordered defecation, due to loss of normal sensory and/or motor control as a result of central neurological disease or damage [4]. The neurogenic function may be (hyper) reflexic, areflexic, or mixed.

(Hyper)Reflexic Bowel Dysfunction

Injuries above the conus medullaris result in upper motor neuron (UMN) bowel syndrome, or (hyper)reflexic bowel, characterized by constipation and fecal retention due to EAS hyperactivity. These patients have an intact anal reflex, characterized by a visible contraction of the anus in response to pinprick of the surrounding skin. The bulbo-anal reflex is positive, i.e., the anus contracts in response to pressure on the glans penis or clitoris. However, there is a loss or impairment of sensory perception of the need of defecation and of voluntary control of the EAS and pelvic floor muscles. Modulation of the colonic motor activity from the brain is lost, resulting in less effective peristalsis. Additionally, discoordination between relaxation of the anal canal and rectal contraction, known as recto-anal dyssynergia, can occur. If the damage is in the thoracic and cervical spinal cord, patient's ability to use the diaphragm and abdominal wall muscles to voluntarily increase abdominal pressure causing a pressure gradient over the anal canal for the evacuation of stool is reduced [3].

Areflexic Bowel Dysfunction

When injuries occur at the conus medullaris and/or cauda equine (at or below the first lumbar vertebra), this results in lower motor neuron (LMN) bowel syndrome, characterized by constipation and fecal incontinence due to an atonic EAS and lack of muscle control [7, 8]. These patients have no anal or bulbo-anal reflex. Like in (hyper)reflexic bowel dysfunction, there is a loss or impairment of sensory perception of the need for defecation, as well as voluntary control of the EAS. In contrast, in areflexic bowel dysfunction, the EAS is denervated and flaccid. Because of the loss of spinal cord-mediated peristalsis and modulation of colonic motility by the brain, colonic transit time increases, resulting in constipation. The constipation is often accompanied by fecal incontinence [7], due to a reduced pressure in the IAS and pelvic floor muscles, allowing sigmoid colon and rectum to descend into the pelvis, reducing the anorectal angle and opening the rectal lumen. Additionally, the loss of voluntary control of the mentioned denervated and flaccid EAS will increase the risk of fecal incontinence. These patients are capable of generating an increase in abdominal pressure. With the paralysis of the pelvic floor muscles, this increase in abdominal pressure will cause the pelvic floor and anus to descend rather than allow feces to pass through the anal canal. Continued resorption of fluid from the feces when these remain in the rectum will cause impaction.

NBD is the dysfunction of the bowel due to disruption of normal modulation of the intrinsic nervous system, resulting in altered blood flow, enzyme secretion, and water and electrolyte transport in the gastrointestinal tract. As a consequence, dysmotility, precipitating increased colonic transit time, increased rectal distension, and symptoms of constipation occur. Symptoms vary according to the severity of the underlying pathology.

Clinical Features of Neurogenic Bowel Dysfunction

Constipation

Although there is no universally agreed definition of constipation, it is suggested to involve two or more of the following symptoms, straining during at least 25% of defecations, lumpy or hard stools, sensation of incomplete evacuation, sensation of anorectal obstruction or blockage, or use of manual maneuvers to facilitate evacuation in at least 25% of defecations (e.g., digital rectal evacuation, support of the pelvic floor), and fewer than three defecations per week. These Rome III criteria should have been fulfilled for the last 3 months with symptom onset at least 6 months prior to diagnosis [9]. Additionally, constipation is associated with rectal and abdominal pain and painful defecation.

Constipation is common in neurogenic bowel dysfunction and occurs in up to 80% of spinal cord injury (SCI) patients [10–13], up to 70% of MS patients [2, 14], and up to 89% of Parkinson's patients [15]. Contributing factors to constipation are slowing of gut transit due to interruption of nerve pathways, disability-associated changes in mobility, spasticity, fatigue, inadequate intake of fiber and fluid, and concomitant use of multiple medications (polypharmacy) [16].

Fecal Incontinence

Fecal incontinence is defined by the International Consultation on Incontinence as "the involuntary loss of flatus, liquid or solid stool that is a social or hygienic problem" [17]. This definition does not contain any prerequisite for duration of symptoms. Whitehead defined fecal incontinence as "recurrent uncontrolled, involuntary, or unplanned passage of fecal material or flatus, for at least 1 month" [18]. Among individuals with central neurological conditions, the majority suffer from fecal incontinence: up to 70% of MS patients, up to 75% in SCI patients [11, 12, 19], and up to 68% in spina bifida patients [20–22].

Fecal Impaction

Although not well defined, fecal impaction is suggested to be described as "copious formed stool in the colon, which is not progressing through the colon or cannot be expelled from the rectum" [23]. Symptoms may include absent or reduced evacuation of stool for a longer period than usual for the individual, abdominal bloating or distention, nausea, and pain. It may be accompanied by diarrhea by loose stool overflowing the impacted stool, resulting in soiling and/or overflow incontinence.

Hemorrhoids

In the lower anal canal, cushion-like vascular tissues contribute to continence. These so-called hemorrhoidal veins (as part of the rectal venous plexus or internal hemorrhoidal plexus) may become dilated and prolapse and could evoke bloody stools and itching. Hemorrhoids are associated with chronic constipation or diarrhea, straining at defecation, prolonged toileting, and low dietary fiber intake and become more common with age. The external hemorrhoidal plexus can also enlarge, sometimes thrombose, and may leave redundant skin, also known as skin tags. These may cause skin irritation due to difficulty in adequate cleaning of the perianal region. Hemorrhoids are quite common and up to 40% of individuals with SCI report having hemorrhoids [10].

Rectal Prolapse

Rectal prolapse refers to three distinct presentations of a protruding mass from the anus. First, a full-thickness rectal wall prolapse may be encountered, usually determined by the concentric circular lines in the mucosa or massive edema. A second presentation is a mucosal prolapse only revealing mucosa, classically determined by radial or linear irregular lines in the mucosa protruding from the anus. The third presentation is an internal prolapsed intestine or intussusception, in which collapsed tissue "telescopes" on itself but remains within the colon. External prolapse often results in fecal incontinence and increased mucosal leakage, leading to soiling. Internal prolapse may cause a feeling of incomplete evacuation [10].

Autonomic Dysreflexia

This term refers to an abnormal sympathetic nervous system response to a noxious stimulus below the level of injury in individuals with SCI above the sixth thoracic vertebra. One of the noxious stimuli can be, e.g., the infusion of fluid into the large bowel during bowel management. Among susceptible individuals, 36% report dysreflexic symptoms occasionally and 9% always when they conduct bowel management [24]. Increased blood pressure without symptoms during bowel management has been recorded, not necessarily requiring treatment [25]. Complaints related to autonomic dysreflexia are flushing, sweating and blotchiness above the lesion, chills, nasal congestion, and headache. Bowel distension caused by impaction, rectal stimulation, suppository insertion, and enemas have all been reported as triggering autonomic dysreflexia of hyperreflexia [26].

The cardinal sign is a rapidly developing headache. Bowel management should be stopped immediately, allowing the complaints to subside. When the dysreflexia persists after stopping the procedure, prompt treatment should be commenced, which usually involves sublingual nifedipine or a glyceryl trinitrate patch or spray. Bowel management should however be continued on a regular basis: local anesthetic gel or ointment should be applied prior to digital interventions, reducing or eradicating the autonomic dysreflexic response during bowel care [27].

Impact on Quality of Life

Loss of voluntary bowel control may cause a lot of anxiety and distress [11, 28] and can potentially have a negative impact on all areas of adult life, such as working, leisure activities, and developing and maintaining personal relationships, thereby significantly reducing the quality of life. The broader effects of disability, including loss of mobility, spasticity, muscle weakness, fatigue, and loss of independence in toileting, in some cases related to cognitive impairment and the use of drugs whose actions may adversely affect bowel function, all contribute to the extent of NBD and its impact on quality of life [29]. It is, however, not just the loss of control that has an impact, the fear or anticipation of incontinence may in itself result in reduced social activity and isolation [7, 16]. Additionally, NBD is associated with hemorrhoids, abdominal complaints, fecal impaction, rectal bleeding, rectal prolapse, anal fissure, abdominal bloating, nausea, autonomic dysreflexia, and prolonged evacuation, which all impact quality of life [12, 19, 30–33]. Quality of life (QoL) reporting is however very heterogeneous for patients with central neurological conditions and bowel dysfunction, and the bowel dysfunction by itself does not necessarily have a negative impact on QoL [1, 34].

Despite these heterogeneous reports, when an affected individual is to maintain or return to an active role in the community, a bowel management program that is effective, timely, and sustainable is essential. Nevertheless, the often time-consuming and arduous active management of the neurogenic bowel that is required to avoid constipation and incontinence also diminishes quality of life, although there are studies that show inconsistencies in such clinical- and patient-reported measures [35].

While QoL has been defined in various ways, an often cited definition is that QoL is "an individual's perception of their position in life in the context of the culture and value systems in which they live, and in relation to their goals, expectations, and concerns" [36]. There are multiple QoL measures (Qualiveen, Fecal Incontinence and Constipation Quality of Life, Adolescent Fecal Incontinence and Constipation Symptom Index, and Quality of Life Tool Relating to Bowel Movement) available and validated for SCI and MS patients, but none are validated in other neurogenic populations [37], thus making the interpretation of the loss of quality of life less reliable. Nevertheless, overall it seems that data from these tests can be extrapolated to other neurogenic populations as well.

Neurogenic Bowel Management

Bowel management in individuals with a central neurologic condition is "the regular delivery of a programme of planned interventions designed to pre-emptively achieve effective bowel evacuation at a specific frequency in individuals with central neurological conditions, reducing its impact on quality of life by avoiding fecal

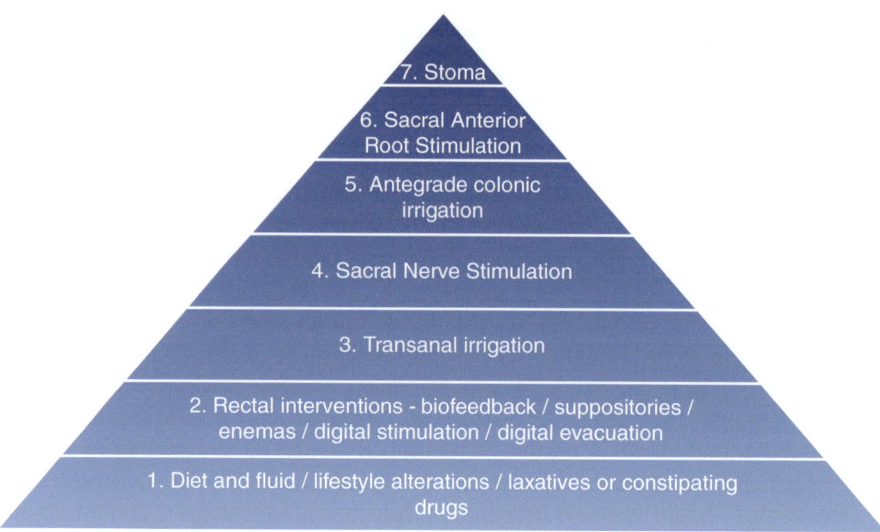

Fig. 1 A proposed stepped approach to management of neurogenic bowel dysfunction (adapted from [38]). NB: Not all levels are appropriate to all individuals and the pyramid does not represent a strict pathway—movement up or down the pyramid is guided by ongoing assessment and evaluation [38]

incontinence and constipation, minimising associated morbidity and facilitating carer input where required" [3]. The management should fit with the lifestyle of the individual, enabling activity without fear of fecal incontinence. It should provide an effective routine that is acceptable to the individual, promoting autonomy, verbal, and where possible, physical independence.

The figure below (Fig. 1) illustrates a generally accepted hierarchy of interventions. It reflects the level of complexity, invasiveness, risk, and reversibility of the various interventions while acknowledging issues of costs and evidence of benefit [3]. Not all levels are appropriate to all individuals, and the pyramid does not represent a strict pathway.

Choice of intervention does not solely depend on the specific bowel dysfunction but will also be determined by patient factors such as mobility, hand function, personal preference, and independence, as well as resource factors such as availability of caretakers and home setting.

Treatment Modalities

As mentioned bowel symptoms are the result of inadequate modulation of the intrinsic nervous system. The resulting dysmotility needs to be addressed by different treatment modalities. Stool consistency needs to be modulated, as well as the promotion of colon transit time and the mechanical evacuation of stool from the rectum at an appropriate time and place [3].

While there is a great deal of information on the causes of NBD, there are few studies that focus on how to practically manage the problem. Although basic advice is to have sufficient fluid intake, a balanced diet, regular planned bowel routine, and as much physical exercise as the neurological condition permits, scientific evidence is limited.

The strategy most commonly applied, therefore, is the establishment of a bowel emptying routine. Bowel care is conducted at a set frequency and time of day and could consist of oral laxative medicines, stimulation of the gastrocolic reflex, abdominal massage, rectal stimulants (suppositories or enema), digital rectal stimulation (DRS) to produce a reflex evacuation of stool, and digital removal of stool [39, 40]. The most effective treatment should always be individualized and will be established after some degree of trial and error. Constipation and incontinence will often coexist in these patients. Unfortunately, any intervention can easily be effective for the one, simultaneously precipitating the other [29].

Conservative Measures

Multiple conservative measures are available in the treatment of NBD. Depending on the severity and type of the NBD ((hyper)reflexic, areflexic, or mixed), the tendency of the individual to be constipated or fecally incontinent, and the available resources surrounding the individual, an individualized bowel management program needs to be established. Examples of conservative NBD treatment are shown in Figs. 2 and 3 [3].

Dietary Manipulations

Although there is little evidence to support dietary manipulations in the treatment or prevention of constipation in patients with central neurological conditions, many individuals change their diet to assist their bowel management [24, 40]. Individuals with (hyper)reflexic bowel function are encouraged to aim for a soft-formed stool consistency (Bristol Scale 4 [41], Fig. 4), while those with areflexic bowel are more likely to avoid fecal incontinence if they aim for firmer stools (Bristol Scale 2–3).

Dietary fiber and their pharmaceutical counterparts, the bulking agents, will absorb fluid within the bowel lumen, thus avoiding both hard and watery stools. There is no evidence that extra fluids reduce a tendency of constipation unless an individual is clinically dehydrated.

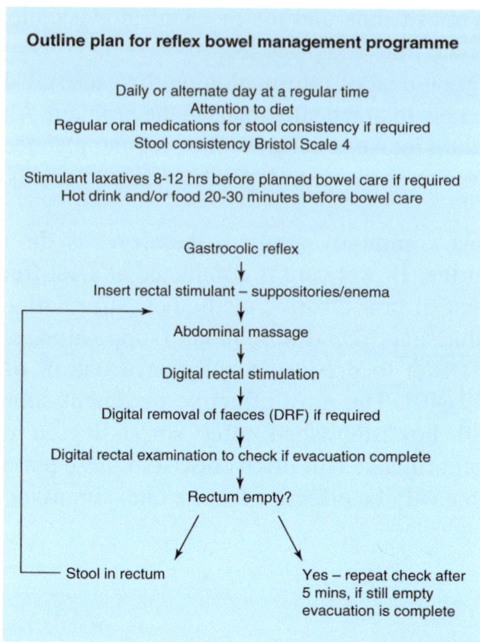

Fig. 2 Bowel management program for reflexic bowel (as presented in [3])

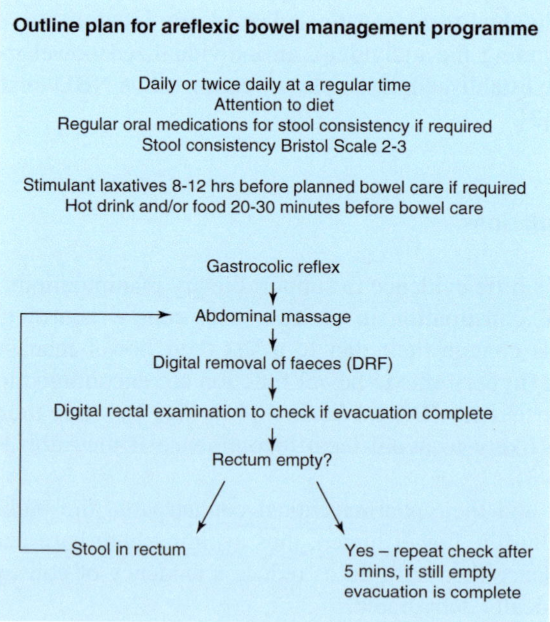

Fig. 3 Bowel management program for areflexic bowel (as presented in [3])

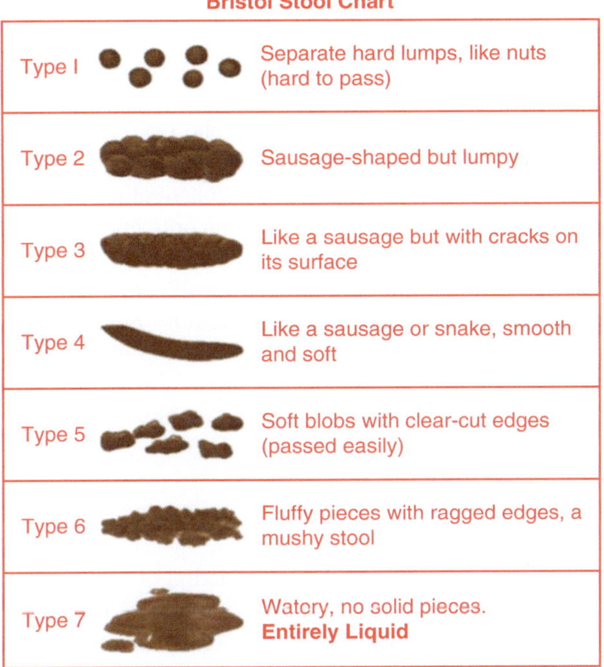

Fig. 4 The Bristol Stool Form Scale (after [41])

Oral Medication

60% of SCI individuals use oral laxatives [24]. Nevertheless, little research has been conducted to evaluate the efficacy of laxatives in NBD management [42, 43]. Medications that are commonly used include stool softeners (i.e., dioctyl), bulking agents (i.e., psyllium), and osmotic laxatives (i.e., polyethylene glycol, macrogol, lactulose), used to modulate the stool consistency and maintaining its predictability, and stimulants (i.e., senna, bisacodyl) that prompt increased bowel activity resulting in the movement of stool.

In a recent Cochrane review, polyethylene glycol (PEG) was shown to be more effective than lactulose, milk of magnesia, and placebo [44]. PEG increases bowel frequency and reduces encopresis without significant side effects [42]. Macrogol [43] as well as psyllium [45] have been reported to increase the number of bowel movements in patients with Parkinson's disease.

So, while osmotic laxatives such as polyethylene glycol and stimulant laxatives such as senna compounds remain the mainstay in NBD treatment, several newer agents that target different mechanisms have been described as being promising. A significant median increase in weekly bowel movements and median decrease in colonic transit time were seen in SCI patients using prucalopride (a systemic entero-kinetic drug which is a selective and specific 5-HT4 agonist targeting serotonin-4 receptors involved in initiating peristalsis) compared to placebo [46]. Side effects were reported in the majority of patients, including gastrointestinal complaints (flatulence, diarrhea, abdominal pain) and headache. Neostigmine-glycopyrrolate (neostigmine is a reversible cholinesterase inhibitor; glycopyrrolate is a selective anticholinergic agent, reducing the cholinergic effect) was shown to reduce the total bowel evacuation time in a small crossover study compared to placebo [47]. However, they should be used with caution given the possible cardiovascular and pulmonary side effects.

Although laxatives are effective in treating constipation, without the use of a regular rectal evacuation, it often results in fecal incontinence [3]. It is paramount to individualize this laxative treatment and add supplementary treatment modalities in order to optimize defecation without the risk of fecal incontinence. In addition, it is important to realize that NBD individuals may require medication for other problems related to their neurological condition that may interfere with bowel management. Some examples are anticholinergics for the treatment of neurogenic bladder, antidepressants, narcotics, and antispasticity medications.

Gastrocolic Reflex

The gastrocolic reflex is a response to the introduction of food and/or drink into the stomach, resulting in an increase in muscular activity throughout the gut [48], which can result in movement of stool into the rectum, ready for evacuation. Although its effect in individuals with NBD is equivocal, it is still considered a useful tool in bowel management. Its strongest effect is 15–30 min after ingestion and usually after the first meal of the day, but it can be stimulated at any time.

Abdominal Massage

It has been demonstrated that abdominal massage produces a measurable response in the rectum and anus [49]. 22–30% of individuals with NBD use abdominal massage [3]. Massage is applied to the abdomen following the usual position of the colon in a clockwise direction, hereby promoting stool transit to the rectum. A recent review stated that abdominal massage can relieve constipation by stimulating peristalsis, decreasing colon transit time, and increasing the frequency of bowel movements [50]. It can reduce feelings of discomfort and pain and induce a feeling of relaxation. It has even been found to improve patient's quality of life [51]. However, evidence concerning its mechanism of action, time required for effectiveness and in whom it is potentially beneficial, is still lacking.

Valsalva Maneuver or Straining

This technique results in a rise in intra-abdominal pressure, creating a pressure gradient for the feces. Some individuals can strain to assist with evacuation; however, straining as the main method of evacuation is associated with a high degree of incontinence, constipation, and other difficulties with evacuation [52] and should be discouraged. Moreover, it can lead to the development of hemorrhoids, rectal prolapse, and even obstructed defecation due to the development of an enterocele. Therefore, in individuals with areflexic bowel, straining should be used with caution, if at all.

Biofeedback

As pelvic floor dyssynergia and an increased threshold for rectal sensation have been reported in neurogenic conditions, biofeedback as sensory awareness may be of additional value in the overall treatment of NBD [40]. Although biofeedback has gained a place in the treatment of constipation and fecal incontinence in the general population, little is published about NBD individuals, and its effect in patients with NBD therefore remains unclear [53, 54]. The best candidates for this type of intervention would be the patient with mild to moderate disability [53], persistent rectal sensation, good motivation, and an absence of significant psychological dysfunction [55].

Rectal Evacuation Therapy

Many NBD patients have lost their ability to control their defecation definitively and little can be done to restore these functions sufficiently. Timely evacuation of feces under controlled conditions however may help to prevent involuntary passages, thus rendering them pseudo-continent and avoiding constipation.

Stimulants

Rectal stimulation is an important part of the bowel management process for many individuals with NBD, providing a trigger for bowel evacuation at a chosen time. This can be achieved by mechanical or pharmaceutical means. Despite the frequent clinical use of suppositories and enemas for this purpose, research evidence for the efficacy of the various products and approaches is seriously lacking [29]. Nevertheless, rectal stimulants continue to be used in bowel management at a large scale, as oral laxatives cannot replace their function. They are said to be used in 32–71% of individuals with NBD [3]. In individuals without full control over their defecation, use of oral laxatives without planned stimulated reflex evacuation, or other method in areflexic bowel function, often results in fecal incontinence.

Available rectal stimulants are glycerin suppositories, bisacodyl suppositories (either polyethylene glycol or hydrogenated vegetable oil based) and small-volume enemas (micro-enema, like sodium citrate or sorbitol). Large-volume phosphate enemas are not used routinely as retention is often not possible and autonomic dysreflexia may be triggered in susceptible individuals [56]. Rectal stimulants alone are seldom sufficient to prompt complete reflex evacuation; most individuals also require digital stimulation or digital removal of stool [24].

Digital Rectal Stimulation (DRS)

The use of digital rectal stimulation (DRS) in individuals with NBD after SCI is reported in 35–50% [24, 31, 32]. DRS is a technique used to increase reflex muscular activity in the rectum, thereby increasing the rectal pressure aiding in expulsion of stool, and to relax the EAS, hereby reducing any outlet resistance [24, 49, 57]. The technique relies upon intact reflex bowel activity; it is only applicable to individuals with reflex bowel dysfunction [3].

DRS is performed by introducing a lubricated, gloved finger through the anal canal into the rectum, slowly rotating the finger in a circular movement, and maintaining contact with the rectal mucosal wall, hereby gently stretching the anal canal while avoiding injuring rectal mucosa [58] or precipitating autonomic dysreflexia [59]. The maneuver is continued until relaxation of the EAS is felt, flatus and/or stool is passed, or tightening of the IAS as a sign of colonic activity is detected. Usually up to 15–20 s will suffice, and longer than 1 min is rarely necessary [7]. DRS can be repeated every 5–10 min until evacuation is complete. There seems to be a considerable variation between individuals as to what is needed. It seems reasonable to repeat the stimulation until either the reflex evacuation is complete, with no fecal retention, or until the reflex has "tired" and is not effective anymore in prompting reflex evacuation. When there is still fecal retention, one should proceed with digital removal of feces. For DRS to function optimally, the stool should have the consistency of Bristol Scale 4 (bulky, soft-formed). Looser stool and constipated stool both result in less effective responses [3].

Digital Removal of Feces

Digital removal of feces involves insertion of a lubricated, gloved finger into the rectum to break up or remove the stool [60]. It is said to be used in 56% of NBD patients [24]. This maneuver is associated with shorter duration of bowel care and fewer episodes of fecal incontinence [24]. The intervention is recommended in the early phase after spinal cord injury, to remove stool from the areflexic rectum to prevent overdistension with consequent damage to later reflex rectal function [61], and is also used in the majority of chronic spinal cord injured individuals, as part of a bowel management routine [62]. It has been reported the method of choice for long-term bowel evacuation in individuals with areflexic bowel dysfunction [7] and for impacted stool removal. Individuals with reflex bowel could also profit from this intervention, when reflex activity alone is insufficient to complete empty the bowel.

Transanal Irrigation (TAI) of the Colon

Transanal irrigation (TAI) involves the introduction of water into the rectum and descending colon using a pumped or gravity-fed system via a cone-shaped device (Qufora ©, MBH International A/S, Denmark) or a rectal catheter with an integral balloon (Peristeen©, Coloplast Ltd., Fig. 5). The cone-shape catheter is less likely to provoke reflex activity, but needs to be held in place during use, requiring adequate balance, grip, and flexibility. The balloon catheter allows the device to be self-retaining and allows for a seal that aids in retention of the irrigant. Around 500 milliliters is a suitable starting point for adults, although the definitive volume varies widely between individuals [38]. After instilling lukewarm tap water, the balloon is deflated, the catheter removed, and the water and other bowel contents are evacuated [63, 64]. Irrigation does not rely upon retention of the fluid for effectiveness, and its effect to clear out the entire left-sided colon probably relies on reflex peristalsis rather than mechanical lavage.

It has been shown to be a safe intervention, and does not seem to provoke autonomic dysreflexia [63], although it is a potential risk. Rectal perforations with the canula appear extremely rare and usually occur in the first few attempts of use [38, 65]. TAI may be used in individuals who experience fecal incontinence, constipation, abdominal pain associated with evacuation, bloating, or prolonged duration of

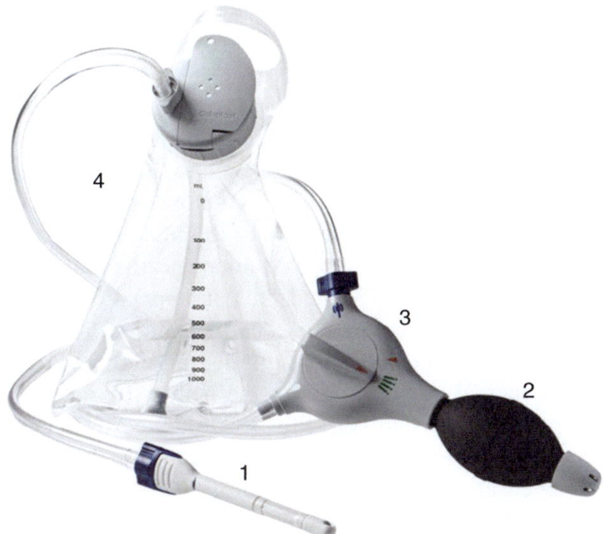

Fig. 5 Peristeen anal irrigation system (1). Coated rectal catheter with a balloon (2). Manual pump (3). Control unit (4). Water bag. The catheter is inserted into the rectum, and the balloon is inflated to hold the catheter in the rectum, while lukewarm tap water is administered with the manual pump. Pressure generated in the bag with the manual pump drives the water into the bowel. Subsequently, the balloon is deflated, and the catheter is removed, followed by bowel emptying of the water and other bowel contents

bowel evacuation [63], although robust criteria for suitability have not been defined. Nevertheless, increasing evidence shows its beneficial effect on constipation and fecal incontinence in patients with unsatisfactorily NBD treatment [63, 64, 66–69], resulting in an improvement of quality of life [16, 64, 67, 69–71]. However, there is currently a lack of evidence in the acute and rehabilitating neurogenic bowel population.

Moreover, the long-term results of TAI seem to be less satisfactory [65]. Some patients give up TAI because of technical problems (such as pain or difficulty inserting the catheter, expulsion of the catheter despite inflated balloon, inadequate seal of the inflated balloon resulting in leakage of irrigation fluid, soiling in between irrigations) and time required for the procedure [64, 65, 72]. If the irrigations are technically impossible but the results of irrigations were adequate, antegrade irrigations are an option although it needs some kind of surgery (see below, antegrade continent enema).

Surgical Measures

Most surgical interventions for NBD are designed to facilitate, rather than replace medical management. It is an adjunct to medical and conservative treatment as opposed to disease progression or failure of medical management [37].

Antegrade Continence Enema (ACE)

The ACE is a nonrefluxing, continent catheterizable stoma formed surgically. Classically the appendix was attached and opened to the abdominal wall and skin. If not available (e.g., because the appendix was removed or used as in a Mitrofanoff appendicostomy to the bladder), a cecal flap or terminal ileum can be used to create an alternative access to the cecum. Dr. Malone was the first urologist using the appendix for antegrade enemas [73], and thus an appendicostomy for antegrade enemas is often called a Malone-stoma or a neo-Malone stoma (in case of a cecal flap) [74]. It gives access to the colon for administration of an enema or irrigation in an antegrade manner. While common in the pediatric practice in spina bifida patients with improvement of quality of life [75, 76], few ACEs have been reported in adult NBD care, and failure rate in some studies is high. Nevertheless, a recent meta-analysis showed an overall success rate of 74.3% in adults with a median follow-up of 39 months [77]. This meta-analysis covers studies of functional constipation and incontinence, as well as patients with NBD. Adult series typically are small and heterogeneous in terms of recruitment, design, and outcome metrics [37]. Although continence rates are high, reaching 93% [78], in the long-term, complications such as stomal stenosis and leakage or failure to effectively treat symptoms lead to revision, reversal, or conversion to stoma in 30–50% of patients [79, 80].

Percutaneous Endoscopic Colostomy/Cecostomy (PEC)

A classic catheterizable appendicostomy is not feasible or preferable in all patients. This could be the case, for instance, when the appendix is not available (missing after appendectomy or preferred usage for a simultaneous Mitrofanoff), obesity, or preference to avoid abdominal surgery or general anesthesia. Access to the colon for antegrade enemas can be achieved by other means as well. An alternative could be an indwelling catheter, placed under colonoscopic insufflation and direct vision. This percutaneous endoscopic cecostomy (PEC) can be replaced by a MicKey button (as in gastrostomy) or by Chait tube after 6 weeks, when the tract has matured. The Chait tube is a low-profile, continent cecostomy "button," held in place by several pigtail coils inside the colon [81]. It has an external "trapdoor" lid that opens to attach to the irrigation tubing. These buttons and Chait tubes are most often placed in the cecum, although some prefer the sigmoid colon as well [82].

A concern regarding the PEC is a possible inconsistent fixation of the cecum to the peritoneum of the abdominal wall, resulting in variably matured percutaneous tracts. This may allow for fecal leakage when disrupted, leading to possible detrimental complications such as peritonitis and infected ventriculoperitoneal shunts. These complications have led some to consider open or laparoscopically assisted procedures, especially when confronted with obesity, prior abdominal surgery, or ventriculoperitoneal shunt revisions [83]. Complications that are encountered in the perioperative period include intra-abdominal or subcutaneous abscesses and ventriculoperitoneal shunt infections. Long-term adverse events include the, frequently occurring, leakage of liquid stool around the tube and associated cellulitis [37]. Minor complications such as leakage and dislodgement occur in up to half of the patients [84]. In general, though validated satisfaction scales are rarely employed, most patients receiving Chait tubes appear satisfied [84].

Stoma Formation

The formation of an enterostomy has for long been regarded a last resort when dealing with NBD and even a failure of rehabilitation services [39, 85]. However, studies have found that formation of an enterostomy can greatly improve quality of life for some individuals [3]. The presence of an enterostomy can result in less time spent on bowel management, a reduction of the number of hospitalizations caused by gastrointestinal problems and bowel care-related complaints, and an increase in independence in bowel care [3, 86–89].

Stomas are however not without complications. Postoperative bowel obstruction, peristomal hernia, stoma prolapse, stenosis, and skin rashes are all known complications, affecting those involved. The discharge of mucus from the remaining dysfunctioning bowel can also be problematic, necessitating the use of pads or even proctectomy for some individuals [3]. Around 2.4% of SCI individuals in the UK have a colostomy formed for bowel management problems [24]. Colostomies, despite their possible complications, do appear to be a valuable therapeutic alternative for patients with NBD not satisfactorily responding to conservative treatment or previously mentioned surgical measurements. In patients with extremely slow colonic passage, an ileostomy may be considered.

Sphincter Reconstruction or Artificial Sphincter Construction

Artificial bowel sphincter construction and graciloplasties have a limited place in the management of NBD. Postoperative evacuation difficulties occur in up to one-half of the patients [90]. Although obstructive symptoms can usually be resolved with laxatives or enemas, it significantly increases the risk of fecal incontinence. The reason for this remains unclear.

An indication for artificial bowel sphincter construction can only be seen in selected individuals, who are highly motivated and well-informed, are able to manipulate the control pump, have sufficient intellectual capacity to understand the functioning of the device, and are willing to actively treat their constipation by transanal irrigation [40]. Infectious complications, necessitating the removal of the device, do occur regularly.

Nerve Stimulation Techniques

Nerve stimulation techniques may result in remarkable improvements in some patients. They are not applied on a large scale since many patients do not benefit sufficiently to omit any other techniques.

Sacral Anterior Root Stimulation (SARS)

SARS has originally been used for bladder management problems after SCI but has been reported to have a beneficial effect on bowel management as well [91, 92]. Electrodes are placed on the second, third, and fourth sacral anterior nerve roots, and high-voltage, short-lived stimulation is applied by an external radio-frequency transmitter several times daily to empty the bladder; the colon is stimulated simultaneously, resulting in increased colon activity, reduced constipation, and sometimes defecation during stimulation [93]. Although its beneficial effect has been shown, implantation of the SAR-stimulators remains rare; in a recent questionnaire on SCI bowel management, only 7 out of 1330 respondents reported using a SARS for bowel management [10].

Sacral Nerve Stimulation (SNS)

SNS uses lower-amplitude, chronic stimulation applied continuously to the sacral plexus and has become a well-established treatment option for urinary dysfunction, as has been used for fecal incontinence and constipation as well. The goal of SNS is to stimulate the nerve supplying the pelvic floor and large bowel and to modulate bowel motility, the afferent sensory pathway, and the spinal reflex. Intact sacral nerves are essential, and therefore SNS is not effective in individuals with complete SCI [94].

Multiple studies in the recent past have reported a significant decrease in fecal incontinence episodes after permanent implantation and an improved quality of life in patients with incomplete spinal cord lesions (traumatic or vascular spinal lesions, MS, spina bifida) [94–97]. SNS has received increasing attention as a treatment option for constipation; however, in patients suffering from fecal incontinence, SNS does not seem to increase frequency of bowel movements. If the cause of fecal incontinence is an incomplete peripheral or central neurologic lesion, this may be a good prognostic indicator for a successful treatment with SNS [98]. It seems advisable to wait at least a year between the acute neurologic lesion and a test stimulation to allow for a possible spontaneous recovery [97].

External Stimulation

There is limited data on less invasive external electrical stimulations. It has been hypothesized that electrical stimulation of the abdominal wall musculature might improve bowel management in patients with tetraplegia, as contraction of the abdominal wall musculature plays an important role in defecation by increasing intra-abdominal pressure, and some spinal cord injury patients may not be able to voluntarily contract these muscles, depending on the level of injury. Korsten in his study on electrical stimulation (abdominal belt with embedded electrodes) in SCI patients showed a significant reduction in bowel care time and reduced time to first stool compared to no electrical stimulation [99]. External electrical stimulation has also been studied in spina bifida patients; however, a randomized trial failed to detect any significant effect on bowel function [100].

Functional magnetic stimulation has also been studied for its effect on bowel function in NBD individuals. It is suggested to stimulate the spinal nerves and contract deep muscles to facilitate bowel evacuation without surgical intervention. Several studies have shown increase in rectal pressure, suppression of hyperactive rectal contractions, and shortened transit time [101–103].

While these external electrical and magnetic stimulations show promising results, additional controlled studies in larger populations are required to determine whether their use is appropriate in NBD management.

Evaluation of Bowel Management

Measuring Effectiveness of Interventions

When initiating bowel management routine, plan it in collaboration with the individual in the context of their goals and intended lifestyle, aiming at promoting autonomy and independence. It is essential that its effectiveness is recorded. Not only does this allow the individual and his/her caregivers to evaluate its effect, it also gives the opportunity to reevaluate when confronted with problems during bowel care and change the routine when time progresses, based on objective measures, and it promotes continuity of care and identifications of problems. When evaluating the bowel management program, use both objective outcome measures and patient perception.

Items such as frequency of bowel care, time of day that care is delivered, the care provider and setting (e.g., toilet, bed), equipment, rectal stimulants and interventions used, and the order in which they are used (abdominal massage, digital rectal stimulation, evacuation, irrigation etcetera) should be recorded. Objective outcome measures such as episodes of fecal incontinence, stool consistency (Bristol Stool Scale), volume of incontinence, duration of bowel care episodes, result, and the Neurogenic Dysfunction Score [104] are essential keys for the evaluation of the program. Specific attention is required to document the condition of the perianal area (hemorrhoids, anal fissure, skin erosions, rectal bleeding, etc.), autonomic symptoms and dysreflexia episodes related to bowel care, abdominal symptoms (bloating, nausea, pain, etc.), and changes to any part of the bowel management program [3].

Impact of Interventions for Neurogenic Bowel Dysfunction on Quality of Life (QoL)

There is limited evidence evaluating interventions for NBD and its impact on QoL. Additionally, the range of reported prevalence of constipation and fecal incontinence in literature is substantial, due to varying definitions used. Adding to this confusion are the multiple scoring systems and QoL assessment tools, such as FICQoL for bowel dysfunction in spina bifida and QoL-BM for SCI and MS. These questionnaires have not been validated in larger, heterogeneous populations, and the correlation of their results with existing overall and disease-specific QoL questionnaires remains unclear [105]. Concerning patient-related outcomes measures (PROM), a standardized assessment tool is needed that is widely accepted and used to adequately assess bowel specific concerns and overall QoL.

Prognosis of NBD

Conservative treatment of NBD appears to be successful in 60–90% of NBD patients [68, 106, 107]. In most conditions the symptoms increase over time and management becomes more demanding. Where conservative methods of management are unsuccessful, the choices remain limited. The use of gut motility stimulants remains largely unexplored. As mentioned, transanal bowel irrigation (TAI) has received increasing attention in the adult literature, and although outcomes have been mainly positive, reliable identification of those patients likely to benefit in the long run remains elusive. The significant proportion of patients who stop using these irrigations merits further investigation [108]. Sacral nerve stimulation still has limited evidence regarding good long-term outcome and is mainly used for specific indications [109]. The use of a colostomy in this context remains limited, but it should be considered earlier than usual in the course of the individual's journey with neurogenic bowel dysfunction [29].

Further trials are required in all aspects of care of NBD including relatively simple elements like the role of fiber and diet but also the use and long-term implications of laxatives and other conservative measurements [29]. Further down the line, all surgical options lack appropriate evidence for their true long-term effect and benefit, particularly in appropriate trials comparing different techniques.

The development and adoption of agreed definitions of constipation and fecal incontinence in individuals with NBD would also greatly improve comparability of studies and facilitate meta-analysis of the findings of smaller trials [29].

References

1. Cameron AP, Rodriguez GM, Gursky A, et al. The severity of bowel dysfunction in patients with neurogenic bladder. J Urol. 2015;194:1336–41.
2. Chia YW, Fowler CJ, Kamm MA, et al. Prevalence of bowel dysfunction in patients with multiple sclerosis and bladder dysfunction. J Neurol. 1995;242(5):105–8.
3. Coggrave M, Ash D, Adcock C et al. Guidelines for management of neurogenic bowel dysfunction in individuals with central neurological conditions. Multidisciplinary Association of Spinal Cord Injured Professionals (MASCIP). 2012. http://www.mascip.co.uk/guidelines.aspx.
4. Chung AL, Emmanuel AV. Gastrointestinal symptoms related to autonomic dysfunction following spinal cord injury. In: Weaver LC, Polosa C, editors. Progress in brain research. New York: Elsevier; 2006. p. 317–33.
5. Christensen J. Normal colonic motor function and relevant structure. In: Holschneider AM, Puri P, editors. Hirschsprung's disease and allied disorders. Berlin, Heidelberg: Springer-Verlag; 2008. p. 79–94.
6. Brading AF, Ramalingham T. Mechanisms controlling normal defaecation and the potential effects of spinal cord injury. In: Weaver LC, Polosa C, editors. Progress in brain research. New York: Elsevier; 2006. p. 345–58.

7. Stiens SA, Bergman SB, Goetz LL. Neurogenic bowel dysfunction after spinal cord injury: clinical evaluation and rehabilitative management. Arch Phys Med Rehabil. 1997;78(3 Suppl):S86–S102.

8. Singal AK, Rosman AS, Bauman WA, Korsten MA. Recent concepts in the management of bowel problems after spinal cord injury. Adv Med Sci. 2006;51:15–22.

9. Longstreth GF, Thompson WD, Chey WG, et al. Functional bowel disorders. Gastroenterology. 2006;130(5):1480–91.

10. Coggrave M, Norton C, Wilson-Barnett J. Management of neurogenic bowel dysfunction in the community after spinal cord injury: a postal survey in the United Kingdom. Spinal Cord. 2009;47(4):323–30.

11. Krogh K, Nielsen J, Djurhuus JC, et al. Colorectal function in patients with spinal cord lesions. Dis Colon Rectum. 1997;40(10):1233–9.

12. Menter R, Weizenkamp D, Cooper D, et al. Bowel management outcomes in long-term spinal cord injuries. Spinal Cord. 1997;35(9):608–12.

13. Roach MJ, Frost FS, Creasey G. Social and personal consequences of acquired bowel dysfunction for persons with spinal cord injury. J Spinal Cord Med. 2000;23(4):263–9.

14. Hinds JP, Eidelman BH, Wald A. Prevalence of bowel dysfunction in multiple sclerosis. A population survey. Gastroenterology. 1990;98(6):1538–42.

15. Cersosimo MG, Benarroch EE. Pathological correlates of gastrointestinal dysfunction in Parkinson's disease. Neurobiol Dis. 2012;46(3):559–64.

16. Emmanuel A. Review of the efficacy and safety of transanal irrigation for neurogenic bowel dysfunction. Spinal Cord. 2010;48(9):664–73.

17. Norton C, Whitehead WE, Bliss DZ, et al. Conservative and pharmacological management of faecal incontinence in adults. In: Abrams P, Cardozo L, Khoury S, Wein A, editors. Incontinence. Plymouth: Health Publications; 2009. p. 1321–86.

18. Whitehead WE, Wald A, Diamant NE, et al. Functional disorders of the anus and rectum. Gut. 1999;45(Suppl 2):1155–9.

19. Harari D, Sarkarati M, Gurwitz J, et al. Constipation-related symptoms and bowel program concerning individuals with spinal cord injury. Spinal Cord. 1997;35:394–401.

20. Malone P, Wheeler R, Williams J. Continence in patients with spina bifida: long term results. Arch Dis Child. 1997;70(2):107–10.

21. McDonnell G, McCann J. Issues of medical management in adults with spina bifida. Childs Nerv Syst. 2000;16(4):222–7.

22. Verhoef M, Lurvink M, Barf HA, et al. High prevalence of incontinence among young adults with spina bifida: description, prediction and problem perception. Spinal Cord. 2005;43:331–40.

23. Coggrave M, Emmanuel A. Neurogenic bowel management. In: Fowler C, Panicker J, Emmanuel A, editors. Pelvic organ dysfunction in neurological disease. Cambridge: Cambridge Medicine, Cambridge University Press; 2010.

24. Coggrave M. Neurogenic continence. Part 3: bowel management strategies. Br J Nurs. 2008;17(11):706–10.

25. Kirshblum SC, House JG, Oçonnor KC. Silent autonomic dysreflexia during a routine bowel program in persons with traumatic spinal cord injury: a preliminary study. Arch Phys Med Rehabil. 2002;83(12):1774–6.

26. Colachis SC. Autonomic hyperreflexia with spinal cord injury. J Am Paraplegia Soc. 1992;15(3):171–86.

27. Cosman BC, Vu TT. Lidocaine anal block limits autonomic dysreflexia during anorectal procedures in spinal cord injury: a randomized, double-blind, placebo-controlled trial. Dis Colon Rectum. 2005;48(8):1556–61.

28. Nanigian DK, Nguyen T, Tanaka ST, et al. Development and validation of the fecal incontinence and constipation quality of life measure in children with spina bifida. J Urol. 2008;180:1770–3.

29. Coggrave M, Norton C, Cody JD. Management of faecal incontinence and constipation in adults with central neurological diseases. Cochrane Database Syst. 2014:CD002115.
30. De Looze D, Van Laere M, De Muynck M, et al. Constipation and other gastrointestinal problems in spinal cord injury patients. Spinal Cord. 1998;36(1):63–6.
31. Han TR, Kim JH, Kwon BS. Chronic gastrointestinal problems and bowel dysfunction in patients with spinal cord injury. Spinal Cord. 1998;36(7):485–90.
32. Correa GI, Rotter KP. Clinical evaluation and management of neurogenic bowel after spinal cord injury. Spinal Cord. 2000;38(5):301–8.
33. Lynch AC, Dobbs BR, Keating J, Frizelle FA. The prevalence of faecal incontinence and constipation in a general New Zealand population; a postal survey. N Z Med J. 2001;114(1142):474–7.
34. Freeman KA, Smith K, Adams E, et al. Is continence status associated with quality of life in young children with Spina Bifida? J Pediatr Rehabil Med. 2013;6(4):215–23.
35. Pardee C, Bricker D, Rundquist J, et al. Characteristics of neurogenic bowel in spinal cord injury and perceived quality of life. Rehabil Nurs. 2012;37(3):128–35.
36. The WHOQOL Group. The World Health Organization quality of life assessment (WHOQOL): position paper from the World Health Organization. Soc Sci Med. 1995;41(10):1403–9.
37. Gor RA, Katorski JAAR, Elliott SP. Medical and surgical management of neurogenic bowel. Curr Opin Urol. 2016;26(4):369–75.
38. Emmanuel AV, Krogh K, Christensen P, et al. Consensus review of best practice of transanal irrigation. Spinal Cord. 2013;51:732–8.
39. Krassioukov A, Eng JJ, Claxton G, et al. Neurogenic bowel management after spinal cord injury: a systematic review of the evidence. Spinal Cord. 2010;48(10):718–33.
40. Paris G, Gourcerol G, Leroi AM. Management of neurogenic bowel dysfunction. Eur J Phys Rehabil Med. 2011;47(4):661–76.
41. Heaton KW, Radvan J, Cripps H, et al. Defaecation frequency and timing, and stool form in the general population: a prospective study. Gut. 1992;33(6):818–24.
42. Rendeli C, Ausili E, Tabacco F, et al. Polyethylene glycol 4000 vs. lactulose for the treatment of neurogenic constipation in myelomeningocele children: a randomized-controlled clinical trial. Aliment Pharmacol Ther. 2006;23:1259–65.
43. Zangaglia R, Martignoni E, Glorioso M, et al. Macrogol for the treatment of constipation in Parkinson's disease. A randomized placebo-controlled study. Mov Disord. 2007;22(9):1239–44.
44. Gordon M, Naidoo K, Akobeng AK, Thomas AG. Osmotic and stimulant laxatives for the management of childhood constipation. Evid Based Child Health. 2013;8:57–109.
45. Ashraf W, Pfeiffer RF, Park F, et al. Constipation in Parkinson's disease: objective assessment and response to psyllium. Mov Disord. 1997;12(6):946–51.
46. Krogh K, Jensen MB, Gandrup P, et al. Efficacy and tolerability of prucalopride in patients with constipation due to spinal cord injury. Scand J Gastroenterol. 2002;37(4):431–6.
47. Rosman AS, Chaparala G, Monga A, et al. Intramuscular neostigmine and glycopyrrolate safely accelerated bowel evacuation in patients with spinal cord injury and defecatory disorders. Dig Dis Sci. 2008;53(10):2710–3.
48. Harari D. Bowel care in old age. In: Norton G, Chelvanayagam S, editors. Bowel continence nursing. Beaconsfield: Beaconsfield Publishers; 2004. p. 132–49.
49. Coggrave M. Neurogenic bowel management in chronic spinal cord injury: evidence for nursing care. Unpublished PhD. King's, College: London; 2007.
50. McClurg D, Hagen S, Hawkins S, Lowe-Strong A. Abdominal massage for the alleviation of constipation symptoms in people with multiple sclerosis: a randomized controlled feasibility study. Mult Scler. 2011;17:223–33.
51. Lämås K. Using massage to ease constipation. Nurs Times. 2011;17(4):26–7.
52. Yim S, Yoon S, Lee I, et al. A comparison of bowel care patterns in patients with spinal cord injury: upper motor neuron bowel vs lower motor neuron bowel. Spinal Cord. 2001;39:204–7.

53. Wiesel PH, Norton C, Roy AJ, et al. Gut focused behavioral treatment (biofeedback) for constipation and faecal incontinence in multiple sclerosis. J Neurol Neurosurg Psychiatry. 2000;69(2):240–3.
54. Yang D-H, Myung S-J, Jung KW, et al. Anorectal function and the effect of biofeedback therapy in ambulatory spinal cord disease patients having constipation. Scand J Gastroenterol. 2010;45:1281–8.
55. Wald A. Biofeedback therapy for fecal incontinence. Ann Intern Med. 1981;95:146–9.
56. Ash D, Harrison P, Slater W. Bowel management. In: Harrison P, editor. Managing spinal cord injury: the first 48 hours: SIA Milton Keynes; 2006. p. 20–1.
57. Korsten M, Singal A, Monga A, et al. Anorectal stimulation causes increased colonic motor activity in subjects with spinal cord injury. J Spinal Cord Med. 2007;30(1):31–5.
58. Wang F, Frsibie JH, Klein MA. Solitary rectal ulcer syndrome (colitis cystica profunda) in spinal cord injury patients: 3 case reports. Arch Phys Med Rehabil. 2001;82:260–1.
59. Kewalramani LS. Autonomic dysreflexia in traumatic myelopathy. Am J Phys Med. 1980;59:1–21.
60. Kyle G, Oliver H, Prynn P. The procedure for the digital removal of feces. Amsterdam: Norgine Ltd; 2005.
61. Consortium for Spinal Cord Medicine. Neurogenic bowel management in adults with spinal cord injury. J Spinal Cord Med. 1998;21:249–91.
62. Coggrave M. Transanal irrigation for bowel management. Nurs Times. 2007;103(26):47–9.
63. Christensen P, Bazzocchi G, Coggrave M, et al. A randomized, controlled trial of transanal irrigation versus conservative bowel management in spinal cord-injured patients. Gastroenterology. 2006;131(3):738–47.
64. Christensen P, Bazzocchi G, Coggrave M, et al. Outcome of transanal irrigation for bowel dysfunction in patients with spinal cord injury. J Spinal Cord Med. 2008;31:560–7.
65. Christensen P, Krogh K, Buntzen S, et al. Long-term outcome and safety of transanal irrigation for constipation and fecal incontinence. Dis Colon Rectum. 2009;52:286–92.
66. Ausili E, Focarelli B, Tabacco F, et al. Transanal irrigation in myelomeningocele children: an alternative, safe and valid approach for neurogenic constipation. Spinal Cord. 2010;48:560–5.
67. Del Popolo G, Mosiello G, Pilati C, et al. Treatment of neurogenic bowel dysfunction using transanal irrigation: a multicenter Italian study. Spinal Cord. 2008;46:517–22.
68. Velde SV, Biervliet SV, Bruyne RD, Winckel MV. A systematic review on bowel management and the success rate of the various treatment modalities in spina bifida patients. Spinal Cord. 2013;51:873–81.
69. Midrio P, Mosiello G, Ausili E, et al. Peristeen® transanal irrigation in paediatric patients with anorectal malformations and spinal cord lesions: a mulicentre Italian study. Colorectal Dis. 2016;18:86–93.
70. Christensen P, Krogh K. Transanal irrigation for disordered defecation: a systematic review. Scand J Gastroenterol. 2010;45(5):517–27.
71. Choi EK, Shin SH, Im YJ, et al. The effects of transanal irrigation as a stepwise bowel management program on the quality of life of children with spina bifida and their caregivers. Spinal Cord. 2013;51:384–8.
72. Faaborg PM, Christensen P, Kvitsau B, et al. Long-term outcome and safety of transanal colonic irrigation for neurogenic bowel dysfunction. Spinal Cord. 2009;47:545–9.
73. Malone PS, Ransley PG, Kiely EM. Preliminary report: the antegrade continence enema. Lancet. 1990;336:1217–8.
74. Chatoorgoon K, Pena A, Lawal T, et al. Neoappendicostomy in the management of pediatric fecal incontinence. J Pediatr Surg. 2011;46:1243–9.
75. Ok J, Kurzrock EA. Objective measurement of quality of life changes after ACE Malone using the FICQOL survey. J Pediatr Urol. 2011;7:389–93.
76. Curry JL, Osborne A, Malone PS. The MACE procedure: experience in the United Kingdom. J Pediatr Surg. 1999;34:338–40.

77. Chan DSY, Delicata RJ. Meta-analysis of antegrade continence enema in adults with faecal incontinence and constipation. Br J Surg. 2016;103:322–7.
78. Randall J, Coyne P, Jaffray B. Follow up of children undergoing antegrade continent enema: experience of over two hundred cases. J Pediatr Surg. 2014;49:1405–8.
79. Gerharz EW, Vik V, Webb G, et al. The value of the MACE (Malone antegrade colonic enema) procedure in adult patients. J Am Coll Surg. 1997;185:544–7.
80. Meurette G, Lehur PA, Coron E, Regenet N. Long-term results of Malone's procedure with antegrade irrigation for severe chronic constipation. Gastroenterol Clin Biol. 2010;34:209–12.
81. Chait PG, Shandling B, Richards HM, et al. Fecal incontinence in children: treatment with percutaneous cecostomy tube placement: a prospective study. Radiology. 1997;203:621–4.
82. Ellison JS, Haraway AN, Park JM. The distal left Malone antegrade continence enema - is it better? J Urol. 2013;190(4 suppl):1529–33.
83. Myers JB, Hu EM, Elliott SP, et al. Reconstructive urology short-term outcomes of Chait trapdoor for antegrade continence enema in adults. Urology. 2014;83:1423–6.
84. Marker DR, Perosi N, Ul Haq F, et al. Percutaneous cecostomy in adult patients: safety and quality-of-life results. J Vasc Interv Radiol. 2015;26:1526–32.
85. Randell N, Lynch AC, Anthony A, et al. Does a colostomy alter quality of life in patients with spinal cord injury? A controlled study. Spinal Cord. 2001;39(5):279–82.
86. Frisbie JH, Tun CG, Nguyen CH. Effect of enterostomy on quality of life in spinal cord injury patients. J Am Paraplegia Soc. 1986;9:3–5.
87. Kelly SR, Shashidharan M, Borwell B, et al. The role of intestinal stoma in patients with spinal cord injury. Spinal Cord. 1999;37:514–8.
88. Rosito O, Nino-Murcia M, Wolfe VA, et al. The effects of colostomy on the quality of life in patients with spinal cord injury: a retrospective analysis. J Spinal Cord Med. 2002;25:174–83.
89. Branagan G, Tromans A, Finnis D. Effect of stoma formation on bowel care and quality of life in patients with spinal cord injury. Spinal Cord. 2003;41:680–3.
90. Wong WD, Congliosi SM, Spencer MP, et al. The safety and efficacy of the artificial bowel sphincter for fecal incontinence. Dis Colon Rectum. 2002;45:1139–53.
91. Creasey GHMCF, Grill JHM, Korsten MAM, et al. An implantable neuroprosthesis for restoring bladder and bowel control to patients with spinal cord injuries: a multicenter trial. Arch Phys Med Rehabil. 2001;82:1512–9.
92. Liu L, Chung E, Coggrave M et al. Sacral anterior root stimulator implants (SARSI): their effect on patterns of bowel management in patients with spinal cord injury. Abstracts of ISCoS 44th Annual Scientific Meeting, Munich and Murnau, Germany, 2005.
93. Chia YW, Lee TK, Kour NW, et al. Microchip implants on the anterior sacral roots in patients with spinal trauma: does it improve bowel function? Dis Colon Rectum. 1996;39(6):690–4.
94. Jarrett M, Mowatt G, Glazener C, et al. Systematic review of sacral nerve stimulation for faecal incontinence and constipation. Br J Surg. 2004;91(12):1559–69.
95. Rosen HR, Urbarz C, Holzer B, et al. Sacral nerve stimulation as a treatment for fecal incontinence. Gastroenterology. 2001;121:536–41.
96. Jarrett ME, Matzel KE, Christiansen J, et al. Sacral nerve stimulation for fecal incontinence in patients with previous partial spinal injury including disc prolapse. Br J Surg. 2005;92:734–9.
97. Holzer B, Rosen HR, Novi G, et al. Sacral nerve stimulation for neurogenic fecal incontinence. Br J Surg. 2007;94:749–53.
98. Gourcerol G, Gallas S, Michot F, et al. Sacral nerve stimulation in fecal incontinence: are there factors associated with success? Dis Colon Rectum. 2007;50:3–12.
99. Korsten MA, Fajardo NR, Rosman AS, et al. Difficulty with evacuation after spinal cord injury: colonic motility during sleep and effects of abdominal wall stimulation. J Rehabil Res Dev. 2004;41(1):95–100.
100. Marshall DF, Boston VE. Altered bladder and bowel function following cutaneous electrical field stimulation in children with spina bifida - interim results of a randomized double-blind placebo-controlled trial. J Urol. 1997;158:1272–6.

101. Lin VWH, Nino-Murcia M, Frost F, et al. Functional magnetic stimulation of the colon in persons with spinal cord injury. Arch Phys Med Rehabil. 2001;82:167–73.
102. Chiu CM, Wang CP, Sung WH, et al. Functional magnetic stimulation in constipation associated with Parkinson's disease. J Rehabil Med. 2009;41:1085–9.
103. Tsai PY, Wang CP, Chiu FY, et al. Efficacy of functional magnetic stimulation in neurogenic bowel dysfunction after spinal cord injury. J Rehabil Med. 2009;41:41–7.
104. Krogh K, Christensen P, Sabroe S, Laurberg S. Neurogenic bowel dysfunction score. Spinal Cord. 2006;44:625–31.
105. Patel DP, Elliott SP, Stoffel JT, et al. Patient reported outcomes measures in neurogenic bladder and bowel: a systematic review of the current literature. Neurourol Urodyn. 2016;35:8–14.
106. Vande Velde S, van Biervliet S, van Laecke E, et al. Colon enemas for fecal incontinence in patients with spina bifida. J Urol. 2013;189(1):300–4.
107. Faleiros-Castro FL, de Paula EDR. Constipation in patients with quadriplegic cerebral palsy: intestinal reeducation using massage and a laxative diet. Rev Esc Enferm USP. 2013;47:836–42.
108. Faaborg PM, Christensen P, Buntzen S, et al. Anorectal function after long-term transanal colonic irrigation. Colorectal Dis. 2010;12(10):e314–9.
109. Lombardi G, Del Popolo G, Cecconi F, et al. Clinical outcome of sacral neuromodulation in incomplete spinal cord-injured patients suffering from neurogenic bowel dysfunction. Spinal Cord. 2010;48(2):154–9.

Part VI
Clinical Entities: Sexual Dysfunction

Erectile Dysfunction and Anejaculation in the Neurologic Patient

Uroš Milenković and Maarten Albersen

Background

A normal erection is a hormonally controlled, combined neurovascular tissue phenomenon. Arterial dilatation, trabecular smooth muscle relaxation, and activation of the corporeal veno-occlusive mechanisms are essential components of the process. The NIH Consensus Development Panel on Impotence defined erectile dysfunction (ED) as the persistent inability to attain and maintain an erection sufficient for satisfactory sexual intercourse. ED is the preferred term since sexual desire and the ability to achieve orgasm may as well be intact, in absence of an erection. While premature ejaculation is probably the most prevalent, ED is without a doubt the most studied male sexual dysfunction and a highly prevalent sexual complaint in men presenting to their healthcare providers. Notwithstanding variations in definitions and methodology, various large-scale studies substantiate the high global prevalence of ED.

Epidemiology

According to the Massachusetts Male Aging Study (MMAS) (the first large prospective observational longitudinal study in healthy, randomly selected men), ED has a high prevalence and incidence worldwide. This pilot, landmark study was performed in different parts of the globe (Boston, Cologne, NHSLS, Brazil, the Netherlands, Taiwan, Ghana, etc.). The highest number reported includes an overall

U. Milenković (✉) · M. Albersen
Department of Urology, University Hospitals, Leuven, Belgium
e-mail: maarten.albersen@uzleuven.be

© Springer International Publishing AG, part of Springer Nature 2018
R. Dmochowski, J. Heesakkers (eds.), *Neuro-Urology*,
https://doi.org/10.1007/978-3-319-90997-4_19

prevalence of 52% in the United States among non-institutionalized men between 40 and 70 years old (17% was minimal, 25% moderate, and 10% included complete ED).

Even though the prevalence of mild ED remained the same (17%) between the ages of 40 and 70 years old, a doubling of moderate ED (34%) and even a tripling of the amount of men reporting complete ED were noticeable.

Reports from men over 65 years old indicate that around 70% are still sexually active, although close to 40% are dissatisfied with their sexual function.

In the European Male Aging Study (EMAS), the mean age of reported ED was 60 years old. About one-third of all patients included in the EMAS showed signs of ED. EMAS is a collaborative effort of eight European centers investigating the effects of aging on general and sexual health in a 40- to 79-year-old male population.

Despite patients in older age groups being more frequently affected by the disease, they are not bothered as much with the presence of ED. An increase in ED in the years to come is to be expected, especially with our rapidly aging population and longer life expectancy. In a short 10 years, it is estimated that about 10% of the world population will be older than 65 years; consequently, the number of men suffering from ED will reach 322 million worldwide.

Erectile Dysfunction as a Harbinger of Cardiovascular Disease

Although ED cannot be viewed as an immediate danger to the health status of the patient, it still can have profound effects on the quality of life, personal well-being of the patient, and sexual partner alike. Notwithstanding the psychological distress, ED is an important independent predictor for cardiovascular morbidity and mortality.

A urological dogma says, "the penis is the antenna of the heart," and as such, the complaint of ED should always trigger further questioning and investigation to identify possible underlying cardiovascular disease or other comorbidities. Hypertension, hyperlipidemia, metabolic syndrome, diabetes mellitus, cardiac disease, and smoking are major predictors of ED and vice versa. The latter occurs in a dose-dependent matter. In the MMAS study, exercise starting from midlife leads to a 70% reduced risk in ED compared to sedentary men.

Other causes with a high prevalence of ED include brachytherapy, radiation, or surgery for prostate cancer or other pelvic malignancies. Alternatively, ED can be caused by a myriad of medications. Psychologically speaking, ED correlates with decreased self-esteem, depression, anxiety, anger, and relationship dissatisfaction.

Of importance to the readers of this book is to be aware that community-based, preclinical, and clinical data have demonstrated a strong and consistent association between LUTS and ED. And so, it should be paramount that elderly men with LUTS get evaluated for ED and vice versa.

Considering this, it should be clear that ED merits attention from the primary care general practitioner, as well as the specialist. It is an important health concern and could be an augur for other serious medical conditions. In this chapter the pathophysiology, diagnostic evaluation, and treatment of ED in men will be discussed.

Prerequisites for Normal Erections and Pathophysiology of ED

Sex drive is the main initiator of penile erection. Therefore, an intact libido, mood, and psychosocial circumstances are of the greatest importance for normal erectile function. Penile erection requires neural transmission of pro-erectile impulses, i.e. the efficacious delivery of the neurotransmitter nitric oxide (NO) to the smooth muscle in the corpus cavernosum by nerve endings and endothelium. Furthermore, an intact arterial blood supply is key for supplying the cavernous erectile tissue with sufficient oxygenated blood. The end organ, the corpus cavernosum, needs to be in good health, containing elastic smooth muscle tissue to successfully expand and compress the subtunical venous plexus during the rigid phase of erection. Lastly, hormonal balance should be in order, considering testosterone is a key mediator of libido and keeps the peripheral effectors, such as cavernous smooth muscle and cavernous nerves, in good shape. ED can develop as a result of failure in one of these systems or, as is commonly the case, a multilevel failure. ED is typically defined as neurogenic, vasculogenic, hormonal, anatomical/structural, drug-induced, or psychogenic. A summary of prevalent causes of ED is given in Table 1.

Diagnostic Evaluation

In the management of ED, it is essential that there is context of a trusting patient/ provider relationship. It requires a detailed medical and sexual history of patients and partners alike. An effort should be made to include the partner on the second, if not the first, visit. Taking a comprehensive medical history may reveal one of the many common disorders associated with ED. As mentioned, the pathophysiology may be vasculogenic, neurogenic, anatomical, hormonal, drug-induced, and/or psychogenic.

Of great importance is creating a relaxed atmosphere during history taking. It can facilitate asking questions about sexual history and erectile dysfunction. One can consider displaying literature in the consultation and waiting rooms, signifying a discrete and nonjudgmental approach toward sexual dysfunction and ED.

The initial evaluation of ED should include a complete medical, psychosocial, and sexual history with the aim of identifying comorbid or underlying disease.

Table 1 Comorbid conditions and causes for ED

Vasculogenic	Cardiovascular disease; atherosclerosis
	Hypertension
	Diabetes mellitus
	Hyperlipidemia
	Smoking
	Major surgery (retroperitoneum)
	Radiotherapy (retroperitoneum)
Neurogenic—central causes	Multiple sclerosis
	Multiple atrophy
	Parkinson's disease
	Tumors
	Stroke
	Intravertebral disc disease
	Spinal cord disorders
Neurogenic—peripheral causes	Diabetes mellitus
	Alcoholism
	Uremia
	Polyneuropathy
	Surgery (pelvis or retroperitoneum, radical prostatectomy)
Anatomical/structural	Peyronie's disease
	Penile fibrosis (following pelvic radiotherapy or pelvic surgery)
	Penile trauma (penile fracture)
	Congenital curvature of the penis
	Micropenis
	Hypospadias, epispadias
Hormonal	Primary hypogonadism (e.g., late-onset hypogonadism)
	Secondary hypogonadism/hypogonadotropic hypogonadism (e.g., hyperprolactinemia)
	Hyper- and hypothyroidism
	Cushing's disease
Drug or substance induced	Antihypertensives (thiazides and beta-blockers are most common)
	Antidepressants
	Antipsychotics
	Antiandrogens
	Antihistamines
	Recreational drugs/smoking
Psychogenic	Generalized type (e.g., lack of arousability and disorders of sexual intimacy)
	Situational type (e.g., partner-related and performance-related issues or due to distress)

Sexual History Taking and Questionnaires

When available, the sexual history should include information about previous and present sexual relations, emotional status of patient and partner, onset and duration of the problem, and significance of this concern for this particular couple. Sexual orientation issues and gender identity should be addressed as well. Descriptive comments on rigidity and duration of nocturnal erections, morning erections, erections during masturbation, and erections during sexual arousal should be made, as they can give clues toward the etiology. The onset and situational factors that ameliorate and exacerbate ED should be documented. For instance, the persistent presence of nocturnal erections and good erectile function during masturbation, with situational or sudden onset of ED hints toward a psychogenic component. Conversely, non-situational ED, gradual onset, and loss of the naturally occurring nocturnal erections are strong clues for an organic cause of ED. The distinction is not always this clear, often a psychogenic factor (e.g., performance anxiety) superposes onto an existing organic disorder. Problems with arousal, ejaculation, and difficulty reaching orgasm should be discussed as well.

The most commonly used validated psychometric questionnaires are the 15-item International Index of Erectile Function (IIEF) and the abridged 5-item version (IIEF-5) (or Sexual Health Inventory for Men (SHIM)), which is more suited for office use. They can serve as an "icebreaker" and help measure certain functions more objectively, such as sexual desire, erectile function, orgasmic function, ejaculation, intercourse, and overall satisfaction. It has a proven strong internal consistency and adequate test-retest reliability.

In cases when clinical depression is suspected, the use of a 2-question scale for depression is recommended: "During the past month, have you often been bothered by feeling down, depressed or hopeless? During the past month have you often been bothered by little interest or pleasure doing thing?"

Screening for hypogonadism is necessary as well as decreased energy, libido, fatigue, and cognitive impairment, as well as symptomatic LUTS. If appropriate, screening questionnaires, such as the International Prostate Symptom Score (IPSS), should be utilized.

Cardiovascular Disease

Patients seeking treatment for sexual dysfunction have a high prevalence of cardiovascular disease. Although arteriogenic ED can be present congenitally or posttraumatically, often it is a part of a wider systemic arterial disease. Epidemiological surveys have confirmed the association between cardiovascular and metabolic risk factors and sexual dysfunction in men and women. Identification of ED can improve the sensitivity of screening for asymptomatic cardiovascular disease in men with (un)diagnosed diabetes mellitus (DM). The third Princeton Consensus (a leading document on the relationship of ED and cardiovascular disease) states that:

Table 2 Cardiovascular risk assessment in ED patients

Low-risk category	Intermediate-risk category	High-risk category
Asymptomatic, <3 risk factors for CAD (excluding sex)	>2 risk factors for CAD (excluding sex)	High-risk arrhythmias
Mild, stable angina (evaluated and/or being treated)	Moderate, stable angina	Unstable or refractory angina
Uncomplicated previous MI	Recent MI (>2, <6 weeks)	Recent MI (<2 weeks)
LVD/CHF (NYHA class I)	LVD/CHF (NYHA class II)	LVD/CHF (NYHA class III/IV)
Post-successful coronary revascularization	Noncardiac sequelae of atherosclerotic disease (e.g., stroke, peripheral vascular disease)	Hypertrophic obstructive and other cardiomyopathies)
Controlled hypertension		Uncontrolled hypertension
Mild valvular disease		Moderate-to-severe valvular disease

CAD coronary artery disease, *CHF* congestive heart failure, *LVD* left ventricular dysfunction, *MI* myocardial infarction, *NYHA* New York Heart Association
Adapted from Nehra A et al. The Princeton III Consensus recommendations for the management of erectile dysfunction and cardiovascular disease

- ED does not only share risk factors with cardiovascular disease but is an independent marker of increased cardiovascular risk (ACCF/AHA Class Ia).
- ED significantly increases the risk of cardiovascular disease, coronary heart disease, stroke, and all-cause mortality.

The recommendations emphasize the testing of exercise ability and stress endurance before prescribing treatment for ED. This highlights the fact that patients with ED may benefit from cardiovascular risk reduction. These patients can be stratified into three cardiovascular risk categories (Table 2) and can be used as a basis for an algorithm for initiating or resuming sexual activity.

As previously mentioned, ED is an independent marker of cardiovascular events (1.5× relative risk) and all-cause mortality (1.2× relative risk) superposed on traditional risk factors (e.g., age, positive family history of cardiovascular events, weight, hypertension, diabetes, hyperlipidemia, and cigarette smoking). Thus, we can strongly recommend further investigation of underlying cardiovascular disease in a patient presenting with ED. Typically, time to coronary artery disease event and ED onset is 2–5 years (Class Ia), and so, it provides an excellent opportunity for cardiovascular risk reduction.

Aging and Systemic Disease

It is well-known that sexual function progressively declines in "healthy" aging. A nonlinear decline is seen in most aspects of sexual function with increased age, with a more pronounced decline in older groups. Relational, psychologic, and organic issues contribute significantly to ED across age groups; however, as men age, organic reasons play a more profound role.

ED appears three times as frequently in men with DM compared to the general population. It approaches 55% at 60 years old and can either be a presenting symptom or a predictor of neurological sequelae. DM can have profound neurovascular effects, thus decreasing the responsiveness of oral PDE-5 inhibitor therapy overtime.

Men with pulmonary disease may have ED because of fear of aggravating dyspnea during sexual intercourse.

Anxiety, depression, or penile arterial insufficiency is relatively common in patients with angina, myocardial infarction (MI), or heart failure and may contribute to ED.

Chronic renal failure as well has been consistently associated with decreased erectile function, impaired libido, and infertility. Many were found to have cavernous artery occlusive disease and veno-occlusive dysfunction. This ED is likely multifactorial, a combination of low serum testosterone, DM, vascular insufficiency, polypharmacy, autonomic and somatic neuropathy, and psychological distress.

Clinical Examination

General Considerations

For many patients, a first sexual clinical examination can be experienced as stressful and embarrassing, while others see it as a potential for alleviation and consolation. A comfortable setting for the physical exam is necessary. Not only is this more convenient for the patient, it leads to more consistent and reliable clinical data. Stress can augment the adrenergic tonus and confound the results, especially in young men where a psychogenic factor is the most important. Explanation of the course of examination is important, as this shows how the proposed examinations can lead to a diagnosis and treatment. Delaying the examination if the patient is too stressed out is a viable option.

Broader Picture

When patients consult a first-line medical care provider for the first time with a complaint of ED, it can be the prelude of a serious, yet undiagnosed, underlying medical condition. For example, it could be an augur for hypogonadotropic hypogonadism and/or a prolactinoma of the pituitary gland.

Physical examination uncommonly leads to the correct diagnosis; nonetheless it can reveal valuable information. The main goal is assessing prostatic disease, cardiovascular or neurological comorbidity, penile deformity or plaques (signifying Peyronie's disease), and signs of hypogonadism.

The best strategy to stratify ED patients who need further cardiovascular work-up is by dividing the patients into risk groups (high, intermediate, and low), according to the SCORE system or Framingham Risk Score. Intermediate-risk patients should undergo an exercise stress test, and high-risk patients need a cardiological referral. A low threshold for additional testing should be handled when in doubt.

General Non-genital Exam

This should include a brief overall health assessment, length and weight to calculate the body mass index (BMI, kg/m^2), blood pressure, and heart rate. Waist circumference is an important measure to assess the risk for abdominal obesity and metabolic syndrome. An easy question for this could be asking about pants size. Palpation of the peripheral arterial pulsation and carotid auscultation can be performed. Physical proportions, pubic and general hair growth, pitch of the voice, and presence of gynecomastia should be assessed.

Neurologic Exam and Spinal Cord Reflexes

Assessment of the perineal and lower limb dermatomes can be performed by tactile and pinprick sensation. More profound testing of reflexes is not advised routinely, but can be executed if spinal cord injuries are suspected.

The somatic S2-S4 innervation can be tested with the perianal reflex or anal wink (stroking the skin around the anus); it causes a reflexive contraction of the external anal sphincter. The bulbocavernosus reflex can be seen in 70% of healthy men, although the validity of this has been recently challenged. It can be provoked by firmly squeezing the glans penis with contraction of the bulbocavernosus muscle between the scrotum and anal sphincter (S2-S3). By the same maneuver, the bulbo-anal reflex can be evoked (S3-S4).

Genital Examination

The penis should be checked for abnormalities in size, stance, and overall appearance. Flaccid penis size ranges from 5 to 10 cm. A very short penis (micropenis) can be the result of a wide array of genetic disorders, such as hypo- or hypergonadotropic hypogonadism or androgen resistance (e.g., Klinefelter or Kallmann syndrome). The glans should be inspected for signs of infection. Palpation of the penis is necessary to determine the presence of fibrous plaques under the skin that can signify the existence of Peyronie's disease. The physician either injects alprostadil to induce an erection during consultation or relies on pictures taken by the patient at home to assess the presence of a deformity.

The bilateral presence of normal-sized testes should be investigated. A normal testis volume is around 12–20 mL and can be measured using an orchidometer or ultrasound. Patients with Klinefelter syndrome have small, firm testes. The investigator should also look for non-tender nodules or masses on the testes that could signify a tumor. A painless testicular swelling could also be a hydrocele, typically visible on transillumination.

Since there is a strong relationship between LUTS and ED, due to the correlation of BPH and sexual dysfunction, a digital rectal exam (DRE) should always be performed. A DRE should be performed in every patient above 40 years old. The presence of noduli or firm irregular zones calls for further prostate assessment.

Laboratory Testing

Laboratory investigation should be tailored to the complaints, risk factors, and pre-test probability of associated conditions. Fasting glucose or HbA1C and lipid profiling are necessary if not completed recently. Hormonal profiling is done by measuring free and total testosterone from a morning sample; it is especially recommended in patients with signs of hypogonadism. However, results should be interpreted with care; for levels >8 nM, the correlation between circulating testosterone and sexual function is very low.

Additional hormonal tests are only indicated when a low testosterone is detected (e.g., FSH, LH, etc.). PSA screening can be performed in patients above 40 years old or when LUTS accompany the ED.

Additional Diagnostic Testing

A myriad of vascular and neurologic diagnostic tests are available to identify the cause of ED and plan treatment for patients with more complex problems. These are not routinely recommended in primary care setting. They can be ordered when there is penile deformity, history of pelvic or perineal trauma, ED of unknown etiology, cases requiring vascular or neurosurgical intervention, endocrinopathy, complicated psychiatric disorders, or complex relationship issues.

Especially in young men with primary ED investigations, intracavernosal injection of vasoactive substances with subsequent color Doppler or duplex of the penile arteries may be helpful to rule out correctable, vascular causes. It may also assist in identifying venous leakage in specific situations. In this way, the neurogenic and hormonal influences are bypassed as the vascular status of the penis is assessed objectively. An erection lasting >10 min is indicative of normal venous function. No conclusions can be made about the arterial status, since men with mild arterial insufficiency may still have sufficient erections.

Nocturnal penile tumescence (NPT) tests have no role in routine evaluation of ED. They are used to distinguish between organic and psychogenic ED. Nocturnal erections occur in 80% of healthy men and are relatively free of psychologically mediated effects.

Clinical Practice: Treatment

Lifestyle Changes and General Principles

Underlying reversible conditions should be tackled and treated before or together with starting up specific ED-directed treatment. The beneficial effects of lifestyle adjustments (total body weight loss of 10% or more by reducing caloric intake and increasing physical activity) were proven in a randomized, single-blind trial of 110 obese men. In the intervention group, the IIEF score improved but remained stable in the control group who were given general considerations about exercise and healthy food. As previously mentioned, ED is closely related to the atherosclerotic coronary and peripheral vascular diseases, as well as the metabolic syndrome. The risk of ED for improving underlying dysfunction can be reduced by a combination of regular exercise, healthy diet, smoking cessation, and limiting the use of alcohol, where applicable.

Another modifiable risk factor for ED might be chronic perineal compression on penile arteries from long-distance cycling. Changing the bicycle seat or riding practices will often lead to ED improvement.

When there is a complaint of sexual dysfunction after taking certain medication, it is useful to determine the exact nature of the problem, whether it is a loss of sexual drive, impaired erection, or rapid/delayed ejaculation. Usually, changing to a different class of medication is a sensible first step. Since antihypertensive agents lower the blood pressure, this has been thought of as the mechanism of occurring ED. Switching to calcium channel blockers and/or angiotensin-converting enzyme (ACE) inhibitors may reverse ED in some cases.

Patients with severe psychological issues as an underlying cause should be referred to a psychologist or sex therapist, since elimination of this condition may result in a cure.

Pharmacotherapy: Phosphodiesterase Type 5 Inhibitors (PDE-5I)

It is necessary to set realistic treatment goals for patients. Current medication does not "cure" ED; it acts solely symptomatic to the underlying cause. However, they can be relied upon to greatly improve erectile function. One should also focus on legitimizing a kind of intimacy that does not only depend on penetrative sexual intercourse. Regaining unassisted potency will not be possible for most ED patients. Nonetheless, a great deal of patients should be able to experience restoration of satisfying sexual encounters, with or without pharmacotherapy.

Currently, the four most well-known selective and approved PDE-5Is; sildenafil (Viagra), vardenafil (Levitra), tadalafil (Cialis), and avanafil (Spedra), have equivalent efficacy in the treatment of ED (several trials have established an on-demand efficacy of 60–70%), are well tolerated, and have similar contraindications and caveats. They have become the preferred first-line therapy for most men with ED, thanks to their high efficacy, excellent safety profiles and ease of use.

During sexual stimulation NO is set free from nerve endings and vascular endothelium cells in the penis, diffusing into vascular and corporal smooth muscle cells. Subsequent stimulation of guanylyl cyclase (GC) raises the amount of intracellular cGMP. The second messenger cascade causes a lowering of intracytoplasmatic calcium, resulting in smooth muscle relaxation, vasodilatation, and penile erection.

PDE-5Is are non-hydrolysable analogs of cGMP and trigger the physiologic erectile response to sexual stimulation and NO and amplify the NO-cGMP pathway by way of competitive inhibition of second-messenger cGMP enzymatic degradation (by PDE-5). So, PDE-5Is potentiate, rather than trigger, the physiologic response to NO and exert their effect regardless of the underlying etiology of ED.

Each of the different molecules has slightly different pharmacokinetics. Effects of vardenafil and sildenafil last up to 5 h, while avanafil has a slightly faster course of action and lasts longer. Tadalafil has a window of 36–48 h in which the patient can rely upon its effect to have sexual intercourse. This means there is less planning and pressure to have intercourse bound to a schedule, resulting in greater convenience.

Adverse events seen with the use of PDE-5Is are limited. In randomized, controlled trials flushing (10%) and vision disturbances were more common in patients using sildenafil or vardenafil, and back pain/myalgia (1–4%) was more frequent in tadalafil users. These were, however, very mild, dissipated with time, and did not lead to a discontinuation of therapy in many patients.

PDE-5 inhibition in the vascular bed or gastrointestinal vessels can cause headaches (15%), flushing, rhinitis (5–10%), slight lowering of blood pressure, dyspepsia, etc.

Since ED is common in men with generalized atherosclerotic disease and coronary disease, there was a safety concern regarding heart disease. Post-marketing studies showed no increased risk of MI or death rates in double-blind, placebo-controlled study designs. As mentioned before, patients should undergo cardiovascular assessment following the Princeton III Consensus. This will determine if the patient is fit enough to have sexual intercourse.

Certain drugs interfere with the usual pharmacokinetics of PDE-5Is through induction or inhibition of liver enzymes of the cytochrome p450 system. Itraconazole, ketoconazole, and protease inhibitors (such as ritonavir) slow down the metabolic breakdown of PDE-5Is by blocking the CYP3A4 pathway and may require a dose reduction. Conversely, agents such as rifampicin, carbamazepine, phenytoin, and phenobarbital induce the CYP3A4 system which leads to enhancement of the breakdown of PDE-5Is and asks for dose escalation.

As an important contraindication, nitroglycerin should not be used within 24 h of intake of sildenafil/vardenafil or 48 h for tadalafil, since a life-threatening hypotensive episode may occur with concurrent use. There is also a warning against use of PDE-5Is in patients with severe cardiovascular diseases, left ventricular outflow obstruction, unstable angina pectoris, recent MI, arrhythmias, and poorly controlled hypertension. Furthermore, concomitant use with some alpha-blockers may cause postural hypotension.

It is recommended to start at highest doses available (100 mg for sildenafil and 20 mg for tadalafil and vardenafil) and lower dosage according to efficacy and adverse events. It is important to stress the fact that sexual stimulation is paramount for the drug to work. Incorrect use and disinformation are the main reasons for therapy failure.

Furthermore, patients with concomitant LUTS are the ideal candidates for daily PDE-5I dosage in the form of 2.5–5 mg tadalafil daily.

Pharmacotherapy: Intracavernous Injection (ICI) and Intra-urethral Administration of Vasodilating Compounds

Nowadays (local) intracavernous and intra-urethral treatment are a second-line treatment option for ED in a group of patients not responding to PDE-5I. Prostaglandin E1 (PGE1) (or the synthetic formulation alprostadil) is the most commonly used compound, as well as the only FDA-approved one. Its working mechanism is independent of the NO-cGMP pathway and thus ideal for PDE-5I non-responders or patients with intolerable side effects. Alprostadil causes smooth muscle relaxation, vasodilatation, and inhibition of platelet aggregation through elevation of intracellular cAMP. After injection, 96% of the compound is metabolized locally within 60 min, and no change in peripheral blood levels is seen.

ICI PGE1 therapy has relatively high success rates when the patients are motivated and well-informed and expectations are realistic. Papaverine is available for ICI as well; however its uses are limited to combination therapy (also known as BiMix or TriMix).

Alprostadil is also available for intra-urethral administration as a pellet (medicated urethral system for erection (MUSE)) and is currently being launched into a cream to be applied into the urethra through the meatus. Topical applications of PGE1 and MUSE are both associated with urethral burning or pain. Vaginal irritation in the partner is also seen; so the use of a condom should be considered.

ICI of PGE1 has several potential advantages for the patient in question, including a rapid onset of action, reduced incidence of systemic complications, limited drug interactions, and reliable efficacy for vascular and nonvascular forms of

ED. Efficacy rates in the general ED population have found to be >70%, as well as in certain subgroups (e.g., diabetes or cardiovascular disease) with reported sexual activity after 94% of the injections and satisfactory rates of 87–93.5% in patients and 86–90.3% in partners.

Complications include penile pain (even though 50% of the patients experienced pain, the pain was only present after 11% of the total amount of injections), small hematoma or bruising, prolonged erections (5%), priapism (1–3%), and fibrosis (1–3%). Systemic side effects are rare to nonexistent.

Despite favorable data and satisfaction, high drop-out rates remain, ranging from 40 to 70% and occurring mostly within the first 2–3 months. Major contributing factors are desired for a permanent solution, lack of a suitable partner, poor response, fear of needles and complications, and lack of spontaneity.

It is imperative that the physician stresses that priapism is a urologic emergency and any erection lasting more than 4 h without sexual stimulus requires urgent medical attention. Most frequently this is caused by rapid dose escalation by the patient, while gradual and progressive dose increases will prevent most cases of priapism. The best treatment is diluted 250–300 µg of phenylephrine every 3–5 min until detumescence while monitoring blood pressure and pulse, especially in patients with cardiovascular disease.

ICI should not be administered in patients with sickle cell anemia, schizophrenia, or a severe psychiatric disorder intake of antipsychotics and severe venous incompetence.

When there is poor manual dexterity, the sexual partner can be instructed to perform the injection.

Vacuum Erection Device (VED)

For some patients, a VED may be the first-line therapy in case of reluctance for medication use or those with contraindications. This is a good option for patients with veno-occlusive disease where PDE-5Is and ICI with PGE1 are not appropriate.

A negative pressure is created within the penis by the device, initiating passive engorgement of the sinusoidal spaces and inducing an erection. A constricting ring is applied to the base of the penis to maintain erection. Due to the resulting cold penis and trapped ejaculation, this may be an undesirable option for younger patients, even though it is effective in 90% of the patients. Other complications include penile pain and numbness, ecchymosis, petechiae, and difficult ejaculation. It is advised to limit the penile constriction for up to 30 min to avoid skin necrosis.

Nonetheless, some patients may prefer this option as it is a one-time investment, whereas this is not the case with PDE-5I and ICI.

Surgery

Surgical implantation of a penile prosthesis may be considered in patients who do not respond to previously mentioned methods or who are considering a more permanent solution. The implanted device can either be malleable or inflatable (two- or three-piece). Non-inflatable devices have the advantage of being lower cost, better mechanical reliability, and ease of use. However, inflatable devices resemble the natural states of a flaccid and erect penis best. The surgical technique is quite straightforward, and asepsis during surgery is of paramount importance. The most commonly used device is the three-piece one, which contains the paired penile cylinders, a scrotal pump, and a suprapubic fluid reservoir. Modern three-piece devices are extremely durable and reliable. Nonetheless, patients should be informed of the 5–15% failure rate within the first 5 years and around 50% after 10 years. Most of the devices will fail within 15 years and will need replacement.

Overall, it has a satisfactory rate of 70–90%, but patients should be aware of the definitive and irreversible nature of this surgery. This means that if the patient is not satisfied or complications occur, there is no other therapeutic option left after the removal of the device.

Other complications include infection (1–3%) and, rarely, erosion. Preventive measures for infection are of the utmost significance. In practice this means that the patient should not have a urinary tract infection or infection elsewhere. No wounds, cutaneous lesions, or dermatitis are allowed in the operative field. Antibiotics covering Gram-positive and Gram-negative bacteria should be provided preoperatively and 24–48 h postoperatively.

Other surgical options for ED include penile revascularization and venous ligation. Outcomes of these surgeries, however, are poor and should be withheld for a selective group of mostly young patients.

Erectile Dysfunction in the Neurologic Patient

Some patients regard the altered sexual experience due to their neurologic disease as the worst facet of their affliction. Neurologic disorders can change the processing of sexual stimuli, including increased or decreased desire, diminish penile engorgement, and spontaneous ejaculation and orgasms.

Owing to the development of noninvasive functional imaging technology in the form of positron emission tomography and magnetic resonance (fMRI), several areas activated during sexual stimulation were identified and studied further. (E.g., erotic images activate the (para)limbic regions in sexually healthy people which are presumed to be essential for sexual motivation.)

An overview for sexual dysfunctions and their treatments in neurological disorders is given in Table 3.

Table 3 Sexual dysfunctions in neurological disorders and treatment options

	Applicability	Randomized controlled trials	Clinical comments
Fatigue or hypersomnolence	TBI, SAH	Methylphenidate	Potential replacement of GH or hypocretin-1
Prefrontal executive dysfunction	TBI	Bromocriptine	
Hypersexuality	TBI, stroke, epilepsy PD		CBT, SSRIs, steroidal antiandrogens (spironolactone, cyproterone, medroxyprogesterone), nonsteroidal antiandrogens (e.g., flutamide), GnRH agonists (leuprorelin, etc.), dopamine antagonists, and atypical antipsychotics (e.g., quetiapine). No data for use of antiandrogens in women) Quetiapine (no dopamine antagonists), avoid high-dose spironolactone (hypotension)
Gonadal axis deficiency	TBI, SAH		Potential replacement of testosterone
Spasticity	TBI, stroke, MS, SCI		Baclofen, tizanidine, sclerosing injections, or Botox injections
Vaginal lubrication	SCI MS	Minor increase from PDE-5I Minor increase from PDE-5I but no improvement to orgasmic capacity or overall sexual response	
Erectile dysfunction	PD, stroke, SCI, MS, PN PD PD PD, stroke, PN SCI MS	PDE-5Is are usually beneficial in PD, enhancement of both reflexes and psychogenic erections, MS Apomorphine (small trial)	Caution with PDE5is in PD, especially MSA, hypotension risk Clinical improvement noted DBS can improve sexuality in men, but not in women Intracavernosal PGE1 if contra-indication for PDE-5I PGE1 is effective for both reflex and psychogenic erections PGE1 is effective

TBI traumatic brain injury, *SAH* subarachnoid hemorrhage, *GH* growth hormone, *CBT* cognitive behavioral therapy, *SSRI* selective serotonin reuptake inhibitor, *MS* multiple sclerosis, *SCI* spinal cord injury, *PD* Parkinson's disease, *MSA* multiple system atrophy, *PN* peripheral neuropathy, *DBS* deep brain stimulation, *PDE5i* phosphodiesterase type 5 inhibitor, *PGE-1* intracavernosal prostaglandin E-1

Adapted from Rees et al. Sexual function in men and women with neurological disorders. The Lancet 2007;369:512–25

Head Trauma

Sometimes the effects of neuronal injury on sexual function can be confounded with general changes in mood or pain from musculoskeletal injury, which can make the assessment of neuron damage alone particularly challenging. In other words, the overall, non-cerebral effects after brain injury might explain the high reported rates (36–54%) of sexual dysfunction in this set of patients, mainly encompassing hypoactive sexual desire disorder. Damage to the prefrontal cortex may either lead to apathy with hyposexuality or, less commonly, disinhibition with hypersexuality (making inappropriate sexual remarks or exhibitionism). Lobar injuries outside of the prefrontal cortex lead to hyposexuality.

Independent determinants of worse sexual well-being include high impact of injury on daily life, low self-esteem, anxiety, and, most importantly, depression. Most common difficulties for women with brain trauma are reduced lubrication, while men must deal with ED and/or ejaculatory dysfunction.

Damage to the hypothalamopituitary area may also cause a central hypogonadism with deficiencies in growth hormone and/or gonadotropin. However, the value of measuring growth hormone, with the purpose of hormonal supplementation, needs to be investigated further.

Late adrenal axis suppression with suppression of testosterone/estrogen from the generalized stress response in answer to the cerebral injury also has major implications.

Hypersomnolence as well has a major impact on sexual function in these patients. It is associated with lower levels of hypothalamic peptidergic neurons of orexin-A (hypocretin-1), which regulates the sleep-wake cycle.

Stroke

There is a large similarity in the high sexual dissatisfaction after brain injury and stroke. A serious stroke will cause difficulties with movement and body positioning, drooling, incontinence, and several other potentially unattractive demeanors. However, stroke patients, who previously had myocardial infarction or diabetes, experienced little change in the sexual satisfaction. Psychosocial issues and depression usually contribute significantly to the sexual disorders as well.

Moreover, many antihypertensive agents given to patients after a stroke cause lowering of the cavernosal arterial pressure, inhibiting erections, and some also decreasing desire (β-blockers).

Epilepsy

Epilepsy is unique in this section, as it may be able to provoke involuntary sexual gestures. Fronto- and/or temporolimbic partial seizures can cause self-fondling, grabbing, scratching of the genital area, masturbatory movements, or pelvic thrusting. Such genital automatisms were seen in 11% of the patients who were submitted to video-electroencephalography for medically refractory seizures. Independent of these automatisms, patients may experience sexual arousal during these seizures and may proceed to an ejaculatory orgasm in men, but ictal orgasm has been seen more commonly in women. However, these women tend to be profoundly hyposexual in between seizures.

The modifiable cause of sexual disorder in epilepsy seems to be the choice of antiepileptic drugs. Sexual dysfunction is linked with induction of the hepatic P450 enzyme (phenytoin, phenobarbitone, primidone, and carbamazepine). Their use is associated with increased serum levels of sex hormone-binding globulin, which in turn causes a decreased bioavailability of free testosterone. However, the possibility of avoiding sexual dysfunction using antiepileptic drugs such as gabapentin, lamotrigine, levetiracetam, pregabalin, or vigabatrin should be studied further, before being promoted as such.

Spinal Cord Injury

Reflex erections remain intact, even after a full, high lesion where the psychogenic erections are lost. Psychogenic erections are mediated by the T12-L2 sympathetic nerves. Low lesions close to the cauda equine significantly impair erectile function, seeing as erotic sensations travel upward next to the spinothalamic tract.

Multiple Sclerosis

Between 50 and 75% of uncontrolled MS, patients must deal with erectile dysfunction, and the spinal cord has been indicated as the major cause. Since initially the deficit is partial, nocturnal and morning erections can be preserved but absent otherwise. Fatigue, depression, spasticity, and anxiety are also major contributors to the sexual dysfunction.

Anejaculation and Infertility in the Neurologic Population

Bilateral sympathectomy at the L2 level may result in ejaculatory failure for about 40% of the patients. Moreover, a high bilateral retroperitoneal lymphadenectomy causes an even higher failure rate.

Normal reproductive function relies not only on appropriate sperm production but also on the adequate transportation and intravaginal delivery of sperm by way of ejaculation. This reflex is highly regulated and dependent of several interacting factors such as spinal cord integrity and pelvic floor musculature. Most severely, neurological diseases or injuries cause anejaculation. This term describes the complete lack of both antegrade and retrograde ejaculation, leading to male infertility despite normal sperm production. Most commonly this is caused by spinal cord injury (SCI) and typically occurs in young men who might want to start a family, thus being of major clinical significance.

Successful emission and ejaculation without orgasm are possible in some patients with spinal cord injury. Detailed history taking of disease or surgery is necessary in determining the difference between emission failure and retrograde ejaculation.

If there is sperm presence in the bladder urine after performing a microscopic examination and a dry ejaculation, retrograde ejaculation is confirmed. If no sperm is found, emission failure is the cause. Retrograde ejaculation is usually caused by dysfunction/relaxation of the internal sphincter or the bladder neck, as seen after radical prostatectomy, alpha-blocker therapy, and diabetic autonomic neuropathy. It can be temporarily remedied by administration of sympathomimetic medication such as imipramine, ephedrine, pseudoephedrine, and phenylpropanolamine, which helps to contract the internal urinary sphincter. If the problem cannot be solved medication-wise, the next step is post-ejaculation harvest of sperm from the bladder.

Ejaculation in the Neurologically Intact Men

Like erection, ejaculation is the end result of the combined input of both psychological and physical/tactile sexual stimulation. The reflex is coordinated by sympathetic nervous input T10-L2 and somatic fibers from S2-S4 regions of the spinal cord.

The somatic input is primarily from the dorsal nerve of the penis (activated by the glans penis) and subsequently through the pudendal nerve, which causes a local reflex arch in the thoracolumbar and sacral spinal cord levels once an excitatory threshold is reached. There are pathways firing upward to the central nervous system (CNS) as well; however their function is poorly understood and likely to be of limited importance.

Before ejaculation, sperm that is stored in the epididymis is transported to the vas deferens by smooth muscle contraction, followed by contractions of the vas mediated by the sympathetic fibers. This moves the sperm to the ejaculatory ducts, which also have an input from the seminal vesicles. Together with the seminal plasma from the prostate and seminal vesicles, it is then transported to the urethra, from which they are expelled. The expulsion is projectile in nature and is orchestrated by somatic nerve fibers to cause a rhythmic contraction of the pelvic/periurethral muscles. During ejaculation, sympathetic fibers prevent retrograde ejaculation by closing the bladder neck.

Given that erection and ejaculation are two separate events coordinated by different neurons, it is very much possible that ejaculation occurs without erection and erections can be present without the ability to ejaculate.

Neurogenic Ejaculatory Dysfunction

Disruption of the reflex arc can lead to complete inability for emission of ejaculate. In less severe cases, neurogenic ejaculatory dysfunction can lead to delayed ejaculation or retrograde ejaculation. In delayed ejaculation, as the name implies, ejaculation can still occur at a higher threshold of sexual stimulation than usual.

Causes of Neurogenic Anejaculation

There is no definitive set of comparable data, but SCI is considered the most common cause of neurogenic anejaculation. An estimated 10% of the men with SCI are unable to ejaculate through normal intercourse or masturbation. It can be evoked by any type of trauma/disease causing damage to the CNS and/or peripheral nerves in and around the pelvic floor.

CNS disorders of note are congenital spinal abnormalities, transverse myelitis, vascular spinal injuries, and multiple sclerosis.

Pelvic trauma or surgery (damaging peripheral nerves), periaortic surgery, and retroperitoneal lymph node dissection (RPLND) (damaging sympathetic ganglia of uprising neurons) are other anejaculation causes.

Poorly controlled diabetes mellitus can eventually lead to peripheral neuropathy, associated with a gradual decline in ejaculatory function (approximately 40% of men with diabetes mellitus I are afflicted). It usually starts with retrograde and/or delayed ejaculation, eventually possibly progressing to anejaculation.

Management of Anejaculation

As with retrograde ejaculation, anejaculation caused by mild neurological disturbances can occasionally be treated by sympathomimetic agents. When the disorders are more serious, assisted ejaculation consisting of penile vibratory stimulation (PVS) or electroejaculation (EEJ) can be considered. When all else fails, surgical sperm retrieval can be attempted.

In PVS, an ejaculation can be induced mechanically in SCI men (FertiCare vibrator). There is a success rate of 88% if the spinal cord lesion is situated above the reflex arc (T10), though it is only 15% with lower injuries. Cortical inhibition can prevent the reflex response; thus the best candidates for PVS are SCI men with complete lesions. Non-SCI men have limited benefits of this device. Patients are considered non-responders after two failed attempts, at least 1 week apart. However, patients with recent lesions may not respond so easily due to the spinal shock phase, and another effort should be made after 1–6 months.

Skin irritation is a rare side effect with prolonged stimulation, since due to the reduced or absent glans sensation, the patient may not notice bruises or abrasions. PVS must also be performed with caution in patients with a penile prosthesis since the vibrator may push the glans onto the implant. Moreover, it can cause a rise in blood pressure, which means it should not be used in patients with severe cardiac disease or untreated hypertension.

More importantly, patients with an injury of T6 or above can experience an uninhibited sympathetic reflex response, called autonomic dysreflexia (AD). It begins as symptoms of hypertension, headache, flushing, and bradycardia and results in stroke, seizure, and death. So, in all patients, healthcare practitioners should be aware of these presymptoms during stimulation.

An electrical current is used in EEJ (Seager Model 14 Electroejaculator) to induce ejaculation and is efficient in both SCI patients and patients suffering from other neurological causes of anejaculation. The device is placed into the patient's rectum with the electrodes facing the seminal vesicles and prostate. Presumably, the reflex is activated by muscular contractions that are induced by the electricity. It is an extremely effective procedure (with success rates reaching 100%) in patients who can endure it and considered a very safe procedure. However, it is more expensive and invasive than PVS, being the less chosen procedure by patients. Contraindications for EEJ include lesions/inflammation of the rectum, bleeding disorders, and anticoagulation therapy. As with PVS, EEJ can cause AD in patients with lesions above T6, and the same limitations and precautions still hold true here.

Lastly, if sperm cannot be acquired with the discussed devices, it can be attempted to retrieve sperm through aspiration or surgical intervention. These are invasive procedures where the sperm is taken directly from the epididymis or testis. Originally this was developed for sperm retrieval from azoospermic men and generally is not the first-line therapy for neurologically induced anejaculation, as PVS and EEJ are much cheaper, less invasive, and result in higher motile sperm count.

Further Reading

Albersen M et al. The future is today: emerging drugs for the treatment of erectile dysfunction. Expert Opin Emerg Drugs. 2010;15(3):467–80. A review on what to expect from the future therapies for ED.

Corona G et al. EMAS Study Group. Age-related changes in general and sexual health in middle-aged and older men: results from the European Male Ageing Study (EMAS). J Sex Med. 2010;7(4 Pt 1):1362–80. One of the capital studies on the epidemiology of ED.

Fode M et al. Penile rehabilitation after radical prostatectomy: what the evidence really says. BJU Int. 2013;112(7):998–1008. Mikkel Fode and coworkers critically revise the evidence for post-prostatectomy penile rehabilitation and conclude that better documentation for current penile rehabilitation and/or better rehabilitation protocols are needed: "One must be careful not to repeat the statement that penile rehabilitation improves erectile function after RP so many times that it becomes a truth even without the proper scientific backing."

Lue TF. Erectile dysfunction. N Engl J Med. 2000;342(24):1802–13. Excellent review on all aspects of ED by one of the pioneers of ED research.

Nehra A et al. The Princeton III Consensus recommendations for the management of erectile dysfunction and cardiovascular disease. Mayo Clin Proc. 2012;87(8):766–78. The Princeton III consensus: first emphasizing the use of exercise ability and stress testing to ensure that each man's cardiovascular health is consistent with the physical demands of sexual activity before prescribing treatment for ED, and second highlighting the link between ED and CVD, which may be asymptomatic and may benefit from cardiovascular risk reduction.

Rees et al. Sexual function in men and women with neurological disorders. The Lancet. 2007;369:512–25. An in-depth look at which brain areas are responsible for sexual sensations and a more detailed overview of all neurologic disorders with their respective sexual disorders.

Part VII
Management: Conservative Approach

Appliances, Catheterisation and Other Aids

Hanny Cobussen-Boekhorst and Shirley Budd

Introduction

People experiencing bladder dysfunction caused by neuropathic conditions often endure complex bladder symptoms. The use of equipment such as absorbent containment products, intermittent catheters, male external catheter (MEC) also known as a sheath and indwelling catheters are an essential management option.

Prior to use of any management equipment, a continence assessment should be completed to identify any concerning signs and symptoms including assessing fluid and diet intake, bladder and bowel function, urinary tract infection (UTI) history and objective assessments (if not already done) including completion of a bladder diary, urinalysis, a bladder scan and physical examination [1, 2].

In this chapter we describe the different management equipment options, according to the latest international literature and guidelines.

Absorbent Containment Products for Urinary and Faecal Incontinence

A frequently chosen management option is to use an absorbent containment system. For more detailed information, access the following link: http://www.cochrane.org/CD007408/INCONT_absorbent-products-for-moderate-heavy-urinary-andor-faecal-incontinence-in-women-and-men [3].

H. Cobussen-Boekhorst (✉)
Department of Urology, Radboudumc, Nijmegen, The Netherlands
e-mail: hanny.cobussen-boekhorst@radboudumc.nl

S. Budd
Great Western Hospital Foundation Trust, Swindon, Wiltshire, UK

© Springer International Publishing AG, part of Springer Nature 2018
R. Dmochowski, J. Heesakkers (eds.), *Neuro-Urology*,
https://doi.org/10.1007/978-3-319-90997-4_20

Much of the evidence regarding efficacy of absorbent products is limited, based on patient experience, and this is over 8 years old. Assessment by an experienced clinician to advise on the most appropriate products is required. Risks experienced by inappropriate absorbent product use include loss of wellbeing and damage to skin integrity such as incontinence-associated dermatitis (IAD) indicating prolonged exposure of the skin to urine and faeces resulting in skin maceration and breakdown. For the best practice principles, access the link: http://www.woundsinternational.com/media/other-resources/_/1154/files/iad_web [4].

A Cochrane report [5] identified that disposable products were more effective at managing incontinence than washable reusable products. Washable reusable products are often made as underwear with a sewn-in washable pad or an insert. However, these products are only for minimal urinary incontinence due to risks of damage to skin integrity and poor efficacy. They were also reported to have limited acceptability. When laundering fabric softener should be avoided as this can decrease absorbency. Disposable absorbent products come in various formats and are also readily available from supermarkets and chemists. National and local area policies vary, and some styles may not be available requiring products to be purchased. Disposable absorbent products may contain only fluff pulp or superabsorbent polymers with pulp. A trial in the Cochrane report [3] identified fewer alterations in skin colour and integrity when using superabsorbent polymers in the pulp, thus maintaining drier skin. There are four main designs for disposable absorbent products:

- Disposable inserts which vary in absorbency from light to heavy incontinence and require close-fitting underwear or manufacturer fixation pants
- Disposable diapers, also known as all in one or slip pads
- T-shaped, belted absorbent products
- Disposable pull-up pant-style products

Disposable products vary in cost, and the pull-up pant style is likely to be the most expensive due to the manufacturing process. Different styles of disposable products are appropriate in different situations depending on the patient's level of incontinence, physical and cognitive ability and time of day. A thorough assessment is required to identify the correct product for an individual. They should be informed of how absorbent products work, how to use them and when to change them.

Intermittent Catheterisation/Dilatation

Introduction

Intermittent (self) catheterisation is a minimally invasive treatment and is currently the preferred method of emptying the bladder in neuro-urological patients [6], with or without antimuscarinics® or Botulinum toxin A® [7].

Intermittent (in/out) catheterisation is defined as drainage or aspiration of the bladder or a urinary reservoir with subsequent removal of the catheter [8].

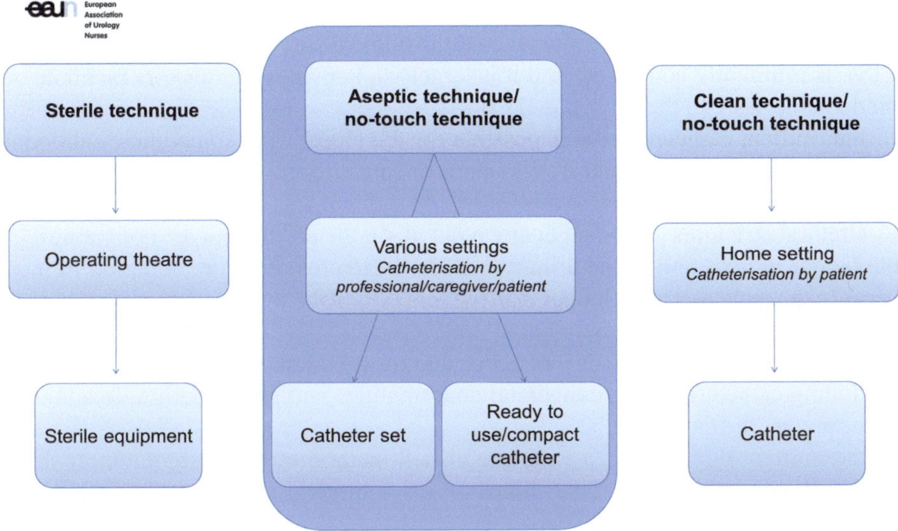

Flowchart 1 Intermittent catheterisation. Techniques—simplified. Adapted with permission from the EAUN guideline 2013 [9]

The guideline of the European Association of Urology Nurses (EAUN) http://nurses.uroweb.org/nurses/guidelines/ [9] describes different intermittent catheterisation techniques (see Flowchart 1).

A clean technique is only used by patients or caretakers in the home setting. A clean technique implies that the setting is non-sterile and the catheter is sterile or reusable and with or without lubricant. Hand hygiene is described as using water and soap; genital hygiene is using water or water and soap, and the catheter can be touched without gloves.

Clean intermittent self-catheterisation (CISC) is used if the technique is performed by the patients themselves. Clean intermittent catheterisation (CIC) is used when the technique is performed by caretakers [9].

Various intermittent catheterisation techniques are described in literature, and despite the same name, the practice may vary. According to current data, it is not possible to state that one catheter type, technique or strategy is better than another [10].

Increasing numbers of patients are advised to perform CISC. Since the introduction of intermittent catheters, nurses have been involved in teaching and coaching patients on how to catheterise and offer continued support and follow-up care. In most countries, nurses teach and coach the technique of CISC or CIC to patients, professionals and carers [11].

The procedure is associated with improved quality of life in patients and is often considered to be both simple and safe [12, 13].

Cobussen-Boekhorst et al. [14] stated that patients are satisfied about the instruction and the follow-up care, but in everyday life, patients describe that the preparation before the handling of the catheter is more difficult than the catheterisation itself and that they felt bounded by catheterisation moments.

Aspects such as gender, age, catheterisation frequency, type of catheter, temporary or long-term catheterisation, technical difficulties, comorbidity, personality and the role of the instructor are important [15, 16]. Furthermore, the 'simplicity' of CISC seems presumed, rather than factual. In clinical studies patient adherence with CISC is minimally addressed, and it is largely unknown which factors facilitate or hinder adherence to the procedure [17].

Intermittent catheterisation is possible for the elderly, but sometimes additional support is needed by community clinicians or carers for this group to achieve better outcomes [18–22].

Urethral strictures can occur at any point along the urethra but are commonest in the bulbar urethra and at the urinary meatus. Strictures are more common in men because the male urethra is longer than the female and the female urethra is straighter than the male.

Urethral strictures/stenosis can occur due to infection, trauma, instrumentation (including catheterisation), congenital abnormalities and inflammation. In addition to the above, the cause can be unknown.

Intermittent dilatation is a well-established method of managing urethral strictures following either a urethral dilatation (as a surgical procedure) or an internal urethrotomy.

When the medical decision is made that a patient would benefit from practising urethral dilatation, the patient is taught to self-dilate within a month of surgery. Ideally the catheter should be a size 16 Ch or 18 Ch. Occasionally the patient may need to commence intermittent self-dilatation (ISD) initially with a smaller Charrière size because the urethra will not accommodate the larger catheter. If this is the case, the Charrière size should be increased over time to a larger diameter catheter if possible.

Urethral dilatation is considered a long-term solution; patients should be informed that they need to continue to dilate intermittently in the long term, unless reconstructive surgery is considered.

The frequency is a medical order. In the early days of learning, frequency should be up to daily. Thereafter, frequency can be less often depending on individual symptoms. The recurrence of strictures is much lower, when urethral dilatation is continued for more than 12 months [9].

Catheter Materials, Types of Catheters and Charrière Gauge

Intermittent catheter materials are made of polyvinyl chloride (PVC), silicone, ethylene vinyl acetate (EVA) or in some countries red rubber catheters or stainless steel if single-use catheters are not available. Be aware that patients with latex allergy need latex-free catheters.

There are several types of catheters and sets available; Flowchart 2 provides an overview of catheter types.

Catheters can be divided into female and male or standard lengths.

Female catheters are between 7 and 25 cm long (see Fig. 1).

Male or standard catheters have a length of about 40 cm (see Figs. 2 and 3).

The external diameter size of intermittent catheters is measured in mm, known as Charrière (Ch) or French (Fr) gauge which measures the circumference.

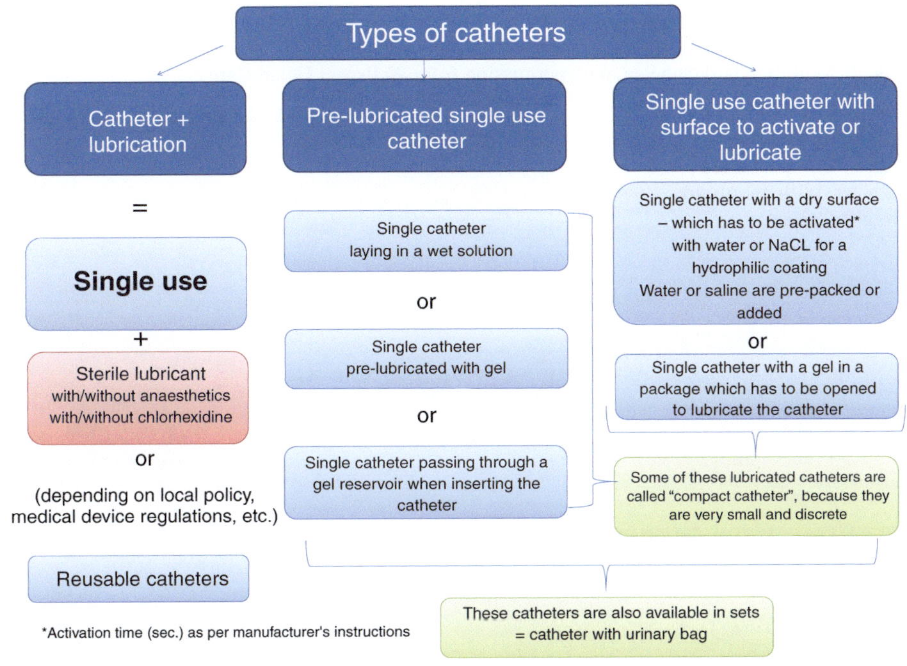

Flowchart 2 Types of catheters. Adapted with permission from the EAUN guideline 2013 [9]

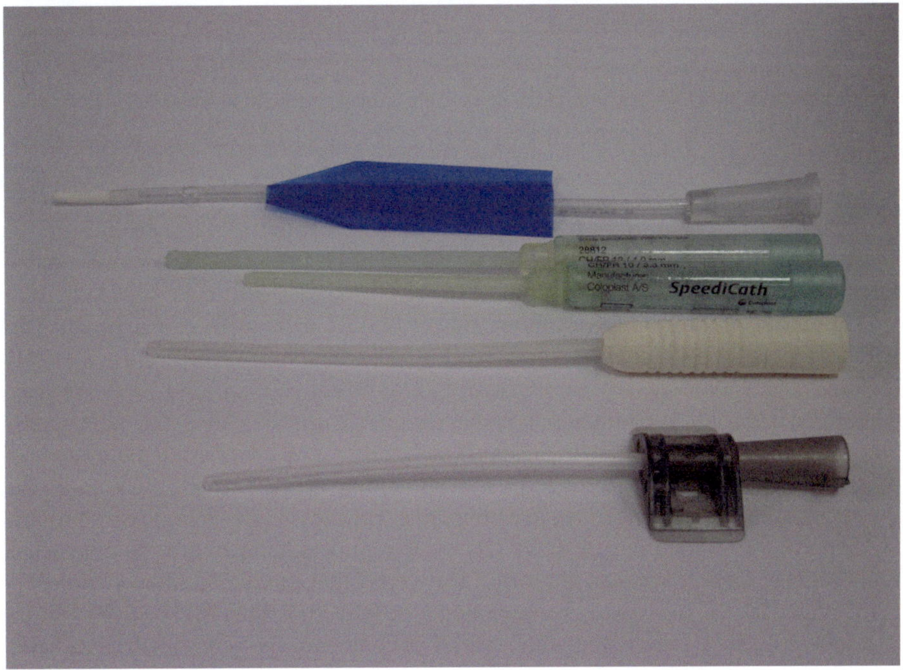

Fig. 1 Few examples of female catheters. Adapted with permission from the EAUN guideline 2013 [9]

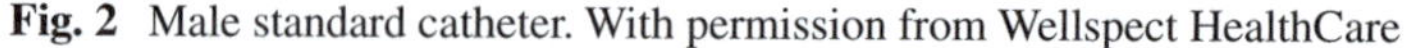

Fig. 2 Male standard catheter. With permission from Wellspect HealthCare

Fig. 3 Compact male catheter. With permission from Coloplast

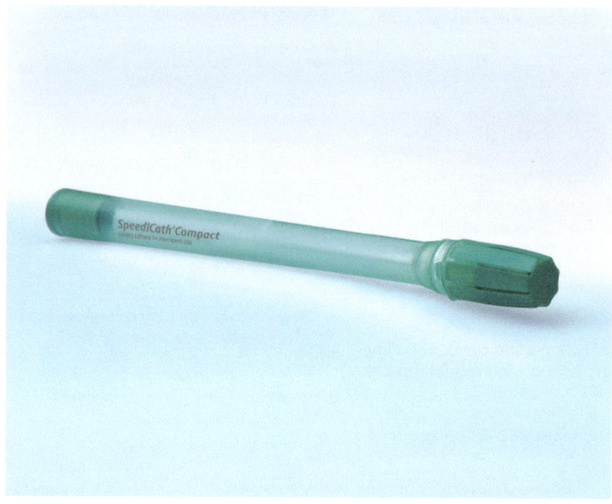

Standard catheter connector colour chart

Catheter size	8	10	12	14	16	18	20
Colour							
Tube diameter	2,7	3,3	4	4,7	5,3	6	6,7

Fig. 4 Standard catheter connector colour chart. Adapted with permission from the EAUN guideline: *Catheterisation, Urethral Intermittent in Adults* (2013) [9]

Sizes range from 6 to 24 Ch. Catheter gauge for children range from 6 to 10, adult female Charrière gauge 10 to 14 Ch and men 12 to 14 Ch. Larger gauge catheters can be used for treating strictures [16–18].

The colour of the connector of the catheter indicates the catheter size or Ch. The colours are an international standard (see Fig. 4).

Single-use catheters may have a hydrophilic or gel coating, or a lubricant may need to be added. Many catheters now have a plastic grip or sleeve to enable a non-touch technique or a sleeve with an additional introducing cover around the catheter tip so the catheter can be introduced without touching the first few millimetres of the urethra. Catheter innovations, such as this, may prevent UTI (see Figs. 5, 6 and 7).

There are also complete catheter sets available; the catheters are pre-connected to a drainage bag. These sets are useful for wheelchair patients or those who catheterise themselves, or by caregivers, in bed (see Figs. 8, 9, and 10).

Catheters are also available with a variety of catheter tips. The standard catheter has a Nelaton tip (soft rounded tip).

Fig. 5 Male catheter
no-touch. With permission
from Wellspect HealthCare

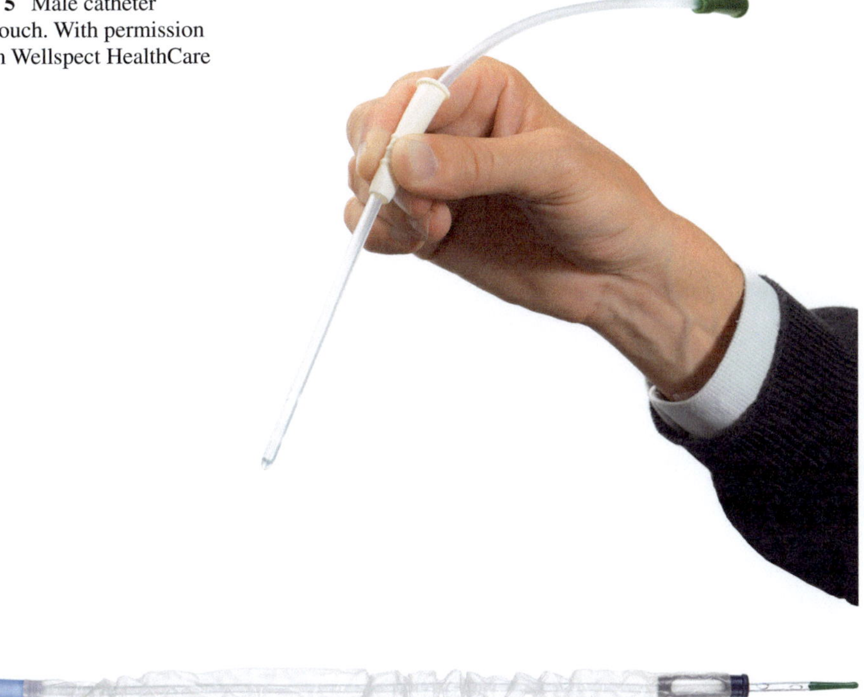

Fig. 6 Male catheter with sleeve. With permission from Teleflex Ltd

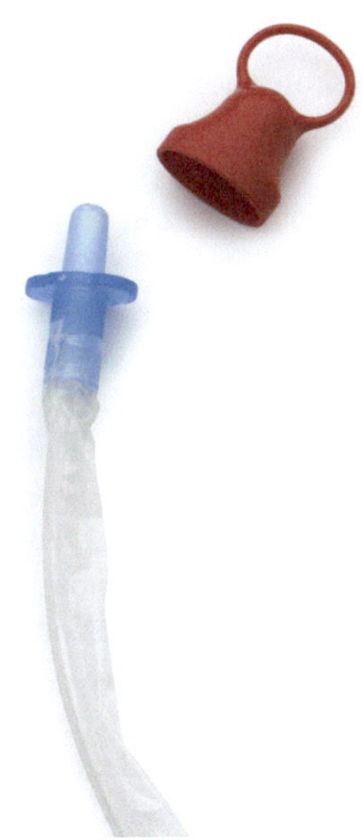

Fig. 7 Male catheter with sleeve and an additional
introducing cover around the catheter tip. With permission
from Hollister

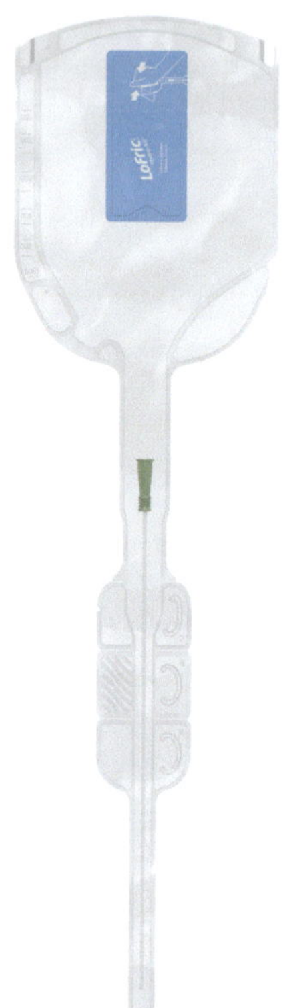

Fig. 8 Example of catheter set. With permission from Wellspect
HealthCare

A Tiemann/Coude tip has a slightly curved and tapered tip and can be used in
patients with prostate obstruction, a steep bladder neck or narrow urethral passage.
The professional teaching the use of this catheter type will require further training
to avoid trauma to the urethra (see Fig. 11).

An Ergothan tip has a flexible rounded catheter tip which increases in size and
can also be used in patients with prostate obstruction or a narrow urethral passage
(see Fig. 12).

The IQ-tip is a pointed flexible tip which ends in a ball and is a stiffer catheter.
This catheter may be used in patients with prostate obstruction or when patients
experience pain at the height of the bladder neck (see Fig. 13).

A flexible catheter with a flexible rounded catheter tip (Coloplast) may also be
used in patients who experience pain at the height of the bladder neck (see Fig. 14).

Urinary bags or a bladder syringe can be attached to the connector of the catheter, or a Luer Lock adapter system (see Fig. 15) can be attached for irrigation or
instillation of medication or solutions into the bladder. A catheter with a Luer Lock
connector is available (see Fig. 16).

There are also catheter insertion aids and support devices available, such as
mirrors, leg spreaders, freehand clothing holders, penile support, and a catheter
handle or cath-hand or ergo-hand, and a special condom/male external catheter
expander tool.

Fig. 9 Example of
catheter set. With
permission from Hollister

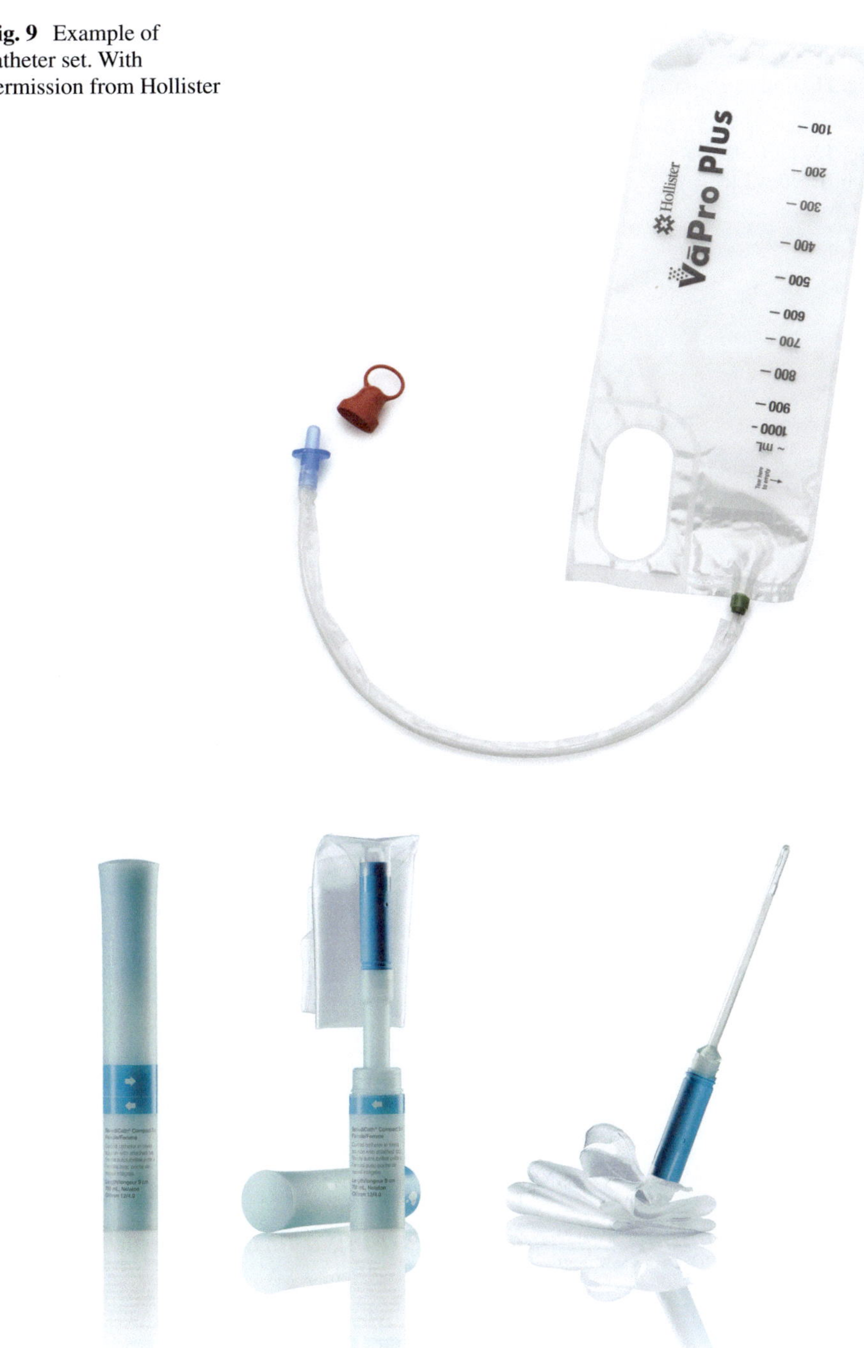

Fig. 10 Example of catheter set. With permission from Coloplast

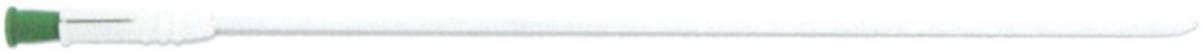

Fig. 11 Catheter with Tiemann tip. With permission from Wellspect HealthCare

Fig. 12 Flexible Ergothan tips with various Charrière gauges. With permission from Teleflex Ltd

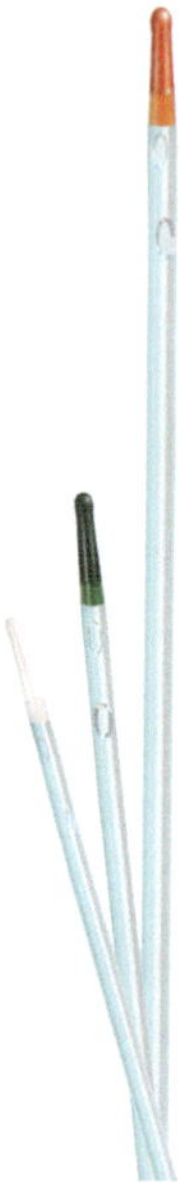

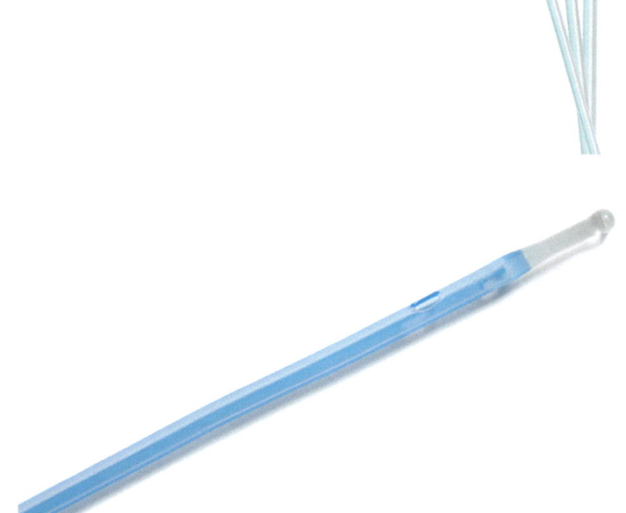

Fig. 13 Flexible pointed IQ-tips with various Charrière gauges. With permission from Manfred Sauer

Patient Education, Explanation, Training and Documentation

Cobussen et al. [18] recommend that patients, who would benefit from CISC, should receive in advance a patient information leaflet. Following this they should receive information and instruction about the treatment by specialised nurses in continence care (continence or urology nurse), preferably during a scheduled (1-h) consultation held at an outpatient clinic, during an admission on a ward or in their own home. At each visit ensure that the patient's privacy and dignity are maintained [15]. During the consultation the patient's history must be assessed; (patho)physiology of the

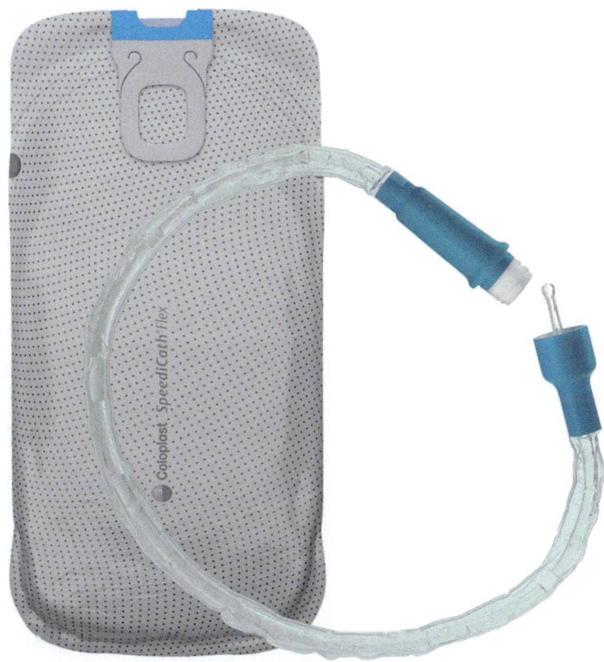

Fig. 14 Male catheter with flexible rounded catheter tip. With permission from Coloplast

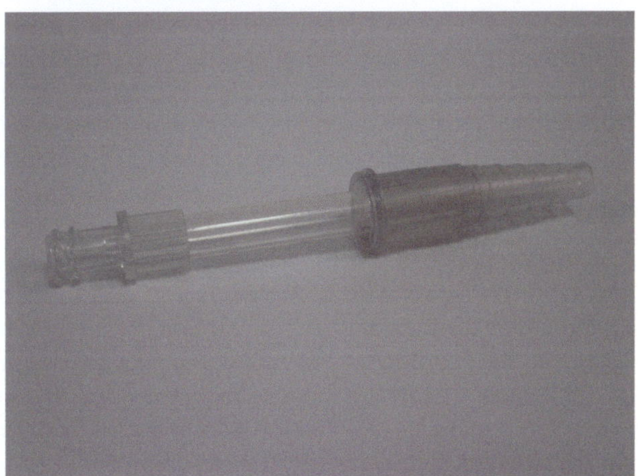

Fig. 15 Example of Luer Lock adaptor. Adapted with permission from the EAUN guideline 2013 [9]

bladder explained; potential problems due to impaired cognitive level or physical disability, if present, discussed; and motivation for catheterisation should be assessed. The procedure must be explained and examples of catheters shown. A catheter type must be chosen, based on the patient's preference and clinical needs taking into consideration disabilities such as physical impairment. The size must be large enough to allow free flow of urine without causing damage to the urethra. The best location for performing catheterisation must be discussed with the patient, e.g. in bed, in a wheelchair or on the toilet. Depending on the situation, the patient or partner/caregiver will perform the catheterisation. The clean technique should be

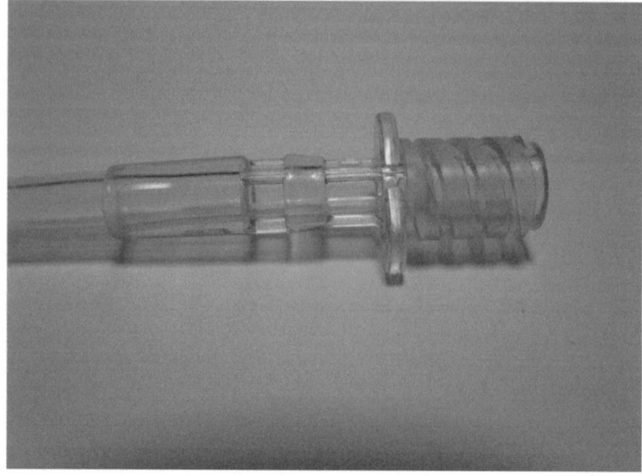

Fig. 16 Example of catheter with Luer Lock connector. Adapted with permission from the EAUN guideline 2013 [9]

explained and instructed [9]. An evaluation and individualised advice on managing catheterisation in the patient's home setting should be undertaken. Samples should be given to the patient to accommodate the first days of catheterisation, and additional materials can be ordered once the most appropriate catheter has been identified. In the rehabilitation centre, the educational instruction is part of the rehabilitation process. Follow-up must take place within or soon after the first week and further follow-up preferably after 3 and 12 months or when patients request support. Patients should be given contact details for support in case of problems or questions.

Frequency of catheterisation per day can vary. In adults, a residual of >500 mL must be avoided, but this depends also on urodynamic findings. If the patient suffers from urinary retention, usually CI(S)C is required 4–6 times per day. If the patient has a post-void residual, the frequency of CI(S)C depends on the residual volume. A bladder diary can be useful to determine the frequency of CI(S)C identifying frequency and volume of voids. In children the age of the child is also important.

For compliance to CI(S)C frequency times, Cobussen et al. [14] stated that it is important to discuss with each patient tips and tricks to simplify the preparation, e.g. where to store the catheter when away from their home environment and how to prepare the handling of the catheter in specific situations or places. In follow-up care a standard evaluation list is recommended to evaluate important adherence issues. This includes satisfaction and concerns with catheterisation and with the chosen catheter, frequency of catheterisation and how to deal with this at different times of the day and successful catheterisation away from the home environment. Also discuss any impact of catheterisation on sexuality and sexual function.

Nurses should to be aware of any problems experienced and if necessary adjust the teaching program when problems occur. This may include cognitive impairment such as in MS patients, lack of motor skills including limited hand function, wheelchair user, problems with compliance due to embarrassment, resistant to sickness role, complexity of the procedure, CI(S)C outside the home, or difficulties with inserting the catheter. Sometimes additional psychological support is necessary, especially for children.

When problems with inserting the catheter occur, this can be related to detrusor sphincter dyssynergia. In these cases sometimes a catheter with a special tip can be helpful and trying different positions such as standing, sitting or lying. Also the patient can take a deep breath whilst inserting the catheter and apply a little pressure. The sphincter often relaxes and allows the catheter to pass after a short while. These problems may occur when the bladder is full, so catheterising at a shorter interval may prevent this.

If patients suffer from recurrent urinary tract infections, CI(S)C can reduce these. Patients need to be instructed about the signs of UTI and how to prevent them. Symptoms that can occur are burning on urination, frequency/urgency, offensive smelling urine and cloudy and dark urine, feeling tired or shaky, fever or chills, haematuria and difficulties inserting the catheter. Urine samples should only be sent for culture and sensitivity if patients have symptoms of UTI [9].

UTI prevention techniques include good hand hygiene, adequate fluid intake (1.5–2 L per day) and prevention of constipation. In neuro-urological patients, constipation is an important issue next to the bladder problems, as constipation can influence CI(S)C and recurrent UTI [9].

In patients with a spinal cord lesion above T6, an overfilled bladder (or bowel) can lead to autonomic dysreflexia; this is a life-threatening condition in which the blood pressure rises very quickly. Patients may experience headache or can perspire above the injury. The bladder needs to be emptied quickly to avoid harm.

The teaching program and follow-up care need to be documented in the patient file alongside the type, length and Charrière of the catheter and frequency of CI(S)C.

If a patient travels abroad, a medical travel document can be useful (example in EAUN guideline Vahr [9]).

When patients have a continent stoma (Mitrofanoff/Monti), the same catheters and sets can be used, but most of the time, a 40 cm length is needed.

When the bladder is augmented, be aware of mucus. Depending on how much mucus the augmented bladder makes, patients need to irrigate/washout the bladder to prevent blockage with mucus. Sometimes a catheter with a greater Charrière is possible. Also catheters with four eyelets are available to facilitate this.

Male External Catheter

Introduction

Male external catheters (MEC), also known as condom catheter, urinary or penile sheaths, are external containment products which provide a management option where treatment has not been effective or the individual chooses to not consent to treatment (see Figs. 17, 18 and 19).

MEC may be a better option for men being more dignified and comfortable compared to absorbent containment products. A detailed analysis of MEC assessment application and drainage systems is available from: http://nurses.uroweb.org/guideline/male-external-catheters-in-adults-urinary-catheter-management/ [23].

For effective application of an MEC, the clinician should attend training and be assessed for competence to avoid failure of the MEC and complications associated with poor fitting, skin integrity and the individual's ability to apply and manage the MEC. These include issues such as cognition, penile retraction and dexterity. Contraindications include high pressure chronic retention, excoriation of skin and

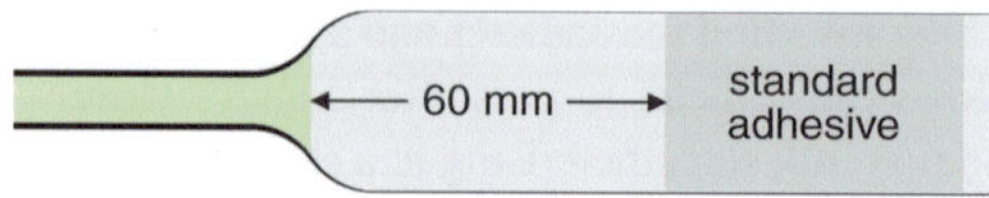

Fig. 17 Example of a male external catheter (MEC). Adapted with permission from the EAUN guideline 2016 [23]

Fig. 18 Example of a male external catheter (MEC). With permission of Coloplast

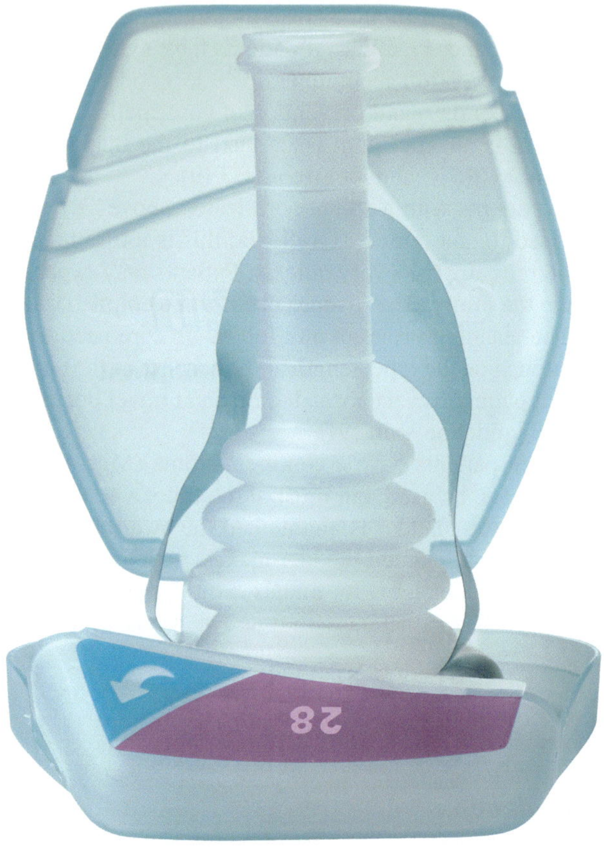

other skin conditions and allergies to the materials of the MEC. Assuming that a continence assessment has been completed and the clinician has decided with the patient that an MEC is an appropriate management option, the following is a guide for assessment and application, managing urine drainage and solutions to avoid MEC failure and skin damage.

Types of MEC

MEC are often made of silicone, latex-free material and latex. They may have an integral inner adhesive lining. Other MECs which include the use of liners and tapes, pubic pressure appliances and a sheath system applied to the glans penis are

Fig. 19 Example of a
male external catheter
(MEC). With permission of
Manfred Sauer

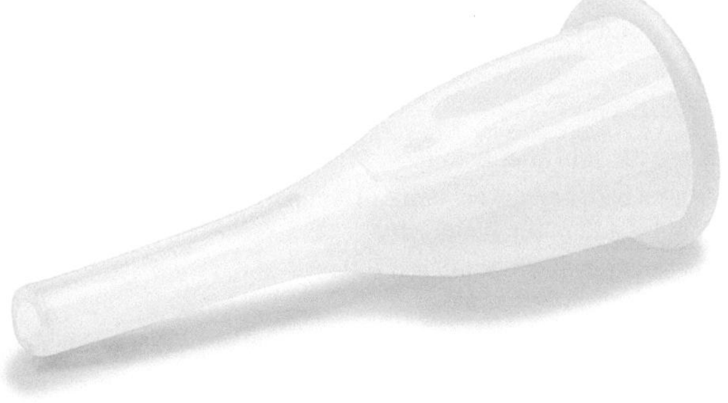

more appropriately assessed for by a specialist nurse. The easier to use MEC have an integral adhesive which adheres to the skin and are rolled on to the penis or may have a pull tab to apply the MEC. There are also differing lengths of MECs and adhesive layers to match different lengths of the penis.

Benefits of MEC are as follows: comfortable to wear, enables urine to drain directly into a drainage system directing urine away from the skin and effective incontinence management. If there is a challenge with the MEC falling off, it is possible for a man to learn how long the MEC will remain effective and use it for this period of time. This may enable a man to go out with confidence.

Negatives of MEC: The MEC may fall off or be pulled off which may result in a loss of confidence and skin damage. Negative pressure may occur as a result of fast urine flow resulting in urine back pressure breaking the adhesive seal and causing MEC failure. If the man is not able to cope with the MEC due to cognitive or dexterity deficit and pulls it off resulting in skin trauma, this is not an appropriate management option. Poorly fitted MEC resulting in either leakage due to creases in the material or the MEC is too tight potentially result in pressure damage.

Assessment for MEC

Gain consent for the use of the MEC by explaining the benefits and challenges of using an MEC. Where the man has cognitive or dexterity challenges, he may require support from carers, relatives and/or healthcare professionals.

Assess for penile retraction by asking the man to sit down and lean forward, and observe the penis retracting backwards into the pubic area. Press gently over the pubic area to see how much pressure is required to extend the penis. This is more likely to occur where the man has had surgery or due to obesity.

Use a company manufactured measuring guide for the MEC that is being fitted as there are variations in sizing. Measure the shaft of the penis at its widest girth. Ask the patient to sit on the edge of a bed or chair with their legs slightly spread. In this free position, both the scrotum and penis are in their natural anatomic orientation and can best be measured.

Table 1 Adapted from Bard: 'Choosing and using your Clear Advantage™ self-adhesive silicone sheath' Ref: 0915/3632 15-099

Do	Don't
Change MEC daily	Use liquid or moisturising soap
Rinse the skin after bathing	Use wet wipes or baby wipes
After a bath or shower, wait 5–10 min to ensure that the skin is completely dry	Use talc or moisturiser cream
Try wrapping a sheet kitchen roll around the penis to absorb excess moisture	Don't retract the foreskin to expose the glans
Leave the foreskin forward to cover the glans penis	Do not shave as this can cause irritation
Use a hair guard to stop hair from being trapped by adhesive	Don't push the penis into the MEC as this may result in urine backflow
After applying the sheath, warm it with the hand for 10 seconds to ensure adhesion	

Application of MEC

Ensure the skin is clean and dry and free from oil or moisturisers.

The man should lie in a semi-reclined position allowing him to see his penis without causing penile retraction. Manufacturers often provide a pubic hair guard so the hair does not get caught under the adhesive of the sheath. The man slides the hair guard along the shaft of the penis and can tuck the pubic hair behind the guard or can trim the hair. Avoid shaving as this can result in skin irritation.

If the man is not circumcised, ensure that the foreskin is forward covering the glans penis. Apply the MEC so it starts to adhere and then pull slightly on the MEC whilst rolling the MEC onto the penis. This prevents wrinkles in the penile skin. Ask the man to place his hand around the MEC to warm up the adhesive for a few seconds. This enhances MEC adhesive bonding to the skin. Apply a suitable drainage system appropriate for the man.

MEC are usually licensed to stay in place for up to 24 h. When removing the MEC, teach the man and any carers to use warm soapy water and a cloth to ease the MEC away from the skin. If this is difficult, an adhesive remover may be used. Advise the man to not pull at the MEC as this may result in skin damage. Table 1 gives a short overview regarding the use of a MEC.

Indwelling Catheters: Urethral and Suprapubic

Introduction

Transurethral indwelling catheterisation or urinary catheterisation is defined as the passage of a catheter into the urinary bladder via the urethra (urethral catheter). (MESH term: https://www.ncbi.nlm.nih.gov/) (see Figs. 20 and 21).

Suprapubic catheterisation is the insertion of a catheter into the bladder via the anterior abdominal wall (see Fig. 22).

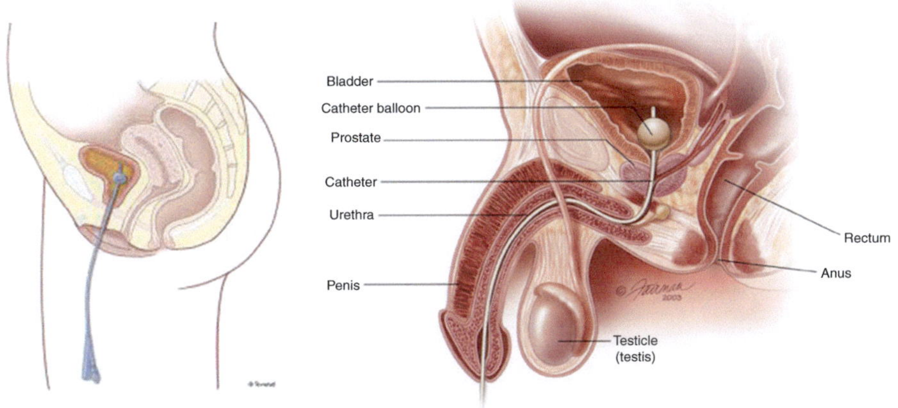

Figs. 20 and 21 Urethral catheterisation female. Adapted with permission from the EAUN guideline 2012 [24] and urethral catheterisation male. Adapted with permission from the American Urological Association

Fig. 22 Suprapubic catheter. Adapted with permission from the EAUN guideline 2012 [24]

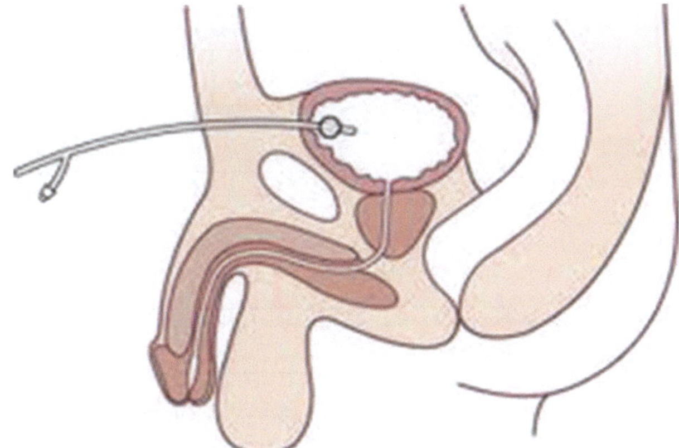

Guidelines for catheterisation procedures and catheter management are available on the internet including: http://nurses.uroweb.org/guideline/catheterisation-indwelling-catheters-in-adults-urethral-and-suprapubic/ [24].

EAUN guidelines on neurogenic lower urinary tract dysfunction recommend, whenever possible, to avoid an indwelling transurethral and suprapubic catheterisation (level 3A) due to a range of complications such as an enhanced risk for catheter-associated UTI (CAUTI), in particular, related to transurethral catheterisation [6].

For other options and alternatives to an indwelling catheter, see flowchart 'Management of incontinence with PVR-decision tree' (see Flowchart 3).

Indications for a suprapubic catheter include problems with urethral catheterisation or when preferred by patients using a wheelchair or sexually active patients.

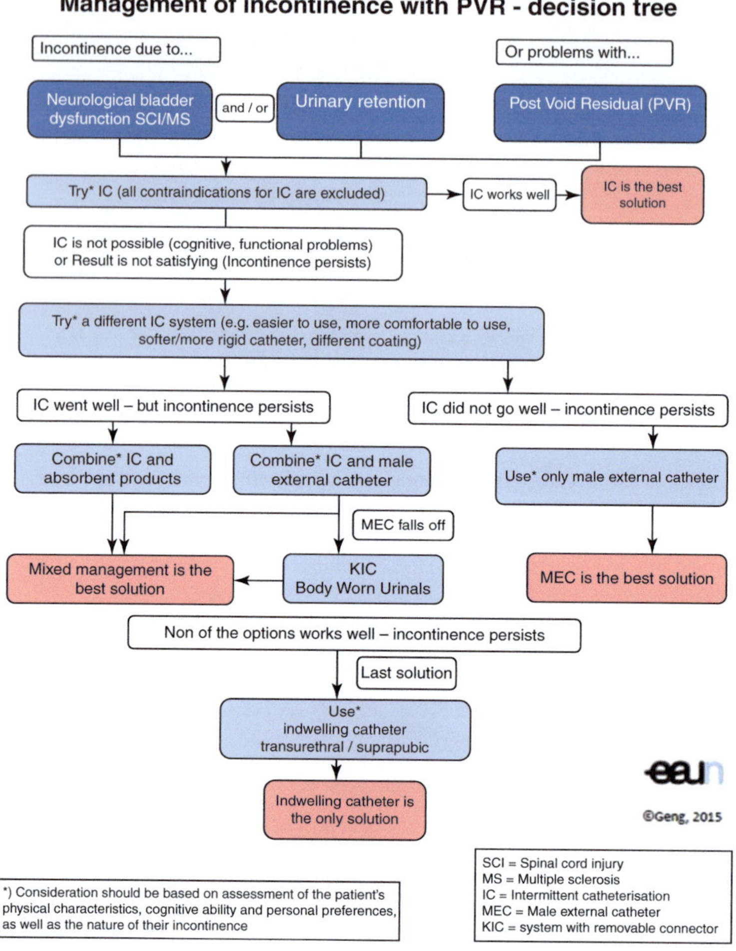

Flowchart 3 Management of incontinence with PVR-decision tree. Adapted with permission from the EAUN guideline 2016 [23], with courtesy V. Geng

Catheter Materials, Types of Catheters and Charrière Gauge

An indwelling catheter consists of a two-way catheter; one channel is used for drainage of urine and one for inflating the (integrated) balloon.

There are different catheter materials, such as latex, silicone, polytetrafluoroethylene (PTFE)-coated, silicone-coated, silicone-elastomer-coated, hydrogel-coated and silver-coated catheters. Silicone catheters are preferred because they are less susceptible to encrustation and because of the high incidence of latex allergy in the neuro-urological patient population [6].

Catheter diameter sizes are measured in Charrière (Ch or CH) also known as French gauge (F, Fr or FG) and indicate the external diameter, 1 mm = 3 Ch, and the sizes range from Ch 6 to 30.

Paediatric	Size 6–10 Ch
Adults	Size 10 Ch clear urine, no debris, no encrustation
	Size 12–14 Ch clear urine, no debris, no encrustation, no haematuria
	Size 16 Ch slightly cloudy urine, light haematuria with or without small clots, none or mild encrustation, none or mild debris.
	Size 18 Ch moderate to heavy encrustation, moderate to heavy debris. Haematuria with moderate clots

Sizes 20–24 used for heavy haematuria and a need for flushing [24]

Charrière 12–16 is recommended by Stohrer [6]

The size of the catheter is marked at the inflation channel as well as with an (international) colour code (see flowchart of connector colours CISC section).

Catheter length of indwelling catheters varies from 25 to 45 cm. In female patients a 25 cm length can be more comfortable and discrete for some women.

The standard catheter tip is round with two drainage eyes and is called a Nelaton tip.

The Tiemann catheter has a curved tip and can be used in male patients or can be helpful in difficult insertions. The 'open-end' catheter is often used for suprapubic indwelling catheterisation but can also be used when problems occur with encrustation or clots.

A 'council' tip catheter may be used when changing a fine-bore suprapubic catheter to a long-term catheter or when changing a long-term suprapubic catheter. This catheter has an open tip and no eyelets and is inserted over a guide wire [24] (Fig. 23).

When the Foley catheter has been placed in the bladder and urine flows, the balloon should be inflated. The balloon size depends on the catheter Charrière gauge and material. Normally this will be between 5 and 15 mL. Always inflate the balloon according to the manufacturer's recommended volume recorded on the packaging and on the inflation valve. Inflation of silicone catheters with water can sometimes lead to water loss from the balloon over time, with an associated risk of the catheter falling out. Some manufacturers recommend filling the balloon with a 5 or 10% aqueous glycerine solution. Some catheter manufacturers provide sterile pre-filled syringes with sterile water or glycerine 5 or 10% inside the package.

The purpose of the retention balloon is to keep the catheter in place in the bladder. The use of a larger balloon size is mistakenly believed to be a solution to bypassing of urine or catheter expulsion. Under- or overinflation can cause occlu-

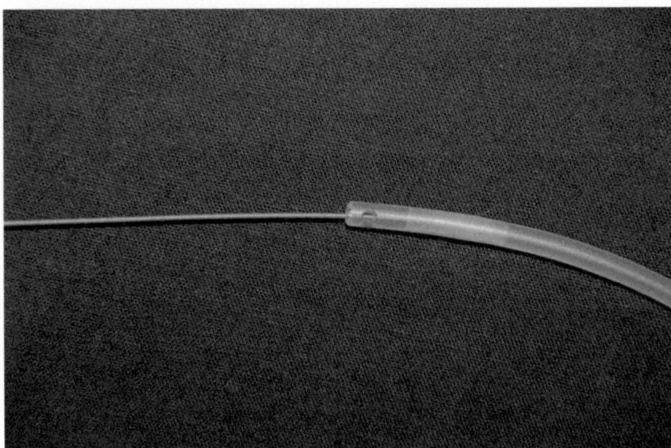

Fig. 23 Open-end catheter with guide wire. Adapted with permission from the EAUN guideline 2012 [24]

sion of drainage eyes, irritate the bladder wall and lead to bladder spasms. Furthermore, larger balloons tend to sit higher in the bladder with the potential for increased residual urine volumes to collect below the catheter eyelets [24].

When the catheter is placed, a drainage bag should be connected and may be connected to the catheter before catheter insertion, so the closed system is maintained to minimise the risk of CAUTI. Pre-connected drainage systems are also available.

Drainage bags are designed with an anti-reflux valve or anti-reflux chamber to prevent reflux of contaminated urine from the bag going into the tubing.

Most drainage bags have a special sampling port designed to obtain urine specimens whilst maintaining a closed system (see Fig. 24). Many companies produce drainage bags with a needle-free sample port to avoid sharp injuries.

During the daytime patients can wear leg bags which are available in different sizes, capacity, tubes, chambers and outlet taps. It is important to select a bag according to the patient's preference, mobility and the intended duration (see Fig. 25).

In patients with limited hand function, an appropriate outlet tap is important for the patient's independence. Different designs are available such as barrel tap, lever tap and push-pull taps (see Fig. 26).

An overnight bag can be used during the night or on long journeys. Capacity of these bags varies from 1.5 to 4 L. The overnight bag can be connected to the leg bag with the outlet tap open so the system isn't disconnected (see Fig. 27).

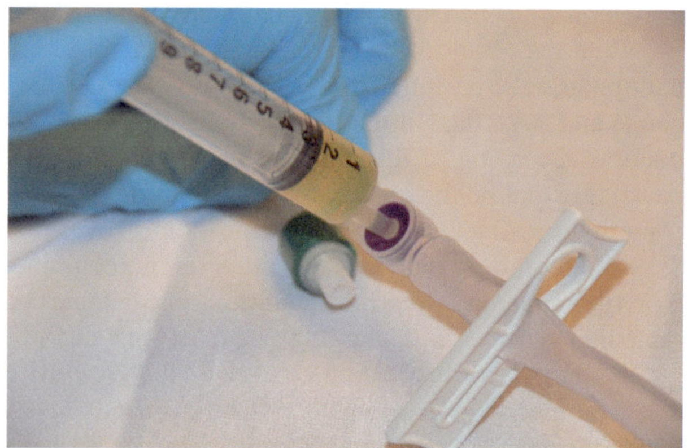

Fig. 24 Catheter with sample port. Adapted with permission from the EAUN guideline 2012 [24]

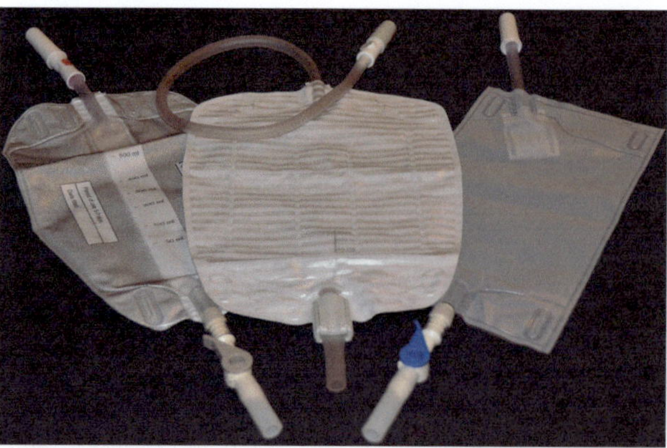

Fig. 25 Examples of different types of leg bags. Adapted with permission from the EAUN guideline 2012 [24]

Fig. 26 Examples of
different types of outlet taps.
Adapted with permission
from the EAUN guideline
2012 [24]

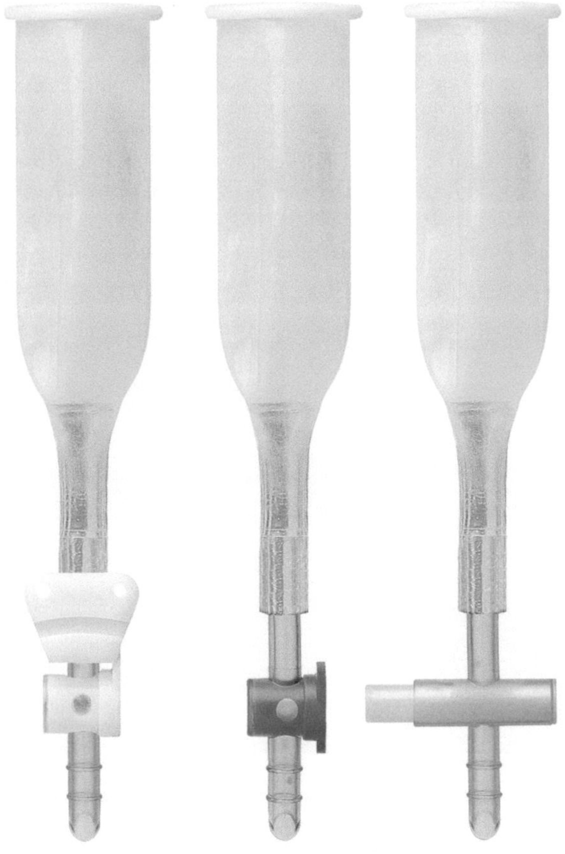

Fig. 27 Examples of
different types of night
bags. Adapted with
permission from the EAUN
guideline 2012 [24]

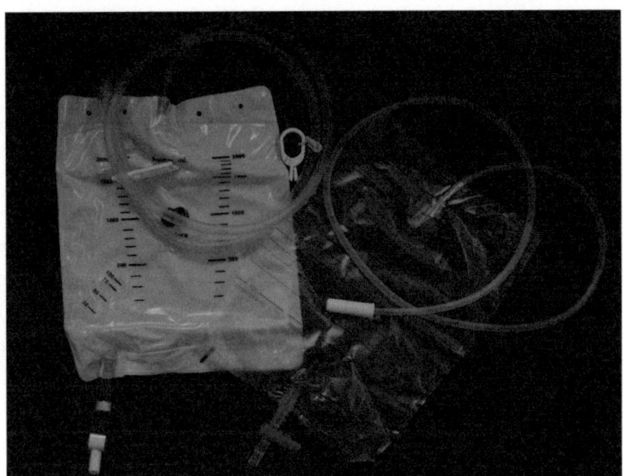

Fig. 28 Examples of different types of catheter valves. Adapted with permission from the EAUN guideline 2012 [24]

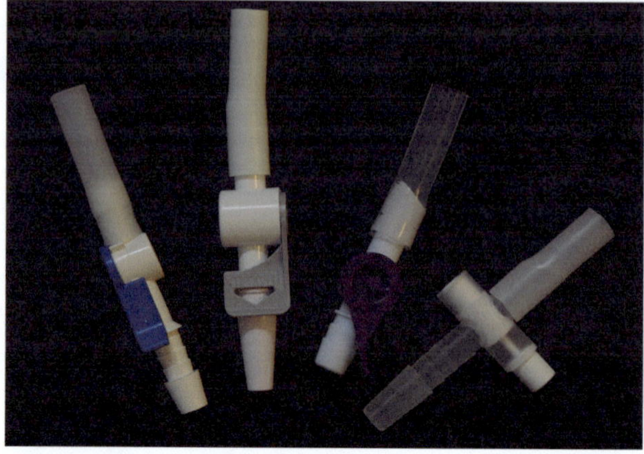

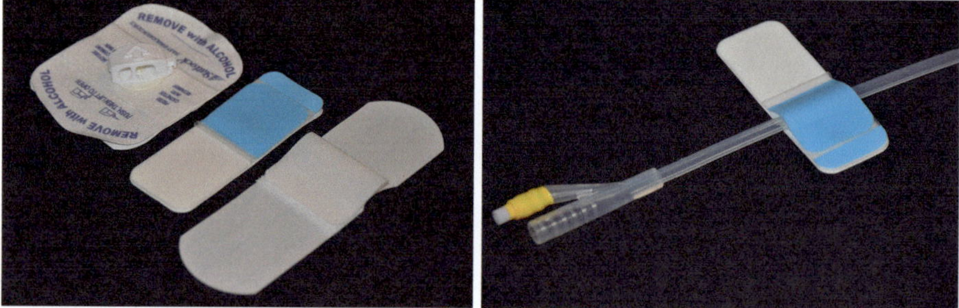

Figs. 29 and 30 Examples of different types of securement devices. Adapted with permission from the EAUN guideline 2012 [24]

In some countries there are single-use drainage bags available. These are without a tap or with a single-use tap and need to be changed when full. In other countries leg and night bags are cleaned and reused for long-term catheters at home [24].

Catheter valves are small devices connected to the catheter outlet instead of a bag and are available in a variety of designs. The catheter valves are an alternative to leg bags which give the patient more freedom to move and more discreet drainage. Most valves are designed to fit with linked systems so it is possible to connect to a drainage bag (see Fig. 28).

Many patients with neuropathic conditions are not able to manipulate a catheter valve and may have overactive bladder symptoms resulting in poor bladder function, and so the valve is not an optimal solution for all patients. Therefore, the nurse specialist has to assess the suitability for each patient. In some countries the use of catheter valve is not approved [25].

Catheter securement devices are designed to prevent excessive traction of the catheter against the bladder neck or inadvertent catheter removal. There are different kinds of securement devices (tape, Velcro™) (see Figs. 29 and 30).

Lubricant is required to assist safe catheterisation and dilates and lubricates the urethra. Four types of lubricants can be distinguished:

1. Water-soluble lubricants
2. Water-soluble lubricants with chlorhexidine (antiseptic)
3. Water-soluble lubricants with anaesthetic lignocaine/lidocaine
4. Water-soluble lubricants with anaesthetic lignocaine/lidocaine and chlorhexidine [24]

Catheter Management

Individual assessment for use of an indwelling catheter should be carried out to identify the risks and benefits. Neuropathy can create challenges for people with indwelling catheters including bladder spasm resulting in bypassing of urine around the outside of the catheter, catheter expulsion and bladder stones in addition to other indwelling catheter issues.

Identify the reason for insertion of an indwelling catheter. If the rationale is not evident, apply the HOUDINI acronym [26] supporting nurses to apply catheter stop orders:

Haematuria visible
Obstruction/inability to empty the bladder
Urological surgery or gynaecology procedures
Decubitus ulcer/open sacral wound
Input/output fluid monitoring haemodynamic instability
Nursing care only/end-of-life care to promote comfort
Immobility

In Table 2 practices to promote successful catheter management and benefits of recommended practice are described.

Catheter management should promote evidence-based practice. The following table (Table 3) identifies some practices that may have been performed previously but are not evidence based or within a manufacturers license.

Table 2 Successful catheter management taken from *Practical Functional Urology* 2016 p. 371 [27]

Practice to promote successful catheter management	Benefits of recommended practice
Routinely assess for catheter removal	Reduce risk of catheter associated UTI (CAUTI), bladder stones, catheter encrustation and catheter blockage
Apply aseptic non-touch technique for catheter insertion	
Advise handwashing technique, and teach the patient and people associated with the catheter handwashing technique	
Maintain the closed drainage system	
Promote adequate fluid intake to pass 50–100 mL/h	

(continued)

Table 2 (continued)

Practice to promote successful catheter management	Benefits of recommended practice
Assess for CAUTI based on two or more symptoms including: New pain in the flank or suprapubic region Frank haematuria, rigours, new onset or worsening of pre-existing confusion or agitation, unusual bladder spasm and bypassing around the catheter Replacing chronic catheters prior to commencement of antibiotics for symptomatic UTI yields greater and faster clinical improvement [24]	Correct use of antibiotics To avoid bacteraemia
Refer patients to urology for bladder stone assessment when catheters are routinely blocking with grit or toothpaste consistency encrustation. Identify this by cutting lengthways the top 5 cm of the catheter to reveal the catheter lumen	Bladder stones are a potential cause of catheters blocking with encrustation
Use appropriate catheter size, e.g. standard/male length for male urethra, suprapubic, and for females where a shorter catheter is uncomfortable, for example, if they have mobility or obesity problems, use the smallest gauge catheter. Use the smallest balloon/10mls. An appropriate length of drainage bag tubing to avoid negative pressure which causes the eyelets to be occluded by bladder mucosa	Reduce risk of CAUTI and trauma Reduces traction and piston effect promoting comfort and free drainage of urine
Apply catheter and drainage system support with abdominal and thigh drainage system support straps, mesh leg sleeves and catheter stands	
Correct volume of gel for insertion female and suprapubic 6 mL, male 11 mL	Reduce risk of trauma. Promote comfortable, easier catheterisation
Follow product license, e.g. long-term Foley catheters 3–12 weeks, drainage bags and catheter valves 5–7 days, single-use 2 L night bags	Patient safety Prevention of CAUTI, encrustation and bladder stones
Assess for appropriate use of catheter valve. Be aware of the impact of the neuropathic bladder; poor compliance and detrusor overactivity can be contraindications for the use of catheter valves	Patient comfort and dignity, reduce risk of CAUTI, catheter blockage and maintain normal bladder function
Adequate bowel action avoiding straining and the passing of large hard stools	Promotes catheter drainage, reduces risk of urine bypassing and catheter expulsion
Treat overactive bladder symptoms that cause bypassing and expelled catheters with anticholinergic medication or β-3-adrenoceptor-agonist	Patient comfort, promote functional catheter management
Provide patient, family and carers with written advice, who to contact for support, what equipment is needed and how to obtain equipment	Patient and carers are independent

Table 3 Practice that is not evidence based [24]

Not recommended	Rationale
Using a 30 mL balloon with the intention that it will help to keep the expelling catheter in the bladder	The 30 mL balloon will be heavy and may cause pressure necrosis. This size balloon is most often used short term for haemostasis to stop or prevent postsurgical haemorrhage within a urology department
Using antimicrobial bladder washouts to treat urine infections or to prevent CAUTI or the blocking catheter, e.g. chlorhexidine	This is not effective, and potentially it will encourage the development of antibiotic-resistant bacteria
Do not use physical force with a citric acid catheter management solution or use a catheter tip syringe to unblock a non-draining catheter unless requested by urology explaining rationale and technique	There is the potential for inappropriate force to be used with a bladder washout syringe which may cause trauma as fluid and debris are forced against the fragile mucosal lining of the bladder
Do not send urine samples for microbiology to assess for CAUTI	It is well accepted that bacterial colonisation with catheterisation is inevitable with some reports estimating the risk to be in the region of 5% per day with almost 100% colonisation Risk at 7–10 days of catheterisation Assess for symptoms of CAUTI, and only send a sample if the person is symptomatic. The sample is to identify the most appropriate antibiotic. Always ensure it is clear on the information for microbiology that the sample is from a catheter
Breaking the closed drainage system more frequently than every 5–7 days	This increases the risk of CAUTI and bladder stones
Disconnecting and then reconnecting the same drainage bag	
Allowing drainage bags to drag or lie on the floor	Will increase the likelihood of a CAUTI and may promote cross infection. May cause traction on the catheter resulting in urethral trauma
Cutting any part of the catheter drainage tube to help removal of the catheter	Potentially the catheter will slide up into the bladder requiring urgent hospital admission. This will breach the product license
Clamping the catheter tubing	May compress the tubing and damage the balloon inflation channel
Do not take a urine sample from a drainage bag	This is likely to be contaminated. Instead use the needle-free sample port
Never use a female length catheter in a male urethra	To avoid urethral trauma, pain, bleeding and potentially patient fatality
Do not use techniques or equipment in a way that is not recommended by the manufacturer	You are legally accountable for your own actions and will be held responsible for your actions. If you use a product in a way that is not the manufacturer guidelines, then your practice may be scrutinised

References

1. Bayliss V, Locke R, Elizabeth S. Continence care pathways. Chichester: Wiley Blackwell; 2009. ISBN: 978-0-470-06143-5.
2. Wound, Ostomy. Continence, Nurses, Society. Reversible causes of acute/transient urinary incontinence: clinical resource guide. Mt. Laurel. 2016.
3. Fader M, Cottenden AM, Getliffe K. Absorbent products for moderate-heavy urinary and/or faecal incontinence in women and men. 2008 Cochrane Library. https://doi.org/10.1002/14651858.CD0074084.
4. Beeckman D. Incontinence associated dermatitis: moving prevention forward. In: Proceedings of the Global IAD Expert Panel. 2015.
5. Fader M, Cottenden AM, Getliffe K. Absorbent products for light urinary incontinence in women. 2007 Cochrane Library. https://doi.org/10.1002/14651858.CD001406.pub2.
6. Stohrer M, Blok B, Castro-Diaz D, Chartier-Kastler E, Del Popolo G, Kramer G, et al. EAU guidelines on neurogenic lower urinary tract dysfunction. Eur Urol. 2009;56(1):81–8.
7. Castel-Lacanal E, Game X, De Boissezon X, Guillotreau J, Braley-Berthoumieux E, Terracol C, et al. Impact of intermittent catheterization on the quality of life of multiple sclerosis patients. World J Urol. 2013;31(6):1445–50.
8. Abrams P, Cardozo L, Fall M, Griffiths D, Rosier P, Ulmsten U, et al. The standardisation of terminology of lower urinary tract function: report from the Standardisation Sub-committee of the International Continence Society. Neurourol Urodyn. 2002;21(2):167–78.
9. Vahr S, Cobussen-Boekhorst H, Eikenboom J, Geng V, Holroyd S, Lester M, Pearce I, Vandewinkel C. Evidence-based guidelines for best practice in urological health care. Catheterisation: urethral intermittent in adults. Dilatation, urethral intermittent in adults. Drukkerij Gelderland. 2013. ISBN: 978-90-79754-59-5.
10. Moore KN, Fader M, Getliffe K. Long-term bladder management by intermittent catheterisation in adults and children. Cochrane Database Syst Rev. 2007(4). https://doi.org/10.1002/14651858.CD006008.pub2.
11. Woodward S, Rew M. Patients' quality of life and clean intermittent self-catheterization. Br J Nurs. 2003;12(18):1066–74.
12. Cravens DD, Zweig S. Urinary catheter management. Am Fam Physician. 2000;61(2):369–76.
13. Kessler TM, Ryu G, Burkhard FC. Clean intermittent self-catheterization: a burden for the patient? Neurourol Urodyn. 2009;28(1):18–21.
14. Cobussen-Boekhorst H, Hermeling E, Heesakkers J, van Gaal B. Patients' experience with intermittent catheterisation in everyday life. J Clin Nurs. 2016;25(9–10):1253–61.
15. Logan K, Shaw C, Webber I, Samuel S, Broome L. Patients' experiences of learning clean intermittent self-catheterization: a qualitative study. J Adv Nurs. 2008;62(1):32–40.
16. Shaw C, Logan K, Webber I, Broome L, Samuel S. Effect of clean intermittent self-catheterization on quality of life: a qualitative study. J Adv Nurs. 2008;61(6):641–50.
17. van Achterberg T, Holleman G, Cobussen-Boekhorst H, Arts R, Heesakkers J. Adherence to clean intermittent self-catheterization procedures: determinants explored. J Clin Nurs. 2008;17(3):394–402.
18. Cobussen-Boekhorst H, Beekman J, van Wijlick E, Schaafstra J, van Kuppevelt D, Heesakkers J. Which factors make clean intermittent (self) catheterisation successful? J Clin Nurs. 2016;25(9–10):1308–18.
19. Bennett CJ, Diokno AC. Clean intermittent self-catheterization in the elderly. Urology. 1984;24(1):43–5.
20. Pilloni S, Krhut J, Mair D, Madersbacher H, Kessler TM. Intermittent catheterisation in older people: a valuable alternative to an indwelling catheter? Age Ageing. 2005;34(1):57–60.
21. Girotti ME, MacCornick S, Perisse H, Batezini NS, Almeida FG. Determining the variables associated to clean intermittent self-catheterization adherence rate: one-year follow-up study. Int Braz J Urol. 2011;37(6):766–72.

22. Parsons BA, Narshi A, Drake MJ. Success rates for learning intermittent self-catheterisation according to age and gender. Int Urol Nephrol. 2012;44(4):1127–31.
23. Geng V, Cobussen-Boekhorst H, Lurvink H, Pearce I, Vahr S. Evidence-based guidelines for best practice in urological health care. Male external catheters in adults—urinary catheter management. 2016. ISBN: 978-90-79754-87-8.
24. Geng V, Cobussen-Boekhorst H, Farrell J, Gea-Sanchez J, Pearce I, Schwennesen T, et al. Evidence-based guidelines for best practice in urological health care catheterisation indwelling catheters in adults urethral and suprapubic 2012. ISBN: 978-90-79754-50-2.
25. Pannek J, Gocking K, Bersch U. To clamp or not to clamp? Bladder management by suprapubic catheterization in patients with neurogenic bladder dysfunction. World J Urol. 2010;28(5):637–41.
26. Bernard MS, Hunter KF, Moore KN. A review of strategies to decrease the duration of indwelling urethral catheters and potentially reduce the incidence of catheter-associated urinary tract infections. Urol Nurs. 2012;32(1):29–37.
27. Heesakkers J, Chapple C, Deridder D, Farag F, editors. Practical functional urology. Cham: Springer; 2016. ISBN: 978-3-319-25430-2.

Pharmacologic Management of Neurogenic Lower Urinary Tract Dysfunction

Casey G. Kowalik, Sophia Delpe, and Roger Dmochowski

Introduction

Normal lower urinary tract function is dependent on precise neural control of storage and emptying of urine. Any alteration of this complex coordination from a neurologic lesion can result in neurogenic lower urinary tract dysfunction (NLUTD), with the extent and location of the neurologic lesion affecting the type and severity of dysfunction.

A prior chapter has described, in -depth, the neurophysiology of micturition, but it will be briefly reviewed below to provide context for the effects of pharmacologic management of neurogenic bladder. Prior to an in-depth exploration of the pharmacologic treatment options, goals of management and assessment of NLUTD will be discussed to offer a complete understanding of the scope of this issue.

Neurologic Control of Micturition

Lower urinary tract function is controlled by the autonomic (parasympathetic and sympathetic) and somatic nervous systems. Parasympathetic pathways are responsible for bladder emptying, while sympathetic nerve activation is involved in bladder storage. Parasympathetic preganglionic nerves originate in the sacral spinal cord, travel in the pelvic nerve, and synapse with parasympathetic postganglionic neurons in the pelvic plexus. Parasympathetic postganglionic neurons release acetylcholine, which binds to M2 and M3 receptors located within the detrusor muscle, to stimulate contraction. Although M2 receptors are present in higher density, M3

C. G. Kowalik · S. Delpe · R. Dmochowski (✉)
Department of Urologic Surgery, Vanderbilt University Medical Center, Nashville, TN, USA
e-mail: casey.kowalik@vanderbilt.edu; sophia.d.delpe@vanderbilt.edu; roger.dochowski@vanderbilt.edu

© Springer International Publishing AG, part of Springer Nature 2018
R. Dmochowski, J. Heesakkers (eds.), *Neuro-Urology*,
https://doi.org/10.1007/978-3-319-90997-4_21

receptors are the principal receptors involved in mediating bladder contraction and are the target of antimuscarinic drugs [1]. Parasympathetic pathways to the urethral sphincter cause relaxation during voiding through release of the inhibitory neurotransmitter, nitric oxide [2].

Sympathetic preganglionic nerves exit the thoracolumbar spinal cord and pass through the hypogastric nerve to synapse with nicotinic receptors on sympathetic postganglionic neurons. Sympathetic postganglionic nerves release norepinephrine to act on adrenergic receptors in the lower urinary tract and facilitate bladder storage. Specifically, norepinephrine acts on β-adrenergic receptors (β1, β2, β3) located within the bladder body to promote relaxation and α1-adrenergic receptors in the bladder base and proximal urethra causing smooth muscle contraction. Bladder relaxation is primarily induced through stimulation of β3 adrenergic receptors and is the target of mirabegron, a β3 agonist, in the treatment of detrusor overactivity [3].

The somatic pudendal nerve originates from Onuf's nucleus in the sacral spinal cord and releases acetylcholine which acts on nicotinic receptors to induce contraction of the striated urinary sphincter and pelvic floor musculature [4].

The pontine micturition center (PMC), also known as Barrington's nucleus, is the regulation center for voluntary control of the bladder and is located in the rostral brainstem. Neurons from the PMC project in descending spinobulbospinal pathways to the intermediolateral cell column of the sacral spinal cord. Activation of this pathway causes urethral relaxation and activation of pelvic parasympathetic nerves and inhibits the sympathetic and pudendal effects on the urethral outlet to promote bladder emptying [5].

During bladder storage, the raphe nuclei of the central nervous system (CNS) send serotonergic inputs to the sympathetic and parasympathetic nerves with resultant inhibition of reflex bladder contractions. A serotonin and norepinephrine reuptake inhibitor has been shown to both increase sphincter activity and decrease bladder contractions in an animal model [6].

On a cellular level, interstitial cells of Cajal (ICCs) are located just below the urothelium within the lamina propria and with the detrusor muscle of the bladder [7]. ICCs act as pacemakers and trigger contractions of adjacent smooth muscle cells, as well as interact with cholinergic and sensory nerve endings [8]. This allows ICCs to act as a channel of information between the autonomic system and sensory nerves with the detrusor muscle. Any disturbance in the ICC signaling may alter detrusor contraction and cause detrusor overactivity and/or may alter bladder sensation and cause bladder pain.

In addition to ICCs, purinergic receptors are present within the lamina propria and may have a role in detrusor overactivity. Adenosine triphosphate released from urothelial cells during filling can stimulate purinergic receptors and help mediate normal detrusor contraction directly [9]. Bladder biopsy specimens from patients with neurogenic detrusor overactivity (NDO) showed higher rates of atropine-resistant contractions compared to stable bladder specimens. These contractions were ameliorated by a purinergic receptor blocker, suggesting not only a direct influence of ATP on NDO but also the possibility for alternative drug developments

[10]. The role of ICCs and purinergic receptors highlights the idea that the urothelium has a function in modulating bladder activity.

Lastly, it is also important to remember that neurologic lesions can be partial and/or multiple, creating the opportunity for multiple combinations of neurologic effects that may not precisely correlate with the location of the lesion(s). Also, neural plasticity following injury can occur, inducing structural and functional changes, over time [11]. Clinically, this can result in evolving neurologic deficits. The neurologic findings present at an initial encounter can alter over time, and continuous and vigilant care is needed.

Goals of Management

Early diagnosis and treatment are paramount to avoiding long-term complications of the neurogenic bladder. Protection of upper tract function is the primary concern with continence being an important, yet secondary, matter. Upper tract preservation is dependent upon maintaining a low-pressure reservoir (detrusor pressure below 40 cmH$_2$O, compliance greater than 12.5 cmH$_2$O/mL), complete emptying, and reducing the risks of urinary tract infection [12, 13]. More recent data in children with myelodysplasia suggested that detrusor leak point pressure <20 cmH$_2$O may be a more sensitive measurement of the risk of upper tract damage [14]. Patients with continuous versus intermittent DSD had an increased incidence of upper urinary tract abnormalities suggesting that duration of elevated bladder pressures is a factor [15]. The proposed treatment, whether medical or surgical, must be acceptable to the patient to ensure compliance. Lastly, quality of life is also an important aspect in the care of these patients and should be continuously assessed.

Assessment of Neurogenic Bladder

Patient assessment should begin with an evaluation of the patient's symptoms. Lower urinary tract symptoms can be categorized into three groups: storage, voiding, and post-micturition [16]. Storage symptoms include frequency, nocturia, urgency, and urinary incontinence. Voiding symptoms include hesitancy, intermittency, and straining. Post-micturition symptoms are the sensation of incomplete emptying and post-micturition dribbling. The symptoms can provide insight into the underlying pathophysiology of the NLUTD. A detailed physical examination, including not only of the genitourinary system but also neurologic findings, is important because this will affect treatment selection. For example, it is prudent to understand the feasibility of performing self-intermittent catheterization prior to initiating treatment that may result in urinary retention. Urinalysis, serum creatinine, and upper tract imaging should also be performed at initial presentation.

Table 1 Functional classification of neurogenic lower urinary tract dysfunction

	Storage dysfunction	Emptying dysfunction
Bladder	Neurogenic detrusor overactivity	Detrusor areflexia
Outlet	Sphincter underactivity	Detrusor sphincter dyssynergia

Videourodynamic evaluation is performed to document the specific dysfunctions of the lower urinary tract. The functional classification system for voiding dysfunction developed by Wein [17] is a practical method to understand the underlying pathophysiology based on urodynamic findings and is shown in Table 1. These abnormalities of the bladder and outlet can occur in isolation, yet in cases of NLUTD, they often occur in combination. This classification system can then direct appropriate treatment options, either medical or surgical, aimed at correcting the functional abnormality.

Patients with neurogenic bladder often also have concomitant neurogenic bowel dysfunction due to a common underlying neurologic process. Also, the side effects of medications used in the treatment of NLUTD can exacerbate constipation. Treatment of neurogenic bowel should not be overlooked as constipation can worsen detrusor overactivity and bladder emptying, while fecal incontinence may increase the risk of urinary tract infections and predispose to skin breakdown. Medical therapy of neurogenic bowel dysfunction is beyond the scope of this chapter, but in general, aggressive treatment of constipation and involvement of gastroenterology specialists early are beneficial [18].

Pharmacologic Management of Neurogenic Lower Urinary Tract Dysfunction

The remainder of this chapter will discuss the pharmacologic management of neurogenic bladder based on the functional classification system shown in Table 1. Patients should additionally be counseled on non-pharmacologic interventions including behavioral management, such as fluid regulation and timed voiding or catheterization, and pelvic floor physical therapy when appropriate.

Detrusor Areflexia

Detrusor areflexia occurs during the period of spinal shock immediately following spinal cord injury (SCI) and in cases of lower motor neuron lesions, such as cauda equina syndrome. Patients with detrusor areflexia may be in urinary retention, or some may be able to void with straining. Initially detrusor areflexia can be managed with indwelling catheterization, but it is important to establish a reliable and acceptable long-term method of bladder emptying. The earliest record for management of bladder emptying was by transurethral bronze tubes, reeds, and palm leaves and dates to 1500 BC [19]. The use of clean, intermittent, self-catheterization was formally reintroduced in the 1970s by Lapides [20]. Clean intermittent catheterization has been shown to preserve bladder compliance in SCI patients [13]. In some instances, intermittent catheterization is not a feasible option, and long-term indwelling catheterization is required, and in these cases, suprapubic tube placement is often preferred over urethral catheterization.

As an alternative to catheterization, women with detrusor areflexia can consider using the inFlow™ device, which is a magnetized valve-pump device inserted into the urethra. During voiding, an activator is held over the pubic bone and turned "on" to open the valve and allow urine flow. Once finished, the "on" button is released and the valve closes. In a multicenter trial, of the women who completed the study, there were significant improvements in the quality of life. Eighty-one subjects withdrew during the active treatment phase with the most commonly reported reasons being discomfort and leakage. Women who completed the study were more likely to have a lower baseline quality of life, more limited ability to ambulate, and poorer manual dexterity [21]. The inFlow™ device is a nonsurgical alternative option to catheterization and may have a bigger role in those patients with poorer quality of life or more difficulty performing self-catheterization.

Bethanechol

Recall that bladder contraction is mediated by parasympathetic pathways via action on muscarinic cholinergic receptors. Bethanechol (Urecholine®) is an oral cholinergic agonist that is resistant to degradation by acetylcholinesterase and acts on the parasympathetic postganglionic neurons. It has been proposed to improve voiding in patients with nonobstructive urinary retention; however, the clinical outcomes in randomized placebo-controlled trials have not shown efficacy [22].

In a study of patients with detrusor areflexia, 9 of 11 patients that responded to electromotive administration of bethanechol subsequently had return of spontaneous voiding with oral bethanechol, suggesting that it may be only patients with some degree of detrusor contractility that derive any benefit from oral bethanechol [23]. Prostaglandin E2 and bethanechol in combination demonstrated limited effectiveness in a group of patients with detrusor underactivity [24].

In summary, there are no pharmacologic agents effective in the treatment of detrusor areflexia, although several have been studied. Given the pharmacologic properties of bethanechol, it seemed promising to treat detrusor underactivity, but clinical studies have been unable to definitively demonstrate effectiveness.

Neurogenic Detrusor Overactivity

Neurogenic detrusor overactivity (NDO) can cause sustained elevated bladder pressures due to a hyperreflexic, overactive detrusor muscle. Subjectively, patients may experience urinary frequency, urgency, and incontinence. In general, initial management includes antimuscarinic medications in combination with intermittent catheterization. Antimuscarinics have been shown to be effective in improving maximum cystometric bladder capacity (MCC) and compliance and reducing detrusor pressure compared to placebo in neurogenic populations [25, 26].

Antimuscarinic Drugs

Antimuscarinic agents that have been studied in the adult neurogenic population for treatment of NDO include oxybutynin, darifenacin, solifenacin, tolterodine, trospium, and propiverine. Clinically, antimuscarinics appear to act primarily on M3 receptors to reduce bladder contractions in the filling phase. With standard dosages, there appears to be minimal effect on bladder contraction during voiding, although urinary retention is a risk factor with higher doses [27]. The most common side effects of antimuscarinics include dry mouth, dry eyes, and constipation. Of concern are also the CNS side effects associated with antimuscarinics including cognitive impairment and poor memory. Contraindications to their use include acute angle glaucoma and gastric retention.

Oxybutynin

Oxybutynin is available in immediate (Ditropan®) and extended-release (Ditropan XL®) formulations. Oral immediate-release oxybutynin 15 mg versus placebo showed significant differences in MCC (125 vs. -10 mL, $p < 0.0001$), maximum detrusor pressure (-35 vs. -4 cmH$_2$O, $p < 0.0001$), and post-void residual (15 vs. 3 mL, $p = 0.012$); however clinical parameters were not measured in this study [26]. A prospective study of extended-release oxybutynin in SCI patients with NDO started treatment at a dosage of 10 mg daily and increased to 30 mg daily. At 12 weeks, voiding diaries showed decreased urinary frequency and incontinence episodes, and urodynamic evaluation demonstrated increased MCC from baseline. There were no adverse events reported indicating that extended-release oxybutynin dosages up to 30 mg daily are safe and well tolerated.

Transdermal oxybutynin (Oxytrol®) is another available route of administration with the benefit of lower incidence of anticholinergic side effects by avoiding first-pass metabolism [28]. In a study of patients with NDO and incontinence between intermittent catheterizations, there were improvements in the number of incontinence episodes and catheterized volumes. Additionally, there was significant increase in MCC and a decrease in detrusor pressure at capacity. The most common adverse event was application site reaction, occurring in 12.5% of the patients [29].

Intravesical administration of oxybutynin has also been studied. Crushed oxybutynin pills are diluted in water or saline and instilled into the bladder via catheterization and allowed to dwell. Compared to oral oxybutynin, intravesical administration has a higher bioavailability by avoiding first-pass hepatic metabolism resulting in higher efficacy and lower rate of side effects [30]. In a randomized controlled trial comparing intravesical administration of 10 mL 0.1% oxybutynin three times daily (TID) to oral 5 mg TID, there was a significant increase in MCC in the intravesical group compared to the oral group (116 vs. 18 mL, $p = 0.0086$). However, there were no significant differences in maximum detrusor pressure, volume at which vesico-ureteral reflex occurred, or bladder compliance. Clinically, there were no differences in the number of incontinence episodes or frequency of catheterization [31]. Oxybutynin is also thought to have potential local anesthetic effects, which may be of some additional benefit in this use [32].

Tolterodine

Tolterodine (Detrol®, Detrol LA®) acts on both M2 and M3 receptors. The immediate-release tablet is generally administered as 2 mg twice daily and the extended-release capsule is 4 mg once daily.

In a dose-ranging study comparing tolterodine (0.5, 1, 2, or 4 mg twice daily) to placebo, there was a dose-dependent improvement in urodynamic variables. Two patients taking the 4 mg twice daily dosing experienced urinary retention, causing the authors to conclude that 1–2 mg twice daily is the optimal dose for NDO [33]. In a small, randomized, double-blind study, tolterodine 2 mg twice daily reduced incontinence episodes and increased catheterized volumes compared to placebo, but there was no difference in MCC [34].

In a single-arm study evaluating the efficacy of extended-release tolterodine 4 mg/day for NDO showed that after 12 weeks of treatment, there were significant improvements in urinary frequency, urgency, and incontinence episodes. Also, patients had increased MCC and bladder compliance [35]. The rate of reported dry mouth was 8%.

A Cochrane review [36] compared oxybutynin to tolterodine, both immediate and extended-release formulations, with the conclusions that there was no difference in clinical outcomes between the drugs, but tolterodine had less dry mouth, reflecting the lower affinity of tolterodine for M3 receptors in the parotid gland, compared to oxybutynin [37]. Also, in general, extended-release formulations had fewer side effects than the immediate release.

Darifenacin

Darifenacin (Enablex®) is a selective M3 receptor antagonist. It is available in an extended-release formulation at 7.5 mg daily. In a randomized placebo-controlled, crossover study, of patients with NSO, darifenacin was found to significantly suppress unstable bladder contractions [38]. In another study of 38 patients with multiple sclerosis and NDO, 12 weeks of treatment with 15 mg of darifenacin resulted in increased MCC and improved bladder compliance as well as an 82% continence rate [39].

Despite darifenacin being a selective M3 receptor, it is not specific to the bladder. Salivary glands, gastrointestinal tract, and other tissues also contain M3 receptors, so side effects of dry mouth and constipation remain.

Solifenacin

Solifenacin (Vesicare®) is a selective M3 receptor antagonist. The initial dose is 5 mg once daily which can be increased to 10 mg daily if tolerated. In a prospective, randomized, placebo-controlled double-blind trial comparing solifenacin 10 mg to placebo in 51 patients with NDO either due to SCI or multiple sclerosis, the treatment group had a greater increase in MCC (360 vs. 232 mL, $p < 0.001$) and bladder volume at first detrusor contraction (216 vs. 131 mL, $p < 0.001$) and leak (230 vs. 141 mL, $p < 0.05$). Maximum detrusor pressure was also lower in the solifenacin group (50 vs. 82 cmH_2O, $p < 0.01$). There was no difference in the number of incontinence episodes in a 24-h period, but there were significant improvements in treatment satisfaction scores and patient perception of bladder condition. The most common reported side effects were dry mouth (8%) and blurred vision (8%) [40].

Trospium

Trospium (Sanctura®, Sanctura XR®, Trosec®) is a quaternary amine with both immediate-release (20 mg twice daily) and extended-release (60 mg daily) formulations. The benefit of the quaternary amine structure is that it should not be able to cross the blood-brain barrier and should have decreased risk of causing cognitive impairment compared to the other antimuscarinic drugs.

A randomized, placebo-controlled trial comparing trospium 20 mg daily for 3 weeks to placebo showed pre- and posttreatment improvements in MCC (mean difference of 138 mL) and bladder compliance (mean difference of 12 mL/cmH_2O) and a decrease in maximum detrusor pressure (mean change of -38 cmH_2O) in the treatment group [41]. The described side effects were low with only one patient reporting constipation.

In a comparison of trospium 20 mg twice daily to oxybutynin 5 mg TID, there was improvement within each arm in MCC, compliance, and maximum voiding pressure. There were no differences between the two groups, suggesting equivalent efficacy between the two medications. However, there was fewer reports of dry mouth in the trospium group (4% vs. 23%) [42].

Menarini and colleagues [43] conducted a prospective double-blind study comparing standard dose (45 mg/day) to adjustable dose (90–135 mg/day depending on urodynamic response) trospium. Results showed that doses up to 135 mg/day appeared to be well tolerated without any differences in adverse effects between the two groups. However, there were also no significant clinical differences between the standard and higher dosing, suggesting that 45 mg/day provides an effective therapeutic response in patients with NDO.

Propiverine

Propiverine (Detrunorm®, Mictoryl®) is a nonselective antimuscarinic that also has some calcium antagonistic actions, although the clinical importance of this is unclear [27]. It is not available in the United States but is available in Canada and Europe in immediate- and extended-release formulations. Adult initial dosing is 30 mg daily with a maximum of 45 mg daily. Propiverine demonstrated superiority to placebo in a neurogenic population of 113 patients where the treatment group had significant increases in MCC (104 vs. −6 mL), maximum detrusor pressure (27 vs. 0.2 cmH_2O), volume at first detrusor contraction, and duration of contractions (−20 vs. −1.6 s) compared to placebo, but there was no difference in bladder compliance between the treatment and placebo groups. Subjectively, 63% of patients in the propiverine group reported subjective improvement compared to 23% in the placebo group. The treatment group reported the expected anticholinergic side effects with dry mouth being the most common in 37% [44].

An investigation of 66 patients with NDO comparing propiverine extended release 45 mg daily to 15 mg immediate-release TID found no differences in urodynamic parameters. There was a 25% improvement in the reduction of incontinence rates in the extended-release group. The total number of adverse events was slightly lower in the extended-release group (42% vs. 36%) with dry mouth being the most common in both treatment arms [45].

In a randomized comparison of oxybutynin 5 mg TID to propiverine 15 mg TID in patients with NDO, both agents improved urodynamic parameters, and there were no differences between the treatment groups [46].

In brief, antimuscarinic drugs have demonstrated improvements in MCC and bladder compliance, as well as decreased maximum detrusor pressure, with oxybutynin being the most extensively studied. The decrease in maximum detrusor pressure to values under $40cmH_2O$ is crucial to prevent upper tract deterioration [12] Although more limited data, there is still support for using darifenacin, solifenacin, trospium, tolterodine, and propiverine. Most of the studies are short duration (<12 weeks), so the long-term efficacy and tolerability of antimuscarinics are largely unknown in this population.

Mirabegron

Mirabegron (Myrbetriq®) is a selective β-3 agonist. Initial starting dose is 25 mg daily and can be increased to 50 mg daily. A retrospective study of 15 patients with NDO demonstrated improvements in urinary frequency and number of incontinence episodes. There were also improvements in urodynamic parameters, including increased MCC and compliance [47].

Since mirabegron has a different mechanism of action from antimuscarinics, combining the treatments may provide additional benefit. In an animal model of rats with SCI, the combination of oxybutynin and mirabegron reduced detrusor contractions and increased bladder compliance to a greater extent than either medication alone [48].

Mirabegron avoids the anticholinergic effects of constipation and dry mouth but can have cardiovascular side effects including mild elevations in blood pressure and small, dose-dependent increases in heart rate [49, 50]. Caution should be used in patients with uncontrolled hypertension and tachycardia.

Imipramine

Imipramine is a tricyclic antidepressant (TCA) that has systemic antimuscarinic effects and inhibits reuptake of noradrenaline and serotonin and may potentially work by both decreasing bladder contractility and increasing outlet resistance. In a study from 1972 of 9 patients, receiving imipramine 1.0–2.5 mg/kg/day, 6 had improved urinary incontinence. No adverse events were reported in this study, but the cardiovascular toxicity of TCAs has been well described, so it should be used with caution [51]. No other studies have been done assessing efficacy of imipramine on NDO.

Combined Medications

Patients not responsive to high-dose single antimuscarinic drug therapy may respond to combined high-dose antimuscarinic therapy with comparable side effects to standard dosing [52]. Multidrug therapy with two or three drugs may provide additional benefit as one study suggests, particularly in those patients who failed a single antimuscarinic drug [53].

Other Medications

Cyclooxygenase inhibitors have shown a benefit in treatment of NDO in animal models through suppression of unmyelinated C fibers [54]. However the potential side effects on the gastrointestinal, renal, and cardiovascular systems have prevented widespread clinical application for this indication. Tramadol is a μ-receptor agonist that has shown inhibition of detrusor contractions in animal studies but has not been specifically studied in patients with NDO [55].

Botulinum Toxin A

Botulinum toxin A (BTX-A) (Botox®) is a potent neurotoxin produced by *Clostridium botulinum*. It works by blocking the release of ACh from both preganglionic and postganglionic parasympathetic nerves at the neuromuscular junction leading to flaccid paralysis of the detrusor muscle. The injection of BTX-A into the detrusor for management of NDO was first described by Schurch and colleagues in 2000 [56]. Six weeks following injection, 89% (17/19) of patients had continence restored. Also, both MCC (216–416 mL) and reflux volume (296–481 mL) significantly increased. Since then, many studies have done showing long-term efficacy and safety. Over a 4-year study, patients with NDO received BTX-A 200 or 300 units as needed for symptom control and on average had a 9-month duration of effect. Improvements in incontinence episodes and quality of life were consistent over the duration of the study, suggesting that subsequent injections do not have decreased efficacy. Urinary tract infection was the most common complication at a rate of 13.2% [57].

In summary, antimuscarinic medications are currently considered first-line medical treatment in the management of NDO [58]. In head-to-head trials, the antimuscarinic medications appear to have equal effect, such that one cannot be recommended over another in the management of NDO. Depending on receptor selectivity, the side effects vary slightly among the medications, with tolterodine and trospium having fewer side effects than oxybutynin. Additionally, the side effect profile favors extended-release formulations over immediate release when possible. It is also necessary to note the administration of antimuscarinics to elderly adults should be done with caution due to risk of development of CNS effects.

More recent data supports the use of mirabegron as effective in improving clinical and urodynamic parameters in the NDO population. Combination of drugs for treatment of NDO may provide additional benefit over monotherapy. BTX A should be considered in patients whose bladder capacity or compliance declines despite optimal medical therapy or patients who are intolerant to the side effects of the medications.

Detrusor Sphincter Dyssynergia (DSD)

Suprasacral lesions can result in detrusor sphincter dyssynergia (DSD) [59]. DSD is diagnosed on urodynamic study and is characterized by increased electromyography activity and a closed sphincter, with secondary ballooning of the posterior urethra, on voiding cystourethrogram during detrusor contraction [60]. Measurement of urethral pressures has also been described in the diagnosis of DSD [61]. Diagnosis and management of DSD are critical to prevent renal dysfunction from impaired bladder compliance. As mentioned, patients with DSD often also have NDO, and in combination, this can lead to a poorly compliant bladder. Additionally, patients with DSD may be at risk for autonomic dysreflexia.

Baclofen

When baclofen, an antispasmodic drug, is delivered intrathecally, it may inhibit neurons of the CNS, in particular, of Onuf's nucleus. In three patients with spastic paraplegia who received continuous intrathecal baclofen, there was resolution of DSD in one patient although all reported significant improvements in urinary symptoms [62]. Other skeletal muscle relaxants, including dantrolene and valium, have also been trialed without any significant success [63].

Alpha Blockers

It was considered that alpha blockers may have a role in the treatment of DSD to induce sphincter relaxation; however, a study of terazosin 5 mg daily did not demonstrate improvements in voiding pressures [64].

Botulinum Toxin A

As mentioned, botulinum toxin A (BTX-A) inhibits the release of ACh from presynaptic neurons at the neuromuscular junction. Its use for the management of DSD was first evaluated by Dykstra and colleagues. They injected the sphincter with a low dose of BTX-A in 11 men once per week for 3 weeks with resultant decreased urethral pressures and post-void residuals, with an average duration of efficacy of 50 days [65]. In a more recent study, significant reductions in urethral pressures and post-void residuals were seem following intrasphincteric injection of 100 units [66].

BTX-A can be injected into the sphincter either transurethrally or transperineally. There is no standard protocol, but the sphincter is usually injected in a few places along the dorsal aspect (between 9 and 3 o'clock) with a total dose of 100 units [61].

A Cochrane review including four trials showed that injection of BTX-A in the sphincter can improve urodynamic parameters, specifically higher voided volumes and lower detrusor pressures [67]. Intrasphincteric injection of BTX-A could be considered an alternative to sphincterotomy given the lower morbidity, although repeated injections are needed when the effects of the BTX-A dissipate.

Potential side effects of intrasphincteric BTX-A injection is spread to adjacent muscles, as seen in the study by Dykstra et al. who noted limb paresthesia that resolved over 2–3 weeks [68]. However, later series did not note any complications [69].

Sphincter Underactivity

Sphincter underactivity causes low outlet resistance and symptoms of stress urinary incontinence. Drugs targeting bladder outlet resistance have not been specifically studied in the neurogenic population. Nonetheless, several classes of medications have been studied for SUI including alpha adrenergic receptor agonists, beta adrenergic receptor agonists, and tricyclic antidepressants; only serotonin-norepinephrine reuptake inhibitors have shown some benefit.

Duloxetine (Cymbalta®) inhibits the presynaptic reuptake of serotonin and nor-epinephrine at the level of the sacral spinal cord. Duloxetine is approved for use in Europe for women with SUI. A systematic review of nine randomized controlled trials comparing duloxetine to placebo showed improvements in incontinence episode frequency and quality of life, but there was no clear difference in objective data causing the authors to conclude that long-term clinical efficacy of duloxetine on SUI is unclear [70]. Overall, the evidence is weak in the female SUI population and not studied in the neurogenic population. Surgical therapy remains the mainstay in the definitive management of an incompetent sphincter in the NDO population.

Adjunct Medical Treatment

Nocturnal Polyuria

Desmopressin (Minirin®, Nocdurna®, Noctiva™) is a synthetic analogue of vaso-pressin, which binds V2 receptors in the renal collecting ducts, resulting in increased water reabsorption, urine concentration, and decreased urine volume [71]. It is currently approved for use in patients with nocturnal polyuria. A meta-analysis on the efficacy of desmopressin in patients with multiple sclerosis showed a significantly lower voiding frequency in the first 6–8 h following administration and reduced nocturnal urine volume [72]. Desmopressin is contraindicated in patients with hyponatremia or renal dysfunction. Given the risk of hyponatremia, baseline and periodic serum chemistry after initiation of treatment are recommended.

Patients with neurologic disease affecting the autonomic system may have loss of diurnal variation in blood pressure due to loss of vascular tone. Fluid redistribution while supine at night can result in a relative hypertension and increased renal blood flow which can lead to increase in urine production or nocturnal polyuria [73]. Additionally altered levels of antidiuretic hormone, with higher concentrations during the day, influence renal filtration of sodium and water, increasing urine production at night relative to daytime, which is the opposite of normal physiology [74].

Autonomic Dysreflexia

Spinal cord injury patients with lesions above the level of T6 are at risk for autonomic dysreflexia, which is the result of unopposed sympathetic discharge that can occur with noxious stimuli, such as bladder distention. The symptoms of autonomic dysreflexia include headache, sweating, flushing above the level of the lesion, hypertension, and reflex bradycardia, although there is a variable spectrum of presentation. If not properly recognized and treated, this can become life-threatening. If the cause of the autonomic dysreflexia is bladder distention, the first step in management is bladder drainage. Several pharmacologic agents can be used for the treatment of autonomic dysreflexia; current recommendation is placement of 2% nitroglycerin paste above the level of the lesion for rapid blood pressure reduction [75].

Terazosin has also been studied in a small group of adult SCI patients for its effect on decreasing the severity and frequency of autonomic dysreflexia. At all follow-up time points (1 week, 1 month, and 3 months), there were significant decreases in the frequency of AD episodes. At 3 months, during an AD episodes, there were improvements in the severity of systolic blood pressure elevation, heart rate, degree of sweating, and duration compared to baseline severity [76].

Management of DSD may also influence frequency and severity of autonomic dysreflexia. Following intrasphincteric injection of BTX-A for DSD, Dykstra et al. also noted improvements in autonomic dysreflexia [65].

Follow-Up of Patients with Neurogenic Bladder

NLUTD is an evolving condition, and lifelong follow-up is necessary in this patient population to prevent the occurrence of complications, particularly renal failure. Periodic assessments must be performed, including upper tract imaging and repeat urodynamic evaluation at least every 1–2 years and sooner if clinical condition warrants [58]. If a patient's bladder function worsens despite optimal medical treatment, surgical intervention should be considered.

Future of Medical Therapy

As understanding of the pathophysiologic mechanisms underlying NLUTD continues to increase, there is potential for new pharmacologic therapies to be developed. The role of ICCs is unfolding, and there is potential for targets of c-kit, a proto-oncogene expressed by ICCs, to aid in the treatment of detrusor overactivity [8]. Additionally, as the field of regenerative medicine continues to expand, the role for tissue engineering may move to clinical applications in patients with NLUTD. Currently, researchers are able to induce urothelial cells from stem cells, but continued work is needed to create a sustainable bladder reservoir capable of filling and emptying [77].

Conclusions

Early diagnosis and treatment are imperative to preventing long-term complications from NLUTD. A multidisciplinary and individualized approach is often necessary in this complex patient population. The success of antimuscarinic therapy for NDO is well documented and when used in combination with other drugs may maximize efficacy. BTX-A injection into the bladder and sphincter has shown great efficacy in the management of NDO and DSD, respectively. In the future, the use of stem cells in bladder tissue engineering may play a bigger role in the management of NLUTD. Close and lifelong follow-up of all patients with NLUTD is essential to prevent secondary complications.

References

1. Mansfield KJ, Liu L, Mitchelson FJ, et al. Muscarinic receptor subtypes in human bladder detrusor and mucosa, studied by radioligand binding and quantitative competitive RT-PCR: changes in ageing. Br J Pharmacol. 2005;144:1089–99.
2. de Groat WC, Griffiths D, Yoshimura N. Neural control of the lower urinary tract. Compr Physiol. 2015;5:327–96.
3. Andersson K-E, Arner A. Urinary bladder contraction and relaxation: physiology and pathophysiology. Physiol Rev. 2004;84:935–86. https://doi.org/10.1152/physrev.00038.2003.
4. Yoshimura N, Chancellor MB. Neurophysiology of lower urinary tract function and dysfunction. Rev Urol. 2003;5:S3–S10.
5. Fowler CJ, Griffiths D, de Groat WC. The neural control of micturition. Nat Rev Neurosci. 2008;9:453–66. https://doi.org/10.1038/nrn2401.
6. Thor KB, Donatucci C. Central nervous system control of the lower urinary tract: new pharmacological approaches to stress urinary incontinence in women. J Urol. 2004;172:27–33. https://doi.org/10.1097/01.ju.0000118381.04432.22.
7. McCloskey KD. Interstitial cells of cajal in the urinary tract. In: Andersson K-E, Michel MC, editors. Urinary tract. Berlin: Springer; 2011. p. 233–54.
8. Juszczak K, Maciukiewicz P, Drewa T, Thor P. Cajal–like interstitial cells as a novel target in detrusor overactivity treatment: true or myth? Cent Eur J Urol. 2013;66:1–5. https://doi.org/10.5173/ceju.2013.04.art5.
9. Chai TC, Birder LA. Physiology and pharmacology of the bladder and urethra. In: Wein AJ, Kavoussi LR, Partin AW, Peters CA, editors. Campbell-Walsh urology, 11th ed. 2016. p. 1631–84.
10. Pakzad M, Ikeda Y, McCarthy C, et al. Contractile effects and receptor analysis of adenosine-receptors in human detrusor muscle from stable and neuropathic bladders. Naunyn Schmiedeberg's Arch Pharmacol. 2016;389:921–9. https://doi.org/10.1007/s00210-016-1255-1.
11. Jean-Xavier C, Sharples SA, Mayr KA, et al. Retracing your footsteps: developmental insights to spinal network plasticity following injury. J Neurophysiol. 2017. https://doi.org/10.1152/jn.00575.2017.
12. McGuire EJ, Woodside JR, Borden TA, Weiss RM. Prognostic value of urodynamic testing in myelodysplastic patients. J Urol. 1981;126:205–9.
13. Weld KJ, Graney MJ, Dmochowski RR. Difference in bladder compliance with time and associations of bladder management with compliance in spinal cord injured patients. J Urol. 2000;163:1228–33.
14. Tarcan T, Sekerci CA, Akbal C, et al. Is 40 cm H$_2$O detrusor leak point pressure cut-off reliable for upper urinary tract protection in children with myelodysplasia? Neurourol Urodyn. 2016;36:759–63. https://doi.org/10.1002/nau.23017.
15. Weld KJ, Graney MJ, Dmochowski RR. Clinical significance of detrusor sphincter dyssynergic type in patients with post-traumatic spinal cord injury. Urology. 2000;56:565–8.

16. Abrams P, Cardozo L, Fall M, et al. The standardisation of terminology of lower urinary tract function: report from the Standardisation Sub-committee of the International Continence Society. Neurourol Urodyn. 2002;21:167–78. https://doi.org/10.1002/nau.10052.

17. Wein AJ. Classification of neurogenic voiding dysfunction. J Urol. 2081;125:605–9.

18. Agrawal S, Agrawal RR, Wood HM. Establishing a multidisciplinary approach to the management of neurologic disease affecting the urinary tract. Urol Clin North Am. 2017;44:377–89. https://doi.org/10.1016/j.ucl.2017.04.005.

19. Feneley RCL, Hopley IB, Wells PNT. Urinary catheters: history, current status, adverse events and research agenda. J Med Eng Technol. 2015;39:459–70. https://doi.org/10.3109/03091902.2015.1085600.

20. Lapides J, Diokno AC, Silber SJ, Lowe BS. Clean, intermittent self-catheterization in the treatment of urinary tract disease. J Urol. 1972;107:458–61.

21. Chen TYH, Ponsot Y, Carmel M, et al. Multi-Centre study of Intraurethral valve-pump catheter in women with a hypocontractile or acontractile bladder. Eur Urol. 2005;48:628–33. https://doi.org/10.1016/j.eururo.2005.04.020.

22. Finkbeiner AE. Is bethanechol chloride clinically effective in promoting bladder emptying? A literature review. J Urol. 1985;134:443–9.

23. Riedl CR, Stephen RL, Daha LK, et al. Electromotive administration of intravesical bethanechol and the clinical impact on acontractile detrusor management: introduction of a new test. J Urol. 2000;164:2108–11.

24. Hindley RG, Brierly RD, Thomas PJ. Prostaglandin E2 and bethanechol in combination for treating detrusor underactivity. BJU Int. 2004;93(1):89–92. https://doi.org/10.1046/j.1464-410X.2004.04563.x.

25. Madhuvrata P, Singh M, Hasafa Z, Abdel-Fattah M. Anticholinergic drugs for adult neurogenic detrusor overactivity: a systematic review and meta-analysis. Eur Urol. 2012;62:816–30. https://doi.org/10.1016/j.eururo.2012.02.036.

26. Madersbacher H, Murtz G, Stohrer M. Neurogenic detrusor overactivity in adults: a review on efficacy, tolerability and safety of oral antimuscarinics. Spinal Cord. 2013;51:432–41. https://doi.org/10.1038/sc.2013.19.

27. Andersson K-E, Wein AJ. Pharmacologic management of lower urinary tract storage and emptying failure. In: Campbell-Walsh urology. 11th ed. Philadelphia: Elsevier; 2016. p. 1836–1874.e23.

28. Davila GW, Daugherty CA, Sanders SW. A short-term, multicenter, randomized double-blind dose titration study of efficacy and anticholinergic side effects of transdermal compared to immediate release oral oxybutynin treatment of patients with urge urinary incontinence. J Urol. 2001;166:140–5.

29. Kennelly MJ, Lemack GE, Foote JE, Trop CS. Efficacy and safety of oxybutynin transdermal system in spinal cord injury patients with neurogenic detrusor overactivity and incontinence: an open-label, dose-titration study. Urology. 2009;74:741–5. https://doi.org/10.1016/j.urology.2009.05.008.

30. Krause P, Fuhr U, Schnitker J, et al. Pharmacokinetics of intravesical versus oral oxybutynin in healthy adults: results of an open label, randomized, prospective clinical study. J Urol. 2013;190:1791–7. https://doi.org/10.1016/j.juro.2013.05.011.

31. Schröder A, Albrecht U, Schnitker J, et al. Efficacy, safety, and tolerability of intravesically administered 0.1% oxybutynin hydrochloride solution in adult patients with neurogenic bladder: a randomized, prospective, controlled multi-center trial. Neurourol Urodyn. 2015;35:582–8. https://doi.org/10.1002/nau.22755.

32. De Wachter S, Wyndaele J. Intravesical oxybutynin: a local anesthetic effect on bladder C afferents. J Urol. 2003;169:1892–5. https://doi.org/10.1097/01.ju.0000049903.60057.4b.

33. van Kerrebroeck PEVA, Amarenco G, Thuroff JW, et al. Dose-ranging study of tolterodine in patients with detrusor hyperreflexia. Neurourol Urodyn. 1998;17:499–512.

34. Ethans KD, Nance PW, Bard RJ, et al. Efficacy and safety of tolterodine in people with neurogenic detrusor overactivity. J Spinal Cord Med. 2004;27:214–8.

35. Watanabe M, Yamanishi T, Honda M, et al. Efficacy of extended-release tolterodine for the treatment of neurogenic detrusor overactivity and/or low-compliance bladder. Int J Urol. 2010;17:931–6. https://doi.org/10.1111/j.1442-2042.2010.02635.x.

36. Madhuvrata P, Cody JD, Ellis G, Herbison GP, Hay-Smith J. Which anticholinergic drug for overactive bladder symptoms in adults. Cochrane Database Syst Rev. 2012;1:CD005429. https://doi.org/10.1002/14651858.CD005429.

37. Nilvebrant L, Andersson KE, Gilberg PG, et al. Tolterodine—a new bladder-selective antimuscarinic agent. Eur J Pharmacol. 1997;327:195–207.

38. Bycroft J, Leaker B, Wood S, et al. The effect of darifenacin on neurogenic detrusor overactivity in patients with spinal cord injury. International Continence Society. 2003.

39. Carl S, Laschke S. Darifenacin is also effective in neurogenic bladder dysfunction (multiple sclerosis). Urology. 2006;68(Suppl):250–1. https://doi.org/10.1016/j.urology.2006.08.736.

40. Amarenco G, Sutory M, Zachoval R, et al. Solifenacin is effective and well tolerated in patients with neurogenic detrusor overactivity: results from the double-blind, randomized, active- and placebo-controlled SONIC urodynamic study. Neurourol Urodyn. 2017;36(2):414–21. https://doi.org/10.1002/nau.22945.

41. Stohrer M, Bauer P, Giannetii BM, et al. Effect of trospium chloride on urodynamic parameters in patients with detrusor hyperreflexia due to spinal cord injuries. Urol Int. 1991;47:138–43.

42. Madersbacher H, Stohrer M, Richter R, et al. Trospium chloride versus oxybutynin: a randomized, double- blind, multicentre trial in the treatment of detrusor hyper- reflexia. Br J Urol. 1995;75:452–6.

43. Menarini M, Del Popolo G, Di Benedetto P, et al. Trospium chloride in patients with neurogenic detrusor overactivity: is dose titration of benefit to patients? Int J Clin Pharmacol Ther. 2006;44:623–32.

44. Stohrer M, Madersbacher H, Richter R, et al. Efficacy and safety of propiverine in SCI-patients suffering from detrusor hyperreflexia—a double-blind, placebo-controlled clinical trial. Spinal Cord. 1999;37(3):196–200.

45. Stohrer M, Murtz G, Kramer G, et al. Efficacy and tolerability of propiverine hydrochloride extended-release compared with immediate-release in patients with neurogenic detrusor overactivity. Spinal Cord. 2013;51:419–23. https://doi.org/10.1038/sc.2012.174.

46. Stöhrer M, Mürtz G, Kramer G, et al. Propiverine compared to oxybutynin in neurogenic detrusor overactivity—results of a randomized, double-blind, multicenter clinical study. Eur Urol. 2007;51:235–42. https://doi.org/10.1016/j.eururo.2006.03.016.

47. Wollner J, Pannek J. Initial experience with the treatment of neurogenic detrusor overactivity with a new beta-3 agonist (mirabegron) in patients with spinal cord injury. Spinal Cord. 2016;54:78–82. https://doi.org/10.1038/sc.2015.195.

48. Wada N, Shimizu T, Takai S, et al. Combinational effects of muscarinic receptor inhibition and β3-adrenoceptor stimulation on neurogenic bladder dysfunction in rats with spinal cord injury. Neurourol Urodyn. 2016;36:1039–45. https://doi.org/10.1002/nau.23066.

49. Nitti VW, Auerbach S, Martin N, et al. Results of a randomized phase III trial of mirabegron in patients with overactive bladder. J Urol. 2013;189:1388–95. https://doi.org/10.1016/j.juro.2012.10.017.

50. Nitti VW, Rosenberg S, Mitcheson DH, et al. Urodynamics and safety of the β3-Adrenoceptor agonist mirabegron in males with lower urinary tract symptoms and bladder outlet obstruction. J Urol. 2013;190:1320–7. https://doi.org/10.1016/j.juro.2013.05.062.

51. Pacher P, Kecskemeti V. Cardiovascular side effects of new antidepressants and antipsychotics: new drugs, old concerns? Curr Pharm Des. 2004;10:2463–75.

52. Amend B, Hennenlotter J, Schäfer T, et al. Effective treatment of neurogenic detrusor dysfunction by combined high-dosed antimuscarinics without increased side-effects. Eur Urol. 2008;53:1021–8. https://doi.org/10.1016/j.eururo.2008.01.007.

53. Cameron AP, Clemens JQ, Latini JM, McGuire EJ. Combination drug therapy improves compliance of the neurogenic bladder. J Urol. 2009;182:1062–7. https://doi.org/10.1016/j.juro.2009.05.038.

54. Tanaka I, Nagase K, Tanase K, et al. Improvement in neurogenic detrusor overactivity by peripheral C fiber's suppression with cyclooxygenase inhibitors. J Urol. 2010;183:786–92. https://doi.org/10.1016/j.juro.2009.09.071.
55. Kumar A, Prabha R, Paul T, et al. Tramadol inhibits the contractility of isolated caprine detrusor muscle. Auton Autacoid Pharmacol. 2012;32:15–22. https://doi.org/10.1111/j.1474-8673.2012.00470.x.
56. Schurch B, Stohrer M, Kramer G, et al. Botulinum-A toxin for treating detrusor hyperreflexia in spinal cord injured patients: a new alternative to anticholinergic drugs? Preliminary results. J Urol. 2000;164:692–7.
57. Rovner E, Kohan A, Chartier-Kastler E, et al. Long-term efficacy and safety of onabotulinumtoxinA in patients with neurogenic detrusor overactivity who completed 4 years of treatment. J Urol. 2016;196:801–8. https://doi.org/10.1016/j.juro.2016.04.046.
58. Pannek J, Blok B, Castro-Diaz D, et al. Guidelines on neurogenic lower urinary tract dysfunction. Eur Urol. 2009;56(1):81–8.
59. Agrawal M, Joshi M. Urodynamic patterns after traumatic spinal cord injury. J Spinal Cord Med. 2015;38:128–33.
60. Blaivas JG, Sinha HP, Zayed AAH, Labib KB. Detrusor-external sphincter dyssynergia. J Urol. 1981;125:542–4.
61. Stoffel JT. Detrusor sphincter dyssynergia: a review of physiology, diagnosis, and treatment strategies. Trans Androl Urol. 2016;5:127–35.
62. Bushman W, Steers WD, Meythaler JM. Voiding dysfunction in patients with spastic paraplegia: urodynamic evaluation and response to continuous intrathecal baclofen. Neurourol Urodyn. 1993;12:163–70.
63. Hackler RH, Broecker BH, Klein FA, Brady SM. A clinical experience with dantrolene sodium for external urinary sphincter hypertonicity in spinal cord injured patients. J Urol. 1980;124:78–80.
64. Chancellor MB, Erhard MJ, Rivas DA. Clinical effect of alpha-1 antagonism by terazosin on external and internal urinary sphincter function. J Am Paraplegia Soc. 1993;16:207–14.
65. Dykstra DD, Sidi AA, Scott AB, et al. Effects of botulinum a toxin on detrusor-sphincter dyssynergia in spinal cord injury patients. J Urol. 1988;139:919–22.
66. Chen S, Bih L, Huang Y, et al. Effect of single botulinum toxin A injection to the external urethral sphincter for treating detrusor external sphincter dyssynergia in spinal cord injury. J Rehabil Med. 2008;40:744–8. https://doi.org/10.2340/16501977-0255.
67. Utomo E, Groen J, Blok BF. Surgical management of functional bladder outlet obstruction in adults with neurogenic bladder dysfunction. Cochrane Database Syst Rev. 2014;(5):CD004927. https://doi.org/10.1002/14651858.CD004927.pub4.
68. Dykstra DD, Sidi AA. Treatment of detrusor-sphincter dyssynergia with Botulinum A toxin: a double-blind study. Arch Phys Med Rehabil. 1990;71(1):24–6.
69. Phelan MW, Franks M, Somogyi GT, et al. Botulinum toxin urethral sphincter injection to restore bladder emptying in men and women with voiding dysfunction. J Urol. 2001;165:1107–10.
70. Mariappan P, Alhasso A, Ballantyne Z, et al. Duloxetine, a serotonin and noradrenaline reuptake inhibitor (SNRI) for the treatment of stress urinary incontinence: a systematic review. Eur Urol. 2007;51:67–74. https://doi.org/10.1016/j.eururo.2006.08.041.
71. Wilson JLL, Miranda CA, Knepper MA. Vasopressin and the regulation of aquaporin-2. Clin Exp Nephrol. 2013;17:751–64. https://doi.org/10.1007/s10157-013-0789-5.
72. Bosma R, Wynia K, Havlikova E, et al. Efficacy of desmopressin in patients with multiple sclerosis suffering from bladder dysfunction: a meta-analysis. Acta Neurol Scand. 2005;112:1–5. https://doi.org/10.1111/j.1600-0404.2005.00431.x.
73. Goh MY, Millard MS, Wong ECK, et al. Diurnal blood pressure and urine production in acute spinal cord injury compared with controls. Spinal Cord. 2017;55:39–46. https://doi.org/10.1038/sc.2016.100.
74. Szollar SM, Dunn KL, Brandt S, Fincher J. Nocturnal polyuria and antidiuretic hormone levels in spinal cord injury. Arch Phys Med Rehabil. 1997;78:455–8.

75. Eldahan KC, Rabchevsky AG. Autonomic dysreflexia after spinal cord injury: systemic pathophysiology and methods of management. Auton Neurosci. 2017;209:1–12. https://doi.org/10.1016/j.autneu.2017.05.002.
76. Chancellor MB, Erhard MJ, Hirsch IH, Stass WE Jr. Prospective evaluation of terazosin for the treatment of autonomic dysreflexia. J Urol. 1994;151:111–3.
77. Chan YY, Sandlin SK, Kurzrock EA, Osborn SL. The current use of stem cells in bladder tissue regeneration and bioengineering. Biomedicine. 2017;5:4. https://doi.org/10.3390/biomedicines5010004.

Part VIII
Management: Surgical Therapy

Minimally Invasive Treatments

Yunliang Gao, Melissa Sanford, Francisco Cruz, and David Ginsberg

Abbreviations

BoNT	Botulinum neurotoxin
BoNT-A	Botulinum neurotoxin type A
BoNT-B	Botulinum neurotoxin type B
CIC	Clean intermittent catheterization
CVA	Cerebrovascular accident
DESD	Detrusor-external sphincter dyssynergia
DO	Detrusor overactivity
IDO	Idiopathic detrusor overactivity
MCC	Maximum cystometric capacity
MDP	Maximal detrusor voiding pressure
NDO	Neurogenic detrusor overactivity
NLUTD	Neurogenic lower urinary tract dysfunction

Y. Gao
Department of Urology, The Second Xiangya Hospital, Central South University,
Changsha, Hunan, China
e-mail: yunliang.gao@csu.edu.cn

M. Sanford
Department of Urology, Texas Tech University, Lubbock, TX, USA
e-mail: Melissa.Sanford@med.usc.edu

F. Cruz
Faculty of Medicine of Porto, Department of Urology, Hospital de São João, Institute for
Molecular and Cell Biology (IBMC), Porto, Portugal
e-mail: cruzfjmr@med.up.pt

D. Ginsberg (✉)
Department of Urology, Rancho Los Amigos National Rehabilitation Center, Downey, CA,
USA

Department of Urology, Keck School of Medicine, University of Southern California,
Los Angeles, CA, USA
e-mail: ginsberg@med.usc.edu

© Springer International Publishing AG, part of Springer Nature 2018
R. Dmochowski, J. Heesakkers (eds.), *Neuro-Urology*,
https://doi.org/10.1007/978-3-319-90997-4_22

387

OAB	Overactive bladder
PD	Parkinson's disease
PVR	Post-voiding residual volume
QOL	Quality of life
RCT	Randomized controlled trial
RTX	Resiniferatoxin
RV	Reflex volume
SNAP-25	Synaptosomal-associated protein 25
TRPV1	Transient receptor potential vanilloid 1
U	Unit/units
UTI	Urinary tract infection
VUR	Vesicoureteral reflux

Introduction

The ability of the lower urinary tract to both store and release urine is mediated by a complex, multilevel process that involves both the central and peripheral nervous system [1]. Neurologic disease can impair these processes and lead to neurogenic lower urinary tract dysfunction (NLUTD). NLUTD is a chronic illness that affects millions of individuals worldwide, impacting morbidity and mortality of these patients as well as quality of life and healthcare costs. First-line treatment for NLUTD often involves oral therapy (antimuscarinics and/or beta-3 agonist) and clean intermittent catheterization (CIC) as needed. Patients that continue to be symptomatic despite pharmacologic management may benefit from further minimally invasive treatments, mainly presented as intravesical pharmacological therapy such as botulinum neurotoxin (BoNT).

Owing to circumventing systemic administration of active compounds, intravesical therapy brings two potential benefits for patients suffering from NLUTD. Intravesical therapy can easily provide high concentrations of pharmacological agents in the bladder tissue with enhanced local effects. Additionally, drugs with bladder-specialized effect, but inappropriate for systemic administration, may be safely used. Attractively, intravesical therapy should be considered as second-line treatment in patients refractory to oral therapy or intolerant to its systemic side effects. Until now two main kinds of minimally invasive, intravesical agents have been studied: (1) BoNT drugs which block the parasympathetic outflow and (2) vanilloid substances which block the sensory input (capsaicin and resiniferatoxin [RTX]). This chapter is aimed to give an overview of these minimally invasive substances currently used for intravesical therapy of NLUTD and their efficacy and limitations.

Botulinum Toxin

BoNT is formed by the Gram-positive, anaerobic spore-forming bacteria *Clostridium botulinum* and is responsible for human botulism. The use of BoNT injection in the lower urinary tract was first studied by Dykstra et al. in 1988 for the treatment of detrusor-external sphincter dyssynergia (DESD) in spinal cord injury (SCI) patients [2]. Following this, the number of investigations regarding urologic applications of BoNT increased dramatically. Ultimately, the FDA approved BoNT for use in neurogenic detrusor overactivity (NDO) in 2011.

Mechanism of Action

BoNT is a two-chain neurotoxic protein consisting of a light and heavy chain joined by a disulfide bond. Eight serotypes, A to H, have been described, with different tertiary structures and significant sequence divergences. Even within the same subgroup, there are distinct properties that do not allow for easy comparison between toxins [3]. Only types A (BoNT-A) and B (BoNT-B) have been used clinically, with BoNT-A being the most extensively studied and the serotype with the longest duration of effect. BoNT-B has been used in few patients, primarily for bladder dysfunction resistant to BoNT-A [4, 5]. Currently the commercially available BoNT-A preparations are onabotulinumtoxinA (Botox®, Allergan Pharmaceuticals, USA), abobotulinumtoxinA (Dysport®, Ipsen Biopharm, France), incobotulinumtoxinA (Xeomin®, Merz Pharmaceuticals, Germany) and rimabotulinumtoxinB (Neurobloc/Myobloc®, Solstice Neurosciences Inc., USA) (Table 1). The various BoNT-A products have different units, and it is not possible to convert units from one product to another; however it is postulated that one unit of onabotulinumtoxinA is equivalent to 3–5 units (U) of abobotulinumtoxinA [6–8].

The molecular target of BoNT-A is synaptosomal-associated protein 25 (SNAP-25). SNAP-25 is a protein that allows for vesicle fusion and mediates release of acetylcholine (and other motor and sensory neurotransmitters) from neuronal axon endings into the neuromuscular junction, ultimately resulting in muscle contraction. BoNT-A cleaves SNAP-25 and prevents release of neurotransmitters (e.g., acetylcholine) at the neuromuscular junction, thus inhibiting detrusor contraction [9].

BoNT-A binds with high affinity to synaptic vesicle protein 2, which is expressed in nearly all healthy human bladder parasympathetic cholinergic fibers and half of

Table 1 Botulinum toxin preparations

Trade name	Drug name	Serotype	Manufacturer	Vial dose
Botox	OnabotulinumtoxinA	A	Allergan	50 100 U 200 U
Dysport	AbobotulinumtoxinA	A	Ipsen	300 U 500 U
Xeomin	IncobotulinumtoxinA	A	Merz	50 U 100 U
Myobloc	RimabotulinumtoxinB	B	Solstice	2500 5000 10,000

sensory fibers. Synaptic vesicle protein 2 is not expressed in urothelial or muscular cells [10]. Likewise, BoNT-A may impact a variety of substances involving both efferent, parasympathetic, afferent, and nociceptive pathways. For example, ATP appears to play a role in both idiopathic and neurogenic detrusor overactivity (DO), and studies indicate that BoNT may inhibit ATP release [11]. In addition, increased afferent activity is thought to be crucial to the pathophysiology of DO and sensory disorders, and increasing evidence is emerging for BoNT-A blocking afferent signaling in the bladder. Suburothelial substances such as transient receptor potential vanilloid 1 (TRPV1), purinergic receptor subtype P2X3, calcitonin gene-related peptide, and substance P appear to have a role in the pathophysiology of DO, and BoNT-A has been shown to decrease these levels [12, 13].

Treatment for NDO

Indications

NDO refers to a urodynamic finding characterized by involuntary detrusor contractions during the filling phase due to a relevant, underlying neurological condition [14]. Patients with spinal cord injury (SCI) and multiple sclerosis (MS) often suffer from NDO, which can lead to symptoms of frequency, urgency, and urinary incontinence. In addition, patients with DESD can develop elevated detrusor pressures, which can cause upper urinary tract deterioration. Therefore, it is important to maintain low bladder storage pressures in order to prevent the dire consequence of irreversible renal insufficiency. BoNT-A is a highly effective treatment for neurogenic patients who have persistent symptoms and NDO despite oral pharmacotherapy.

Outcomes

The effectiveness of BoNT-A injections into the detrusor smooth muscle to treat NDO has been reported in several studies (Table 2). Schurch et al. published the first pilot study evaluating and demonstrating the successful application of onabotulinumtoxinA (200 or 300 IE; BOTOX®) in NDO patients in 2000 [15]. In this prospective, nonrandomized trial study, a total of 21 patients with SCI underwent detrusor injection. All of the patients had NDO and UI despite a high dose of anticholinergic medication. Nineteen of 21 patients underwent a complete examination 6 weeks after onabotulinumtoxinA injections, and 17 of these 19 cases achieved complete continence and were able to either stop or significantly reduce their anticholinergic medication. Overall, several urodynamic parameters were improved, including increased maximum cystometric capacity (MCC) (from 296.3 to 480.5 mL), increased mean volume to the first reflex detrusor contraction (RV) (from 215.8 to 415.7 mL), and decreased maximal detrusor voiding pressure (MDP) (from 65.6 to 35 cm water). The effect lasted for at least 9 months and no side

Table 2 Randomized controlled trials of botulinumtoxinA to treat neurogenic detrusor overactivity (NDO)

Study	Reference number	Gender (M/F)	Causes for NDO	T/C	No. of patients	UI change	MCC change	MDP change	QOL change	Duration of effect
1	[17]	36/23	SCI (53), MS (6)	Placebo	21	0.2	+45.0	−10.1	Significant improvement in onabot-treated groups	NA
				200 U onabot	19	−0.9	+182.1	−44.4		> 24 weeks
				300 U onabot	19	−1.5	+169.1	−62.2		> 24 weeks
2	[73]	33/23	SCI (50), MS (6)	Placebo	NA	NA	NA	NA	Significant improvement in onabot-treated groups	NA
				200 U onabot						
				300 U onabot						
3	[28]	17/14	SCI (20), MS (6), myelomeningocele (2), trauma (2), unclear (1)	Placebo	14	NA	+10	−12	Significant improvement in abobot-treated groups	NA
				500 U abobot	17		+180	−52		26 weeks
4	[74]	34/23	SCI (38), MS (19)	Placebo	29	+0.73	−29	+13	Significant improvement in onabot-treated group	NA
				300 U onabot	28	−1.75	+224	−27.5		>36 weeks
5	[18]	120/155	SCI (121), MS (154)	Placebo	92	−13.2	+ 2.8	+6.4	Significant improvement in onabot-treated group	13.1 weeks
				200 U onabot	92	−21.8	+ 150.8	−28.5		42.1 weeks
				300 U onabot	91	−19.4	+ 157.2	−26.9		42.1 weeks
6	[19]	171/245	SCI (189), MS (227)	Placebo	149	−8.8	+ 15.5	−2.4	Significant improvement in onabot-treated group	92 days
				200 U onabot	135	−21	+ 151.2	−35.1		256 days
				300 U onabot	132	−22.7	+ 167.7	−33.3		254 days

T treatment group, *C* control group, *M* male, *F* female, *MCC* maximum cystometric capacity, *MDP* maximum detrusor pressure, *SCI* spinal cord injury, *MS* multiple sclerosis, *QOL* quality of life, *NA* not available

effects were observed. The author recommended a dose of 300 U for detrusor hyper-reflexia. Similar results were found in a retrospective, multicenter European study of 200 individuals with severe NDO that found significant improvement of bladder function with corresponding continence and subjective satisfaction in patients treated with onabotulinumtoxinA [16].

In addition to conducting the first prospective open-labeled study, Schurch et al. also performed the first randomized placebo-controlled study evaluating the use of BoNT-A (BOTOX®) to treat NDO. A total of 59 patients (53 SCI and 6 MS) were treated with intradetrusor injections of placebo (saline) or onabotulinumtoxinA (200 or 300 U) [17]. Compared to placebo, both doses of onabotulinumtoxinA groups showed significant decreases in incontinence episodes (approximately 50%), improved urodynamic outcomes (improvements in MCC, RV, and MDP), and improvements in QOL. No statistically significant difference was found between the 200 and 300 U doses, possibly due to the few number of subjects.

Subsequently, several other studies also proved the effectiveness of BoNT-A in patients with neuro-urological disorders in placebo-controlled trails (2013). Among them, two pivotal phase III studies by Cruz et al. and Ginsberg et al. resulted in FDA approval of onabotulinumtoxinA to treat NDO refractory to antimuscarinic therapy [18, 19]. In those trials a total of 691 patients were randomized to 30 intradetrusor injections of 200 U, 300 U, or placebo. In the two studies, patients receiving 200 U and 300 U had significantly less UI episodes per week compared to placebo (200 U, -21 to -21.8; 300 U, -19.4 to -22.7; placebo, -8.8 to -13.2 at week 6, $p < 0.01$); there was no significant difference between the two treatment doses. At week 6, more patients receiving onabotulinumtoxinA (36–38% of 200 U and 40–41% of 300 U) were fully continent compared to the placebo group (8–10%). Patients receiving onabotulinumtoxinA additionally demonstrated significantly improved MCC, MDP during first DO, and I-QOL scores. Of note, 42% of patients receiving 300 U initiated intermittent catheterization (IC) compared to 30–35% and 10–12% in the 200 U group and placebo group, respectively. The most common side effect noted in both studies was urinary tract infection (UTI). Based on similar efficacy and a greater need for CIC with the higher dose, the FDA-approved dose for NDO is 200 U onaBoNT-A.

It is important to note that while BoNT-A was approved based on trials including patients with SCI and MS, onabotulinumtoxinA is FDA-approved for use in any patients with UI and NDO associated with any neurologic condition (not limited to SCI or MS). Anderson et al. described the results of 100 U of onabotulinumtoxinA in patients (12 men and 8 women) with NDO secondary to Parkinson's disease (PD) [20]. In this study, 59% of patients reported moderate to marked symptom relief at 3 months and a 50% incontinence decrease over 6 months compared to baseline. These results suggested that low-dose onabotulinumtoxinA is a potential long-term management strategy for patients with PD and UI who fail oral antimuscarinic agents. The low-dose treatment at 100 U is effective, safe, and comes with a lesser risk for urinary retention in NDO patients that are voiding spontaneously at baseline and want to minimize the risk of postinjection CIC. Apart from PD, onabotulinum-toxinA can also effectively inhibit the occurrence of NDO related to cerebrovascular accident (CVA). Kuo et al. used 200 U (rather than 300 U which was often the standard dose for NDO at the time the study was completed), in order to minimize the risk of retention requiring CIC as this can be more difficult for the elderly CVA population [21]. However, after treatment only 50% of the patients with CVA had increased bladder capacity and improved incontinence compared to 91.6% of SCI patients. The authors theorized that a weak sphincter and impaired bladder wall contractility could contribute to the lower efficacy.

To evaluate long-term efficacy and safety of BoNT-A injections for NDO, Kennelly et al. published a 3-year, prospective, multicenter extension study on 387 patients focusing on the results of repeated treatment for up to five treatment cycles [22]. Among them, 387, 336, 241, 113, and 46 patients received 1, 2, 3, 4, and 5 onabotulinumtoxinA treatments, respectively. Compared with baseline, the UI episodes per week were consistently reduced after repeated onabotulinumtoxinA treatment. The proportion of $\geq$50% and 100% "dry" (100% reduction) patients were 73–94% and 36–55%, respectively. The time to patients request for repeat treatment over cycles 1 and 2 remained consistent (~36 weeks). An increased mean volume per void and increased QOL were additionally noted after repeat treatment. Urinary tract infections (UTI) and urinary retention were the most common adverse events, with no change in the adverse event profile over time. A more recent study by Rovner et al. also demonstrated long-term durability of treatment effect by examining NDO patients who had completed 4 years of treatment with onabotulinumtoxinA [23]. In this study, the median duration of effect of 200 U onabotulinumtoxinA was 9.2 months, and most patients only needed 1.5 treatments per year. Re-treatment was equally as effective as the initial treatment with consistent year-to-year reductions in UI episodes per day and improvement in QOL, without new safety signals.

While a large number of patients respond well to BoNT-A, only a few studies have evaluated predictors of success or failure in this population. As shown by Alvares et al., several baseline urodynamic parameters appeared to be correlated with successful onabotulinumtoxinA treatment, including higher MCC, higher RV, and better compliance [24]. However, pooled analyses of the above two phase III studies found similar improvements in UI regardless of bladder compliance, etiology, and concomitant anticholinergic use [25, 26]. Additionally, most studies found that antimuscarinics could be discontinued in a significant number of patients after onabotulinumtoxinA injection. What is not clear is whether or not antimuscarinics could potentially be used concomitantly to achieve better outcomes or added toward the end of the cycle to allow for greater duration of effect.

At this point only onabotulinumtoxinA has an FDA indication to treat NGB/NDO; however, studies evaluating the use of the other two BoNT-A compounds to treat NDO have been done. Del Popolo et al. performed a retrospective review of their 8-year experience using abobotulinumtoxinA (Dysport®) in 199 patients with NDO [27]. MCC, RV, and bladder compliance improved significantly after treatment compared with baseline values, and no significant differences in effectiveness were noted between the higher and lower doses of Dysport® (500, 750, or 1000 U). Among these 199 patients, 39 with a mean duration of efficacy after each injection >12 months (very good responders), 80 with 10–12 months (good responders), 60 with <10 months (responders), and 20 with <6 months (low responders). Ehren et al. conducted a randomized, placebo-controlled study that compared the effects of abobotulinumtoxinA (Dysport®, 500 U) to placebo in 31 patients with NDO [28]. Compared to placebo, abobotulinumtoxinA treatment leads to significantly decreased UI, decreased mean detrusor pressure, and improved QOL. Particularly, the cystometric bladder capacity was significantly higher in the abobotulinumtoxinA treated group at both 6 and 12 weeks postinjection compared to placebo. This difference was present at the end of the study at 26 weeks despite no longer being statistically significant. Similar to onabotulinumtoxinA treatment, those receiving abobotulinumtoxinA had a significant decrease of anticholinergic intake compared to placebo. In general a conversion rate of 1:2 or 1:3 is recommended for onabotulinumtoxinA to abobotulinumtoxinA, and incobotulinumtoxinA has a conversion of 1:1 with onabotulinumtoxinA; however, it is important to note this calculation is based on all uses of the products for all indications and no direct comparator studies have been done in the lower urinary tract [29].

Treatment for Detrusor-External Sphincter Dyssynergia

Detrusor-external sphincter dyssynergia (DESD) refers to a spastic and uncoordinated contraction of the external sphincter upon voiding which can occur in patients with suprasacral spinal cord lesions. DESD can result in incomplete emptying, thus increasing the risks of UTI and upper urinary tract damage. BoNT-A injection into the external sphincter was the earliest urologic indication evaluated [2]. Multiple small trials have studied its use in patients with SCI or MS with a dose of 100–200 U, resulting in a "pharmacologic sphincterotomy." For example, a small randomized controlled trial (RCT) comparing onabotulinumtoxinA 100 U to lidocaine showed improvements in post-voiding residual volume (PVR) at 30 days after postinjection in SCI patients with DSD [30]. Similarly, another RCT compared onabotulinumtoxinA 100 U to placebo via single transperineal injection in MS patients. In this study, voiding volume and MDP were significantly increased in patients with onabotulinumtoxinA injections, despite no significant difference in PVR [31]. A further meta-analysis also demonstrated that SCI patients with onabotulinumtoxinA injection showed a decrease PVR from 251.8 to 153.0 mL lasting up to 6 months as well as reduced UTI episodes [32]. Currently, quality data is still lacking, and further research is needed before making more definitive recommendations.

Treatment in Children

Accumulating evidence has emerged and demonstrated the important role of BoNT-A therapy in pediatric NGB patients [33–35]. Most studies noted that a dose of 10–12 U/kg of onabotulinumtoxinA can lead to both clinical and urodynamic improvements. For example, Schulte-Baukloh and colleagues reported a preliminary study of 17 children with urodynamically verified NDO due to myelomeningocele [36]. Intravesical injection significantly improved urodynamic parameters, including increased RV and MCC and decreased MDP. The beneficial effects of onabotulinumtoxinA lasted up to 6 months without side effects.

SCI and MS are the common etiologies of NDO in adult patients, whereas myelomeningocele is the most common cause of NDO in children. Compared to adults, these pediatric patients have a greater potential for abnormal bladder compliance, which, if not treated, could lead to upper tract damage. Several studies have evaluated the use of BoNT-A in the treatment of poor bladder compliance in these patients. As shown by Horst et al., 3 months after the first injection, the bladder compliance increased by 28% from 7 ± 3.5 to 9 ± 6 mL/cmH$_2$O [37]. Similarly, Altaweel et al. found that bladder compliance significantly increased from 5.2 ± 2.6 to 13 ± 6.9 mL/cmH$_2$O. And at an average of 8.1 months after the first injection, bladder compliance remained increased from 6.0 ± 3.1 to 15.1 ± 5.2 mL/cmH$_2$O [38]. Additionally, BoNT-A injection can reduce vesicoureteral reflux (VUR) associated with poor compliance which ultimately reduces the rate of UTI and incidence of renal damage in children who have failed conservative management [33, 35]. Follow-up urodynamics are indicated for any patients undergoing BoNT-A with abnormal compliance to ensure appropriate improvement and safe storage pressures.

Administration and Injection Technique

Pre-procedure Considerations

Patients should be formally evaluated prior to undergoing BoNT-A injection with a basic urologic work-up and demonstration of prior failed conservative therapy. A urinalysis should be performed, and patients presenting with UTI should be treated appropriately prior to injection. Patients should be fully counseled about the risks of injection. Given the risk of retention, some providers recommend that patients learn CIC prior to injection to demonstrate their ability should they experience voiding difficulty postinjection. While anticoagulant medication is not a contraindication, it should be noted preoperatively, and providers can consider using less injection sites to reduce the risk of bleeding.

Technique

The procedure of BoNT-A injection can be performed using either a rigid or flexible cystoscope under general, spinal, or local anesthesia. A variety of needles for each type of scope are available. There are also rigid cystoscopes specifically designed for needle injection, which are small and quite tolerable to the patient with only local anesthesia. Possible needle variables to consider include cost, working length, tip length, tip sharpness, and flexibility. The optimal needle gauge should be between 4 and 8 mm with a tip length of 22–27 mm.

Proper mixing of BoNT-A is of the utmost importance to keep the toxin effective. Prior to reconstitution, vials of onabotulinumtoxinA should be stored in a refrigerator (2–8 °C) or freezer (at or below −5 °C). After reconstitution vials can be stored in the refrigerator and should be used within 24 h. OnabotulinumtoxinA vials come in 50, 100, and 200 U doses, and each vial is under a vacuum. Vials should be diluted with 10 mL of saline and then gently mixed.

There is currently no universally accepted protocol regarding the location and number of injections. During the FDA approval trials, 200 U of onabotulinumtoxinA was diluted in 30 mL of preservative-free saline (NDO) and then injected in 1 mL increments separated by a distance of 1–1.5 cm, approximately 2 mm into the detrusor, avoiding the trigone. The need for a 30 mL dilution was to allow for 30 injection of 1 mL for all arms of the study (placebo and both 200 and 300 U) to maintain blinding; most providers presently dilute each vial with 10 mL, so if 200 U is to be injected, a total of 20 injections would be performed. Generally, the target layer within the bladder wall for cystoscopic intravesical injection is the detrusor muscle. Penetration of the bladder wall and an injection into the perivesical tissues should be avoided. Injections to the trigone have traditionally been spared out of concern for producing VUR. However, several authors have shown trigonal injections to be safe and effective without evidence of VUR [39, 40]. Based on a recent meta-analysis comparing trigonal and extratrigonal injection technique, patient-specific factors and dosing likely matter more for response to BoNT-A than location of injection [41]. The use of suburothelial injection compared to intradetrusor injection was evaluated in the study of Krhut et al. with 32 NDO patients secondary to SCI. No significant difference was noted between the two techniques [42]. The most recent studies suggest efficacy may be maintained with fewer injections. Denys et al. had similar outcomes comparing 15–30 injections, and Avallone et al. had appropriate outcomes using a total of 1–3 injections (though unfortunately there was not a comparison to placebo or standard number of injection sites) [43, 44].

Generally, intravesical instillation is not presently a viable option mainly due to the high molecular weight of injected preparations. However, an alternative delivery technique using BoNT-A encapsulated in liposomes achieved significant clinical improvements in cystitis rats [45]. A recent pilot study involving 24 patients showed significant reductions in OAB symptom scores, micturition frequency, and urgency episodes at 4 weeks [46]. The liposomal BoNT-A has several advantages, including lower risk of hematuria, pain, urinary retention, and UTI. However, the depth of penetration of liposomal BoNT-A is yet unknown, possibly reaching only the urothelium and suburothelium. No data are currently available for NDO patients and require further researches.

Post-procedure

Patients should receive a dose of antibiotics at the time of injection for antimicrobial prophylaxis, but no additional therapy is indicated. AUA guidelines recommend fluoroquinolones for endoscopic procedures (though this recommendation did come out prior to the FDA black box warning related to quinolone use) [47]. Significant bleeding is rarely encountered during the injection even in patients on anticoagulants, but patients should be informed that they can see blood in the urine for a day and have dysuria with voiding for up to 48 h due to urethral manipulation. Patients who do rely on bladder emptying by CIC should follow-up in 2 weeks to check a post-void residual and ensure adequate emptying as the full effect of injection may not be noticed until that time.

Safety

Nearly all studies reported an excellent safety profile of BoNT-A intradetrusor injection. The adverse events secondary to intradetrusor injection of BoNT-A can be divided into two groups: local and systemic side effects.

The most common local adverse events were UTI and hematuria, mainly related to the procedure. Based on the phase III data, the risk of UTI was 24% (compared to 17% for placebo) in NDO patients treated with onabotulinumtoxinA 200 U. UTI was primarily based on a positive urine culture, irrespective of symptoms. However, many NDO patients may have colonization due to CIC and did not have a symptomatic infection requiring treatment. Hematuria may also occur and, if it does occur, is usually mild in nature. Urinary retention can be the most problematic complication of BoNT-A injection in patients with spontaneous voiding. Intradetrusor injections of BoNT-A could lead to excess weakness or relaxation of the muscles resulting in detrusor underactivity with temporary increased risk of urinary retention requiring catheterization (CIC vs indwelling). Based on the phase III data, the risk of new-onset CIC was ~25% in NDO patients treated with onabotulinumtoxinA 200 U (35% for onabotulinumtoxinA and 10% for placebo).

Systemic events could occur due to migration of toxin beyond the detrusor muscle, leading to muscle weakness or hyposthenia in nontargeted adjacent muscles or distal ones. Thankfully, this is rarely an issue with the doses used for NDO and is usually transient and mild [27]. However, this should always be discussed with patients. When treating patients who receive onabotulinumtoxinA for other indications, the total dose needs to be monitored. It is recommended that the total dose of onabotulinumtoxinA does not exceed 360 U in a 3-month period.

Capsaicin and RTX

The demonstration that capsaicin suppressed detrusor overactivity in chronic spinalized cats, but had no effect in voiding contractions of normal cats, had two consequences [48]. One was the demonstration of the key role of bladder C fibers in the micturition reflex that emerges after spinal cord transection. The other was the possibility of using C-fiber desensitization with topical intravesical vanilloids like capsaicin or resiniferatoxin as a treatment for neurogenic detrusor overactivity. Capsaicin is a spice commonly used in the diet of many countries, and its application is not related to any adverse event besides a transient burning pain in the mouth. Resiniferatoxin, extracted from the latex of cactus-like plants, was used in the traditional medicine of North African populations as a pain killer [49].

Capsaicin and resiniferatoxin bind a specific receptor, TRPV1. Activation of these channels by capsaicin induces massive Ca^{2+} and Na^+ inward currents that can be completely blocked by capsazepine. Inward currents evoked by capsaicin are strong in amplitude but short lasting, while those evoked by RTX are weak yet long lasting [50]. Desensitization follows TRPV1 excitation by capsaicin or resinifera-toxin. A progressive decrease in the amplitude of the inward currents is observed after consecutive applications. This is accompanied by a decreased responsiveness of the TRPV1-expressing sensory neurons to natural stimuli. It is, therefore, desensitization, and not excitation, that offers potential for clinical application. Between the two vanilloids, RTX offers the best therapeutic profile as it induces a low-intensity excitation phase but a prolonged desensitization effect.

The C-fiber micturition reflex was shown to enhance in patients with chronic spinal cord lesions above sacral segments [48] in those with chronic bladder outlet obstruction [51] and in those with idiopathic detrusor overactivity (IDO) [49]. In the bladders of NDO patients, the enhancement of the micturition reflex is accompanied by an increase in the number of sub-urothelial C fibers expressing TRPV1 [52]. Increase in sub-urothelial C-fiber innervation expressing neuropeptides [53] or TRPV1 [54] was also reported in patients with sensory urgency. In IDO patients, responders to intravesical RTX are closely associated with the overexpression of the receptor in the bladder mucosa [54]. In women with sensory urgency, TRPV1 mRNA expressed in trigonal mucosa was not only increased but also inversely correlated with the bladder volume at first sensation of filling during cystometry, further indicating that TRPV1 plays a role in premature bladder sensation [55].

NDO patients who responded better to intravesical RTX exhibited a significant decrease in the density of TRPV1-immunoreactive fibers, whereas non-responders experience a nonsignificant variation [52]. A decrease in TRPV1 expression in urothelial cells of NDO patients was also demonstrated after intravesical application of RTX [56, 57].

Intravesical Capsaicin

Intravesical capsaicin for NDO was studied in six non-controlled [58–63] and one controlled clinical trial [64]. Capsaicin was dissolved in 30% alcohol, and 100–125 mL (or half of the bladder capacity if lower than that volume) of 1–2 mM solutions were instilled into the bladder and left in contact with the mucosa for 30 min. Best clinical results were found among patients with incomplete spinal cord lesions, in whom clinical improvement could be observed in up to 70–90% of patients [59, 62, 63]. In patients with complete spinal cord lesions, the success rate was usually much lower [60]. One small randomized controlled study compared capsaicin against 30% ethanol, the vehicle solution. Ten patients received capsaicin and found a significant regression of the incontinence and urge sensation. In contrast, only one among the ten patients that received ethanol had clinical improvement [64].

The pungency of alcoholic capsaicin solutions has prevented the widespread use of this compound. In particular, the possibility of triggering autonomic dysreflexia in patients with higher spinal cord lesions has progressively restrained the capsaicin use. In 2006 de Séze et al. [2006] evaluated a glucidic capsaicin formulation. They conducted a double-blind placebo-controlled study using the glucidic solution of capsaicin in 33 NDO patients. The glucidic-capsaicin-treated group showed improvement both in symptoms and urodynamic parameters above the comparator arm. The global tolerance of this new capsaicin formulation was excellent [65]. However, subsequent trials of this compound have not been published.

Intravesical RTX

RTX has the advantage over capsaicin as being much less pungent [62]. Intravesical RTX application in NDO patients was evaluated in five small open-label studies [62, 66–69]. Different RTX concentrations, 10 nM, 50 nM, 100 nM, and 10 μM, were tested. RTX brought a rapid improvement or disappearance of urinary incontinence in up to 80% of the selected patients and a 30% decrease in their daily urinary frequency. Furthermore, RTX also increased the volume to first detrusor contraction and maximum cystometric capacity. In general, in patients receiving 50–100 nM RTX, the effect was long-lasting, with a duration of more than 6 months being reported. In patients treated with 10 μM doses, transient urinary retention may occur [66].

In one placebo-controlled study, the urodynamic effects of RTX in NDO patients were specifically evaluated. A significant increase in volume at first detrusor contraction and maximum cystometric capacity was found in the RTX arm [70]. RTX also caused a significant improvement in urinary frequency and incontinence [70, 71].

RTX 600 nM was compared against 300 U onabotulinumtoxinA in a study involving 25 patients with NDO due to chronic spinal cord injury. Both neurotoxins were capable of significantly reducing the number of daily incontinence episodes and improving maximum bladder capacity, although onabotulinumtoxinA turned out to be more effective [72].

Conclusions

Intravesical therapy serves as a valuable surrogate treatment for NLUTD patients who either failed or are unable to tolerate oral therapy. With the advent of BoNT-A, the practitioner has an important tool when treating NLUTD, particularly for refractory NDO. BoNT-A injection is an effective, safe, and well-tolerated option for the patient and is regarded as the current mainstay of intravesical therapy. Future studies will likely continue to explore the mechanism of action, the optimal delivery method, and the alternative techniques for injection therapy.

Acknowledgment   Conflict of interest: None

References

1. de Groat WC, Griffiths D, Yoshimura N. Neural control of the lower urinary tract. Compr Physiol. 2015;5(1):327–96. https://doi.org/10.1002/cphy.c130056.
2. Dykstra DD, Sidi AA, Scott AB, Pagel JM, Goldish GD. Effects of botulinum A toxin on detrusor-sphincter dyssynergia in spinal cord injury patients. J Urol. 1988;139(5):919–22.
3. Aoki KR, Ranoux D, Wissel J. Using translational medicine to understand clinical differences between botulinum toxin formulations. Eur J Neurol. 2006;13(Suppl 4):10–9. https://doi.org/10.1111/j.1468-1331.2006.01649.x.
4. Pistolesi D, Selli C, Rossi B, Stampacchia G. Botulinum toxin type B for type A resistant bladder spasticity. J Urol. 2004;171(2 Pt 1):802–3. https://doi.org/10.1097/01.ju.0000108844.10235.f1.
5. Reitz A, Schurch B. Botulinum toxin type B injection for management of type A resistant neurogenic detrusor overactivity. J Urol. 2004;171(2 Pt 1):804.; ; discussion 804–5. https://doi.org/10.1097/01.ju.0000108407.53880.6a.
6. Sampaio C, Ferreira JJ, Simoes F, Rosas MJ, Magalhaes M, Correia AP, Bastos-Lima A, Martins R, Castro-Caldas A. DYSBOT: a single-blind, randomized parallel study to determine whether any differences can be detected in the efficacy and tolerability of two formulations of botulinum toxin type A—Dysport and Botox—assuming a ratio of 4:1. Mov Disord. 1997;12(6):1013–8. https://doi.org/10.1002/mds.870120627.
7. Odergren T, Hjaltason H, Kaakkola S, Solders G, Hanko J, Fehling C, Marttila RJ, Lundh H, Gedin S, Westergren I, Richardson A, Dott C, Cohen H. A double blind, randomised, parallel group study to investigate the dose equivalence of Dysport and Botox in the treatment of cervical dystonia. J Neurol Neurosurg Psychiatry. 1998;64(1):6–12.
8. Ranoux D, Gury C, Fondarai J, Mas JL, Zuber M. Respective potencies of Botox and Dysport: a double blind, randomised, crossover study in cervical dystonia. J Neurol Neurosurg Psychiatry. 2002;72(4):459–62.
9. Moore DC, Cohn JA, Dmochowski RR. Use of botulinum toxin A in the treatment of lower urinary tract disorders: a review of the literature. Toxins (Basel). 2016;8(4):88. https://doi.org/10.3390/toxins8040088.
10. Coelho A, Dinis P, Pinto R, Gorgal T, Silva C, Silva A, Silva J, Cruz CD, Cruz F, Avelino A. Distribution of the high-affinity binding site and intracellular target of botulinum toxin type A in the human bladder. Eur Urol. 2010;57(5):884–90. https://doi.org/10.1016/j.eururo.2009.12.022.
11. Khera M, Somogyi GT, Kiss S, Boone TB, Smith CP. Botulinum toxin A inhibits ATP release from bladder urothelium after chronic spinal cord injury. Neurochem Int. 2004;45(7):987–93. https://doi.org/10.1016/j.neuint.2004.06.001.
12. Apostolidis A, Popat R, Yiangou Y, Cockayne D, Ford AP, Davis JB, Dasgupta P, Fowler CJ, Anand P. Decreased sensory receptors P2X3 and TRPV1 in suburothelial nerve fibers following intradetrusor injections of botulinum toxin for human detrusor overactivity. J Urol. 2005;174(3):977–82.; ; discussion 982–3. https://doi.org/10.1097/01.ju.0000169481.42259.54.
13. Rapp DE, Turk KW, Bales GT, Cook SP. Botulinum toxin type a inhibits calcitonin gene-related peptide release from isolated rat bladder. J Urol. 2006;175(3 Pt 1):1138–42. https://doi.org/10.1016/S0022-5347(05)00322-8.
14. Abrams P, Cardozo L, Fall M, Griffiths D, Rosier P, Ulmsten U, Van Kerrebroeck P, Victor A, Wein A, Standardisation Sub-committee of the International Continence

Society. The standardisation of terminology of lower urinary tract function: report from the Standardisation Sub-committee of the International Continence Society. Neurourol Urodyn. 2002;21(2):167–78.

15. Schurch B, Stohrer M, Kramer G, Schmid DM, Gaul G, Hauri D. Botulinum-A toxin for treating detrusor hyperreflexia in spinal cord injured patients: a new alternative to anticholinergic drugs? Preliminary results. J Urol. 2000;164(3 Pt 1):692–7.

16. Reitz A, Stohrer M, Kramer G, Del Popolo G, Chartier-Kastler E, Pannek J, Burgdorfer H, Gocking K, Madersbacher H, Schumacher S, Richter R, von Tobel J, Schurch B. European experience of 200 cases treated with botulinum-A toxin injections into the detrusor muscle for urinary incontinence due to neurogenic detrusor overactivity. Eur Urol. 2004;45(4):510–5. https://doi.org/10.1016/j.eururo.2003.12.004.

17. Schurch B, de Seze M, Denys P, Chartier-Kastler E, Haab F, Everaert K, Plante P, Perrouin-Verbe B, Kumar C, Fraczek S, Brin MF, Botox Detrusor Hyperreflexia Study Team. Botulinum toxin type a is a safe and effective treatment for neurogenic urinary incontinence: results of a single treatment, randomized, placebo controlled 6-month study. J Urol. 2005;174(1):196–200. https://doi.org/10.1097/01.ju.0000162035.73977.1c.

18. Cruz F, Herschorn S, Aliotta P, Brin M, Thompson C, Lam W, Daniell G, Heesakkers J, Haag-Molkenteller C. Efficacy and safety of onabotulinumtoxinA in patients with urinary incontinence due to neurogenic detrusor overactivity: a randomised, double-blind, placebo-controlled trial. Eur Urol. 2011;60(4):742–50. https://doi.org/10.1016/j.eururo.2011.07.002.

19. Ginsberg D, Gousse A, Keppenne V, Sievert KD, Thompson C, Lam W, Brin MF, Jenkins B, Haag-Molkenteller C. Phase 3 efficacy and tolerability study of onabotulinumtoxinA for urinary incontinence from neurogenic detrusor overactivity. J Urol. 2012;187(6):2131–9. https://doi.org/10.1016/j.juro.2012.01.125.

20. Anderson RU, Orenberg EK, Glowe P. OnabotulinumtoxinA office treatment for neurogenic bladder incontinence in Parkinson's disease. Urology. 2014;83(1):22–7. https://doi.org/10.1016/j.urology.2013.09.017.

21. Kuo HC. Therapeutic effects of suburothelial injection of botulinum a toxin for neurogenic detrusor overactivity due to chronic cerebrovascular accident and spinal cord lesions. Urology. 2006;67(2):232–6. https://doi.org/10.1016/j.urology.2005.08.016.

22. Kennelly M, Dmochowski R, Ethans K, Karsenty G, Schulte-Baukloh H, Jenkins B, Thompson C, Li D, Haag-Molkenteller C. Long-term efficacy and safety of onabotulinumtoxinA in patients with urinary incontinence due to neurogenic detrusor overactivity: an interim analysis. Urology. 2013;81(3):491–7. https://doi.org/10.1016/j.urology.2012.11.010.

23. Rovner E, Kohan A, Chartier-Kastler E, Junemann KP, Del Popolo G, Herschorn S, Joshi M, Magyar A, Nitti V. Long-term efficacy and safety of onabotulinumtoxinA in patients with neurogenic detrusor overactivity who completed 4 years of treatment. J Urol. 2016;196(3):801–8. https://doi.org/10.1016/j.juro.2016.04.046.

24. Alvares RA, Araujo ID, Sanches MD. A pilot prospective study to evaluate whether the bladder morphology in cystography and/or urodynamic may help predict the response to botulinum toxin a injection in neurogenic bladder refractory to anticholinergics. BMC Urol. 2014;14:66. https://doi.org/10.1186/1471-2490-14-66.

25. Rovner E, Dmochowski R, Chapple C, Thompson C, Lam W, Haag-Molkenteller C. OnabotulinumtoxinA improves urodynamic outcomes in patients with neurogenic detrusor overactivity. Neurourol Urodyn. 2013;32(8):1109–15. https://doi.org/10.1002/nau.22376.

26. Ginsberg D, Cruz F, Herschorn S, Gousse A, Keppenne V, Aliotta P, Sievert KD, Brin MF, Jenkins B, Thompson C, Lam W, Heesakkers J, Haag-Molkenteller C. OnabotulinumtoxinA is effective in patients with urinary incontinence due to neurogenic detrusor overactivity [corrected] regardless of concomitant anticholinergic use or neurologic etiology. Adv Ther. 2013;30(9):819–33. https://doi.org/10.1007/s12325-013-0054-z.

27. Del Popolo G, Filocamo MT, Li Marzi V, Macchiarella A, Cecconi F, Lombardi G, Nicita G. Neurogenic detrusor overactivity treated with english botulinum toxin a: 8-year experience of one single centre. Eur Urol. 2008;53(5):1013–9. https://doi.org/10.1016/j.eururo.2007.09.034.

28. Ehren I, Volz D, Farrelly E, Berglund L, Brundin L, Hultling C, Lafolie P. Efficacy and impact of botulinum toxin A on quality of life in patients with neurogenic detrusor overactivity: a randomised, placebo-controlled, double-blind study. Scand J Urol Nephrol. 2007;41(4):335–40. https://doi.org/10.1080/00365590601068835.

29. Scaglione F. Conversion ratio between Botox(R), Dysport(R), and Xeomin(R) in clinical practice. Toxins (Basel). 2016;8(3). https://doi.org/10.3390/toxins8030065.

30. de Seze M, Petit H, Gallien P, de Seze MP, Joseph PA, Mazaux JM, Barat M. Botulinum a toxin and detrusor sphincter dyssynergia: a double-blind lidocaine-controlled study in 13 patients with spinal cord disease. Eur Urol. 2002;42(1):56–62.

31. Gallien P, Reymann JM, Amarenco G, Nicolas B, de Seze M, Bellissant E. Placebo controlled, randomised, double blind study of the effects of botulinum A toxin on detrusor sphincter dyssynergia in multiple sclerosis patients. J Neurol Neurosurg Psychiatry. 2005;76(12):1670–6. https://doi.org/10.1136/jnnp.2004.045765.

32. Mehta S, Hill D, Foley N, Hsieh J, Ethans K, Potter P, Baverstock R, Teasell RW, Wolfe D, Spinal Cord Injury Rehabilitation Evidence Research Team. A meta-analysis of botulinum toxin sphincteric injections in the treatment of incomplete voiding after spinal cord injury. Arch Phys Med Rehabil. 2012;93(4):597–603. https://doi.org/10.1016/j.apmr.2011.11.020.

33. Neel KF. Total endoscopic and anal irrigation management approach to noncompliant neuropathic bladder in children: a good alternative. J Urol. 2010;184(1):315–8. https://doi.org/10.1016/j.juro.2010.01.058.

34. Zeino M, Becker T, Koen M, Berger C, Riccabona M. Long-term follow-up after botulinum toxin A (BTX-A) injection into the detrusor for treatment of neurogenic detrusor hyperactivity in children. Cent Eur J Urol. 2012;65(3):156–61. https://doi.org/10.5173/ceju.2012.03.art12.

35. Marte A. Onabotulinumtoxin A for treating overactive/poor compliant bladders in children and adolescents with neurogenic bladder secondary to myelomeningocele. Toxins (Basel). 2012;5(1):16–24. https://doi.org/10.3390/toxins5010016.

36. Schulte-Baukloh H, Michael T, Schobert J, Stolze T, Knispel HH. Efficacy of botulinum-A toxin in children with detrusor hyperreflexia due to myelomeningocele: preliminary results. Urology. 2002;59(3):325–7. discussion 327-328

37. Horst M, Weber DM, Bodmer C, Gobet R. Repeated botulinum-A toxin injection in the treatment of neuropathic bladder dysfunction and poor bladder compliance in children with myelomeningocele. Neurourol Urodyn. 2011;30(8):1546–9. https://doi.org/10.1002/nau.21124.

38. Altaweel W, Jednack R, Bilodeau C, Corcos J. Repeated intradetrusor botulinum toxin type A in children with neurogenic bladder due to myelomeningocele. J Urol. 2006;175(3 Pt 1):1102–5. https://doi.org/10.1016/S0022-5347(05)00400-3.

39. Abdel-Meguid TA. Botulinum toxin-A injections into neurogenic overactive bladder—to include or exclude the trigone? A prospective, randomized, controlled trial. J Urol. 2010;184(6):2423–8. https://doi.org/10.1016/j.juro.2010.08.028.

40. Karsenty G, Elzayat E, Delapparent T, St-Denis B, Lemieux MC, Corcos J. Botulinum toxin type a injections into the trigone to treat idiopathic overactive bladder do not induce vesicoureteral reflux. J Urol. 2007;177(3):1011–4. https://doi.org/10.1016/j.juro.2006.10.047.

41. Davis NF, Burke JP, Redmond EJ, Elamin S, Brady CM, Flood HD. Trigonal versus extratrigonal botulinum toxin-A: a systematic review and meta-analysis of efficacy and adverse events. Int Urogynecol J. 2015;26(3):313–9. https://doi.org/10.1007/s00192-014-2499-2.

42. Krhut J, Samal V, Nemec D, Zvara P. Intradetrusor versus suburothelial onabotulinumtoxinA injections for neurogenic detrusor overactivity: a pilot study. Spinal Cord. 2012;50(12):904–7. https://doi.org/10.1038/sc.2012.76.

43. Denys P, Del Popolo G, Amarenco G, Karsenty G, Le Berre P, Padrazzi B, Picaut P, Dysport Study G. Efficacy and safety of two administration modes of an intra-detrusor injection of 750 units dysport(R) (abobotulinumtoxinA) in patients suffering from refractory neurogenic detrusor overactivity (NDO): A randomised placebo-controlled phase IIa study. Neurourol Urodyn. 2016;36:457. https://doi.org/10.1002/nau.22954.

44. Avallone MA, Sack BS, El-Arabi A, Guralnick ML, O'Connor RC. Less is more—a pilot study evaluating one to three intradetrusor sites for injection of OnabotulinumtoxinA for neu-

rogenic and idiopathic detrusor overactivity. Neurourol Urodyn. 2016;36:1104. https://doi.org/10.1002/nau.23052.

45. Chuang YC, Tyagi P, Huang CC, Yoshimura N, Wu M, Kaufman J, Chancellor MB. Urodynamic and immunohistochemical evaluation of intravesical botulinum toxin A delivery using liposomes. J Urol. 2009;182(2):786–92. https://doi.org/10.1016/j.juro.2009.03.083.

46. Kuo HC, Liu HT, Chuang YC, Birder LA, Chancellor MB. Pilot study of liposome-encapsulated onabotulinumtoxina for patients with overactive bladder: a single-center study. Eur Urol. 2014;65(6):1117–24. https://doi.org/10.1016/j.eururo.2014.01.036.

47. FDA. FDA Drug Safety Communication: FDA updates warnings for oral and injectable fluoroquinolone antibiotics due to disabling side effects. 2016. http://www.fda.gov/Drugs/DrugSafety/ucm511530.htm.

48. de Groat WC. A neurologic basis for the overactive bladder. Urology. 1997;50(6A Suppl):36–52; discussion 53–6

49. Silva C, Ribeiro MJ, Cruz F. The effect of intravesical resiniferatoxin in patients with idiopathic detrusor instability suggests that involuntary detrusor contractions are triggered by C-fiber input. J Urol. 2002;168(2):575–9.

50. Cruz F. Vanilloid receptor and detrusor instability. Urology. 2002;59(5 Suppl 1):51–60.

51. Chai TC, Gray ML, Steers WD. The incidence of a positive ice water test in bladder outlet obstructed patients: evidence for bladder neural plasticity. J Urol. 1998;160(1):34–8.

52. Brady CM, Apostolidis AN, Harper M, Yiangou Y, Beckett A, Jacques TS, Freeman A, Scaravilli F, Fowler CJ, Anand P. Parallel changes in bladder suburothelial vanilloid receptor TRPV1 and pan-neuronal marker PGP9.5 immunoreactivity in patients with neurogenic detrusor overactivity after intravesical resiniferatoxin treatment. BJU Int. 2004;93(6):770–6. https://doi.org/10.1111/j.1464-410X.2003.04722.x.

53. Smet PJ, Moore KH, Jonavicius J. Distribution and colocalization of calcitonin gene-related peptide, tachykinins, and vasoactive intestinal peptide in normal and idiopathic unstable human urinary bladder. Lab Invest. 1997;77(1):37–49.

54. Liu HT, Kuo HC. Increased expression of transient receptor potential vanilloid subfamily 1 in the bladder predicts the response to intravesical instillations of resiniferatoxin in patients with refractory idiopathic detrusor overactivity. BJU Int. 2007;100(5):1086–90. https://doi.org/10.1111/j.1464-410X.2007.07151.x.

55. Liu L, Mansfield KJ, Kristiana I, Vaux KJ, Millard RJ, Burcher E. The molecular basis of urgency: regional difference of vanilloid receptor expression in the human urinary bladder. Neurourol Urodyn. 2007;26(3):433–8 ; discussion 439; discussion 451–3. https://doi.org/10.1002/nau.20326.

56. Apostolidis A, Brady CM, Yiangou Y, Davis J, Fowler CJ, Anand P. Capsaicin receptor TRPV1 in urothelium of neurogenic human bladders and effect of intravesical resiniferatoxin. Urology. 2005;65(2):400–5. https://doi.org/10.1016/j.urology.2004.10.007.

57. Apostolidis A, Gonzales GE, Fowler CJ. Effect of intravesical Resiniferatoxin (RTX) on lower urinary tract symptoms, urodynamic parameters, and quality of life of patients with urodynamic increased bladder sensation. Eur Urol. 2006;50(6):1299–305. https://doi.org/10.1016/j.eururo.2006.04.006.

58. Fowler CJ, Jewkes D, McDonald WI, Lynn B, de Groat WC. Intravesical capsaicin for neurogenic bladder dysfunction. Lancet. 1992;339(8803):1239.

59. Fowler CJ, Beck RO, Gerrard S, Betts CD, Fowler CG. Intravesical capsaicin for treatment of detrusor hyperreflexia. J Neurol Neurosurg Psychiatry. 1994;57(2):169–73.

60. Geirsson G, Fall M, Sullivan L. Clinical and urodynamic effects of intravesical capsaicin treatment in patients with chronic traumatic spinal detrusor hyperreflexia. J Urol. 1995;154(5):1825–9.

61. Das A, Chancellor MB, Watanabe T, Sedor J, Rivas DA. Intravesical capsaicin in neurologic impaired patients with detrusor hyperreflexia. J Spinal Cord Med. 1996;19(3):190–3.

62. Cruz F, Guimaraes M, Silva C, Rio ME, Coimbra A, Reis M. Desensitization of bladder sensory fibers by intravesical capsaicin has long lasting clinical and urodynamic effects in patients with hyperactive or hypersensitive bladder dysfunction. J Urol. 1997;157(2):585–9.

63. De Ridder D, Chandiramani V, Dasgupta P, Van Poppel H, Baert L, Fowler CJ. Intravesical capsaicin as a treatment for refractory detrusor hyperreflexia: a dual center study with long-term followup. J Urol. 1997;158(6):2087–92.
64. de Seze M, Wiart L, Joseph PA, Dosque JP, Mazaux JM, Barat M. Capsaicin and neurogenic detrusor hyperreflexia: a double-blind placebo-controlled study in 20 patients with spinal cord lesions. Neurourol Urodyn. 1998;17(5):513–23.
65. de Seze M, Gallien P, Denys P, Labat JJ, Serment G, Grise P, Salle JY, Blazejewski S, Hazane C, Moore N, Joseph PA. Intravesical glucidic capsaicin versus glucidic solvent in neurogenic detrusor overactivity: a double blind controlled randomized study. Neurourol Urodyn. 2006;25(7):752–7. https://doi.org/10.1002/nau.20296.
66. Lazzeri M, Beneforti P, Turini D. Urodynamic effects of intravesical resiniferatoxin in humans: preliminary results in stable and unstable detrusor. J Urol. 1997;158(6):2093–6.
67. Lazzeri M, Spinelli M, Beneforti P, Zanollo A, Turini D. Intravesical resiniferatoxin for the treatment of detrusor hyperreflexia refractory to capsaicin in patients with chronic spinal cord diseases. Scand J Urol Nephrol. 1998;32(5):331–4.
68. Silva C, Rio ME, Cruz F. Desensitization of bladder sensory fibers by intravesical resiniferatoxin, a capsaicin analog: long-term results for the treatment of detrusor hyperreflexia. Eur Urol. 2000;38(4):444–52.
69. Kuo HC. Effectiveness of intravesical resiniferatoxin in treating detrusor hyper-reflexia and external sphincter dyssynergia in patients with chronic spinal cord lesions. BJU Int. 2003;92(6):597–601.
70. Silva C, Silva J, Ribeiro MJ, Avelino A, Cruz F. Urodynamic effect of intravesical resiniferatoxin in patients with neurogenic detrusor overactivity of spinal origin: results of a double-blind randomized placebo-controlled trial. Eur Urol. 2005;48(4):650–5. https://doi.org/10.1016/j.eururo.2005.04.012.
71. Dinis P, Silva J, Ribeiro MJ, Avelino A, Reis M, Cruz F. Bladder C-fiber desensitization induces a long-lasting improvement of BPH-associated storage LUTS: a pilot study. Eur Urol. 2004;46(1):88–93.; ; discussion 93–4. https://doi.org/10.1016/j.eururo.2004.01.016.
72. Giannantoni A, Di Stasi SM, Stephen RL, Bini V, Costantini E, Porena M. Intravesical resiniferatoxin versus botulinum-A toxin injections for neurogenic detrusor overactivity: a prospective randomized study. J Urol. 2004;172(1):240–3. https://doi.org/10.1097/01.ju.0000132152.53532.5d.
73. Schurch B, Denys P, Kozma CM, Reese PR, Slaton T, Barron RL. Botulinum toxin A improves the quality of life of patients with neurogenic urinary incontinence. Eur Urol. 2007;52(3):850–8. https://doi.org/10.1016/j.eururo.2007.04.026.
74. Herschorn S, Gajewski J, Ethans K, Corcos J, Carlson K, Bailly G, Bard R, Valiquette L, Baverstock R, Carr L, Radomski S. Efficacy of botulinum toxin A injection for neurogenic detrusor overactivity and urinary incontinence: a randomized, double-blind trial. J Urol. 2011;185(6):2229–35. https://doi.org/10.1016/j.juro.2011.02.004.

The Artificial Urinary Sphincter AMS 800™ (Boston Scientific, Boston, MA, USA) in Neurogenic Patients

Christine Reus and Emmanuel Chartier-Kastler

Abbreviations

AUS	Artificial urinary sphincter
DO	Detrusor overactivity
CIC	Clean intermittent catheterization
ISC	Incontinence Society Consensus
ISD	Intrinsic sphincter deficiency
NSUI	Neurogenic stress urinary incontinence
PPUI	Post-prostatectomy urinary incontinence
PRB	Pressure regulating balloon
SCI	Spinal cord injury

Introduction

"Neurogenic bladder" is a general, non-specific terminology used in the literature, to describe neurological bladder dysfunctions, ranging from noncontractile bladders to detrusor overactivity (DO) [1]. Patients with spinal cord injury (SCI) involving the infra-sacral spinal cord, with associated lower motor neuron disorder, will suffer de-innervation of the urethral sphincters (internal and/or external), resulting in neurogenic stress urinary incontinence (NSUI) by intrinsic sphincter deficiency (ISD) [2, 3].

The etiology includes posttraumatic causes such as lower spinal column, sacral or pelvic fractures and post-laminectomy complications, neurologic diseases—the

C. Reus
Karolinska Institute, Department of Molecular Medicine and Surgery, Section of Urology, Stockholm, Sweden and Academic Hospital Pitié Salpétrière, Paris, France

E. Chartier-Kastler (✉)
Department of Urology, Academic Hospital Pitié Salpétrière, AP-HP, Médecine Sorbonne Université, Paris, France
e-mail: emmanuel.chartier-kastler@upmc.fr

R. Dmochowski, J. Heesakkers (eds.), *Neuro-Urology*,
https://doi.org/10.1007/978-3-319-90997-4_23

most common being myelomeningocele (spina bifida) and cauda equina syndrome—and finally denervation following pelvic cancer surgery [3].

The reported incidence of neurogenic bladder dysfunction in adults associated with SCI is 69% and 31% with spina bifida [4]. Hunt and colleagues also report that 68% of children in school age affected by spina bifida suffer from NSUI due to ISD [5].

Optimal treatment modalities for these patients are complex. The main therapeutic objective is to preserve renal function [6]. There are currently no ideal international guidelines available for the surgical management of adult patients suffering from neurogenic urinary incontinence due to ISD. The latest available Incontinence Society Consensus (ISC) group report was more focused on non-neurogenic urinary incontinence [7]. Intermittent self-catheterization is central in obtaining continence in patients with NSUI. When this fails, other options may involve procedures such as bladder neck closure, urethral lengthening, urethral slings, and bulking agents [2]. However the artificial urinary sphincter (AUS) AMS 800ta is still considered the gold standard for the treatment of ISD in male neurogenic bladder dysfunction today [3], LoE [3], Grade A recommendation (EAU guidelines 2015, International Consultation on Incontinence or ICI 2012). Initially designed to treat postprostatectomy urinary incontinence (PPUI) 40 years ago, little data is available in the literature on AUS implantation in patients with NSUI secondary to ISD.

We will address the specificities of ISD management with AMS 800™ implantation in this particular patient group and underline the questions arising from the current literature on the subject. We will also highlight the surgical technique challenges in both male and female patients and explore novel AUS trends and future perspectives. Regardless of the gender, the central part of the surgical indication, patient counseling and post-operative follow-up will revolve around the necessity to perform CIC in the majority of this population, in order to achieve adequate voiding phase with minimal impact on the upper urinary tract.

History of the Artificial Urinary Sphincter

The artificial urinary sphincter (AUS) development attempts date back to antiquity [8]. Rosen designed the first model of AUS in 1976. However, 100% of hydraulic failure rates and fistula formation saw this project abandoned [9, 10].

In 1976 Mr. Scott developed the AMS 721(American Medical Systems, Minnetonka, MN), with a reported 79% success rate published in 1978, marking the history of the first successful artificial urinary sphincter device [11]. Other improved variations of the AMS followed, the AMS 742, providing an automatic cuff closure after cuff decompression (Campbell 10th edition, Chapter 79, p. 2291). The AMS 791 and AMS 792 used silicone cuff and a deactivation button [12]. The final version, the AMS 800™, still in use today, incorporates a deactivation button to the control pump. The narrow-back designed cuff introduced in 1987 improved pressure transmission from the cuff to the underlying urethral tissues, thereby significantly decreasing the incidence of erosion and tissue atrophy [13].

Finally, the latest improvement to the AMS 800™ in April 2008, called InhibiZone®, consisted in adding an antibiotic coating to the existing artificial urinary sphincter.

However, some authors [14, 15] as well as the AUS report of the latest Consensus Conference [16, 17] failed to prove its superiority over the non-coated version. It is not used, labeled, and available worldwide.

Historically, Jakobsen and colleagues reported an overall survival rate of 55% at 7 years for model AS 742, while a 4-year survival rate of 90% for AS791/792 models was reported in a cohort of 33 patients with neurogenic urinary incontinence over a 10-year period. A 76% continence rate (defined as complete continence or "slight but socially inconvenient incontinence") is reported by the same authors [18], results that are comparable to those obtained with the AMS 800™ in a similar population today [2].

Description of the AMS 800™ Device

To date, the AMS 800™ (Boston Scientific, Boston, MA, USA) AUS remains the "gold standard" for the treatment of severe non-neurogenic male UI (represented in Fig. 1). This three-piece device is composed of a fluid-filled inflatable cuff placed around the bladder neck or bulbar urethra, a hydraulic control pump located in the scrotum or labia majora (in women), and a pressure-regulating balloon (PRB) inserted pre- or intraperitoneally. These units, made primarily from silicone elastomer, are connected with kink-resistant tubings during surgery. Fluid transfer from cuff to the PRB is achieved by active manual pumping. Refilling occurs passively by pressure gradient from the PRB through a resistor located in the pump. This valve-like mechanism prevents acute pressure transmission from reservoir to cuff.

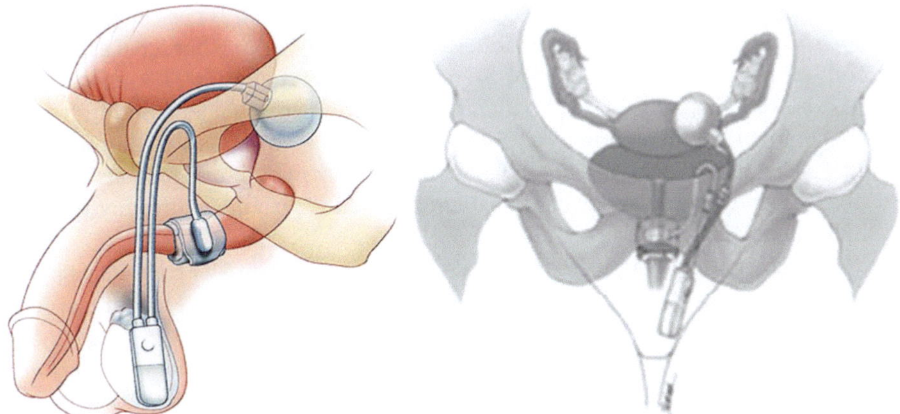

Fig. 1 The AMS Sphincter 800TM urinary prosthesis. Courtesy of American Medical Systems, Inc., Minnetonka, Minnesota. Illustrations by Michael Schenk. www.visitAMS.com

The main advantage of the AMS800™ is that the patient has a preserved voiding sensation. Although AUS surgery has proven its efficacy, it continues to have high complication and revision rates [19]. Furthermore, the system applies a constant pressure around the urethra, causing urethral injuries and is not user-friendly. Although some high-volume centers have reported good long-term results for AMS 800™ in females [20, 21], it remains a limited practice worldwide and is still branded an off-label use, according to the 2015 ICS Consensus conference report [16, 17].

Problems Arising from the Literature on AMS 800™ Implantation for NSUI

1. *Paucity of data in adult neurogenic patients and heterogeneity of the reported population*
   The data on AUS implantation in adults with ISD secondary to NSUI is scarce.

   The literature available on AMS 800™ surgery in patients with neurogenic bladder dysfunction stems mainly from pediatric population studies. Levesque et al. published pediatric data with the longest follow-up, reporting continence rates of 70% and an overall continence rate with a functioning AUS of 47% at 10 years [22].

   Another retrospective cohort of 107 children, with a mean follow-up of 61 months, the majority affected by spina bifida, reported an overall success rate of 77% with a complete continence rate of 83% and a revision rate of 19% [23]. We will discuss the results from adult studies in more specific details in another paragraph, as the difference between men and women needs to be examined more closely.

   Many reported studies mix neurological patients in the same series as non-neurological patients. There are few data available which focus on a homogeneous adult neurological population. One such study from Chartier-Kastler and coll. on a retrospective cohort of 51 male patients reported a 74% functioning AUS at 10 years with 86% of patients performing CIC, 39% benefitting from a concomitant augmentation cystoplasty, and finally a postoperative morbidity of 19%. The authors emphasize the importance of having a homogeneous population in a study, as it enables better patient counseling prior to confirming surgical indication [4].

   Bersch et al. also published data on AUS implantation in SCI patients, another homogeneous cohort, although their data referred to a modified technique, rendering comparison with other techniques more difficult [24].

2. *The lack of evidence-based material*
   Although AMS 800™ is considered the "golden standard" for NSUI management; the current practice lacks state-of-the-art evidence. A recent systematic review on quality assessment of NSUI surgical treatment outlines the absence of randomized clinical trials on this topic [2]. This review highlights the need to

improve evidence-based medicine in neurogenic patient groups, in order to offer the best care possible in accordance with today's scientific demands. This is essential in order for the clinician to offer appropriate counseling to the patient.

All 30 studies reviewed by the authors show level 3 of evidence and are cohort-prospective or retrospective studies, with an overall reporting quality rate varying from 43 to 81%. Studies published between 2002 and 2013 are of higher standard than those produced in the 1990s. Furthermore, from a statistical point of view, the exact P-value is provided in only 17% of the studies (the majority after 2002). Potential sources of bias and study limitations were also taken into account in 37% of the studies. This review highlights the heterogeneous nature of the analyzed articles, demonstrating how difficult it is to unify surgical outcomes with an adequate systematic meta-analysis.

Randomized controlled trials are required in order to comply with contemporary standards. However their realization is costly, and it is difficult to conduct studies involving a statistically significant cohort in this particular group of patients. In addition, future studies will not only have to take into account the use of validated questionnaires but also consider other factors specific to the neurogenic patient, such as general condition, bladder compliance, upper urinary tract status, cognitive function, degree of mobility, and hand dexterity. In the meantime, the urologist will combine the current literature resources with expert opinion available in a handful of reference centers. Moreover nobody knows which comparator has to be used for such study.

3. *The issue of nonstandardized definitions for primary outcome criteria*
As observed in AUS implantation for male non-neurogenic incontinence studies [19], there is a lack of standardization with regard to outcome criteria and reoperation rates. Some authors don't make the distinction between "perfect continence" and "moderate continence" as primary outcome criteria or define "moderate continence" as "social continence." Moreover male vs. female results in the neurogenic population should not be mixed. This result accounts for a great disparity in outcomes seen in the literature. Reported continence rates with a functioning AUS range between 57 and 92% [6, 25–29]. These results must also be interpreted by taking into consideration the global bladder-sphincter balance of each individual, which is not always clearly reported in the literature [4].

4. *Subjectivity in surgical indications*
There is a great deal of subjectivity in terms of surgical indications, i.e., whether a bladder neck procedure should or should not be indicated in a given patient with NSUI due to ISD. Video-urodynamic studies, if at all available, are of great help in diagnosing ISD, without however being definitive [3]. It is common practice for urologists to perform bladder neck surgery during augmentation cystoplasty in order to protect the upper urinary tract, when ISD is suspected, aimed for optimal functional results and for bladder augment development. This practice has mainly been described in a pediatric neuro-urologic population [22, 25, 26, 30]. This has led to selection bias in the literature [3]. It is recommended to treat refractory neurogenic detrusor overactivity (DO) with bladder augmentation.

However, detrusor myectomy is also an acceptable alternative in highly selected cases (EAU guidelines 2015, LE (3), Grade B recommendation).

5. *AUS in female neurogenic bladders*

A recent review of mechanical devices concluded that there was insufficient evidence to support the use of AUS in women [15]. The current EAU guidelines recommend the use of an autologous urethral sling in women with neurogenic stress urinary incontinence (NSUI) able to perform ISC (EAU guidelines 2015, LE (4), Grade B recommendation). The underlying idea is that any attempt to avoid a prosthesis has to be made to decrease morbidity (infection and device failure).

Preoperative Assessment Considerations in Neurogenic Patients

The complexity of the treatment of NSUI/ISD lies in the fact that it must be tailored for each case, taking into account the individual's neurological and urodynamic status, as well as their social and psychological requirements. It is essential to assess the mental and physical ability of the patient and evaluate their capacity to perform intermittent self-catheterization themselves or if the gesture is carried out by a third party. This assessment can only be achieved by thorough history taking and clinical examination.

Augmentation and substitution cystoplasty as well as AMS 800™ implantation have a role in the management of NSUI, where bladder hypo-compliance and hyper-reflexia may coexist with intrinsic sphincter deficiency [6, 31]. Both gestures may be performed concomitantly in some selected patients [4, 32]. The choice of the surgical technique is important when counseling the patient.

Furthermore, favoring the periprostatic placement of the AUS cuff (shown in Fig. 2) in these patients is based on four arguments [4]:

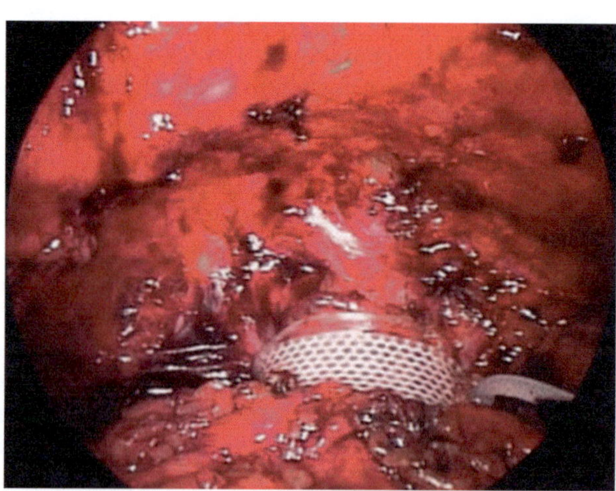

Fig. 2 Peri-prostatic AMS 800™ placement in a male patient with NSUI

1. Reducing the risk for bulbar urethral erosion due to regular CIC, thus reducing AUS explanation risks.
2. Wheelchair dependency increases perineal pressure sores, therefore increasing infection risks in peribulbar AUS placements.
3. Open bladder necks are often associated with sacral lesions. The urine-engorged prostatic urethra is an additional infection source should the sphincter be placed around the bulbar urethra.
4. Neurogenic patients are prone to bladder stone formation, which may require litholapaxy with a cystoscope greater than Charrière17, invariably inducing a peribulbar cuff erosion.

Surgical Technique Specificities

1. *Bladder neck AMS 800™ implantation in female patients and peribulbar implantation in males with NSUI*

   AUS implantation for non-neurogenic ISD in women is less performed compared to men in the same category and is limited to 19 centers worldwide [33]. Implanting an AMS 800™ in women is rarely used as a first treatment intention and is usually reserved to severe SUI refractory to previous less invasive surgical management. Consequently, these patients often present with anatomical modifications, rendering AUS surgery even more challenging, associated with decreased success rates [34, 35]. Furthermore, the technique requires a minimum of 20 implantations per year to maintain surgical skills, which is why this procedure should be reserved to highly specialized centers.

   Interestingly Farag et al. reported higher complication rates in males (20%) compared to females (10%) with AUS for neurogenic UI, a trend previously reported in earlier studies for non-neurogenic series. These results should in fact encourage further AUS placement in women with NSUI. The reason why this isn't the case is explained by the complexity of the surgical technique, by the fact that these patients have many comorbidities and have had previous multiple surgeries.

   The current literature provides very little guidance on the precise indications and ideal timing for AUS insertion in women with non-neurogenic SUI. Even less is written on AUS implantation in women with neurogenic SUI. This area is still the realm of surgical expertise rather than evidence-based medicine. The few available data originate largely from non-neurogenic cohorts. All studies analyzing AUS implantation in neurological bladder dysfunction in both genders only include a limited number of women.

   The largest prospective study involving 376 AMS 800™ implantations in women was published by Costa and colleagues [35]. Like many other published data, this single-center cohort mixed results from both non-neurogenic and neurogenic SUI in 344 women, with a mean age of 57 years, over a 20-year follow-up period. The reported proportion of patients suffering from neurogenic bladder dysfunction was 15%. The mean reported AUS survival rate was 14.7 years, longer than the device longevity observed in men. Previously published mean device survival was 6.9 years in men compared to 11.2 years in women [36]. Over 80% of AUS implanted in women remained functional and in place after 100 months [37].

The difference in AUS survival explanation is three-fold. Firstly, the anatomic bladder neck location of the cuff in women is more secure compared with the peribulbar placement of the cuff in men, a more superficial structure prone to injuries. As a matter of fact, a higher postoperative surgical complication rate in males (20%) compared to female patients (10%) was reported in the latest systematic review [2].

Secondly, the cuff size inserted in women is larger (6 cm in average), while in men 4–4.5 cm cuffs are routinely used. Thirdly, the control pump is more mobile and prone to skin erosion or kinks in the scrotum than in the labia majora [35].

It is surprising to see that Farag et al.'s systematic review of NSUI showed no correlation between gender and overall success rates (77 ± 16%) in AUS implantation nor was success correlated with neurogenic deficit subtypes and augmentation cystoplasty prior or simultaneous to AUS surgery.

2. *Periprostatic AMS 800™ implantation for NSUI*

Periprostatic AMS 800™ implantation for NSUI secondary to ISD is a more invasive technique, contraindicated after radical prostatectomy and reserved for highly specialized reference centers. It may be offered to men with urinary incontinence secondary to NSUI associated with myelomeningocele or other neurological disorders where the prostate is intact [38]. Sometimes it may be discussed carefully for patients suffering exstrophy or epispadias. The main objective of this technique is to decrease urethral erosion rates in patients using CIC and usually wheel chaired. Periprostatic cuff placement allows the wheelchair-bound patient to continue to perform frequent CIC without increasing the risk of infection or cuff erosion (through urethral trauma), particularly when a cystoscopy for bladder stone retrieval is required, a common occurrence in this population. Like bladder neck AUS in women, cuff sizes are larger than those usually fitted around the bulbar urethra, in average between 6 and 8 cm. The pressure-regulating balloon (PRB) remains the same, 61–70 cmH$_2$O [4]. The most common postoperative complication specific to this approach is an overestimation of the cuff size by a less experienced surgeon, a problem well described in pediatric literature [23]. The patient typically never regains continence in spite of the device being in situ. A refitting of the cuff 6 months later usually resolves the issue. Overall refitting rates range from 10 to 57% depending on the series, mostly occurring in the first 2 years following implantation of the device [4]. The largest retrospective multicenter study of 51 adult males with neurogenic bladder dysfunction undergoing periprostatic AUS with a 20-year follow-up was presented by Chartier and colleagues [4].The authors defined perfect continence as "at least a 4-hour period between catheterizations without urinary incontinence episodes" in 60% of patients. They also reported a 48% surgical revision rate including removal and/or replacement of the AUS. Mean device survival amounted to 6 years in this group, illustrating the average limited life span of the AMS 800™ in this particular indication compared to non-neurogenic groups.

Some high-volume centers have initiated robotically assisted periprostatic AUS implantation, which can now be performed as a day-case procedure; however long-term results are required [39].

3. *AMS 800™ implantation with simultaneous enterocystoplasty: yes or no?*

As previously mentioned, a thorough preoperative assessment in a patient with neurogenic bladder and ISD is important. However, in spite of it, vesical modifications may occur [22, 23, 25–28, 30, 40, 41]. Surgeons often tend to perform bladder neck surgery during augmentation cystoplasty, when ISD is suspected, in order to protect the upper urinary tract. The aim is to achieve good functional results [22, 25, 26, 30]. The overall reported enterocystoplasty frequency in neurogenic patients fitted with an AUS is heterogeneous and varies from 33 to 75% [6, 22, 23, 25, 40].

Increased infection and erosion frequency rating from18 to 50% were reported in two studies where enterocystoplasty was performed concomitantly with AMS 800™ implantation [36, 38]. However, both studies involved a small number of patients with a short follow-up. Other authors [6, 23, 25, 28, 42, 43] strongly favor simultaneous AUS and augmentation cystoplasty procedures, as most patients continue to perform CIC postoperatively. Another study with a follow-up of 20 years reported 39% of patients who underwent augmentation cystoplasty, of which 21.6% had simultaneous AMS 800™ insertion [4].

Results

1. *Overall success rate*

AMS 800™ implantation in NSUI for ISD has an overall success rate of 64% (lower compared to non-neurogenic series) and complication rates of 20% (higher compared to non-neurogenic patients) in a median follow-up of 48 months, independently from gender or neurological deficit type [2]. There is also a higher reoperation rate of 51% compared to 27% in non-neurogenic cases, and device longevity is also shown to be significantly lower in the neurogenic group due to previous incontinence surgery prior to AUS implantation [35]. A literature review confirms these findings reporting a revision rate in patients with neurogenic bladders to be 30% higher at 5 years than in patients with non-neurogenic SUI [28, 35, 40].

2. *Failure rates*

Compared with other existing techniques for UI, AMS 800™ was shown to be superior to urethral bulking agent injections (27 ± 20%) but not significantly different to slings (58 ± 25%) at 72 ± 18-month follow-up. However, failure rates were the highest with bulking agents (50 ± 16%), while no significant difference between AUS (10 ± 11%) and slings (22 ± 20%) was observed. AUS shows higher reoperation rates (51 ± 25%) when compared to slings (7 ± 9%). This percentage is superior when compared to the non-neurogenic population where it is reported to be 27% [4]. Patients should be informed about the success rates but also the reoperation and failure rates. The question of undertreatment of patients affected by NSUI may be reasonably raised in view of these findings. Finally AUS or sling implantation at the bulbar urethra show statistically higher complication rates (45 ± 14%) compared to bladder neck implantation (16 ± 21%), $p = 0.04$ [2].

3. *Mechanical failure*

   The AMS 800™ is prone to mechanical failure requiring replacement of some or the entirety of the device components. Once more, a disparity is observed in re-intervention reporting, depending on the team and how closely follow-ups are conducted. Some studies use the "rate of total procedures per year per patient," while others use the "rate of patients needing at least a new procedure" instead [4]. The reported post-prostatectomy AUS insertion revision rates are 50% at 5 years secondary to erosions, mechanical failure, infection, or urethral atrophy [44, 45]. Revision rates are even higher in patients with neurogenic bladder. Murphy et al. compared the functional durability of AMS 800™ in non-neurogenic as opposed to neurogenic ISD. Surprisingly, 85% neurogenic ISDs underwent surgical revision compared to 59% in the non-neurogenic group after 6-year follow-up.

   Definitive AUS removal rates in both adults and pediatric neurogenic populations range between 18 and 40% [26, 28–30].

   The literature is unclear which factors are associated with lower AUS lifespan. Some authors reported pediatric cohorts implicating previous bladder neck surgery and enterocystoplasty as increased risk factors [40, 46]. However this surgical technique correlation was not found in adults NSUI series, probably due to the fact that pediatric neurogenic cases are often mixed with anatomical malformations such as bladder exstrophy.

   Neurogenic patients are far younger (20–30 years) compared with the non-neurogenic group (70–75 years). The former is more likely to undergo more revisions due to their longer life expectancy. Furthermore the device is known to have a limited lifespan of 10 years. This explains the higher revision rates in the younger NSUI group. Another reason is provided by the fact that neurogenic patients are more fragile, with multiple comorbidities (such as hydrocephalus, recurrent UTIs), and have often undergone prior urethral or bladder neck surgery in infancy.

4. *Quality of life*

   QoL measurement is challenging in patients with spinal cord injuries or other neurological diseases. There are few disease-specific validated tools at hand, and there is no standardized QoL available in the current literature specifically designed for non-neurogenic AUS implantation [4]. Despite high revision rates in patients with neurogenic bladder dysfunction, patient satisfaction rates are often higher than complete continence rates. This attests for the fact that in spite of being incompletely continent, patients express satisfaction nonetheless with their continence improvement [47].

Future Perspectives

Newer AUS experimental devices have been designed over the years to address the limitations of the existing AMS 800™. The future AUS, as stated in the Report of the 2015 ICS Consensus Conference on the AMS 800™ (American Medical Systems, Minnetonka, MN, USA), should be a simple, cost-effective, robust design, with ease of manipulation/inactivation, safely implantable, using minimally invasive technique, with adaptable occlusive pressure in real time. The aim is once again to decrease erosion rates in this particularly vulnerable patient category.

However increasingly restrictive quality and regulatory directives, as well as new requirements of the latest ICS Consensus for novel AUS, are currently changing the landscape of the development process of innovative implantable medical devices.

Among the latest developments, some novel devices using Bluetooth technology to improve patient ergonomy are currently in preclinical development phase. For example, the "novel remotely controlled artificial urinary sphincter" (Montreal, QC, Canada) has recently been developed. This hydromechanical, remote-controlled four-piece AUS device, using Bluetooth technology compatible with the existing AMS 800™ tubings, cuff, and balloon, is composed of a small electronic pump implanted beside the AMS reservoir. The pump is designed to minimize energy consumption and mechanical failure and to be cost-effective. The authors claim to overcome the manual dexterity issue, decrease revision rates due to mechanical failure, and offer ease of implantation and adaptable periurethral pressure. It is also claimed that the device can be checked remotely on a daily base and can be used in women [48]. However, further animal in vitro and in vivo studies for biocompatibility and efficacy are still required.

Ludwig et al. presented another illustrating novel AUS device example, for both men and women. Although still in development, this new potentially more ergonomic sphincter harbors hopes for patients with SCI. The activation of the cuff is achieved via a small implant located at inguinal level. The opening is triggered through a remote control allowing patients to urinate easily. A surgical interface enables the medical staff to adjust in an individualized and noninvasive fashion the required postoperative adjustments over time. The advantage of this device is to theoretically decrease the application of a constant urethral pressure by applying sequential pressures instead. This device is hoping to revolutionize the novel AUS market.

It has been implanted on six cadaveric models (three males and three females), demonstrating the technique's feasibility and ease of implantation. Further results from pilot studies are awaited for efficacy and safety outcome assessment [49].

In a more realistic timeframe, the possibility to perform AUS implantation using robotic technology in a day-case setting is within grasp. Long-term results are awaited.

An open bladder neck in patients with SCI fills the prostatic urethra with urine, providing a potential infection source when patients are fitted with a bulbar urethral cuff. Robotic-assisted surgery addresses this particular issue and offers a promising solution. Recently, a very select number of highly specialized centers, with an experienced robotic surgeon with over 500 urological robotic procedures, assisted by a highly experienced AUS surgeon, have applied this innovative technique to AUS

Table 1 Level of evidence and recommendations (2015 EAU guidelines)

Summary of evidence	Level of evidence	Grade of recommendation
In male patients with neurogenic stress incontinence, AUS should be used	3	A
Implantation of an artificial urinary sphincter in women with SCI	3/4	A/B (?)
Warn women receiving AUS that, even in expert centers, there is a high risk of complications, mechanical failure, or a need for explanation	3	A (?)
In female patients with neurogenic stress urinary incontinence who are able to self-catheterize, placement of an autologous urethral sling should be used	4	B
Artificial urinary sphincter can be used to treat neurogenic stress incontinence	3	A
In order to treat refractory neurogenic detrusor overactivity, bladder augmentation is recommended. Detrusor myectomy is an acceptable alternative in highly selected cases	3	A

insertion in men with NSUI. The advantages of the robot are its precision, 3D high-definition vision, and EndoWrist instrumentation facilitating suturing in narrow male pelvis. Six male patients with SCI and a median age of 51.5 years underwent this procedure in one of those units [39]. The mean operating time was 195 min with no intraoperative complications. Mean hospital length of stay was 4 days, and all six patients had a functioning device after a median follow-up of 13 months. The authors reported no early erosion, device infection, or malfunction. Two patients developed a Clavien, one minor complication in the form of epididymitis. A 7.5–8 cm cuff was positioned around the bladder neck, and not the bulbar urethra, for the reasons we have outlined earlier. The main technical difficulty described was the challenging dissection of Retzius space in patients who underwent previous urine incontinence surgery.

Biardeau et al. have also recently prospectively collected published data on robot-assisted laparoscopic AUS implantation in 11 women with non-neurogenic SUI. 5.5–8 cm cuff was positioned around the bladder neck. 72.7% had a successful implantation and 87.5% complete continence rates at 17.6 months mean follow-up. The intraoperative complications were higher compared to open techniques. These results are promising. However the technique needs to be standardized and a greater number of patients are required for assessment. Finally, the costs may be a limiting factor [50]. As a summary of what is known and more accepted worldwide, Table 1 reports levels of evidence and recommendations issued from EAU guidelines.

Conclusion

AMS 800™ implantation in patients with NSUI is feasible, safe, with acceptable success rates. It is however associated with high reoperation rates. Bladder neck AUS positioning should be preferred in neurogenic patients male or female.

Complication rates are lower in women with NSUI. The absence of RCT and high-level designed studies accounts for the scarcity of available data on AUS in NSUI.

One should emphasize the importance of informed consent in appropriate decision-making. More state-of-the-art studies taking into account the specifics of the neurogenic population, such as general physical status, bladder compliance, upper urinary tract quality, cognitive function, and manual dexterity, are required.

Every urologist should be able to offer the best level of care possible based on today's standard of evidence-based medicine to this complex group of patients.

References

1. Ruffion A, Castro-Diaz D, Patel H, Khalaf K, Onyenwenyi A, Globe D, et al. Systematic review of the epidemiology of urinary incontinence and detrusor overactivity among patients with neurogenic overactive bladder. Neuroepidemiology. 2013;41(3–4):146–55.
2. Farag F, Koens M, Sievert K-D, De Ridder D, Feitz W, Heesakkers J. Surgical treatment of neurogenic stress urinary incontinence: a systematic review of quality assessment and surgical outcomes. Neurourol Urodyn. 2016 Jan;35(1):21–5.
3. Myers JB, Mayer EN, Lenherr S, Neurogenic Bladder Research Group (NBRG.org). Management options for sphincteric deficiency in adults with neurogenic bladder. Transl Androl Urol. 2016;5(1):145–57.
4. Chartier Kastler E, Genevois S, Gamé X, Denys P, Richard F, Leriche A, et al. Treatment of neurogenic male urinary incontinence related to intrinsic sphincter insufficiency with an artificial urinary sphincter: a French retrospective multicentre study. BJU Int. 2011;107(3):426–32.
5. Hunt GM. Spina bifida: implications for 100 children at school. Dev Med Child Neurol. 1981 Apr;23(2):160–72.
6. Singh G, Thomas DG. Artificial urinary sphincter in patients with neurogenic bladder dysfunction. Br J Urol. 1996;77(2):252–5.
7. Biardeau X, Aharony S, Campeau L, Corcos J. Overview of the 2015 ICS consensus conference. Neurourol Urodyn. 2016;35(4):437–43.
8. Schultheiss D, Höfner K, Oelke M, Grünewald V, Jonas U. Historical aspects of the treatment of urinary incontinence. Eur Urol. 2000;38(3):352–62.
9. Rosen M. A simple artificial implantable sphincter. Br J Urol. 1976;48(7):675–80.
10. Rosen M. Proceedings: a simple artificial sphincter. Br J Urol. 1976;48(2):154.
11. Scott FB. The artificial sphincter in the management of incontinence in the male. Urol Clin North Am. 1978 Jun;5(2):375–91.
12. Scott FB. The artificial urinary sphincter. Experience in adults. Urol Clin North Am. 1989 Feb;16(1):105–17.
13. Light JK, Reynolds JC. Impact of the new cuff design on reliability of the AS800 artificial urinary sphincter. J Urol. 1992;147(3):609–11.
14. de Cógáin MR, Elliott DS. The impact of an antibiotic coating on the artificial urinary sphincter infection rate. J Urol. 2013;190(1):113–7.
15. De Cógáin M, Elliott D. The impact of inhibizone® on artificial urinary sphincter infection rate. J Urol. 2013;189(4):e562.
16. Biardeau X, Aharony S, Campeau L, Corcos J, AUS Consensus Group. Artificial urinary sphincter: report of the 2015 consensus conference. Neurourol Urodyn. 2016;35(Suppl 2):S8–24.
17. Biardeau X, Aharony S, Campeau L, Corcos J, AUS Consensus Group. Artificial urinary sphincter: executive summary of the 2015 consensus conference. Neurourol Urodyn. 2016;35(Suppl 2):S5–7.
18. Jakobsen H, Hald T. Management of neurogenic urinary incontinence with AMS artificial urinary sphincter. Scand J Urol Nephrol. 1986;20(2):137–41.

19. Van Der Aa F, Drake MJ, Kasyan GR, Petrolekas A, Cornu J-N. The artificial urinary sphincter after a quarter of a century: a critical systematic review of its use in male non-neurogenic incontinence. Eur Urol. 2013;63(4):681–9.
20. Roupret M, Chartier-Kastler E, Richard F. [Artificial urinary sphincters in women: indications, techniques, results]. Prog Urol. 2005;15(3):489–93.
21. Phé V, Benadiba S, Rouprêt M, Granger B, Richard F, Chartier-Kastler E. Long-term functional outcomes after artificial urinary sphincter implantation in women with stress urinary incontinence. BJU Int. 2014;113(6):961–7.
22. Levesque PE, Bauer SB, Atala A, Zurakowski D, Colodny A, Peters C, et al. Ten-year experience with the artificial urinary sphincter in children. J Urol. 1996;156(2 Pt 2):625–8.
23. Simeoni J, Guys JM, Mollard P, Buzelin JM, Moscovici J, Bondonny JM, et al. Artificial urinary sphincter implantation for neurogenic bladder: a multi-institutional study in 107 children. Br J Urol. 1996;78(2):287–93.
24. Bersch U, Göcking K, Pannek J. The artificial urinary sphincter in patients with spinal cord lesion: description of a modified technique and clinical results. Eur Urol. 2009;55(3):687–93.
25. Gonzalez R, Merino FG, Vaughn M. Long-term results of the artificial urinary sphincter in male patients with neurogenic bladder. J Urol. 1995;154(2 II Suppl):769–70.
26. Catti M, Lortat-Jacob S, Morineau M, Lottmann H. Artificial urinary sphincter in children—voiding or emptying? An evaluation of functional results in 44 patients. J Urol. 2008;180(2):690–3; discussion 693
27. Spiess PE, Capolicchio JP, Kiruluta G, Salle JP, Berardinucci G, Corcos J. Is an artificial sphincter the best choice for incontinent boys with spina bifida? Review of our long term experience with the AS-800 artificial sphincter. Can J Urol. 2002;9(2):1486–91.
28. López Pereira P, Somoza Ariba I, Martínez Urrutia MJ, Lobato Romero R, Jaureguizar Monroe E. Artificial urinary sphincter: 11-year experience in adolescents with congenital neuropathic bladder. Eur Urol. 2006;50(5):1096–101.
29. Kryger JV, Barthold JS, Fleming P, González R. The outcome of artificial urinary sphincter placement after a mean 15-year follow-up in a paediatric population. BJU Int. 1999;83(9):1026–31.
30. Hafez AT, McLorie G, Bägli D, Khoury A. A single-centre long-term outcome analysis of artificial urinary sphincter placement in children. BJU Int. 2002;89(1):82–5.
31. McRae P, Murray KHA, Nurse DE, Stephenson TP, Mundy AR. Clam enterocystoplasty in the neuropathic bladder. Br J Urol. 1987;60(6):523–5.
32. Mundy AR, Shah PJ, Borzyskowski M, Saxton HM. Sphincter behaviour in myelomeningocele. Br J Urol. 1985;57(6):647–51.
33. Chartier-Kastler E, Van Kerrebroeck P, Olianas R, Cosson M, Mandron E, Delorme E, et al. Artificial urinary sphincter (AMS 800) implantation for women with intrinsic sphincter deficiency: a technique for insiders? BJU Int. 2011;107(10):1618–26.
34. Costa P, Mottet N, Rabut B, Thuret R, Ben Naoum K, Wagner L. The use of an artificial urinary sphincter in women with type III incontinence and a negative Marshall test. J Urol. 2001;165(4):1172–6.
35. Costa P, Poinas G, Ben Naoum K, Bouzoubaa K, Wagner L, Soustelle L, et al. Long-term results of artificial urinary sphincter for women with type III stress urinary incontinence. Eur Urol. 2013;63(4):753–8.
36. Petero VG, Diokno AC. Comparison of the long-term outcomes between incontinent men and women treated with artificial urinary sphincter. J Urol. 2006;175(2):605–9.
37. Chung E, Cartmill RA. 25-year experience in the outcome of artificial urinary sphincter in the treatment of female urinary incontinence. BJU Int. 2010;106(11):1664–7.
38. Herndon CDA, Rink RC, Shaw MBK, Simmons GR, Cain MP, Kaefer M, et al. The Indiana experience with artificial urinary sphincters in children and young adults. J Urol. 2003;169(2):650–4; discussion 654
39. Yates DR, Phé V, Rouprêt M, Vaessen C, Parra J, Mozer P, et al. Robot-assisted laparoscopic artificial urinary sphincter insertion in men with neurogenic stress urinary incontinence. BJU Int. 2013;111(7):1175–9.

40. Kryger JV, Leverson G, Gonzalez R. Long-term results of artificial urinary sphincters in children are independent of age at implantation. J Urol. 2001;165(6 II Suppl):2377–9.
41. Light JK, Pietro T. Alteration in detrusor behavior and the effect on renal function following insertion of the artificial urinary sphincter. J Urol. 1986;136(3):632–5.
42. Venn SN, Mundy AR. Long-term results of augmentation cystoplasty. Eur Urol. 1998;34(Suppl. 1):40–2.
43. Viers BR, Elliott DS, Kramer SA. Simultaneous augmentation cystoplasty and cuff only artificial urinary sphincter in children and young adults with neurogenic urinary incontinence. J Urol. 2014;191(4):1104–8.
44. Kim SP, Sarmast Z, Daignault S, Faerber GJ, McGuire EJ, Latini JM. Long-term durability and functional outcomes among patients with artificial urinary sphincters: a 10-year retrospective review from the University of Michigan. J Urol. 2008;179(5):1912–6.
45. Wang R, McGuire EJ, He C, Faerber GJ, Latini JM. Long-term outcomes after primary failures of artificial urinary sphincter implantation. Urology. 2012;79(4):922–8.
46. Castera R, Podestá ML, Ruarte A, Herrera M, Medel R. 10-Year experience with artificial urinary sphincter in children and adolescents. J Urol. 2001;165(6 Pt 2):2373–6.
47. Murphy S, Rea D, O'Mahony J, McDermott TED, Thornhill J, Butler M, et al. A comparison of the functional durability of the AMS 800 artificial urinary sphincter between cases with and without an underlying neurogenic aetiology. Ir J Med Sci. 2003 Sep;172(3):136–8.
48. Corcos J, Hached S, Loutochin O, Sawan M. 1375 novel, remotely-controlled, artificial urinary sphincter: a retro-compatible device. J Urol. 2013;189((4):e562.
49. Ludwig TA, Reiss P, Wieland M, Becker A, Fisch M, Chun FK, et al. The ARTUS device: the first feasibility study in human cadavers. Can J Urol. 2015;22(6):8100–4.
50. Biardeau X, Rizk J, Marcelli F, Flamand V. Robot-assisted laparoscopic approach for artificial urinary sphincter implantation in 11 women with urinary stress incontinence: surgical technique and initial experience. Eur Urol. 2015;67(5):937–42.

Sacral Dorsal Rhizotomy and Sacral Anterior Root Stimulation in Neurogenic Patients: The Brindley Procedure

Frank M. J. Martens and John Heesakkers

Introduction

The bladder and the closing mechanism of the bladder have an opposite function in people with a normal function of the lower urinary tract. During the filling phase of the voiding cycle, the bladder relaxes and the urethral sphincter contracts to store urine at a low intravesical pressure. During micturition, the urethral sphincter relaxes and the bladder contracts.

Spinal cord injury is one of the neurological conditions that cause a neurogenic bladder [1]. Patients with damage at the sacral level or to more peripheral nerves mostly suffer from a hypocontractile detrusor. Suprasacral injury to the spinal cord will result in detrusor overactivity. Moreover, coordination between the bladder and sphincter can dysfunction which results in detrusor-external sphincter dyssynergia.

Detrusor overactivity, especially in combination with detrusor-external sphincter dyssynergia, might cause high intravesical pressures and incomplete bladder emptying. Subsequent reflux and urinary tract infections can cause renal deterioration. Detrusor overactivity can trigger autonomic dysreflexia, which can lead to malignant hypertension. Therefore, a major goal in spinal cord injury patient is protection of the upper urinary tract to preserve renal function.

The Brindley procedure combines two procedures for management of multiple organ dysfunction by controlling not only micturition but also defecation and erections in males. Firstly, sacral anterior root stimulation (SARS) of efferent nerves [2] enables micturition, defecation, and erections. Secondly, a dorsal rhizotomy treats detrusor overactivity, prevents detrusor-external sphincter dyssynergia during stimulation, and diminishes autonomic dysregulation by transecting afferent nerves [3].

F. M. J. Martens · J. Heesakkers (✉)
Department of Urology, Radboudumc, Nijmegen, The Netherlands
e-mail: Frank.martens@radboudumc.nl; John.Heesakkers@radboudumc.nl

© Springer International Publishing AG, part of Springer Nature 2018   421
R. Dmochowski, J. Heesakkers (eds.), *Neuro-Urology*,
https://doi.org/10.1007/978-3-319-90997-4_24

The technique, selection of patients, and clinical results are discussed in this chapter [4, Reprinted in adapted form].

Brindley Stimulator

The Brindley system is composed of an external and implanted part. The implanted part consists of electrodes, connecting cables, and a receiver block (Fig. 1). The receiver does not contain a battery. Electrical stimuli are evoked by radiofrequency waves. Patients have to position an external stimulating device on the skin over the implanted receiver to evoke these stimuli (Figs. 1b and 2). With the availability of separate stimulation of the sacral levels and various stimulation settings, it is possible to set various stimulation programmes to optimize micturition, defecation, and penile erections or vaginal lubrication.

A tripolar electrode cuff is used for intradural stimulation of the sacral anterior roots (Fig. 1a, b). A three-channel implant is composed of two books. The upper book contains three parallel slots: one slot for S3 roots and two slots for S2 roots (two slots at one channel). The lower book contains one slot for S4 roots. Each slot contains one cathode in the centre and an anode at each of the two ends to avoid stimulation of tissue structures outside the slot. The two-channel implant allows stimulation of two root levels or sets of root levels. The four-channel implant has the same configuration as the three-channel implant but allows independent stimulation of four sets of roots. The choice for the number of channels depends on the number of different rootlet combinations that have to be stimulated. Usually, the three-channel implant is used. Each channel is connected to the subcutaneous receiver block by a silicone-coated cable.

Extradural electrodes (Fig. 1c) are used in patients in whom intradural electrodes could not be placed due to, for example, arachnoiditis or a previous intradural electrode implantation that failed. Some centres prefer to use extradural electrodes primarily for nearly all patients. The extradural implant has helical electrodes at its end, which are also configured with a cathode between two anodes. The number of helical electrodes can differ depending on the number of different rootlet combinations that have to be stimulated comparable to the intradural electrodes.

Dorsal Rhizotomy of the Sacral Nerves

Sauerwein structurally expanded SARS with a dorsal rhizotomy (deafferentation) of sacral roots S2 till S5 [3]. A dorsal rhizotomy is important because it suppresses neurogenic detrusor overactivity and detrusor-external sphincter dyssynergia [3, 5]. This results in a low-pressure bladder without reflex contractions of the detrusor and subsequently continence. Moreover, it reduces autonomic dysreflexia [5, 6]. Therefore, a dorsal rhizotomy can also be applied

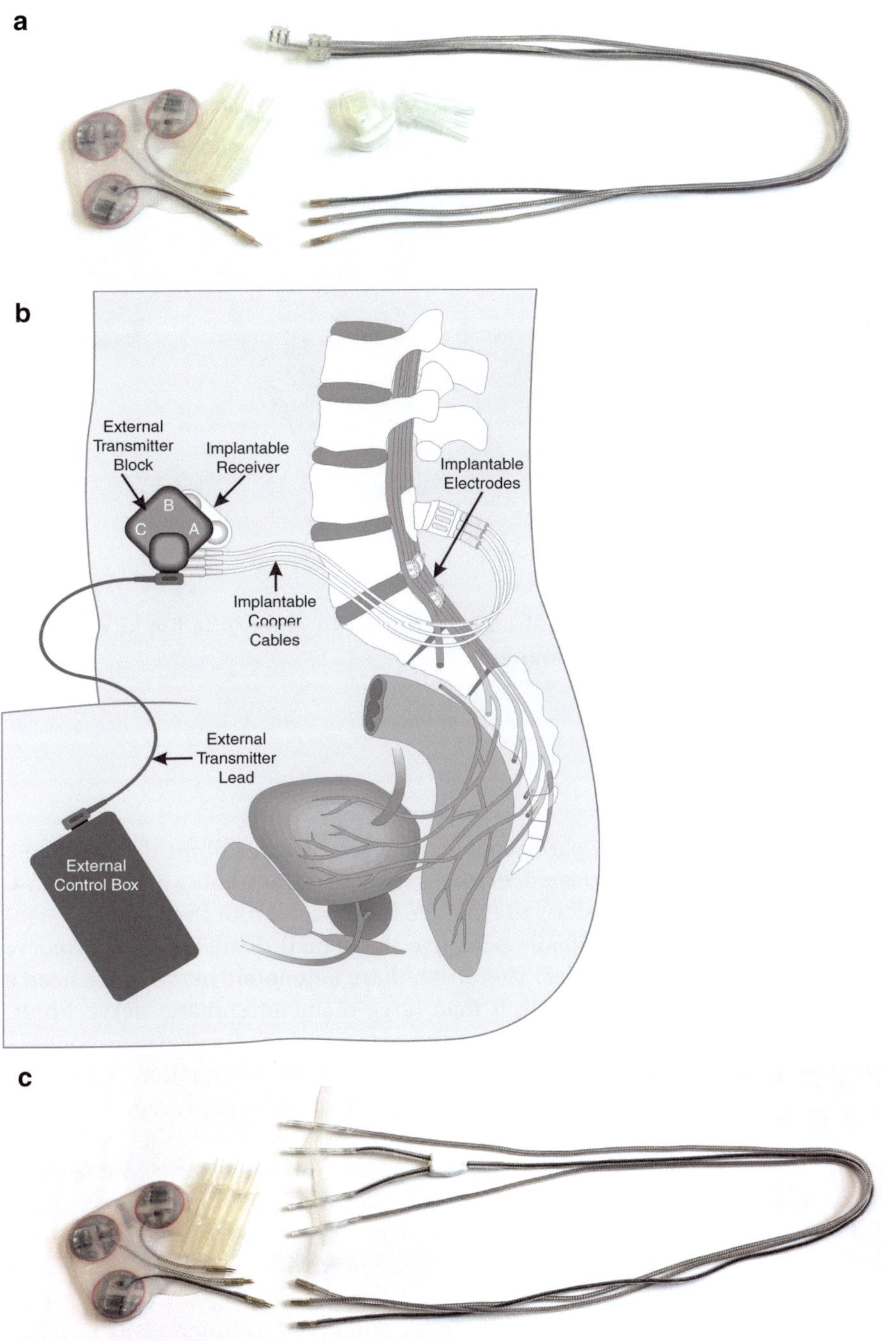

Fig. 1 (**a**) Components of the implanted part for intradural stimulation including a three-channel book and receiver block. (**b**) Implanted and external components for intradural stimulation in situ. (**c**) Components of the implanted part for extradural stimulation including four stimulation electrodes with a two-channel receiver block (Reprinted with permission of Finetech Medical Ltd.)

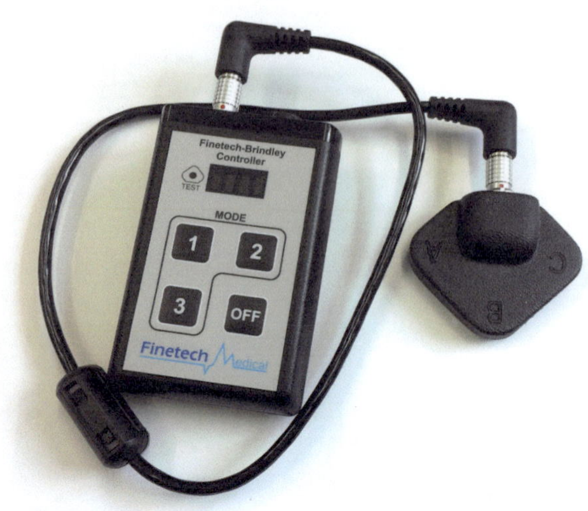

Fig. 2 External stimulator that can be programmed with different stimulation settings to enable the patient to stimulate for micturition, defecation, and erections separately. Signals are transmitted to the subcutaneous receiver block (Fig. 1) by the external stimulation block (Reprinted with permission of Finetech Medical Ltd.)

in combination with intermittent catheterization to empty the bladder without implantation of a Brindley stimulator [6].

Poststimulus Voiding

Most of the small-diameter parasympathetic efferent nerve fibres that innervate the detrusor muscle are located in the sacral anterior roots, mainly S3-S4. Somatic motor nerve fibres derived from the same sacral root levels are substantially larger and more electrically sensitive than small-diameter efferent nerve fibres that innervate the bladder. Therefore, these autonomic nerve fibres need a higher stimulus for their activation than large-diameter somatic nerve fibres. Consequently, electrical stimulation of the anterior roots for detrusor contraction also causes contraction of the urethral sphincter due to simultaneous stimulation of somatic nerve fibres to the urethral sphincter. This prevents adequate emptying of the bladder. To overcome this problem, poststimulus voiding is used. Smooth muscle of the bladder relaxes more slowly than striated muscle of the urethral sphincter. When intermittent stimulation pulse trains are applied with gaps of no stimulation, the difference in muscle relaxation time can be used to achieve a sustained detrusor muscle contraction within intervals of urethral sphincter relaxation [2]. This results in poststimulus voiding with an intermittent flow pattern of micturition during the stimulation-free intervals (Fig. 3). A comparable mechanism has been used for defecation.

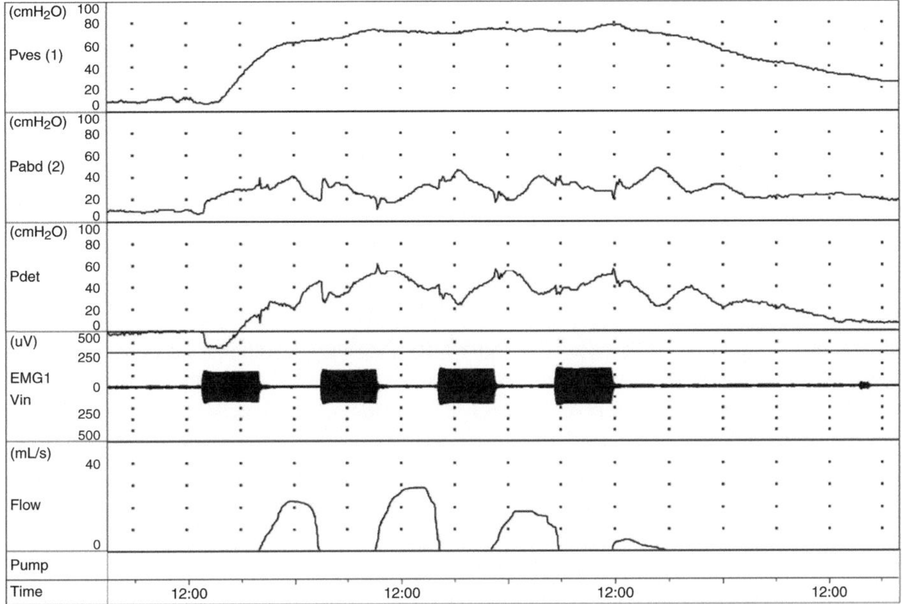

Fig. 3 Example of poststimulus voiding using a Brindley stimulator. The three upper traces show the intravesical (Pves), intra-abdominal (Pabd), and detrusor (Pdet) pressures during stimulation with a Brindley stimulator. The increase in EMG signal reflects the activation of the stimulus during 5 s. Stimulation is activated every 12 s. The intermittent stimulation pattern allows the urethral sphincter to relax while the detrusor pressure remains elevated. This results in an intermittent flow pattern, which is shown in the lower trace

Patient Selection

The Brindley procedure is suitable for a selected group of skeletally mature patients with stable, complete spinal cord injury and with intact spinal reflexes, who do not respond adequately to conservative treatments of neurogenic detrusor overactivity. Especially, patients with severe autonomic dysreflexia or detrusor-external sphincter dyssynergia will benefit from a dorsal rhizotomy. Patients with incomplete injury will lose their sensory function due to the dorsal rhizotomy and risk to experience pain sensation during stimulation due to an incomplete rhizotomy.

Patients need to have intact efferent nerve pathways to the bladder and a bladder that is able to contract. Contractions of at least 50 cmH$_2$O in males or 30 cmH$_2$O in females need to be present during filling cystometry [7]. If no sufficient spontaneous contraction occurs, suitable patients can be selected by rectal stimulation according to electro-ejaculation procedures or direct needle stimulation of the sacral roots to provoke bladder contractions.

Preoperative magnetic resonance imaging is used to exclude arachnoiditis at the level of the conus and cauda equine or other neurological disorder of the spinal cord. Patients with active or previous arachnoiditis are not suitable for intradural electrode implantation.

Surgical Procedure

The surgical procedure consists of a rhizotomy of the dorsal sacral roots and implantation of electrodes. Both parts of the procedure can be done intradurally as well as extradurally [8].

For an intradural rhizotomy and intradural implantation of the electrode cuff, a laminectomy is done from L3-L4 to S1-S2. The dura and arachnoid are opened at midline to expose the sacral nerve roots. Sacral root levels can be identified intradurally by electrical stimulation of the roots while monitoring blood pressure and observing somatic motor responses, including anal sphincter activity, pelvic floor activity, limb muscles activity, and especially bladder activity. The next step after identification of the sacral root levels is to separate the roots into anterior (efferent nerves) and posterior (afferent nerves) components. S2-4 posterior roots have a nearly white colour compared to the darker, pinkish grey colour of the anterior roots. Correct separation can be checked by electrical stimulation again. Only anterior roots should result in somatic motor responses, whereas stimulation of the dorsal roots will result in a rise in blood pressure. S5 roots are thin and not always present or able to separate into anterior or posterior components. If less than 10 cmH$_2$O bladder pressure is obtained, it should be crushed. The anterior sacral roots are positioned into the slots of the electrode cuff. The dura incison is closed to prevent cerebrospinal fluid leakage. Cables from the electrodes are tunnelled to a subcutaneous pocket and connected to the receiver.

An extradural implantation of electrodes requires a laminectomy from L5-S1 to S3-S4. The dorsal rhizotomy is done at the conus medullaris or extradurally at the level of the ganglia. The identity of the sacral roots and anterior and dorsal components are determined by electrical stimulation tests as described in the paragraph before. The extradural electrode is implanted and fixated to the anterior nerve bundle by a strip of reinforced silicone surrounding the nerve. The connecting cables and the receiver are implanted the same way as the intradural procedure.

Clinical Results

Table 1 shows an overview of publications on the clinical results of the Brindley procedure [6–7, 9–26]. These results comprise both the Brindley stimulator, which enables stimulation for micturition, defecation, and erections, and the dorsal rhizotomy to achieve continence.

The Brindley stimulator is used for micturition in 73–100% of patients during follow-up. However, it should be noted that stimulation is not always completely successful while this includes patients who use additional methods to empty their bladder. Percentages of patients that have residual urine of 50 mL or less are lower than the percentages of patients that use the stimulator for micturition. Additional

Table 1 Clinical results

Author	Patients in follow-up	Rhizotomy (intradural/ extradural)	Implantation (intradural/ extradural)	Follow-up (years)	Autonomic dysreflexia (before/after)	Use for voiding (% of patients)	Continence (% of patients)	Bladder capacity (% of increase)	Residual urine (% of patients)	UTI incidence (% of patients or incidence/ year)	Use for defecation (% of patients)	Use for erections (% of males)
Brindley et al. [7]	38 ♂ 12 ♀	17/0 (S2 and/or S3)	50/0	1–9	0/1 (during stimulation)	86%	62%	–	80% <60 mL	–	–	68%
Madersbacher et al. [16]	1 ♂ 6 ♀	7/0	7/0	–	- (1 during stimulation)	100%	100%	122%	100% <40 mL	After 0%	29%	100%
Robinson et al. [18]	20 ♂ 2 ♀	–	–	–	–	73%	68%	–	–	–	–	30% (0% of ♂ used stimulation for sexual intercourse)
MacDonagh et al. [15]	9 ♂ 3 ♀	9/0	12/0	2.2	–	100%	–	–	–	–	50% complete emptying with stimulation	–
Sauerwein et al. [20]	5 ♂ 6 ♀	0/12	0/12	–	–	82%	64%	–	100% <50 mL	–	–	–
Van Kerrebroeck et al. [23]	90 ♂ 94 ♀ **	–	166/18	–	26/10	92%	86%	–	82% <30 mL	Before 88% After 17%	70%	74% (32% of ♂ used stimulation for sexual intercourse)

(continued)

Table 1 (continued)

Author	Patients in follow-up	Rhizotomy (intradural/ extradural)	Implantation (intradural/ extradural)	Follow-up (years)	Autonomic dysreflexia (before/after)	Use for voiding (% of patients)	Continence (% of patients)	Bladder capacity (% of increase)	Residual urine (% of patients)	UTI incidence (% of patients or incidence/ year)	Use for defecation (% of patients)	Use for erections (% of males)
Madersbacher et al. [17]	8 ♂ 22 ♀	–	27/4	–	–	97%	93%	–	90% <50 mL	–	–	–
Sarrias et al. [19]	1 ♂ 6 ♀	7/0	0/7	–	–	100%	100%	–	100% <50 mL	–	100%	–
Brindley [10]	271 ♂ 229 ♀ **	–	≤477/≥23	4	– (3 during stimulation)	86%	–	–	–	–	–	–
Van Kerrebroeck et al. [6]	29 ♂ 18 ♀	47/0	47/0	3.5	7/5 (2 during stimulation)	96%	91%	–	87% <50 mL	Before 4.2/ year After 1.4/year	87%	62% (21% of ♂ used stimulation for sexual intercourse)
Schurch et al. [21]	3 ♂ 7 ♀	10/0	10/0	3.4	6/6 (during stimulation)	100%	80%	213%	100% <50 mL	Before 80% After 60%	–	–
Egon et al. [12]	68 ♂ 28 ♀	0/0	90/9	5.4 ♂ 5.8 ♀	22/0	90%	89%	134% ♂ 375% ♀ (range 300–600)	86% <50 mL	Before 100% After 31%	55% (41% of these had complete evacuation with stimulation alone)	75% (26% of ♂ used stimulation for sexual intercourse)
van der Aa et al. [22]	33 ♂ 4 ♀	37/0	37/0	0.3–12	–	100%	84%	–	73% <30 mL	–	73%	88%

Bauchet et al. [9]	6 ♂ 14 ♀	20/0	20/1	4.5	3/0	90%	90%	142%	95% <50 mL	–	40%	–
Creasey et al. [11]	16 ♂ 7 ♀	23/0	0/23	>1	8/2	78%	87%	–	79% <50 mL	Before 3/ year After 2/year	100%	–
Vastenholt et al. [24]	32 ♂ 5 ♀	37/0	37/0	7.2	–	87%	57%	–	–	–	60%	65% (0% of ♂ used stimulation for sexual intercourse)
Hamel et al. [13]	4 ♂	4/0	0/4	–	–	100%	75%	–	100% <50 mL	–	50%	75% (0% of ♂ used stimulation for sexual intercourse)
Kutzenberger et al. [14]	440 ♂ + ♀	Almost all intradural	Almost all intradural	6.6	187/2	95%	83%	172%	–	Before 6.3/ year After 1.2/ year	91%	–
Krasmik et al. [25]	81 ♂ 56 ♀	137/0	137/0	14.8	84/3	78%	62%	74%	–	Before 6.2 After 2.5	–	–
Castaño-Botero et al. [26]	95 ♂ 9 ♀	0/104	0/104	–	69/6	–	86%	–	91% <50 mL	Before 91% After 15%	88%	59%

This overview includes several multicentre studies (**) which include overlapping results with the reports of various single centre studies. Therefore, no accumulation of results is possible. (−), unreported data or incomplete data for calculation; *UTI* urinary tract infection

methods comprise intermittent catheterization, abdominal straining (Valsalva manoeuvre), abdominal compression (Credé manoeuvre), or suprapubic tapping for reflex contractions.

Continence is achieved in 57–100% of patients, and bladder capacity increased. However, continence is not only achieved by a dorsal rhizotomy. Results on continence also included additional treatments, like anticholinergics and stress incontinence surgery.

Overall, percentages of patients having urinary tract infections and frequency of urinary tract infections decrease after the Brindley procedure compared to preoperative treatment.

The Brindley stimulator is used for defecation in 29–100% of patients in different degrees. Not all patients achieve complete evacuation of defecation using only stimulation. Some patients need laxatives in addition to prevent constipation or enable defecation. Many patients only use the stimulator to get the defecation into the rectum, to enable digital evacuation.

Erections can be evoked in a substantial number of patients, but results vary considerably. This can be explained by the relatively low number of patients that actually use the stimulator to evoke erections for sexual intercourse (0–32%), due to qualitatively inadequate erections for sexual intercourse or deterioration of the stimulation effect over time.

Autonomic dysreflexia mostly decreased after the Brindley procedure as a result of the dorsal rhizotomy. Only a few studies reported stimulation-induced autonomic dysreflexia.

Current and Future Perspectives

The ultimate treatment of neurogenic disorders of the lower urinary tract would be resolvement of the neurogenic disorder that causes the bladder dysfunction to restore the innervations of the bladder. As long as this causal treatment is not available, symptomatic treatment options are required.

Intravesical botulinum toxin A injections are nowadays commonly used, mostly in combination with (intermittent) catheterization. However, the Brindley procedure has several advantages for suitable patients compared to Botulinum toxin A, especially if not only the urological properties of the treatments are taken into account. Spinal cord injury comprises a variety of coherent, physical problems. Therefore, management of multiple organ dysfunctions should be advocated. The Brindley procedure does not only enable continence and micturition but also complete defecation or improvement of defecation pattern, penile erections, and reduction of autonomic dysreflexia and spasms. Patients become less dependent because they do not need assistance for intermittent catheterization anymore and can empty their bladder wherever and whenever. When the treatment options are discussed with a patient, this more extensive application of the Brindley procedure should be mentioned.

The Brindley procedure generally shows good clinical results for restoration of function in spinal cord injury patients with multiple organ dysfunction, including bladder, bowel, and erectile dysfunction. Moreover, the Brindley procedure improves quality of life [24, 27]. However, it is not a procedure that is easy to apply in clinical practice. Firstly, not every patient is suited for the procedure, and the success depends on selection of appropriate patients. Prerequisites are a complete spinal cord lesion since neurostimulation can cause pain in incomplete spinal cord lesions, an intact sacral motor neuron pathway enabling stimulation of the bladder, and a detrusor muscle that is capable to contract on stimulation. Secondly, a dorsal rhizotomy and implantation of a Brindley stimulator is complex and not a routine procedure for urologists and should be reserved for specialized centres. Thirdly, the technique is also prone to failures, including the external and implanted components. Analysis of the external components is easy to apply. Currently, a straightforward solution for analysis and revision of the implanted system without major surgery is not available in every country. This can be explained by national legislation with respect to certain aspects of the surgical procedure for revision of the implant, like burning the insulation of the implanted electrode cables. This excludes these patients from the thorough analysis of the implanted components and revision surgery to restore function of their stimulator. Nowadays, most patients have become increasingly familiar with intermittent catheterization and bowel rinsing. They accept the dysfunction of the stimulator more frequently because they remain continent due to their dorsal rhizotomy in combination with controlled emptying of their bladder and bowels.

Main issues for patients who consider a Brindley procedure are the irreversibility of the rhizotomy and the possibility that future treatment options are not within reach anymore. Although SARS can restore penile erections after a rhizotomy, qualitative useful stimulation of erections is not possible in a substantial number of patients. Therefore, the dorsal rhizotomy should be replaced by a less invasive procedure to abolish detrusor overactivity. Continuous or conditional neuromodulation could be one of the solutions [28, 29]. Sacral posterior and anterior root stimulation combines neuromodulation and SARS without a rhizotomy of the dorsal roots for micturition. These new developments are, however, not generally introduced as a standard treatment. Sacral posterior and anterior root stimulation effectively suppress DO but do not result in complete emptying in all patients due to persisting detrusor-external sphincter dyssynergia [30]. This requires development of techniques that prevent backward stimulation when the anterior roots are stimulated to enable selective detrusor stimulation, like selective anodal block and high-frequency block [31–34].

Conclusion

The Brindley procedure consists of a stimulator for sacral anterior-root stimulation and a rhizotomy of the dorsal sacral roots to abolish neurogenic detrusor overactivity. Stimulation of the sacral anterior roots enables micturition, defecation, and erections. The Brindley procedure is suitable for a selected group of patients with complete spinal cord injury and detrusor overactivity. Overall, the Brindley procedure shows good clinical results and improves quality of life. However, to remain a valuable treatment option for the future, the technique needs some adequate changes to enable analysis of the implanted parts, to improve revision techniques of the implanted parts, and to abolish the sacral dorsal rhizotomy.

References

1. Weld KJ, Dmochowski RR. Association of level of injury and bladder behavior in patients with post-traumatic spinal cord injury. Urology. 2000;55(4):490–4.
2. Brindley GS. An implant to empty the bladder or close the urethra. J Neurol Neurosurg Psychiatry. 1977;40(4):358–69.
3. Sauerwein D. Surgical treatment of spastic bladder paralysis in paraplegic patients. Sacral deafferentation with implantation of a sacral anterior root stimulator. Urologe A. 1990;29(4):196–203.
4. Martens FMJ, Heesakkers JPFA. Clinical results of a brindley procedure: sacral anterior root stimulation in combination with a rhizotomy of the dorsal roots. Adv Urol. 2011. https://doi.org/10.1155/2011/709708.
5. Hohenfellner M, Pannek J, Bötel U, et al. Sacral bladder denervation for treatment of detrusor hyperreflexia and autonomic dysreflexia. Urology. 2001;58(1):28–32.
6. Van Kerrebroeck PEV, Koldewijn EL, Rosier PF, Wijkstra H, Debruyne FMJ. Results of the treatment of neurogenic bladder dysfunction in spinal cord injury by sacral posterior root rhizotomy and anterior sacral root stimulation. J Urol. 1996;155(4):1378–81.
7. Brindley GS, Polkey CE, Rushton DN, Cardozo L. Sacral anterior root stimulators for bladder control in paraplegia: the first 50 cases. J Neurol Neurosurg Psychiatry. 1986;49(10):1104–14.
8. The Finetech-Brindley bladder controller notes for surgeons and physicians. Revision 2002.
9. Bauchet L, Segnarbieux F, Martinazzo G, Frerebeau P, Ohanna F. Neurosurgical treatment of hyperactive bladder in spinal cord injury patients. La Neurochirurgie. 2001;47(1):13–24.
10. Brindley GS. The first 500 patients with sacral anterior root stimulator implants: general description. Paraplegia. 1994;32(12):795–805.
11. Creasey GH, Grill JH, Korsten M, et al. An implantable neuroprosthesis for restoring bladder and bowel control to patients with spinal cord injuries: a multicenter trial. Arch Phys Med Rehabil. 2001;82(11):1512–9.
12. Egon G, Barat M, Colombel P, Visentin C, Isambert JL, Guerin J. Implantation of anterior sacral root stimulators combined with posterior sacral rhizotomy in spinal injury patients. World J Urol. 1998;16(5):342–9.
13. Hamel O, Perrouin-Verbe B, Robert R. Brindley technique with intradural deafferentation and extradural implantation by a single sacral laminectomy. La Neurochirurgie. 2004;50(6):661–6.
14. Kutzenberger J, Domurath B, Sauerwein D. Spastic bladder and spinal cord injury: seventeen years of experience with sacral deafferentation and implantation of an anterior root stimulator. Artif Organs. 2005;29(3):239–41.

15. Macdonagh RP, Sun WM, Smallwood R, Forster D, Read NW. Control of defecation in patients with spinal injuries by stimulation of sacral anterior nerve roots. Br Med J. 1990;300(6738):1494–7.
16. Madersbacher H, Fischer J, Ebner A. Sacral root stimulator (Brindley): experiences especially in women with neurogenic urinary incontinence. Neurourol Urodyn. 1988;7(6):593–601.
17. Madersbacher H, Fischer J. Sacral anterior root stimulation: prerequisites and indications. Neurourol Urodyn. 1993;12(5):489–94.
18. Robinson LQ, Grant A, Weston P, Stephenson TP, Lucas M, Thomas DG. Experience with the Brindley anterior sacral root stimulator. Br J Urol. 1988;62(6):553–7.
19. Sarrias M, Sarrias F, Borau A. The "Barcelona" technique. Neurourol Urodyn. 1993;12(5):495–6.
20. Sauerwein D, Ingunza W, Fischer J, et al. Extradural implantation of sacral anterior root stimulators. J Neurol Neurosurg Psychiatry. 1990;53(8):681–4.
21. Schurch B, Rodic B, Jeanmonod D. Posterior sacral rhizotomy and intradural anterior sacral root stimulation for treatment of the spastic bladder in spinal cord injured patients. J Urol. 1997;157(2):610–4.
22. van der Aa HE, Alleman E, Nene A, Snoek G. Sacral anterior root stimulation for bladder control: clinical results. Arch Physiol Biochem. 1999;107(3):248–56.
23. Van Kerrebroeck PE, Koldewijn EL, Debruyne FM. Worldwide experience with the Finetech-Brindley sacral anterior root stimulator. Neurourol Urodyn. 1993;12(5):497–503.
24. Vastenholt JM, Snoek GJ, Buschman HPJ, Van Der Aa HE, Alleman ERJ, Ijzerman MJ. A 7-year follow-up of sacral anterior root stimulation for bladder control in patients with a spinal cord injury: quality of life and users' experiences. Spinal Cord. 2003;41(7):397–402.
25. Krasmik D, Krebs J, Van Ophoven A, Pannek J. Urodynamic results, clinical efficacy, and complication rates of sacral intradural deafferentation and sacral anterior root stimulation in patients with neurogenic lower urinary tract dysfunction resulting from complete spinal cord injury. Neurourol Urodyn. 2014;33:1202–6.
26. Castaño-Botero JC, et al. Extradural implantation of sacral anterior root stimulator in spinal cord injury patients. Neurourol Urodyn. 2016;35:970–4.
27. Martens FM, den Hollander PP, Snoek GJ, Koldewijn EL, van Kerrebroeck PE, Heesakkers JP. Quality of life in complete spinal cord injury patients with a Brindley bladder stimulator compared to a matched control group. Neurourol Urodyn. 2011;30(4):551–5.
28. Hansen J, Media S, Nøhr M, Biering-Sørensen F, Sinkjaer T, Rijkhoff NJM. Treatment of neurogenic detrusor overactivity in spinal cord injured patients by conditional electrical stimulation. J Urol. 2005;173(6):2035–9.
29. Kirkham APS, Shah NC, Knight SL, Shah PJR, Craggs MD. The acute effects of continuous and conditional neuromodulation on the bladder in spinal cord injury. Spinal Cord. 2001;39(8):420–8.
30. Kirkham APS, Knight SL, Craggs MD, Casey ATM, Shah PJR. Neuromodulation through sacral nerve roots 2 to 4 with a Finetech-Brindley sacral posterior and anterior root stimulator. Spinal Cord. 2002;40(6):272–81.
31. Boger A, Bhadra N, Gustafson KJ. Bladder voiding by combined high frequency electrical pudendal nerve block and sacral root stimulation. Neurourol Urodyn. 2008;27(5):435–9.
32. Brindley GS, Craggs MD. A technique for anodally blocking large nerve fibres through chronically implanted electrodes. J Neurol Neurosurg Psychiatry. 1980;43(12):1083–90.
33. Rijkhoff NJ, Wijkstra H, Van Kerrebroeck PE, Debruyne FM. Selective detrusor activation by electrical sacral nerve root stimulation in spinal cord injury. J Urol. 1997;157(4):1504–8.
34. Seif C, Braun PM, Bross S, et al. Selective block of urethral sphincter contraction using a modified brindley electrode in sacral anterior root stimulation of the dog. Neurourol Urodyn. 2002;21(5):502–10.

Neuromodulation in Neurourology

Paholo G. Barboglio Romo and Priyanka Gupta

Introduction

Neuromodulation is a minimally invasive intervention that is widely used as a third-line therapy to address refractory overactive bladder symptoms and non-neurogenic urinary retention. Contemporary research has focused on improving surgical technique and outcomes and enhancing its potential therapeutic effect by exploring new applications in other groups of patients suffering from overactive bladder, urinary retention, and pain, including patients with neurologic disease.

Neurogenic patients encompass a wide spectrum of disease processes which can alter bladder and bowel function depending on the location of the neurologic lesion. Neurologic disorders affect both storage and voiding functions. Management of neurogenic lower urinary tract dysfunction can involve a combination of several treatment modalities including behavioral modification, intermittent catheterization, indwelling catheterization, medical therapy, botulinum toxin injection, bladder augmentation, urinary diversion, and neuromodulation.

In this chapter the mechanism of action of sacral and peripheral neuromodulation, the operative technique, and its use in the neurogenic population is explored.

P. G. Barboglio Romo · P. Gupta (✉)
Division of Neurourology and Pelvic Reconstruction, Department of Urology,
University of Michigan, Ann Arbor, MI, USA
e-mail: guptapr@med.umich.edu

© Springer International Publishing AG, part of Springer Nature 2018
R. Dmochowski, J. Heesakkers (eds.), *Neuro-Urology*,
https://doi.org/10.1007/978-3-319-90997-4_25

History of Neuromodulation and Mechanism of Action

The application of electrical stimulation to address bladder dysfunction was first described in 1878 by Saxtorph and almost a century later [1] in the 1970s by Tanagho and Schmidt who presented significant advances in this field using canine models [2]. They performed a dorsal rhizotomy and selective ventral neurotomy in dog models. They then performed sacral nerve stimulation using an electrical implant which led to autonomic efferent activation and subsequent restoration of normal bladder emptying. It was determined that the S3 nerve was responsible for innervation to the bladder, pelvic floor muscles, and external urethral sphincter [3, 4]. This study was the pillar for the development of the "bladder pacemaker" that could simultaneously generate and modulate detrusor, pelvic floor, and urethral sphincter contraction [2].

The first implantable neuroprosthesis (Pisces Quad foramen electrode) was developed by Medtronic (Minneapolis, MN) during a multicenter phase II trial. Dissection and division of the lumbodorsal fascia and paraspinous musculature through a paraspinal incision was necessary to place the needle into the S3 foramen. The electrode was then sutured to the posterior sacral periosteum and tunneled to the generator which was implanted into the abdominal wall. The results from the US study showed complete symptom improvement in 6/12 patients who had permanent implantation. The European results showed greater than 50% symptom improvement in 19/23 patients. The results led to the FDA approval of the device for urge incontinence in 1997 [5].

The mechanism of action of how neuromodulation precisely works is not completely understood and involves multiple neural pathways that lead to responses in the bladder, gastrointestinal system, and pelvic floor. Sacral neuromodulation (SNM) is thought to activate efferent fibers to the genitourinary tract and afferent spinal pathways to the pontine micturition center. It may also involve local sacral reflexes [6]. Two main principles are widely accepted to support the effect of SNM: (1) direct activation of efferent fibers to the striated urethral sphincter triggers inhibition of detrusor contraction, and (2) selective activation of afferent fibers causes inhibition of intraspinal and supraspinal signals for micturition.

Neuromodulation can be performed via the sacral nerve or peripherally via the posterior tibial nerve. We will review the operative technique for both approaches, the outcomes, and the adverse events associated with each technique.

Sacral Neuromodulation

This is a technique via which the S3 nerve is percutaneously targeted via a tined electrode that is placed through the S3 foramen. Currently there is one device on the market that has been FDA approved for the treatment of nonobstructive urinary retention and overactive bladder in 1997 and fecal incontinence in 2011 (InterStim®, Medtronic Inc., Minneapolis, MN).

Sacral Neuromodulation Operative Technique

This procedure is performed via a two-stage process. The first stage can be performed as an office-based procedure called a percutaneous nerve evaluation (PNE) or in the operating room as a first-stage lead placement (FSLP). Both methods allow the patient to test the clinical effectiveness of the stimulation prior to having the full device and battery implanted. We will review the operative steps for a PNE, FSLP, and stage II implantation.

Percutaneous Nerve Evaluation (PNE) [7]
1. Position the patient prone.
2. Identify the S3 foramen using anatomic landmarks.
3. Inject a local anesthetic at the needle insertion point.
4. Insert the needle at a 30–60° angle.
5. Confirm lead placement by asking the patient to report the location of the sensation of stimulation. Stimulation should be felt in the vaginal, scrotal, or rectal area. They may exhibit flexion of the big toe.
6. A temporary electrode is passed through the needle and taped to the skin.
7. Repeat on the opposite side.
8. Connect the lead to an external temporary pulse generator for 3–7 days while completing voiding diaries and symptom scores.

First-Stage Lead Placement (FSLP) [7]
1. Position the patient prone.
2. Intravenous sedation is administered.
3. With the assistance of fluoroscopy, a directional guidewire is used to locate the midline which is marked with a vertical line. The intersection of the sacroiliac joint and the spinous process is then identified and marked with a transverse line. This defines the area of the S3 foramen (Fig. 1).
4. If the S3 foramen is clearly visible on fluoroscopy in the anterior/posterior view, then mark the upper medial aspect of the foramen (Fig. 2).
5. If the S3 foramen is not identified due to overlying bowel contents, then start approximately 2 cm lateral and 3 cm superior to the point where the two lines cross (see step #3). Mark this on the right and left sides (Fig. 2).
6. Pass the needle at a 60° angle into the entrance point to access the foramen, and advance it to the edge of the inferior sacral bone plate (Fig. 3).
7. Perform electrical stimulation. The ideal response is a bellow contraction of the pelvic floor followed by flexion of the great toe that occurs with less than 2 V of stimulation. A S2 stimulation would be suggested by plantar flexion of the entire foot with heel rotation, and a S4 stimulation would result in a bellow contraction alone.

8. Fluoroscopy with motor response can help confirm the appropriate foramen. In Fig. 7, imaging first shows the skin location to be too high, then too low, and then just right. On the lateral view, the target area should be about 1 cm above the S3 hillock. The hillock is the anterior protrusion of the bone from the anterior surface of the sacrum at the level of S3 as seen on the lateral X-ray (Fig. 4).

9. The directional guidewire is then placed through the cannula, and the tract is dilated using an introducer sheath. The introducer should not be advanced beyond the inferior bone plate.

10. The tined lead with the curved stylet positioned inferior and lateral is then deployed under fluoroscopic guidance. It has four cylindrical electrodes numbered 0 to 3. Leads 2 and 3 should straddle the bone edge. Each electrode is then stimulated individually. The motor responses are assessed with the goal to achieve response on all four electrodes under low voltage (ideally less than 2 V).

11. Lead position is confirmed with fluoroscopy in the lateral and anterior–posterior positions (Figs. 5 and 6).

12. The potential site of the IPG is identified on the ipsilateral buttock, and a 1 cm incision is made and a subcutaneous pocket created. The IPG will be placed here if the test stage is successful.

13. The percutaneous extension lead is connected to the tined lead, which is tunneled out of the contralateral buttock and connected to the external neuromodulation system (ENS) and programming parameters are set.

14. The incision is closed and the external portions of the leads are secured with sterile 4 × 4 dressings and a bandage.

15. Using the ENS, the patient trials various stimulation parameters during the 7–14-day test period and maintains voiding diaries and symptom scores to assess improvement.

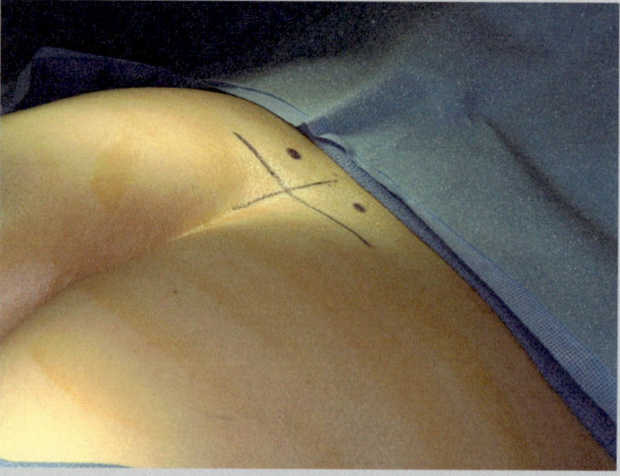

Fig. 1 FSLP landmarks identified

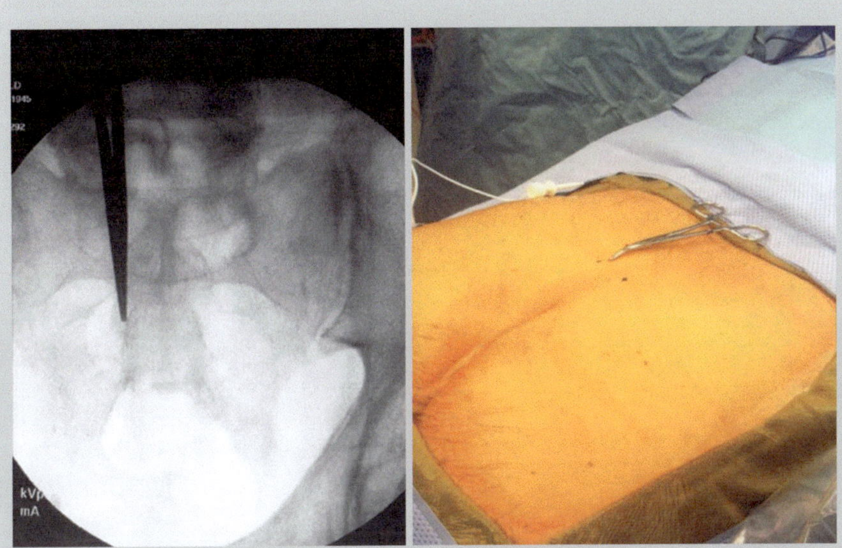

Fig. 2 Marking medial edge of S3 foramen

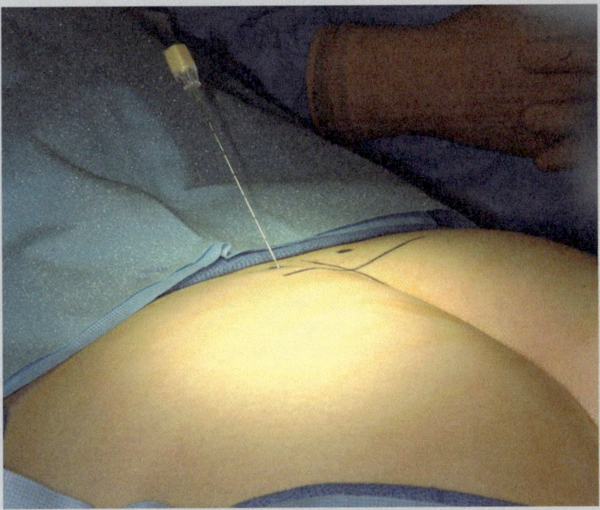

Fig. 3 Needle placement for SNM

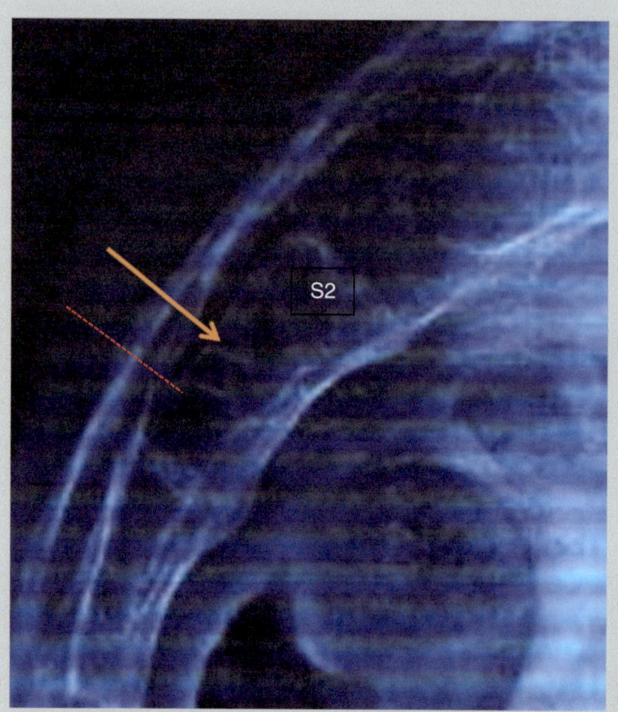

Fig. 4 Determining ideal lateral location

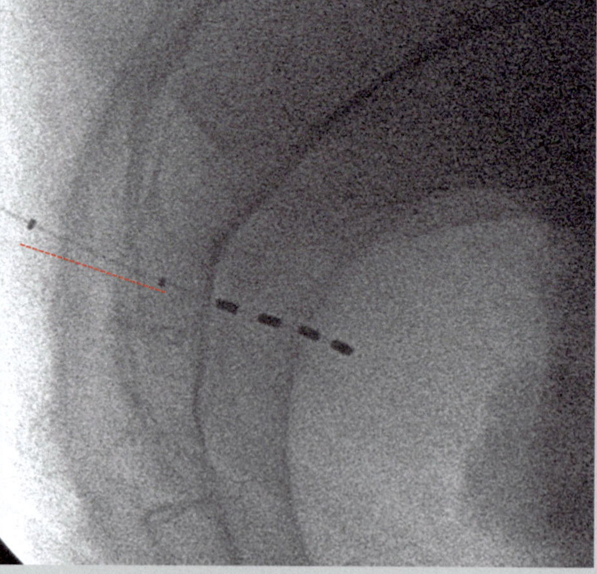

Fig. 5 Ideal lateral X-ray

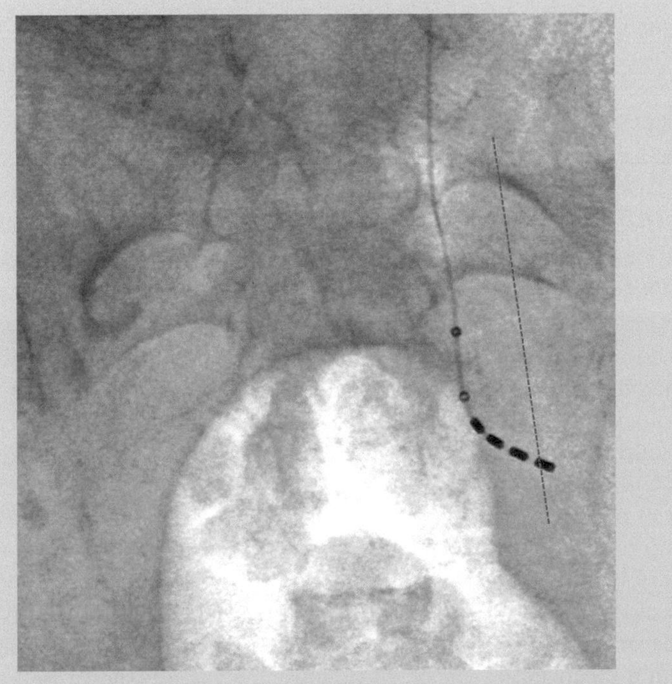

Fig. 6 Ideal anterior–posterior X-ray

Second-Stage Placement of Permanent Implantable Pulse Generator (IPG) [7]
1. Patients experiencing a greater than 50% improvement in their symptoms are considered responders and should undergo a stage II implant.
2. The previous pocket site is reopened and the incision is enlarged. The lead is then connected to the permanent IPG.
3. The device connections are tested and confirmed in the operating room. The pocket incision is closed with absorbable sutures.
4. Specific stimulation programs are tested and then programmed into the device postoperatively to achieve optimal device settings.

Sacral Neuromodulation Outcomes

In the United States, SNM is approved for the treatment of refractory overactive bladder and nonobstructive urinary retention and recommended by the American Urological Association as a third-line therapy in selected patients who have failed

Table 1 Meta-analysis urinary outcomes from SNM in neurogenic bladder

Success rates for specific urinary outcomes [9]		
	Testing phase	Last follow-up
Urinary retention	56% (67/119)	73% (65/89)
Urgency incontinence	60% (46/77)	74% (62/84)
Urinary frequency	75% (6/8)	86% (12/14)

prior behavioral (first) and or drug (second) treatments, or when patients are not candidates for second-line therapy and are willing to undergo a surgical procedure [8].

In the late 1990s this therapy was expanded to the treatment of neurogenic urinary tract symptoms. However, the data supporting the use of SNM for neurogenic bladder is weak and limited to small and heterogeneous studies. This population is particularly difficult to investigate as neurogenic bladder encompasses a wide variety of neurologic etiologies with differing symptom profiles. The literature includes largely retrospective data that assesses heterogeneous populations and different outcomes and is limited to few neurologic ailments.

A meta-analysis published in 2010 reported on combined data from 26 trials with a mean follow-up of 26 months. Only six of the included trials were prospective studies, and half of these had a very small sample size of less than ten patients [9]. The overall success (pooled) rate was 68% in 256 and 92% in 224 patients with neurologic lower urinary tract disease during the test and implantation phases, respectively, with a mean follow-up of 26 months. Results are shown in Table 1 below for specific urinary outcomes.

Analysis of outcomes during both testing and permanent phases suggested a stable and improved success with SNM therapy over time with the caveat of patient drop-off over time during the testing period compared to permanent implantation. More contemporary prospective studies not included in the prior meta-analysis have reported durable and favorable outcomes in frequency, urgency, and urgency incontinence episodes as described in Table 2.

Peters et al. reported outcomes from 71 patients with neurogenic bladder during 2004–2012 with a rate of 89% (63/71) for permanent implantation in those with more than 50% clinical improvement. Outcomes were compared to a cohort of non-neurogenic patients. Stroke, MS, and Parkinson's disease represented the most common etiologies. Objective outcomes were measured using 3-day voiding diary. There was a statistically significant improvement in urinary frequency and urgency at 3, 6, 12, and 24 months. Urinary incontinence episodes improved during the first 12 months but not at 24 months in the neurogenic group when compared to baseline. Validated questionnaire data showed improvement in the non-neurogenic patients and mixed results in the neurogenic group [10].

In 2016 a smaller sample study reported very favorable short-term outcomes in patients with incomplete spinal cord injury (SCI). Complete continence rates in 80% (21/26) on voiding diary and up to 40% of patients were able to stop anticholinergic treatment at 6 months after implantation. The same study also evaluated 11

Table 2 Urinary symptom outcomes from SNM in patients with neurogenic bladder

Author	Etiology	Success test (phase I)	Follow-up	Urinary retention (CIC) Mean baseline—postop, improvement (%)	Urinary frequency Mean baseline—postop, improvement (50%)	Urinary incontinence Mean baseline—postop, improvement (50%)
Wallace 2007 [15]	Various	$N = 28/33$ (85%)	12	3.8–1.6 ± 1.9 ($p < 0.02$) $N = 8/16$ (50%)	10.5–6 ± 1.4 ($p < 0.0001$)	4–1.3 ± 2.4 ($p < 0.0001$)
Daniels 2010 [16]	DM	$N = 26/32$ (81%)	29	$N = 6/9$ (66.7%)	$N = 12/14$ (85.7%)	$N = 18/26$ (69.2%)
Marinkovic 2010 [17]	MS	$N = 12/14$ (86%)	52	$N = 12/14$ (86%)	NA	NA
Chabaane 2011 [12]	Various	$N = 41/62$ (66%)	52	$N = 28/37$ (76%)	NA	NA
Minardi 2011 [18]	MS	$N = 15/25$ (60%)	49	3.3 ± 1.3–1.2 ± 0.7 ($N = 9$)	17.7 ± 3.5–9 ± 0 ($N = 6$)	13 ± 2.6–3.3 ± 31 ($N = 6$)
Peters 2013 [10]	Various	$N = 63/71$ (88.7%)	24	NA	11.6 ± 4.1–10.2 ± 3.9 ($p = 0.02$)	6.7 ± 5.3–5.5 ± 4.8 ($p = 0.06$)
Lombardi 2013 [19]	SCI (incomp)	$N = 36/85$ (42%)	61	$N = 13/13$ (100%)	13.5 ± 2.1–7.4 ± 0.9 ($p < 0.05$)	$2.5 \pm \underline{0}.19$–0.7 ± 0.8 ($p < 0.05$)
Wollner 2016 [11]	Various	$N = 35/50$ (70%)	16	NA	9.9 ± 4.2–5.7 ± 1.5 ($p < 0.05$)	NA

highly functional SCI patients with urinary retention and found that all subjects were able to void spontaneously after device implantation [11].

Another study from 2011 assessed neurogenic bladder outcomes in 62 patients with neurogenic detrusor overactivity (NDO) (34) and urinary retention (28) secondary to a variety of neurologic diseases. They reported a significant improvement in urinary urgency, frequency, and incontinence episodes via 3-day voiding diary data (mean test duration 17 ± 10 days). The testing phase was successful in 41 (66%), and 37 underwent an implant, of which 28/37 (76%) reported a persistent improvement after 4 years. Subgroup analysis suggested that patients with peripheral neuropathy responded better than those with Parkinson's disease. The authors comment that half of the patients with a loss of efficacy had MS and recommended that SNM only be considered in MS patients with relapsing–remitting disease who have not had a relapse for 2 years [12].

Spinelli and Chartier's groups reported on their prospective study and found improvement in both incomplete emptying (up to 66% not doing CIC at 6 months) [13] and overactive urinary symptoms (over 50% improvement in all patients and 5/9 were dry) [14]. Other clinical studies with small sample sizes have followed; however, in the last 30 years, there has not been a large sample trial that has been able to provide level one data for the efficacy of SNM in neurogenic patients.

Future individualization of neurologic diseases and analysis of more specific groups are needed to allow us to understand who will benefit from neuromodulation.

Multiple Sclerosis

Multiple sclerosis is a progressive neurologic disorder that is classified into four major subtypes depending on evolution timeline of the disease, the stage of neurologic impairment, and the location of the neurologic lesions. Bladder symptoms affect up to 80% of patients with MS and are usually associated with spinal lesions and correlated with symptoms affecting lower extremities. Urinary symptoms can oscillate from overactive bladder dry or wet symptoms to incomplete emptying [20].

Bosch and Groen were one of the pioneers in this field investigating stable and slow progressive MS patients. In 1996 they reported more than 50% improvement in urinary incontinence episodes in 4/5 patients with SNM [21]. Success test phase rates are comparable to nonspecific neurogenic bladder outcomes and oscillate from 50 to 84% [9, 12, 18]. Based on limited available data, patients with stable relapsing–remitting MS disease and overactive bladder symptoms appear to be the ideal candidates for this therapy [9].

Data on urinary retention is controversial. Marinkovic and Gillen retrospectively studied a group of 14 patients with MS and reported an 86% success rate for urinary retention in 12/14 subjects after a mean follow-up of 9 years. All patients were doing CIC before SNM and success was defined as no use of catheter afterward. Mean postoperative post-void residual was well below 100 mL. Those with successful outcomes were ambulatory compared to the two patients who did not improve and were wheelchair-bound at baseline. Interestingly, the authors reported only 40% underwent battery replacement despite the long follow-up period of this study [17]. A study by Minardi on 25 patients with a mean follow-up of 4 years showed that 10/25 patients did not pass testing phase and all 10 had urinary retention. Although the number of clean intermittent catheterization significantly decreased from 3 to 1, only 1/9 patients who were originally doing CIC were able to void without the need of CIC. Authors also reported improvement in urinary incontinence and increase in both number of voids and voided volume despite the presence of detrusor sphincter deficiency [18].

It is important to consider the implications of disease progression when considering SNM since this has been reported to range from 16 to 33% [9]. Initial symptoms of urinary urgency and frequency may progress to incontinence and ultimately evolve into urinary retention, and SNM may no longer provide the expected goal. Counseling about the potential need for clean intermittent catheterization and possible future hand dexterity impairment is fundamental. The need for future MRI should be cleared with the neurologist prior to proceeding with SNM.

Spinal Cord Injury

Urinary symptoms from SCI depend on the lesion level, the ASIA classification, and more recently even the timing of the injury. Available data is compromised by heterogeneous groups with complete and incomplete lesions and different SCI levels. Overall success ranges 29–40% in the testing phase and 58–80% in the permanent phase [9].

Meta-analysis results from Kessler and colleagues showed a test phase success rate of 35% depending on ASIA classification. Success rates were 29% for incomplete, 40% for complete, and 44% for undetermined types. Authors reported on relatively lower outcomes (77%) in those who underwent permanent implant when compared to overall neurogenic bladder population (92%). Those with complete SCI had the most benefit from SNM with 83% improvement [9, 11].

Lombardi and colleagues performed a retrospective review on 13 patients with urinary retention, 11 of whom had incontinence. Outcomes were evaluated with voiding diaries and urodynamics, and median follow-up was 61 months. Patients with urinary retention had over 50% decrease in mean number of CIC episodes per day from 3.7 ± 1 to 0.6 ± 0.7 at first postop check and 0.7 ± 0.8 at last follow-up [22]. The same group reported their updated results in 2014 showing a moderate success rate of 42% after testing 85 high-functioning patients with nonobstructive retention (73% traumatic, 25% myelitis, 3% vascular). Patients who experienced sensation during urodynamic on filling phase were more likely to have a positive testing response ($p < 0.05$). In 11/34 (32%) patients with inconsistent improvement, a contralateral lead was implanted. Subsequently the authors placed a lead in the S4 foramen on two subjects who failed prior contralateral placement. After reimplantation patients had improvement on both subjective and objective (urodynamics) parameters. Most of the failures occurred after 3 years, and the cause of failure was often not known, with displacement of the lead representing a minority of cases. The author postulated "nerve fatigue" as a possible source of failure since all subjects who failed their initial implants achieved improvement of symptoms with a new contralateral implant [19].

Recent data supported by Medtronic (Minneapolis, MN) have reported promising results with early use of SNM in patients with complete SCI. Sievert and colleagues were able to prevent the development of NDO and reported a low-pressure acontractile bladder with no evidence of incontinence with the use of early SNM. Subjects had ASIA T2-11 injury and underwent bilateral two electrode lead placement within 4.5 months of the initial injury compared to a similar SCI control group. No individuals in the SNM group developed NDO on urodynamics, poor compliance with detrusor pressures over 30 cmH_2O, or urinary incontinence. Additionally, the SNM group demonstrated decreased infection rates, better quality of life, and improved erectile and bowel function [23]. This study was supported by the stimulator manufacturer, and these results have not been yet reproduced. Due to the success of this study, a multicenter trial is underway to assess the role of SNM in the acute phase of complete SCI [24].

Other Neurologic Diseases

A retrospective review compared the role of SNM in 32 patients undergoing spinal surgery (various levels) mostly performed to address compressive disc disease with 102 non-neurogenic controls. Successful test phase was 63% after spinal surgery compared to 75% in the control group. Sub-analysis of urinary symptoms showed that neurogenic bladder was associated with lower implantation rate when assessing urgency incontinence 60% vs. 90%. There was no difference when assessing explantation rates [25].

Daniels and colleagues studied 32 patients with neurogenic lower urinary tract symptoms from diabetes mellitus and compared them to 211 non-neurogenic and nondiabetic patients. They reported favorable long-term success in the neurogenic patients that was comparable to the controls. There was no difference in the explant rate 38% (9/24) in diabetic versus 26% (36/141) in non-DM ($P = 0.224$) patients. However, when examining the reason for explantation, infectious etiology was higher in diabetic patients (16.7%) compared to nondiabetic patients (4.3%; $P = 0.018$) [16].

Data on cerebral palsy is scarce with mostly few case reports suggesting a high rate for successful test phase as well as good implant results. Since these results are based on limited and very well-selected cases, we caution not to generalize these outcomes and counsel appropriately [10, 12, 26].

Table 3 Adverse events associated with SNM implantation in patients with neurogenic bladder

Study	N	Follow-up (months)	Revision surgery	Battery replacement	Infection	Explant
Wallace 2007 [15]	28/33	12	NR	NR	NR	(3/28) 11%
Daniels 2010 [16]	24/32	29	NR	(1/24) 4%	(4/24) 17%	(9/24) 37.5%
Marinkovic 2010 [17]	12/14	52	NR	(5/12) 40%	NR	NR
Chabaane 2011 [12]	28/37	52	(8/37) 22%	(2/37) 5%	(2/37) 5%	NR
Minardi 2011 [18]	5/25	49	0	NR	NR	NR
Lombardi 2013 [19]	24/24	61	(5/24) 21%	(4/24) 17%	(1/24) 4%	NR
Peters 2013 [10]	63	24	(5/63) 8%	NR	(1/63)1.6%	(6/63) 9.5%
Wollner 2015 [11]	35/50	16	(6/35) 17%	NR	(2/35) 5.7%	(2/35) 5.7%

Adverse Events

Adverse events after SNM are infrequent but these are not rare (Table 3). Meta-analysis showed a pooled complication rate of zero and 24% for the test and the implantation phases which corresponded to 69 patients who reported at least one adverse event. Lead migration (15/224), pain at the site of the implanted permanent generator (12/224), and infection at the site of implantation (11/224) were the most common complications. Explantation of both the lead and permanent device was performed in 25/224 and the lead only in 8/224 [9]. Peters reported similar adverse event rates for neurogenic and non-neurogenic patients in his trial of 11%, lead revision in 8%, and explantation in 10% [10]. In the presence of DM, the infection and explant rate can increase up to 38% [16].

Neurogenic Bowel Outcomes

Neuromodulation was also introduced for the treatment of idiopathic fecal incontinence in 1995 [27]. The operative technique is the same as for urinary symptoms with electrode placement through the S3 sacral foramina. A 50% improvement in fecal incontinence episodes is accepted as a successful outcome. Stimulation parameters are adopted from urinary treatment data (pulse with of 210 μs, a frequency of 15 Hz, and the amplitude set individually usually in the range between 0.1 and 10 V) [28]. This is another area of interest in neurogenic patients.

Small sample studies have shown an improvement in fecal incontinence ranging from 60 to 92% in patients with incomplete SCI [28]. The effects of SNM on

Table 4 Bowel symptom outcomes from SNM in patients with neurogenic bowel

Study	Mean age	Follow-up (months)	Etiology	Fecal incontinence improvement	Constipation
Ganio 2001 [29]	10	19	Various	$N = 6/10$ (60%)	NA
Rosen 2001 [30]	15	15	Various	$N = 11/15$ (73%)	NA
Jarret 2005 [31]	13	12	Various	$N = 12/13$ (92%)	NA
Holzer 2007 [32]	25	12	Various	$N = 18/25$ (72%)	NA
Gstaltner 2008 [33]	11	12	Cauda equina	$N = 8/11$ (73%)	NA
Lombardi 2009 [22]	23	38	SCI	$N = 11/11$ (100%)	$N = 12/12$ (100%)

anorectal physiology in patients with neurogenic bladder are still controversial, and it remains unclear who is the ideal candidate for this therapy. Table 4 displays the success outcomes after SNM in the neurogenic setting.

Holzer and colleagues performed a retrospective review of 36 patients with neurogenic bladder, of which 29 (81%) underwent a permanent implant with a median follow-up of 35 (range 3–71) months. Etiologies of neurogenic bladder were complications after surgical intervention to address spinal stenosis, spinal protrusion, or spinal trauma [32]. Significant continence improvement was seen in 28/29 subjects. Incontinence to solid or liquid stool decreased from a median of 7 (range 4–15) to 2 (range 0–5) episodes in 21 days ($P = 0.002$). Saline retention time increased from a median of 2 (range 0–5) to 7 (range 2–15) min ($P = 0.002$). Maximum resting and squeeze anal canal pressures increased compared with preoperative values. Significant improvement in quality of life was noted among all patients with permanent implant which remained at 2 years of follow-up [32].

Myelomeningocele can result in both fecal and urinary disorders. Ten myelomeningocele patients underwent SNM, and 3/10 reported over 50% improvement during a 3-week testing period and went onto permanent implantation. The authors commented that peripheral stimulation of the nerve was not possible in two candidates during testing (phase I) and in one patient during permanent placement (phase II) [34].

The potential benefit from SNM may be when utilized early after SCI as suggested by Sievert study previously described where improvement in bowel symptoms was also reported. It is important to avoid significant colonic distension to preserve integrity of colon anatomy at the time of early SNM after SCI to preserve overall gastrointestinal and colonic function.

Posterior Tibial Nerve Stimulation (PTNS) [7]

PTNS is an alternative neuromodulation modality for patients who are not interested in direct sacral lead placement or who may not be good candidates for SNM. American Urological Association Guidelines support the use of PTNS as a third-line therapy to address overactive bladder symptoms.

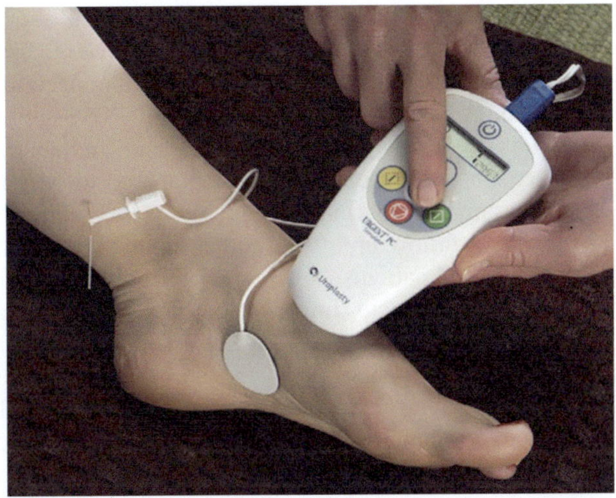

Fig. 7 Posterior tibial nerve stimulation (picture obtained from Kenneth Peters, MD)

PTNS Operative Technique

This procedure is performed in the office or ambulatory setting and requires no anesthesia; it has been previously described and consists of placing a 34-gauge needle about three fingerbreadths above the medial malleolus. The depth may need to be adjusted based on the patient's response and patient's subcutaneous tissue. The device is turned on and amplitude is titrated to patient's sensation (tingling sensation in ankle, foot, or toes) or motor stimulation (great toe flexion and/or fanning or plantar toe flexion of toes 2 through 5) as illustrated in Fig. 7. Once this is achieved, the stimulation session is delivered for 30 min [35].

PTNS Outcomes

Literature supporting PTNS is also limited by few numbers of studies, small sample size, retrospective type, variable neurologic etiologies, and heterogeneous outcomes. A meta-analysis was performed to assess the outcomes of PTNS for urinary symptoms, and there were three studies that evaluated neurogenic bladder of the total 32 included. Outcomes in neurogenic bladder ranged from 40 to 100% and varied among different neurologic diseases [36].

Kabay's group has particularly investigated PTNS outcomes in patients with MS and Parkinson's disease after 12 consecutive weeks. There was improvement in delaying NDO (124 ± 38 to 217.5 ± 66 mL; $p < 0.001$) and increased cystometric capacity (200 ± 29 to 267 ± 37 mL; $p < 0.0001$) in MS patients [37], and similar results were found in those with Parkinson's disease [38]. Another study reported on 3 months' outcomes after weekly PTNS on 70 patients with refractory urinary symptoms who had improvement in urinary urgency (83%); half of the patients had complete resolution of urgency. There were 62% patients who reported significant improvement in incontinence, and 45% had complete resolution of incontinence [39].

Relatively strong data is available from a small sample randomized control trial of neurogenic patients after ischemic cerebrovascular event. Twenty-four subjects without prior urinary symptoms were randomized to PTNS twice weekly for 6 weeks or general advice (control group). PTNS showed improvement in urinary symptoms, reducing urinary urgency and frequency, and reported subjective improvement after treatment when compared to baseline. When compared to the control group, only urinary frequency was superior. This effect persisted after 12 months of follow-up [40]. Another randomized control trial analyzed the effect of PTNS in SCI patients. A hundred patients with complete SCI were randomized to PTNS or solifenacin. Improvement in all bladder diary parameters was statistically significant in both groups at 2 and 4 weeks ($p < 0.05$), and there was no difference between the two groups. The authors commented that PTNS was not associated with any adverse events, whereas 5% of patients complained of side effects in the solifenacin group which led to withdrawal of two subjects [41].

PTNS therapy is contraindicated in patients with pacemakers, implantable defibrillators, or coagulopathy or who are pregnant [35]. PTNS therapy is well tolerated with minimal side effects. The main disadvantage is the time associated with weekly ambulatory sessions. It has shown to be promising in neurogenic patients, but more research is needed to better understand its efficacy for various neurologic disorders.

In summary, data suggests that PTNS can improve neurogenic bladder symptoms in the ambulatory setting after 3 months of therapy with a minimal risk profile.

References

1. Madersbacher H. Konservative Therapie der neurogenen Blasendysfunctktion. Urologe. 1999;38:24–9.
2. Tanagho EA, Schmidt RA, Orvis BRNeural stimulation for control of voiding dysfunction: a preliminary report in 22 patients with serious neuropathic voiding disorders. J Urol [Internet]. 1989;142(2 Pt 1):340–5. http://www.ncbi.nlm.nih.gov/pubmed/2787411.
3. Bross S, Braun ÆPM, Weiß ÆJ, Martinez FJ, Thomas PÆ, Seif C, et al. The role of the carbachol test and concomitant diseases in patients with nonobstructive urinary retention undergoing sacral neuromodulation. World J Urol. 2003:346–9.
4. Fisch M, Wammack R, Hohenfellner R. The sigma rectum pouch (Mainz pouch II). World J Urol [Internet]. 1996 [cited 2016 Feb 12];14(2):68–72. http://www.ncbi.nlm.nih.gov/pubmed/8731120.
5. Dijkema HE, Weil EH, Mijs PT, Janknegt RA. Neuromodulation of sacral nerves for incontinence and voiding dysfunctions. Clinical results and complications. Eur Urol [Internet]. 1993;24(1):72–6. http://www.ncbi.nlm.nih.gov/pubmed/8396034.
6. Groat WC De Griffiths D, Yoshimura N. Neural control of the lower urinary tract. Compr Physiol [Internet]. 2015;5(1):327–96. http://www.ncbi.nlm.nih.gov/pmc/articles/PMC4480926/pdf/nihms697977.pdf.
7. Bartley JM, Killinger KA, Boura JA, Gupta P, Gaines N, Gilleran JP, et al. The impact of prior back surgery on neuromodulation outcomes: a review of over 500 patients. Neurourol Urodyn. 2017;36(6):1535–42.

8. Appell RA, Dmochowski RR, Blaivas JM, Gormley EA, Karram MM, Juma S, et al. Guideline for the surgical management of female stress urinary incontinence: 2009 update. AUA Guidel. 2009;799.
9. Kessler TM, La Framboise D, Trelle S, Fowler CJ, Kiss G, Pannek J, et al. Sacral neuromodulation for neurogenic lower urinary tract dysfunction: systematic review and meta-analysis. Eur Urol. 2010;58(6):865–74.
10. Peters KM, Kandagatla P, Killinger KA, Wolfert C, Boura JA. Clinical outcomes of sacral neuromodulation in patients with neurologic conditions. Urology [Internet]. 2013;81(4):738–43. https://doi.org/10.1016/j.urology.2012.11.073.
11. Wöllner J, Krebs J, Pannek J. Sacral neuromodulation in patients with neurogenic lower urinary tract dysfunction. Spinal Cord [Internet]. 2016;54(2):137–40. http://www.ncbi.nlm.nih.gov/pubmed/26215913.
12. Chaabane W, Guillotreau J, Castel-Lacanal E, Abu-Anz S, De Boissezon X, Malavaud B, et al. Sacral neuromodulation for treating neurogenic bladder dysfunction: clinical and urodynamic study. Neurourol Urodyn [Internet]. 2011;30(4):547–50. http://www.ncbi.nlm.nih.gov/pubmed/21488095.
13. Spinelli M, Bertapelle P, Cappellano F, Zanollo A, Carone R, Catanzaro F, et al. Chronic sacral neuromodulation in patients with lower urinary tract symptoms: results from a national register. J Urol. 2001;166(2):541–5.
14. Chartier-Kastler EJ, Ruud Bosch JL, Perrigot M, Chancellor MB, Richard F, Denys P. Long-term results of sacral nerve stimulation (S3) for the treatment of neurogenic refractory urge incontinence related to detrusor hyperreflexia. J Urol. 2000;164(5):1476–80.
15. Wallace PA, Lane FL, Noblett KL. Sacral nerve neuromodulation in patients with underlying neurologic disease. Am J Obstet Gynecol [Internet]. 2007;197(1):96.e1–5. http://www.ncbi.nlm.nih.gov/pubmed/17618775.
16. Daniels DH, Powell CR, Braasch MR, Kreder KJ. Sacral neuromodulation in diabetic patients : success and complications in the treatment of voiding dysfunction. Neurourol Urodyn. 2010;29(4):578–81.
17. Marinkovic SP, Gillen LM. Sacral neuromodulation for multiple sclerosis patients with urinary retention and clean intermittent catheterization. Int Urogynecol J. 2010;21(2):223–8.
18. Minardi D, Muzzonigro G. Sacral neuromodulation in patients with multiple sclerosis. World J Urol. 2012;30(1):123–8.
19. Lombardi G, Musco S, Celso M, Del Corso F, Del Popolo G. Sacral neuromodulation for neurogenic non-obstructive urinary retention in incomplete spinal cord patients: a ten-year follow-up single-centre experience. Spinal Cord [Internet]. 2014;52(August 2013):1–5. http://www.ncbi.nlm.nih.gov/pubmed/24394604.
20. Nortvedt MW, Riise T, Frugård J, Mohn J, Bakke A, Skår AB, et al. Prevalence of bladder, bowel and sexual problems among multiple sclerosis patients two to five years after diagnosis. Mult Scler [Internet]. 2007;13(1):106–12. http://www.ncbi.nlm.nih.gov/pubmed/17294618.
21. Bosch JLHR, Groen J. Early reports. Treatment of refractory urge urinary incontinence with sacral spinal nerve stimulation in multiple sclerosis patients. The Lancet. 1996;348:717–9.
22. Lombardi G, Del Popolo G. Clinical outcome of sacral neuromodulation in incomplete spinal cord injured patients suffering from neurogenic lower urinary tract symptoms. Spinal Cord. 2009;47(6):486–91. https://doi.org/10.1038/sc.2008.172
23. Sievert K-D, Amend B, Gakis G, Toomey P, Badke A, Kaps HP, et al. Early sacral neuromodulation prevents urinary incontinence after complete spinal cord injury. Ann Neurol [Internet]. 2010;67(1):74–84. http://www.ncbi.nlm.nih.gov/pubmed/20186953.
24. Knüpfer SC, Liechti MD, Mordasini L, Abt D, Engeler DS, Wöllner J, et al. Protocol for a randomized, placebo-controlled, double-blind clinical trial investigating sacral neuromodulation for neurogenic lower urinary tract dysfunction. BMC Urol [Internet]. 2014;14(1):65. http://www.pubmedcentral.nih.gov/articlerender.fcgi?artid=4139491&tool=pmcentrez&rendertype=abstract.
25. Arlen AM, Powell CR, Kreder KJ. Sacral neuromodulation for refractory urge incontinence is less effective following spinal surgery. Sci World J [Internet]. 2011;11:142–6. http://www.ncbi.nlm.nih.gov/pubmed/21258757.

26. Sanford MT, Suskind AM. Neuromodulation in neurogenic bladder. Transl Androl Urol [Internet]. 2016;5(1):117–26. http://www.pubmedcentral.nih.gov/articlerender. fcgi?artid=PMC4739974.

27. Matzel KE, Stadelmaier U, Hohenfellner M, Gall FP. Electrical stimulation of sacral spinal nerves for treatment of faecal incontinence. Lancet (London, England) [Internet]. 1995;346(8983):1124–7. http://www.ncbi.nlm.nih.gov/pubmed/7475602.

28. Worsøe J, Rasmussen M, Christensen P, Krogh K. Neurostimulation for neurogenic bowel dysfunction. Gastroenterol Res Pract. 2013;2013:1.

29. Ganio E, Luc AR, Clerico G, Trompetto M. Sacral nerve stimulation for treatment of fecal incontinence: a novel approach for intractable fecal incontinence. Dis Colon Rectum. 2001;44(5):619–29.

30. Rosen HR, Urbarz C, Holzer B, Novi G, Schiessel R. Sacral nerve stimulation as a treatment for fecal incontinence. Gastroenterology. 2001;121:536–41.

31. Jarrett MED, Matzel KE, Christiansen J, Baeten CGMI, Rosen H, Bittorf B, et al. Sacral nerve stimulation for faecal incontinence in patients with previous partial spinal injury including disc prolapse. Br J Surg [Internet]. 2005;92(6):734–9. http://www.ncbi.nlm.nih.gov/ pubmed/15838899.

32. Holzer B, Rosen HR, Novi G, Ausch C, Hölbling N, Schiessel R. Sacral nerve stimulation for neurogenic faecal incontinence. Br J Surg. 2007;94(6):749–53.

33. Gstaltner K, Rosen H, Hufgard J, Märk R, Schrei K. Sacral nerve stimulation as an option for the treatment of faecal incontinence in patients suffering from cauda equina syndrome. Spinal Cord [Internet]. 2008;46(9):644–7. http://eutils.ncbi.nlm.nih.gov/entrez/eutils/elink.fcgi? dbfrom=pubmed&id=18317481&retmode=ref&cmd=prlinks%5Cnpapers3://publication/ doi/10.1038/sc.2008.6

34. Lansen-Koch SMP, Govaert B, Oerlemans D, Melenhorst J, Vles H, Cornips E, et al. Sacral nerve modulation for defaecation and micturition disorders in patients with spina bifida. Color Dis. 2012;14(4):508–14.

35. Gupta P, Ehlert MJ, Sirls LT, Peters KM. Percutaneous tibial nerve stimulation and sacral neuromodulation: an update. Curr Urol Rep [Internet]. 2015;16(2):4. http://www.ncbi.nlm.nih. gov/pubmed/25630918.

36. Gaziev G, Topazio L, Iacovelli V, Asimakopoulos A, Di Santo A, De Nunzio C, et al. Percutaneous Tibial Nerve Stimulation (PTNS) efficacy in the treatment of lower urinary tract dysfunctions: a systematic review. BMC Urol [Internet]. 2013;13:61. http://www.pubmedcentral.nih.gov/articlerender.fcgi?artid=4222591&tool=pmcentrez&rendertype=abstract.

37. Kabay S, Kabay SC, Yucel M, Ozden H, Yilmaz Z, Aras O, et al. The clinical and urodynamic results of a 3-month percutaneous posterior tibial nerve stimulation treatment in patients with multiple sclerosis-related neurogenic bladder dysfunction. Neurourol Urodyn [Internet]. 2009;28(8):964–8. http://www.ncbi.nlm.nih.gov/pubmed/19373898.

38. Kabay SC, Kabay S, Yucel M, Ozden H. Acute urodynamic effects of percutaneous posterior tibial nerve stimulation on neurogenic detrusor overactivity in patients with Parkinson's disease. Neurourol Urodyn [Internet]. 2009;28(1):62–7. http://www.ncbi.nlm.nih.gov/ pubmed/18837432.

39. de Sèze M, Raibaut P, Gallien P, Even-Schneider A, Denys P, Bonniaud V, et al. Transcutaneous posterior tibial nerve stimulation for treatment of the overactive bladder syndrome in multiple sclerosis: results of a multicenter prospective study. Neurourol Urodyn [Internet]. 2011;30(3):306–11. http://www.ncbi.nlm.nih.gov/pubmed/21305588.

40. Monteiro ÉS, De Carvalho LBC, Fukujima MM, Lora MI, Do Prado GF. Electrical stimulation of the posterior tibialis nerve improves symptoms of poststroke neurogenic overactive bladder in men: a randomized controlled trial. Urology. 2014;84(3):509–14.

41. Chen G, Liao L, Li Y. The possible role of percutaneous tibial nerve stimulation using adhesive skin surface electrodes in patients with neurogenic detrusor overactivity secondary to spinal cord injury. Int Urol Nephrol. 2015;47(3):451–5.

Index

A

Abdominal massage, 296
Abnormal sympathetic nervous system, 290
Abrams-Griffiths nomogram, 223
Acquired immune deficiency syndrome
  (AIDS), 108
Actionable bladder symptom and screening
  tool (ASST), 60
Active reflux, 245
Acute cystitis, 254, 255
Acute prolonged bladder overdistention
  (ApBO), 216
Acute pyelonephritis
  clinical symptoms, 268
  diagnosis, 268
  differential diagnosis, 268
  etiology, 267
  pathology, 267
  severity, 268
  treatment, 268–270
Adaptive immunity, 256
Afferent axons transmit information, 3, 4
Afferent spinal pathways, 28
Alpha-adrenergic receptors, 145–146, 210
Alprostadil, 324
Ambulatory urodynamics, 87
American Spinal Injury Association (ASIA),
  84
Anal manometry, 187
Anal reflex, 17
Anal sphincter, 184
Anal wink (S4/S5) stimulation, 159
Anatomic checkpoints, 235
Anatomic obstruction, 217

Anejaculation
  causes, 331
  EEJ, 331
  neurogenic ejaculatory dysfunction, 331
  neurologically intact men, 330
  PVS, 331
Anogenital stimulation, 202
Antegrade continence enema (ACE), 300
Anterior cingulate gyrus (ACG), 27
Anterior cord syndrome (ACS), 31
Antibiotic prophylaxis, 264
Anticholinergic drugs, 47
Antimicrobial prophylaxis
  antibiotic prophylaxis, 264
  cranberry prophylaxis, 265
  methenamine salts, 265
Antimuscarinic agents, 64
  darifenacin, 371, 372
  oxybutynin, 370
  propiverine, 373
  solifenacin, 372
  tolterodine, 371
  trospium, 372
Areflexic bowel dysfunction, 288
Arginine vasopressin (AVP), 144
Artificial urinary sphincter (AUS)
  AMS 800™ device
    advantages, 408
    bladder neck implantation, 411, 412
    data, 408
    enterocystoplasty, 413
    evidence-based material, 408
    failure rates, 413, 414
    in female neurogenic bladders, 410

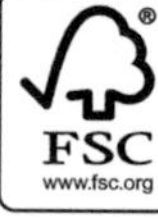